ANCIENT MEDICINE

Selected Papers of Ludwig Edelstein

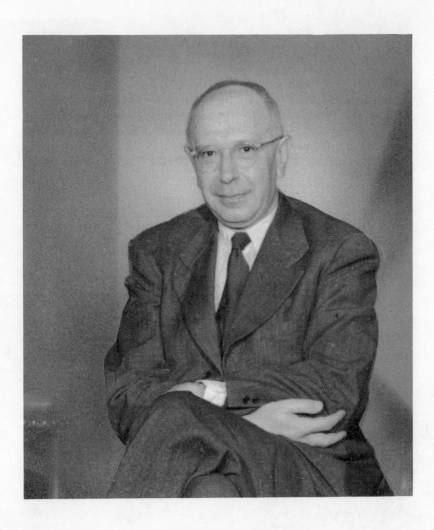

ANCIENT MEDICINE

SELECTED PAPERS OF LUDWIG EDELSTEIN

Edited by
OWSEI TEMKIN
and
C. LILIAN TEMKIN

Translations from the German by C. Lilian Temkin

THE JOHNS HOPKINS PRESS: BALTIMORE

Copyright © 1967 by The Johns Hopkins Press,
Baltimore, Maryland 21218

Printed in the United States of America

Library of Congress Catalog Card Number 67–12425

CONTENTS

PART ONE

PART TWO

PART THREE

PART FOUR

EDITORS' INTRODUCTION

A few years before his death, Ludwig Edelstein began to make plans for the publication of a volume of collected essays on ancient medicine. The volume was to contain English translations of a large portion of his German publications, as well as reprints of most of his English essays on the subject. The Johns Hopkins Press agreed to bring out such a book, Edelstein selected the articles that were to go into it, and C. Lilian Temkin declared her willingness to serve as translator of the German material. In its scope and arrangement, therefore, this book is essentially the work of Edelstein. The tasks that fell upon the editors and the translator will be discussed below.

As it now appears, this volume offers an insight into the contribution of Ludwig Edelstein to our knowledge of ancient medicine. The impact of this contribution was strong owing to the boldness of the author's approach, his skill in the use of the method he chose, and the concentration on his goal. Whatever Edelstein approached he visualized anew, with little regard for established opinion. He was a master of interpretation, guided by what his sources told him and little swayed by general assumptions. His aim was to study the attitudes of Greek physicians toward religion, philosophy, and ethics that made them differ from us, and to elucidate the ties that bind them to us. Edelstein's occupation with ancient medicine was but a part of his study of antiquity. The other part was devoted to Greek philosophy, with Plato, Aristotle, Posidonius as central figures. Together, these parts were his way of gaining insight into man as a moral being who thinks and acts under conditions to which he is subjected, but which he must not allow to dominate him. Edelstein confronts us as a philologist and a historian whose ethos was that of the humanist who wishes to understand man and who lives the life of a teacher. Edelstein was a great teacher, as all those will attest who were privileged to listen to him. But his teaching went far beyond the walls of the institutions with which he was connected. Through his writings he taught a way of looking at the past and of forcing the reader to measure himself against that past. Significantly enough, much of his time during his late years was dedicated to a history of the idea of progress in antiquity.

Ludwig Edelstein was born in Berlin, on April 23, 1902.[1] His father was the owner of a large business, and Edelstein grew up in affluent circumstances. He received his education first from private tutors and then at the humanistic Joachim Friedrich Gymnasium. The private tutoring was believed necessary for reasons of health. The early contact with disease and doctors was often repeated in later years, especially during the prolonged illness of his father and then again that of his wife. His own state of health required frequent hospitalization during the years preceding his death. These personal experiences helped to form Edelstein's views of the art of healing and of the duties of doctors. Such interest as he had in medicine largely originated from this source and from his long exposure to the environment of medical schools.

The education imparted by the humanistic Gymnasium stressed languages and literature, above all Latin, Greek, and the German classics. Afterward, Edelstein turned to the study of philosophy and of classical philology. Philology to him was an object as well as a tool: an object because of his love for ancient Greek civilization and for a literature which formed the basis of Western culture; a tool because it represented the most highly developed art of disciplined interpretation.

Edelstein began the study of philosophy and classics at the University of Berlin, above all with Werner Jaeger and Eduard Spranger. These studies were continued in Heidelberg, where Karl Jaspers, Karl Meister, Alfred Weber, and Otto Regenbogen were his teachers.

In Heidelberg he met Emma J. Levy, a fellow student of classics, whom he married in 1928 and with whom he remained united in a close relationship of love, devotion, and common work until her death in 1958. Here, too, he entered the circle around Marianne Weber, the widow of Max Weber, and formed friendships with the philosopher Erich Frank and the Indologist Heinrich Zimmer.

---

[1] For further biographical data, see the obituaries by Harold Cherniss in the *Year Book of The American Philosophical Society*, 1965, pp. 130–38, and by Owsei Temkin in the *Bulletin of the History of Medicine*, 1966, *40:* 1–13. The latter includes a tentative bibliography of the writings of Edelstein as published at the time of his death. See also the obituaries by George Boas, *Rockefeller University Review*, Nov.–Dec., 1965; Hans Diller, *Gnomon*, 1966, *38:* 429–32; and Fridolf Kudlien, Detlev W. Bronk, and Lloyd G. Stevenson, *Journal of the History of Medicine and Allied Sciences*, 1966, *21:* 173–83.

Edelstein's teacher Regenbogen suggested that he analyze the Hippocratic writing, *On airs, waters and places*. This analysis formed the first part of his dissertation, for which he received the Ph.D. degree in 1929. In revised and extended form, this dissertation appeared in 1931 under the title of *Peri aerōn und die Sammlung der hippokratischen Schriften*. Its publication had several immediate consequences. It attracted much attention, mainly of an antagonistic nature, hindering rather than furthering his career as a philologist and making him receptive to opportunities in the field of the history of medicine. The antagonism was largely due to the uncompromising manner in which Edelstein treated Hippocrates and his teachings. He traced the gradual rise to pre-eminence of the "father of medicine," who, to his contemporaries, was but one among other famous physicians. He denied that Plato, in the *Phaedrus*, made Hippocrates insist on the study of the universe as a requisite for medical knowledge. He depicted the Hippocratic physicians as craftsmen who had to compete for their existence and for whom prognosis was a means of furthering their reputation rather than a form of scientific interest. And he insisted that a mass of anonymous medical writings of the fifth and fourth centuries was gradually ascribed to Hippocrates as his fame grew.

All this was provoking to classicists, historians, and physicians alike. Most of Edelstein's writings, then and later, ran counter to accepted views. To mention only contributions from his German period: he defended the ancient account that credited Erasistratus and Herophilus not only with the dissection of cadavers but also with the vivisection of criminals condemned to death. He ascribed to the school of the Empiricists leanings toward the Academy and made the Methodists the true Aenesidemean skeptics. Not Themison but Thessalus was the real founder of the latter school, a contention that implied a radical redating.

Edelstein's constant deviation from accepted views put him under suspicion of being a *frondeur* for whom opposition was vital. Such an impression was enhanced by his presentation of his arguments as cogent demonstrations with inescapable results, a feature particularly noticeable in his history of anatomy in antiquity. Indeed, Edelstein's was a strong personality which would not tolerate appeasement of what he considered wrong. Nor was he without an ambition which made him look to the very great as his masters. But above all, he had an aversion to repeating oft-told tales and kept silent where he had nothing new to offer. The number of his publications is not large. *Multum, non multa* was the motto which he shared with Schopenhauer, who had been the philosopher of his youth. Edelstein's reluctance to repeat what had already been said was paired with an unshakable faith in truth, at which the scholar must always aim. There was no excuse for superficiality. The review of a book received the same attention as an independent essay. Indeed some of Edelstein's important points were made in his reviews of the books by Jaeger, Petersen, and Pohlenz.

The rise of Hitler denied Edelstein the position he had obtained at the Berlin institute of the history of medicine under Paul Diepgen. It compelled him to liquidate the paternal business, and it drove him into emigration from Germany. In 1934, after one year in Italy, the Edelsteins came to Baltimore, and he stayed at the Johns Hopkins Institute of the History of Medicine until 1947, when Henry E. Sigerist, the director of the Institute, left the United States. To this second period belong two books: *The Hippocratic Oath*, and the two volumes on *Asclepius*. The first volume of *Asclepius*, the collection and translation of the testimonies, was mainly the work of his wife, while he was responsible for the second volume, the interpretation of the testimonies.

The Hippocratic Oath filled a gap in Edelstein's previous picture of Hippocratic medicine. How did this document of the physician who swore to maintain "purity and holiness" in his life and his art fit into the reality reflected by the other Hippocratic works? Edelstein's answer assigned the *Oath* to a particular group of physicians, followers of Pythagorean principles; it dated the *Oath* relatively late and doubted its widespread influence during the centuries preceding the Christian era.

The same surprising originality is also found in the interpretation of the testimonies of *Asclepius*. There was practical unanimity that Asclepius was a chthonic deity. Edelstein broke with this view: Asclepius was a patron saint of the itinerant Greek physician and became a healing god only later. The sanctuaries of Asclepius had nothing to do with the training of the Greek physicians. On the other hand, there was no enmity between secular medicine and religious healing; the Greek physician might send patients to the god when his own art had reached its limits. This attitude toward religion, in contrast to the physician's rejection of magic, had been dealt with in Edelstein's essay on "Greek medicine in its relation to religion and magic," which also falls in this period.

After leaving Baltimore, Edelstein spent the next four years teaching classics, first at the University of Washington and then in Berkeley at the University of California. In 1951 he returned to the Johns Hopkins University where, in 1952, he was appointed Professor of Humanistic Studies and Lecturer in the History of Medicine. This return was prompted by the controversy over the oath which the Regents of the University of California imposed upon the faculty. With his return, Edelstein also resumed work in medical history. During this second phase of his stay in Baltimore, he published three important articles. "On the relation of ancient philosophy to medicine" defends and explains the thesis that medical science was essentially a philosophical pursuit to which only a small elite of philosopher-physicians was dedicated. With this thesis Edelstein put himself in opposition to those who attributed to medical experience a formative influence on Greek philosophy. Scientifically, medicine was the recipient, even though it fell upon medical men to elaborate anatomy, physiology, and other sciences which the sect of the Dogmatists considered essential for medical knowledge. For medicine's contribution to philosophy Edelstein looked elsewhere: the tantalizing rule of the physician over man's body. The thesis of this essay broadened what Edelstein had said about the formation of the medical sects. At the same time, it complemented the essay on "Recent trends in the interpretation of ancient science," which appeared in the same year. Together, these two essays lead to Edelstein's major preoccupation during his last years when he was considering ancient science as a whole rather than medicine.

In *The Hippocratic Oath* Edelstein had tried to establish the date, provenience, and significance of this document. Now, in "The professional ethics of the Greek physician," he attempted an account of the whole of ancient medical ethics. The problem that presented itself was the development of an ethics determined by the character of medicine, in contrast to earlier forms where general ethical principles were merely applied to medicine. This problem could be solved only against the background of the development of professional ethics as such. Here again, the contribution to the history of medicine also became a contribution to the history of philosophy. It also showed how far Edelstein had traveled in the twenty-five years between the publication of his dissertation and the appearance of this essay. In his dissertation, the emphasis lay on the social circumstances of the Hippocratic doctor, his relatively low social status and the means he used to establish and maintain his reputation. This ran counter to the widespread view of the Hippocratic physician as a scientist-philosopher, trying to live up to the lofty principles of the Hippocratic Oath. Edelstein did not turn his back upon the work of his youth; but twenty-five years later he was able to see another side of the Greek doctor—his striving for a moral standard which imposed upon him, as a healer, obligations and restrictions particularly his own.

In 1958 Edelstein's wife died, a blow from which it took him years to recover if, indeed, he can be said ever to have recovered from it; and in 1960 his second Baltimore period came to an end when he moved to New York to accept a position at what is now the Rockefeller University. Shortly before moving, in March, 1960, he delivered the Garrison Lecture at the annual meeting of the American Association for the History of Medicine in Charleston, South Carolina. This lecture on "The distinctive Hellenism of Greek medicine," which was to be his last contribution to medical history proper, in many ways summarized Edelstein's views. It looks once more on subjects dealt with before, and it touches on matters he had not been able to discuss previously. Thus it serves as an unintentional résumé of his work in the history of ancient medicine. Restricted to one field and on a small scale, it reflects what Edelstein, in his younger years, had hoped to write eventually: a history of Greek culture as it should be written in a time so different from that in which Jacob Burckhardt lived, whose *Griechische Kulturgeschichte* was his venerated ideal.

The present volume contains those essays available after his death which Edelstein himself had considered for inclusion. It presents them in the four sections under which he had subsumed them.[2] His arrangement obviously was guided by systematic considerations. The first section deals with his work on the Hippocratics and other physicians down to the Methodists. It was to start out with a long article on Hippocrates that had appeared in the *Realenzyklopädie* of Pauly-Wissowa. But Edelstein allowed himself to be persuaded to substitute two chapters from his doctoral dissertation. His book on *The Hippocratic Oath* has been placed at the head of this section, because it seems to provide a fitting opening to his essays on Hippocratic medicine.

[2] With the exception of *The Hippocratic Oath*, on which he had not reached a decision.

The second group of articles discusses a number of special topics. If Edelstein had lived longer, he would have included an essay on "The concept of disease in ancient medicine." As it is, only notes were found after his death.

The third section contains those essays, of the second Baltimore period, in which he discusses ancient medicine in relation to professional ethics and to philosophy and views its distinctive Hellenistic character. Of the last of these, a revised manuscript of the text was found among his papers. At the time of his death he was still working on the footnotes. The article was published posthumously in 1966. In the present volume, it closes not only the third section but also those contributions specifically devoted to ancient medicine, for the last section gathers a number of articles which, though outside ancient medicine, add perspective to Edelstein's work in this area. The charming little exercise on "Sydenham and Cervantes" stands apart from all these considerations. But its author was rightly fond of it, and he wished it included.

In his will, Ludwig Edelstein had designated Professor Harold Cherniss of the Institute for Advanced Study as his literary executor. In consultation between Professor Cherniss, The Johns Hopkins Press, and Owsei and C. Lilian Temkin, it was agreed that the last two named should act as co-editors of the present volume, C. Lilian Temkin having already taken the translation of the German articles upon herself.

As previously explained, selection and arrangement of the articles were guided by Edelstein's own wishes and suggestions. The title under which the volume now appears was chosen posthumously. Moreover, it was decided to leave those articles that had appeared in English in their original form with some minor adaptations only, such as numbering all reference marks consecutively within each item, identifying the source of original publication in an asterisk footnote, and adjusting the style of *The Hippocratic Oath* to that of an article.

However, the articles that had originally appeared in German posed a number of questions which demanded decisions by the translator and the editors.

The first drafts of all translations had been submitted to Edelstein during his lifetime. He had revised them, sometimes deviating rather markedly and intentionally from the German wording. Such purposeful deviations had, of course, to be respected by the translator. Revised versions of the articles were then submitted to the translator and were adjusted in discussions between her and the author. This was done with all translations except that of "Die Geschichte der Sektion in der Antike," where Edelstein's revised manuscript reached the translator only after his death and in a form suggesting that he had not yet given it his final attention. In accordance with a previous decision, the Greek quotations in the body of the text were replaced by English versions (the original had German translations in the footnotes). But many places merely showed gaps where the Greek text had stood. As far as possible, these gaps were filled by translations from the Loeb Classical Library. Similarly, following Edelstein's lead, Latin quotations were left in the text in the few cases only where neither English translation nor a paraphrase made them expendable. Obviously, Edelstein had tried to adapt the translation to an audience of readers different from the German audience of some thirty years ago. Alerted by this experience, the editors found that in handling the two chapters from his dissertation Edelstein had progressively eliminated Greek citations from the body of the text, replaced Greek titles by English ones, etc. The editors have tried to extend this policy uniformly over both chapters of the dissertation.

The translator has also tried to help the English reader by expanding some of the abbreviations of titles on the assumption that he might not, for instance, easily identify GGA with *Göttingische Gelehrte Anzeigen.*

There were many other instances, too numerous and too trifling to be listed, where the editors had to take Edelstein's place and try to act as they think he would have acted had he been able to see this collection through the press.

In his work on this volume, Edelstein was helped by his secretary, Miss Caroline Clauser. The editors feel that he would have wished to acknowledge her assistance had he been alive.

Note: Bracketed page references followed by an asterisk, e.g. [3*], refer to pages in this volume.

PART ONE

THE HIPPOCRATIC OATH:
TEXT, TRANSLATION AND INTERPRETATION*

In memoriam Albert Fraenkel

* *Supplements to the Bulletin of the History of Medicine,* no. 1, Baltimore: The Johns Hopkins Press, 1943.

INTRODUCTION

That for centuries the so-called Hippocratic Oath was the exemplar of medical etiquette and as such determined the professional attitude of generations of physicians, no one will doubt. Yet when it is asked what historical forces were instrumental in the formulation of this document, no answer can be given that is generally agreed upon. Uncertainty still prevails concerning the time when the Oath was composed and concerning the purpose for which it was intended. The dates proposed in modern debate vary from the sixth century B.C. to the first century A.D. As for the original intent of the manifesto, it is maintained that the Oath was administered in family guilds of physicians; or that it formed the statute of societies of artisans which perhaps were organized in secret; or that it was an ideal program designed without regard for any particular time or place.

In my opinion it is not necessary to resign oneself to leaving the issue undecided. If some data provided by the text itself are evaluated in their true import and are combined with others the proper meaning of which has previously been established, it seems possible to determine the origin of the Hippocratic Oath with a fair degree of certainty. At any rate, it is with this aim in mind that I propose to re-examine the document.

In so doing I shall scrutinize the Hippocratic text sentence by sentence—the treatise is short enough to allow completeness of interpretation—for it is only in this way that the adequacy or inadequacy of the thesis to be offered can be tested. Moreover, I shall give in full the testimony of ancient authors on which I depend in my inquiry. The material used is scattered and in some cases difficult of access, and it should be at hand if the cogency of the argument is to be judged. Such a method of investigation necessarily results in a certain copiousness, but this hardly needs justification in view of the importance of the Hippocratic Oath, both for the history of medicine and of ethics.

TEXT*

ΟΡΚΟΣ

Ὀμνύω Ἀπόλλωνα ἰητρὸν καὶ Ἀσκληπιὸν καὶ Ὑγείαν καὶ Πανάκειαν καὶ
θεοὺς πάντας τε καὶ πάσας ἵστορας ποιεύμενος ἐπιτελέα ποιήσειν κατὰ δύναμιν
καὶ κρίσιν ἐμὴν ὅρκον τόνδε καὶ ξυγγραφὴν τήνδε·
5 ἡγήσασθαί τε τὸν διδάξαντά με τὴν τέχνην ταύτην ἴσα γενέτῃσιν ἐμοῖσιν
καὶ βίου κοινώσασθαι καὶ χρεῶν χρηίζοντι μετάδοσιν ποιήσασθαι καὶ γένος τὸ ἐξ
αὐτοῦ ἀδελφεοῖς ἴσον ἐπικρινέειν ἄρρεσι καὶ διδάξειν τὴν τέχνην ταύτην, ἢν
χρηίζωσι μανθάνειν, ἄνευ μισθοῦ καὶ ξυγγραφῆς, παραγγελίης τε καὶ ἀκροήσιος
καὶ τῆς λοιπῆς ἁπάσης μαθήσιος μετάδοσιν ποιήσασθαι υἱοῖσί τε ἐμοῖσι καὶ τοῖσι
10 τοῦ ἐμὲ διδάξαντος καὶ μαθηταῖσι συγγεγραμμένοις τε καὶ ὡρκισμένοις νόμῳ
ἰητρικῷ, ἄλλῳ δὲ οὐδενί.

διαιτήμασί τε χρήσομαι ἐπ' ὠφελείῃ καμνόντων κατὰ δύναμιν καὶ κρίσιν
ἐμήν· ἐπὶ δηλήσει δὲ καὶ ἀδικίῃ εἴρξειν.

οὐ δώσω δὲ οὐδὲ φάρμακον οὐδενὶ αἰτηθεὶς θανάσιμον οὐδὲ ὑφηγήσομαι
15 ξυμβουλίην τοιήνδε· ὁμοίως δὲ οὐδὲ γυναικὶ πεσσὸν φθόριον δώσω. ἁγνῶς δὲ καὶ
ὁσίως διατηρήσω βίον ἐμὸν καὶ τέχνην ἐμήν.

οὐ τεμέω δὲ οὐδὲ μὴν λιθιῶντας, ἐκχωρήσω δὲ ἐργάτῃσιν ἀνδράσιν πρήξιος
τῆσδε.

ἐς οἰκίας δὲ ὁκόσας ἂν ἐσίω, ἐσελεύσομαι ἐπ' ὠφελείῃ καμνόντων ἐκτὸς ἐὼν
20 πάσης ἀδικίης ἑκουσίης καὶ φθορίης τῆς τε ἄλλης καὶ ἀφροδισίων ἔργων ἐπί τε
γυναικείων σωμάτων καὶ ἀνδρείων ἐλευθέρων τε καὶ δούλων.

ἃ δ' ἂν ἐν θεραπείῃ ἢ ἴδω ἢ ἀκούσω ἢ καὶ ἄνευ θεραπηίης κατὰ βίον ἀνθρώπων,
ἃ μὴ χρή ποτε ἐκλαλέεσθαι ἔξω, σιγήσομαι ἄρρητα ἡγεύμενος εἶναι τὰ τοιαῦτα.

ὅρκον μὲν οὖν μοι τόνδε ἐπιτελέα ποιέοντι καὶ μὴ ξυγχέοντι εἴη ἐπαύρασθαι
25 καὶ βίου καὶ τέχνης δοξαζομένῳ παρὰ πᾶσιν ἀνθρώποις ἐς τὸν αἰεὶ χρόνον, παρα-
βαίνοντι δὲ καὶ ἐπιορκοῦντι τἀναντία τούτεων.

Titulus: ἱπποκράτους ὅρκος M V R U *Mg.* ᾱ´ V   2 ὄμνυμι R U   3 ἅπαντας V τε]
om. V   *Supra* ἵστορας *scr.* μάρτυρας U, *m. rec.* R   ποίησιν V   4 συγγραφὴν *supra scr.*
ξ V, *supra add.* συμφωνίαν U, *m. rec.* R   5 τε] V, δὲ M R U, μὲν *Littré* ἴσα γενέτῃσιν]
ἴσα καὶ γενέτοισιν R U   ἐμοῖσι R U   6 χρέους U, χρέος? *Diels* χρήζοντι V καὶ
γένος — ποιήσασθαι (9) *om.* V   7 αὐτοῦ] *Ermerins*, ἑωυτέου M R, ὠυτέου U ἀδελφοῖς U
ἀποκρινέειν U, *sed corr.*   8 *Supra* ξυγγραφῆς *scr.* συμφωνίας U, *m. rec.* R   *Supra*
παραγγελίης *scr.* παρακλῇ *m. rec.* R, παρακλήσεως U   9 τοῖσι] *in Mg. transiens* U
10 *supra* συγγεγραμμένοις *scr.* συμφωνίαν δοῦσι R   τε] euan. V   ὠρκιζομένοις M, *sed corr.*
13 *Supra* δηλήσει *scr.* βλάβῃ U   14 *supra* ὑφηγήσομαι *scr.* ὑποβαλῶ *m. rec.*, *mg.* ὑπο-
θήσομαι συμβουλεύσω R   15 φθόριον δώσω πεσσόν R U   16 ἐμὸν] τὸν ἐμὸν R U   ἐμήν]
τὴν ἐμὴν R U   17 *post* δὲ *lac. statuit Diels* ἀνδράσιν] M, ἀνδράσι V R U   πρήξεος
V   19 ἐς] V, εἰς M R U   καμνόντων] κα- *in ras.* U   21 ἀνδρείων] V M², ἀνδρίων M,
ἀνδρώων R U   22 *pr.* ἢ *om.* V   θεραπηίης U   23 ἐκκαλέεσθαι U   τὰ τοιαῦτα εἶναι V
24 ποιέοντι] -έο- *in ras mai.* U   25 εἰς M R U   *In fine:* ὅρκος M V

* Text and Apparatus Criticus are taken from *Hippocratis Opera*, ed. I. L.
Heiberg, *Corpus Medicorum Graecorum* I, 1, 1927, pp. 4–5.

5

TRANSLATION

OATH

I swear by Apollo Physician and Asclepius and Hygieia and Panaceia and all the gods and goddesses, making them my witnesses, that I
will fulfil according to my ability and judgment this oath and this
covenant:

To hold him who has taught me this art as equal to my parents
and to live my life in partnership with him, and if he is in need of money
to give him a share of mine, and to regard his offspring as equal to my
brothers in male lineage and to teach them this art—if they desire to
learn it—without fee and covenant; to give a share of precepts and oral
instruction and all the other learning to my sons and to the sons of him
who has instructed me and to pupils who have signed the covenant and
have taken an oath according to the medical law, but to no one else.

I will apply dietetic measures for the benefit of the sick according
to my ability and judgment; I will keep them from harm and injustice.

I will neither give a deadly drug to anybody if asked for it, nor will
I make a suggestion to this effect. Similarly I will not give to a woman
an abortive remedy. In purity and holiness I will guard my life and my
art.

I will not use the knife, not even on sufferers from stone, but will
withdraw in favor of such men as are engaged in this work.

Whatever houses I may visit, I will come for the benefit of the sick,
remaining free of all intentional injustice, of all mischief and in particular of sexual relations with both female and male persons, be they free
or slaves.

What I may see or hear in the course of the treatment or even outside of the treatment in regard to the life of men, which on no account
one must spread abroad, I will keep to myself holding such things shameful to be spoken about.

If I fulfil this oath and do not violate it, may it be granted to me to
enjoy life and art, being honored with fame among all men for all time
to come; if I transgress it and swear falsely, may the opposite of all this
be my lot.

INTERPRETATION

The Hippocratic Oath clearly falls into two parts. The first speci-
fies the duties of the pupil toward his teacher and his teacher's family
and the pupil's obligations in transmitting medical knowledge.[1] The
second gives a number of rules to be observed in the treatment of diseases, a short summary of medical ethics as it were.[2] Most scholars consider these two sections to be only superficially connected or at least
determined by different moral standards.[3] Be this as it may, the two
parts certainly diverge in their subject matter, and, for the purpose of
analyzing their content, it is advantageous first to discuss them sepa-
rately and then to ask how they are related to each other. Again for the
sake of convenience, I shall deal with the so-called ethical code first, the
main question being whether the historical setting in which these rules
of conduct were conceived can be ferreted out.

Modern interpreters are wont to see in the ethical provisions of the
Oath the expression of certain general principles the recognition of
which is demanded by human decency or by the responsibilities inherent in the physician's art. In this sense timeless validity is usually
attributed to the moral law here established.[4] At best such an evaluation
is qualified by the admission that the Oath represents only the ancient
ideal of the physician. Justice is enjoined upon him, it is said, in contrast
to charity that motivates the Christian doctor, and in contrast to duty
toward the community that determines the doctor of today.[5] Even if
such characterizations were correct, it would not be superfluous to ask
when and where this supposedly general attitude toward medicine and
its tasks was codified. Besides, it is only by uncovering the specific

---

[1] Cf. above, p. 5, 5–11. [2] Cf. above, p. 5, 12–23.

[3] Cf. e.g., W. H. S. Jones, *The Doctor's Oath*, 1924, p. 56; K. Deichgräber, Die
ärztliche Standesethik des hippokratischen Eides, *Quellen u. Studien z. Geschichte d.
Naturwissenschaften u. d. Medizin*, III, 1932, p. 34. Cf. also below, p. 50.

[4] Cf. e.g., Jones, *op. cit.*, p. 46: "Custom and convenience, to say nothing of the
human conscience, would sooner or later lay down most of the rules of conduct comprised in *Oath* . . ."; cf. also p. 50: ". . . the appeal to his (*sc.* the Greek doctor's)
better feelings." Cf. also O. Körner, *Der Eid des Hippokrates*, 1921, p. 20: "Alle diese
Gelöbnisse dienen allein dem Wohle der Kranken und keinen Sonderinteressen der
Ärzte. Erschöpfend umfassen sie in grossen Zügen, was der Arzt dem Kranken
schuldet."

[5] Cf. Deichgräber, *op. cit.*, pp. 38 ff.; esp. pp. 41 ff. ("Die Idee des δίκαιος ιατρός
ist in den Bestimmungen des Eides Gestalt geworden, wenn man so will, die Idee
des apollinischen Arztes" [p. 42]).

7

ethical agents which brought about this formulation that the origin of the Oath can be ascertained.

Unfortunately, most of the statements contained in the document are worded in rather general terms; they are vague in their commending of justice, of purity and holiness, concepts which in themselves do not imply any distinct meaning but may be understood in various ways. Yet there are two stipulations that have a more definite character and seem to point to the basic beliefs underlying the whole program which is here evolved: the rules concerning the application of poison and of abortive remedies. Their interpretation should therefore provide a clue for a historical identification of the views embodied in the Oath of Hippocrates.

I. THE ETHICAL CODE

A. *Rules Concerning Poison and Abortion*

"I will neither give a deadly drug to anybody if asked for it, nor will I make a suggestion to this effect. Similarly I will not give to a woman an abortive remedy. In purity and holiness I will guard my life and my art"—such is the vow made.[6] It concerns the physician not so much in his capacity as the healer of diseases but rather in that of the pharmacist who is in possession of the drugs which he prescribes. Poison is a drug and so is the pessary.[7] The physician agrees not to deliver either one to his patient. The term used in both instances is the same; just as he will not *give* the pessary to a woman who comes to seek his help, he will not *give* poison to anyone who is under his care.[8]

Why regulations concerning cases of abortion are introduced into the document is immediately understandable. Under ancient conditions the physician was often presented with the problem as to whether he should give an abortive remedy.[9] But what about the physician's supplying poison? Did he so frequently have occasion to give poison that it seemed worth while to ordain what he should do in such instances? What exactly is the situation referred to in the Oath?

All modern interpreters assume that the interdiction of the supplying of poisons means that the physician is charged not to assist his patient in a suicide which he might contemplate. Some interpreters claim that here the physician is also, or even primarily, asked to refrain from any criminal attempt on his patient's life. Cases of poisoning, they say,

[6] Cf. above, p. 5, 14–16.

[7] E. Littré, *Œuvres complètes d'Hippocrate*, IV, 1844, pp. 622 ff., has shown that this clause presupposes a state of affairs in which the physician was his own apothecary. This he was even in those centuries in which pharmacies existed, cf. e.g., Galen, *Opera*, ed. C. G. Kühn, XIV, 1827, pp. 5 ff. For the pessary, a "Stäbchen . . . mit bestimmten φάρμακα bestrichen," cf. Deichgräber, *op. cit.*, n. 10.

[8] As far as I am aware, Littré was the first to suggest another meaning of the sentence in question. He says, *op. cit.*, IV, p. 630, n. 12, in commenting on δώσω— the word I have translated by *give*—: "Les traducteurs rendent δώσω par *propinabo* (*sc.* in the first stipulation); mais δώσω, qui, un peu plus bas (*sc.* in the second instance), est joint à πεσσός, et qui là ne peut se rendre par *administrer*, montre que dans les deux cas il s'agit d'une substance malfaisante remise à des tiers. . . ." Littré seems to have believed that no physician could possibly give a pessary to his patient directly. But as C. Daremberg, *Œuvres choisies d'Hippocrate*², 1855, p. 9, later pointed out, ancient physicians did do so, and it is in connection with the Hippocratic Oath that it was discussed whether this was right; cf. below, pp. 14 f. Littré's reasoning for his interpretation then is not valid.

[9] For abortion as a general practice in antiquity, cf. below, p. 13.

were very frequent in antiquity; the law, though of course it threatened punishment for murder, was of little avail because the lack of proper scientific methods made it impossible to ascertain whether poison had been administered or not. As a means of strengthening civil jurisdiction, therefore, a clause was introduced into the ancient medical code which today would be entirely out of place.[10] I shall not argue that the Greeks could hardly have been aware of that inability to cope with the situation under discussion which resulted from their ignorance of *post-mortem* examinations and modern chemistry. As a matter of fact they were convinced that they were quite capable of detecting such a crime as poisoning and the criminal who had perpetrated it.[11] More important, if the prohibition were instigated by the wish of society to defend itself against a pernicious assault, then the rules given would be concerned not with the doctor's attitude toward his patient but toward a third party. For the patient himself certainly would not ask his doctor for the poison with which he is to be murdered, and yet the physician vows not to give poison when asked to do so. There is no evidence, however, that the Oath refers to anybody except patient and physician.[12] The words in question, then, can mean only that the doctor promises not to supply his patient with poison if asked by him to do so nor to suggest that he take it. It is the prevention of suicide, not of murder that is here implied.[13]

[10] Cf. Littré, *op. cit.*, IV, pp. 622 ff.; Deichgräber, *op. cit.*, p. 36 (Deichgräber apparently accepts Littré's conception of the motive as well as his explanation). It is often overlooked that Littré admits the probability that suicide is also referred to here, but cf. *op. cit.*, IV, p. 630, n. 12. Jones, *op. cit.*, p. 50, is the only one who seems to exclude the latter possibility.

[11] Cf. L. Lewin, *Die Gifte in der Weltgeschichte*, 1920, pp. 37 ff., where ancient methods of determining cases of poisoning are discussed. Besides, torture of those who were suspected was an excellent substitute for scientific inquiry into the case, cf. Apuleius, *Metamorphoses*, X, 10. Note moreover the harshness of Plato, *Laws*, XI, 932 e ff., in dealing with such a crime, especially when committed by a doctor. As understood by most interpreters the stipulation of the *Oath* would be a useless duplication of the existing laws.

[12] Cf. above, n. 8. Littré is well aware of the fact that his interpretation necessitates a reference to a third person (*op. cit.*, IV, p. 623–24); cf. also J. E. Pétrequin, *Chirurgie d'Hippocrate*, I, 1877, p. 185. Deichgräber, *loc. cit.*, and Jones, *loc. cit.*, do not discuss at all the problem as to whom this stipulation refers. Nor have the modern interpreters pondered over the difficulty that on their assumption, according to which the clause concerns suicide as well as murder, the statement is logically incoherent; for in one instance the patient would be referred to, in the other somebody outside the physician's practice.

[13] Cf. Daremberg, *op. cit.*, p. 9: ". . . l'ensemble de la phrase ne me laisse aucun doute sur cette interprétation." The old Latin and Arabic translations of the *Oath*

But was suicide an instance to be reckoned with in medical practice? Could the doctor ever advise such an act to his patient? In antiquity this was indeed the case. If the sick felt that their pains had become intolerable, if no help could be expected, they often put an end to their own lives. This fact is repeatedly attested and not only in general terms; even the diseases are specified which in the opinion of the ancients gave justification for a voluntary death.[14] Moreover, the taking of poison was the most usual means of committing suicide, and the patient was likely to demand the poison from his physician who was in possession of deadly drugs and knew those which brought about an easy and painless end.[15] On the other hand, such a resolution naturally was not taken without due deliberation, except perhaps in a few cases of great distress or mental strain. The sick wished to be sure that further treatment would be of no avail, and to render this verdict was the physician's task. The patient, therefore, consulted with him, or urged his

reproduced by Jones, op. cit., p. 35; p. 31, seem to presuppose the same meaning. (It is hardly necessary to add that in regard to the issue at stake one cannot possibly draw any conclusion from an undated pharmacological poem whose dependence on the Hippocratic Oath cannot be proved, as Deichgräber himself admits, op. cit., p. 36, n. 33.) Most important: Scribonius Largus urges that the physician should not murder anyone, not even his enemy (p. 2, l. 19 ff. Helmreich). In confirmation of such a postulate he quotes the Hippocratic Oath in the following way: "Hippocrates, conditor nostrae professionis, initia disciplinae ab iureiurando tradidit, in quo sanctum est, ne praegnati quidem medicamentum, quo conceptum excutitur, aut detur aut demonstretur a quoquam medico, longe praeformans animos discentium ad humanitatem. qui enim nefas existimaverit spem dubiam hominis laedere, quanto scelestius perfecto iam nocere iudicabit" (p. 2, l. 27–p. 3, l. 2)? It would be meaningless for Scribonius to argue in such a complicated and indirect manner, if the Oath outlined a criminal assault expressis verbis.

[14] Cf. e.g., Aristotle, E. E., 1229 b 30: ". . . οὔτ' εἰ φεύγοντες τὸ πονεῖν, ὅπερ πολλοὶ ποιοῦσιν, οὐδὲ τῶν τοιούτων οὐδεὶς ἀνδρεῖος, καθάπερ καὶ Ἀγάθων φησί· 'φαῦλοι βροτῶν γὰρ τοῦ πονεῖν ἡσσώμενοι/θανεῖν ἐρῶσιν.' ὥσπερ καὶ τὸν Χείρωνα μυθολογοῦσιν οἱ ποιηταὶ διὰ τὴν ἀπὸ τοῦ ἕλκους ὀδύνην εὔξασθαι ἀποθανεῖν ἀθάνατον ὄντα." The reference to Chiron and his disease makes it certain that the term τὸ πονεῖν means "to suffer bodily pains," cf. also below, pp. 16 f. Cf. also Pliny, Nat. Hist., XX, 199: "Sic scimus interemptum P. Licini Caecinae praetorii viri patrem in Hispania Bavili, cum valetudo inpetibilis odium vitae fecisset; item plerosque alios." For the diseases in question cf. Pliny, Nat. Hist., XXV, 23: "Qui (sc. morbi) gravissimi ex his sint, discernere stultitiae prope videri possit, cum suus cuique ac praesens quisque atrocissimus videatur. et de hoc tamen iudicavere aevi experimenta, asperrimi cruciatus esse calculorum a stillicidio vesicae, proximum stomachi, tertium eorum, quae in capite doleant, non ob alios fere morte conscita."

[15] For poison commonly used in suicide, cf. Lewin, op. cit., p. 139; p. 65. For instances where poison is demanded from the physician, cf. e.g., Scriptores Historiae Augustae, Vita Hadriani, 24, 13; Tacitus, Annals, XV, 64; Apuleius, Metamorphoses,

11

friends to speak to the doctor. If the latter, in such a consultation, confirmed the seriousness or hopelessness of the case, he suggested directly or indirectly that the patient commit suicide.[16]

Of course, I do not mean to claim that everybody whose illness had become desperate thought of ending his own life. Even if human aid was no longer effectual, recourse to the gods was still possible, and men did seek succor in the sanctuaries; even if the pain was excruciating and relief was to be had neither from human nor from divine physicians, men could, and did go on living in spite of all their suffering.[17] Yet the fact remains that throughout antiquity many people preferred voluntary death to endless agony. This form of "euthanasia" was an everyday reality.[18] Consequently it is quite understandable that the Oath deals with the attitude which the physician should take in regard to the possible suicide of his patient. From a practical point of view it was no

---

X, 9. Even Theophrastus, *Hist. Plant.*, IX, 16, 8, speaks of men who invented especially efficacious and painless poisons for suicide; since he says that these people were also versed in all other branches of medicine it is not necessary to understand with Littré, *op. cit.*, IV, p. 622, that they were merely vendors of drugs. They may just as well have been physicians.

[16] Cf. Pliny, *Epistulae*, I, xxii, 7 ff.: "Mirareris, si interesses, qua patientia hanc ipsam valitudinem toleret, ut dolori resistat, ut sitim differat, ut incredibilem febrium ardorem inmotus opertusque transmittat. nuper me paucosque mecum quos maxime diligit advocavit rogavitque ut medicos consuleremus de summa valitudinis, ut, si esset insuperabilis, sponte exiret e vita, si tantum difficilis et longa, resisteret maneretque: dandum enim precibus uxoris, dandum filiae lacrimis, dandum etiam nobis amicis ne spes nostras, si modo non essent inanes, voluntaria morte desereret. id ego arduum in primis et praecipua laude dignum puto. nam impetu quodam et instinctu procurrere ad mortem commune cum multis, deliberare vero et causas eius expendere, utque suaserit ratio, vitae mortisque consilium vel suscipere vel ponere ingentis est animi. et medici quidem secunda nobis pollicentur." This passage, the importance of which is rightly stressed by A. W. Mair, *Encyclopaedia of Religion and Ethics*, s. v. suicide, XII, pp. 31–32, certainly is tinged with Stoic feeling. But there is no reason to doubt that earlier generations were as cautious and responsible in making their decisions as were the Romans.

[17] For the seeking of religious help in hopeless cases, cf. L. Edelstein, Greek Medicine in its Relation to Religion and Magic, *Bulletin of the History of Medicine*, V, 1937, pp. 238 ff. For instances of rejection of suicide cf. below, p. 16.

[18] Strangely enough none of the interpreters of the *Oath* has pointed to this fact. Deichgräber, the only one to mention the problem of euthanasia, *op. cit.*, p. 36, even denies that it had any importance for the ancients. The writers on suicide, on the other hand, though they refer to voluntary death on account of illness, do not mention the *Oath*, cf. e.g., R. Hirzel, Der Selbstmord, *Archiv f. Religionswissenschaft*, XI, 1908, pp. 75 ff.; 243 ff.; 417 ff.; *E. R. E.*, s. v. suicide, XII, pp. 26 b ff.

less important to tell the ancient doctor what to do when faced with such a situation than it was to advise him about cases of abortion.[19]

The relevance of the "pharmacological rules" for a medical oath having been established, one may now ask why the Oath forbids the physician to assist in suicide or in abortion. Apparently these prohibitions did not echo the general feeling of the public. Suicide was not censured in antiquity.[20] Abortion was practiced in Greek times no less than in the Roman era, and it was resorted to without scruple. Small wonder! In a world in which it was held justifiable to expose children immediately after birth, it would hardly seem objectionable to destroy the embryo.[21] Why then should the physician not give a helping hand to those of his patients who wanted to end their own lives or to those who did not wish to have offspring?

For a moment one might harbor the idea that the interdiction of poison and of abortive remedies was simply the outgrowth of medical ethics. After all, medicine is the art of healing, of preserving life. Should the physician assist in bringing about death?[22] I do not propose to discuss this issue in general terms. It suffices here to state that in antiquity many physicians actually gave their patients the poison for which they were asked. Apparently *qua* physicians they felt no compunction about doing so.[23] Although in later centuries some refused to participate in an attempt on men's lives, because, as they said, it was unfitting for their

---

[19] In my opinion it is the neglect of the question of euthanasia that gave currency to the belief that in the *Oath* not only suicide but also manslaughter are forbidden (cf. Deichgräber, *op. cit.*, p. 36: "*Da* das Euthanasieproblem, an das der moderne Mensch denken könnte, in der Antike unbekannt ist, *kann* es sich hier *nur* um den Giftmord und als einen besonderen Fall, den durch Gift herbeigeführten Selbstmord sowie um die Beihilfe zu beidem handeln." [Italics mine.]).

[20] Cf. above, pp. 11 ff., and below, pp. 15 ff.

[21] Cf. in general A. E. Crawley, *E. R. E., s. v.* foeticide, VI, pp. 54 b ff. For the parental power over children of which exposure after birth and destruction of the embryo are the consequences, cf. Wilamowitz, *Staat u. Gesellschaft der Griechen, Die Kultur der Gegenwart*, II, IV, 1², 1923, p. 36.

[22] It is permissible to say that this is the most commonly accepted explanation of the rules, cf. e.g., Körner, *op. cit.*, p. 12: "Seine (*sc.* the physician's) höchste Aufgabe ist Heilen, und sein schlimmstes Verbrechen wäre also Töten oder Vorschubleisten zu Mord, Selbstmord und Kindesabtreibung."

[23] Cf. e.g., Tacitus, *Annals*, XV, 64; cf. also Apuleius, *Metamorphoses*, X, 9, where the physician is approached for poison by a slave, and since he becomes suspicious, gives him a harmless drug only. But he is not astonished about the demand made, nor does he refuse it on general grounds. This can easily be explained, for

sect "to be responsible for anyone's death or destruction,"[24] it is not
reported that they ever employed the same reasoning in cases of self-
murder.[25] As for abortions, many physicians prescribed and gave
abortive remedies. Medical writings of all periods mention the means
for the destruction of the embryo and the occasions where they are to
be employed.[26] In later centuries some physicians rejected abortion
under all circumstances; they supported their decision with a reference
to the prohibition in the Hippocratic Oath and added that it was the
duty of the doctor to preserve the products of nature. Soranus, the
greatest of the ancient gynaecologists, had little patience with these
colleagues of his. In agreement with many other physicians he contended that it was necessary to think of the life of the mother first, and
he resorted to abortion whenever it seemed necessary, much as he
deprecated it if performed for no other reason than the wish to preserve
beauty or to hide the consequences of adultery.[27] In short, the strict
attitude upheld by the Oath was not uncontested even from the medical
point of view. In antiquity it was not generally considered a violation
of medical ethics to do what the Oath forbade. An ancient doctor who

---

those suffering from incurable diseases were doomed to die anyhow; the only issue
was, whether they should be condemned to an unnecessarily protracted suffering.
Moreover, death seemed desirable to the sick, and even the Hippocratic maxim "to
help, or at least not to do harm" (*Epidemiae*, I, 11, *Hippocratis Opera*, ed. H. Kuehlewein, I, 1894, p. 190) could not restrain the physician when he was face to face
with those who believed that they would be helped rather than harmed by annihila-
tion.

[24] Cf. Apuleius, *Metamorphoses*, X, 11; note that these are the words of the same
physician who before (X, 9, cf. preceding note) did not reject the giving of poison
to a suicide.

[25] This assertion, of course, is not refuted by the fact that in Oxyrhynchus
Papyrus 437 (III, 77, third century A.D.) the giving of poison is rejected as incompatible with the art by a quotation from the *Oath;* cf. Deichgräber, *op. cit.*, n. 42.
Through this document the interdiction of poison became part of medical ethics;
that does not mean, however, that originally it was the outgrowth of medical considerations.

[26] Cf. R. Hähnel, Der künstliche Abortus im Altertum, *Archiv f. Geschichte d.
Medizin*, XXIX, 1937, pp. 224 ff. J. Ilberg, Zur gynäkologischen Ethik der Griechen,
Archiv f. Religionswissenschaft, XIII, 1910, pp. 12 ff., holds that the Greek physicians
did not apply abortive remedies; but this thesis is untenable in view of the facts now
conveniently surveyed by R. Hähnel, *loc. cit.;* cf. also Deichgräber, *op. cit.*, n. 37;
P. Diepgen, *Die Frauenheilkunde der Alten Welt*, 1937, p. 301.

[27] Cf. Soranus, ed. J. Ilberg, *C. M. G.*, IV, 1927, p. 45, 8 ff. Incidentally the passage in Soranus proves that the rejection of abortion as advocated in the *Oath* is laid
down without qualification (contrary to the assumption made by F. J. Dölger,
Antike u. Christentum, IV, 1934, p. 8).

accepted the rules laid down by "Hippocrates" was by no means in agreement with the opinion of all his fellow physicians; on the contrary, he adhered to a dogma which was much stricter than that embraced by many, if not by most of his colleagues. Simple reflection on the duties of the physician, on the task of medicine alone, under these circumstances, can hardly have led to the formulation and adoption of the "pharmacological stipulations."

In my opinion, the Oath itself points to other, more fundamental considerations that must have been instrumental in outlining the prohibitions under discussion. For the physician, when forswearing the use of poison and of abortive remedies, adds: "In purity and in holiness I will guard my life and my art."[28] It might be possible to construe purity as a quality insisted upon by the craftsman who is conscious of the obligations of his art. The demand for holiness, however, can hardly be understood as resulting from practical thinking or technical responsibility. Holiness belongs to another realm of values and is indicative of standards of a different, a more elevated character.

Yet certainly not such purity and holiness are meant as might accrue to men from obedience to civil law or common religion. Ancient jurisdiction did not discriminate against suicide; it did not attach any disgrace to it, provided that there was sufficient reason for such an act. And self-murder as a relief from illness was regarded as justifiable, so much so that in some states it was an institution duly legalized by the authorities.[29] Nor did Greek or Roman law protect the unborn child. If, in certain cities, abortion was prosecuted, it was because the father's

---

[28] Cf. above, p. 5, 15–16. It is interesting to note that Körner who sees in these stipulations the expression of medical ethics (cf. above, n. 4) translates ἁγνῶς δὲ καὶ ὁσίως with "ohne Fehl und unbescholten" (op. cit., p. 5), a translation which in no way does justice to the meaning of the words. All other interpreters in their rendering rightly reflect the notions of holiness and purity.

[29] Cf. Hirzel, op. cit., pp. 264 ff.; E. R. E., loc. cit. The special regulations for the burial of a suicide in Athens (Aristotle, N. E., 1138 a 9 ff.) have been rightly explained by Hirzel, ibid. p. 264; 271, as directed against those who committed suicide when still able to bear arms; the same is true of Rome (ibid., p. 266). This fact has been overlooked by Deichgräber, op. cit., p. 36, n. 35. Note moreover that not even these people were deprived of burial. For city regulations concerning the delivery of poisons to suicides, cf. E. R. E., loc. cit., pp. 28 ff. Temporary legislation against suicide (cf. Hirzel, ibid., p. 275) indicative of the frequency of such occurrences was never directed against suicide on account of illness. Thebes was the only city where, according to late evidence, suicide was forbidden (cf. Hirzel, ibid., p. 268); for the explanation of this fact, cf. below, n. 49.

right to his offspring had been violated by the mother's action.[30] Ancient religion did not proscribe suicide. It did not know of any eternal punishment for those who voluntarily ended their lives.[31] Likewise it remained indifferent to foeticide. Its tenets did not include the dogma of an immortal soul for which men must render account to their creator.[32] Law and religion then left the physician free to do whatever seemed best to him.

From all these considerations it follows that a specific philosophical conviction must have dictated the rules laid down in the Oath. Is it possible to determine this particular philosophy? To take the problem of suicide first: Platonists, Cynics and Stoics can be eliminated at once. They held suicide permissible for the diseased. Some of these philosophers even extolled such an act as the greatest triumph of men over fate.[33] Aristotle, on the other hand, claimed that it was cowardly to give in to bodily pain, and Epicurus admonished men not to be subdued by illness.[34] But does that mean that the Oath is determined by Aris-

[30] For lawsuits based on the father's claim to his children, cf. e.g., Lysias, *Fr·* X, p. 333 [Thalheim], and Cicero, *Pro Cluentio*, XI, 32 (for more material, especially for the Roman centuries, cf. Dölger, *op. cit.*, pp. 37 ff.). Even Dölger, *ibid.*, p. 13, admits that in these cases the wish to protect the life of the embryo is not involved, though he is inclined to believe that the Greeks at least knew of laws against abortion. But the so-called laws of Solon and Lycurgus, quoted only in a Ps. Galenic book of unknown date and origin (*An animal sit id quod in utero est* XIX, p. 179 K.; cf. K. Kalbfleisch, *Abh. Berl. Akad.*, 1895, p. 11, n. 1), to which Dölger refers, *ibid.*, pp. 10 ff. (cf. also W. Aly, *R. E.*, III A, p. 963), cannot prove this thesis. They are late inventions, determined by the thought of the Christian era. Dölger himself, *ibid.*, p. 14, admits such a falsification in the case of Musonius, *Fr.* XVa, p. 77H, the only other passage which in general terms speaks of laws against abortion.

[31] This has been shown conclusively by Hirzel, *op. cit.*, pp. 76 ff.; p. 276; on later changes under the influence of Jewish-Christian ideas, cf. *ibid.*, p. 277, and below, n. 45. In *E. R. E.*, XII, pp. 30 b ff., after an elaborate proof that according to the evidence available suicide was not stigmatized by ancient religious dogma, it is nevertheless assumed that popular religious feeling opposed it. This is due to a non-permissible identification of popular religion with the tenets of one particular sect (the Orphics), cf. below, n. 38.

[32] Cf. Dölger, *op. cit.*, pp. 15 ff. Here again as in the case of laws against abortion the first indication of its rejection on religious grounds is found in the first century A.D. Cf. O. Weinreich, Stiftung u. Kultsatzungen eines Privatheiligtums in Philadelphia in Lydien, *S. B. Heidelb.*, 1919.

[33] For Plato, cf. *Laws*, IX, 873c, and Hirzel, *op. cit.*, p. 279, n. 1; for the Cynics, cf. Hirzel, *ibid.*, pp. 279–80; for the Stoics, cf. especially *Stoicorum Veterum Fragmenta*, ed. H. v. Arnim, III, 1923, pp. 187 ff., and in general E. Benz, Das Todesproblem in der stoischen Philosophie, *Tübinger Beiträge z. Altertumswissenschaft*, VII, 1929, pp. 54 ff. The Cyrenaics too permitted suicide, cf. Hirzel, *op. cit.*, p. 422.

[34] For Aristotle, cf. *N. E.*, 1116 a 12 ff.; for Epicurus, cf. *Fr.* 138 [Usener]. It is debatable whether Epicurus opposed suicide at all, cf. Diogenes Laertius, X, 119,

totelian or Epicurean ideas? I shall not insist that it is hard to imagine a physician resisting the adjurations of his patients if he has nothing but Aristotle's or Epicurus' exhortations to courage to quote to them and to himself. It is more important to stress the fact that the Aristotelian and Epicurean opposition to suicide did not involve moral censure. If men decided to take their lives, they were within their rights as sovereign masters of themselves. The Aristotelian and Epicurean schools condoned suicide. Later on the Aristotelians even gave up their leader's teaching, and under the onslaught of the Stoic attack withdrew their disapproval of self-murder.[35] At any rate, Aristotelianism and Epicureanism do not explain a rejection of suicide which apparently is based on a moral creed and a belief in the divine.

Pythagoreanism, then, remains the only philosophical dogma that can possibly account for the attitude advocated in the Hippocratic Oath. For indeed among all Greek thinkers the Pythagoreans alone outlawed suicide and did so without qualification. The Platonic Socrates can adduce no other witness than the Pythagorean Philolaus for the view that men, whatever their fate, are not allowed to take their own lives. And even in later centuries the Pythagorean school is the only one represented as absolutely opposed to suicide.[36] Moreover, for the Pythagorean, suicide was a sin against god who had allocated to man his position in life as a post to be held and to be defended. Punishment threatened those who did not obey the divine command to live; it was considered neither lawful nor holy to seek release, "to bestow this blessing upon oneself."[37] Any physician who accepts such a dogma naturally must abstain from assisting in suicide or even from suggesting it. Otherwise he would be guilty of a crime, he no less than his patient, and in this moral and religious conviction the doctor can well find the courage to remain deaf to his patient's insistence, to his sufferings, and even to

---

and A. Kochalsky, *Das Leben u. die Lehre des Epikur*, 1914, n. 111; in general Hirzel, *op. cit.*, p. 422; p. 282.

[35] Cf. in general Hirzel, *op. cit.*, p. 422. For the later Aristotelians, cf. R. Walzer, Magna Moralia und aristotelische Ethik, *Neue Philologische Untersuchungen*, VII, 1929, p. 192.

[36] Cf. *Phaedo*, 61 d ff., and Hirzel, *op. cit.*, p. 278, who is right in saying that this concept is so emphatically formulated because it is expressed here for the first time. Note that the stipulation is laid down even for those οἷς βέλτιον τεθνάναι ἢ ζῆν (62a). For later Pythagoreans, cf. Athenaeus, IV, 157 C (Euxitheus).

[37] Cf. *Phaedo*, 61 d: τὸ μὴ θεμιτὸν εἶναι ἑαυτὸν βιάζεσθαι . . . 62 a: μὴ ὅσιον αὐτοὺς ἑαυτοὺς εὖ ποιεῖν . . . 62 b: ὁ μὲν οὖν ἐν ἀπορρήτοις λεγόμενος περὶ αὐτῶν λόγος, ὡς ἔν τινι φρουρᾷ ἐσμεν οἱ ἄνθρωποι καὶ οὐ δεῖ δὴ ἑαυτὸν ἐκ ταύτης λύειν οὐδ' ἀποδιδράσκειν . . .

the clamor of the world which disagrees almost unanimously with the stand taken by him. It seems safe to state this much: the fact that in the Hippocratic Oath the physician is enjoined to refrain from aiding or advising suicide points to an influence of Pythagorean doctrines.[38]

In my opinion the same can be asserted of the rule forbidding abortion and rejecting it without qualification. Most of the Greek philosophers even commended abortion. For Plato, foeticide is one of the regular institutions of the ideal state. Whenever the parents are beyond that age which he thinks best for the begetting of children, the embryo should be destroyed.[39] Aristotle reckons abortion the best procedure to keep the population within the limits which he considers essential for a well-ordered community.[40]

To be sure, one limitation apparently is recognized by ancient philosophers. Aristotle advocates that abortion should be performed before the foetus has attained animal life; after that time he no longer considers abortion compatible with holiness.[41] But such a restriction is based on the biological notion that the embryo from a certain time on partakes in animal life. Other philosophers and scientists, in fact most of them, including the Platonists and the Stoics, denied that such was the case. Animation, they thought, began at the moment of birth. Therefore, in their opinion, abortion must have been permissible throughout pregnancy.[42]

It was different with the Pythagoreans. They held that the embryo

[38] I say Pythagorean doctrines. How far this dogma is influenced by Orphism or even dependent upon it, is not for me to decide. J. Burnet, *E. R. E.*, *s. v.* Pythagoras and Pythagoreanism, X, 526 a–b, holds that Philolaus' view as represented by Plato is different from Orphic beliefs and characterizes as Pythagorean the "higher side" of this teaching, that is, its moral implications. But cf. also I. M. Linforth, *The Arts of Orpheus*, 1941, esp. pp. 168 ff. At any rate, one cannot claim on the basis of the words ἐν ἀπορρήτοις which Plato uses that the rejection of suicide is Orphic rather than Pythagorean (contrary to S. Reinach, Ἄωροι βιαιοθάνατοι, *Archiv f. Religionswissenschaft*, IX, 1906, p. 318). For the present purpose the expression "Pythagorean doctrines" seems justified by the fact that the teaching under discussion is directly ascribed to the Pythagoreans by Plato and other writers; cf. below, pp. 20 f.

[39] Cf. *Republic*, V, 461 c; *Laws*, V, 740 d, and for the interpretation of the latter passage, Diepgen, *op. cit.*, p. 297.

[40] Cf. Aristotle, *Politics*, VII, 1335 b 20 ff.

[41] Cf. Aristotle, *Politics*, VII, 1335 b 25: τὸ γὰρ ὅσιον καὶ τὸ μὴ διωρισμένον τῇ αἰσθήσει καὶ τῷ ζῆν ἔσται. Cf. also Dölger, *op. cit.*, pp. 7 ff.

[42] Cf. *Stoicorum Veterum Fragmenta*, II, p. 213 [Arnim], and also Herophilus (H. Diels, *Doxographi Graeci*, 1929, V, 15, p. 426). Concerning the Platonists and Neo-Platonists who denied animation of the embryo because the soul enters the body from without, cf. Kalbfleisch, *op. cit.*, pp. 5 ff.

was an animate being from the moment of conception. That they did so is expressly attested by a writer of the third century A.D.[43] The same can be concluded from the Pythagorean system of physiology as it was outlined in the Hellenistic period by Alexander Polyhistor: the germ is a clot of brain containing hot vapors within it, and soul and sensation are supposed to originate from this vapor. Similar views were previously accepted by Philolaus in the fourth century B.C.[44] Consequently, for the Pythagoreans, abortion, whenever practiced, meant destruction of a living being. Granted that the righteousness of abortion depends on whether the embryo is animate or not, the Pythagoreans could not but reject abortion unconditionally.[45]

Furthermore, abortion was irreconcilable with their ethical beliefs no less than with their scientific views. In their ascetic rigorism, in their strictness concerning sexual matters and regarding matrimony in particular, they went further than any other sect. They banned extramarital relations. Even in matrimony coitus was held justifiable only for the purpose of producing offspring.[46] Besides, children to them were

[43] Cf. Ps. Galen, Πρὸς Γαῦρον περὶ τοῦ πῶς ἐμψυχοῦται τὰ ἔμβρυα, p. 34, 20 [Kalbfleisch]: εἰ δὲ δυνάμει ζῷον ὡς τὸ δεδεγμένον τὴν ἕξιν ἢ μᾶλλον ζῷον ἐνεργείᾳ ἦν τὸ ἔμβρυον, δύσκολον μὲν τὸν καιρὸν ἀφορίσαι τῆς εἰσκρίσεως καὶ πολύ γε τὸ ἀπίθανον ἔξει καὶ πλασματῶδες ὁποῖος ἂν εἶναι ἀφορισθῇ, τοῦ μὲν ὅταν καταβληθῇ τὸ σπέρμα τὸν καιρὸν τοῦτον ἀποδιδόντος ὡς ἂν μηδ' οἴου τε ὄντος ἐν τῇ μήτρᾳ γονίμως κρατηθῆναι μήτι γε ψυχῆς ἔξωθεν τῇ εἰσκρίσει ἑαυτῆς τὴν σύμφυσιν ἀπεργασαμένης—κἀνταῦθα πολὺς ὁ Νουμήνιος καὶ οἱ τὰς Πυθαγόρου ὑπονοίας ἐξηγούμενοι . . . The author of the book is Porphyry, cf. Kalbfleisch, ibid., p. 25.

[44] Cf. Diogenes Laertius, VIII, 28–9. Kalbfleisch, op. cit., p. 80 ad p. 34, 26 (cf. E. Zeller, Die Philosophie d. Griechen, III, 2³, 1881, pp. 89 f.; p. 96) referred to this passage as a parallel to the Galenic statement. The tradition which Diogenes follows is ascribed to the early Peripatos by Diels (H. Diels–W. Kranz, Die Fragmente d. Vorsokratiker, 1934⁵, 58 B 1a). For the similarity of such views with theories of Philolaus (44 A 27 [Diels-Kranz]), cf. in general M. Wellmann, Hermes, LIV, 1919, pp. 232 ff.

[45] Deichgräber, op. cit., p. 37, n. 38, has stated that opposition to abortion is in line with certain philosophical ideas, without saying, however, which ideas these are. As his only reference he quotes Phocylides, ll. 184–5. But this poem was written by a Hellenistic Jew at the beginning of the Christian era, cf. W. Christ–W. Schmid, Geschichte d. griechischen Literatur, II⁶, 1920, p. 621 f. Concerning the general importance of the agreement between Pythagorean and Jewish-Christian theories, cf. Dölger, op. cit., p. 23, who refers to Philo and Josephus, cf. also below, pp. 62 f.

[46] Cf. in general 58 D 8, pp. 476, 7 ff.; 477, 7 ff. [Diels-Kranz] (from Aristoxenus), and Zeller, op. cit., III, 1, p. 143, n. 3; cf. ibid. I, 1⁵, p. 462, n. 2. Cf. especially p. 476, 4 [Diels-Kranz]: ὑπελάμβανον δ', ὡς ἔοικεν, ἐκεῖνοι οἱ ἄνδρες περιαιρεῖν μὲν δεῖν τάς τε παρὰ φύσιν γεννήσεις καὶ τὰς μεθ' ὕβρεως γιγνομένας, καταλιμπάνειν δὲ τῶν κατὰ φύσιν τε καὶ μετὰ σωφροσύνης γινομένων τὰς ἐπὶ τεκνοποιίᾳ σώφρονί τε καὶ νομίμῳ γινομένας. It is sometimes claimed that Aristoxenus' report is reminiscent of Platonic ethics, cf. E. Rohde, Kleine Schriften, II, 1901, p. 162. Yet in regard to the matter under dis-

19

more than future members of a community or citizens of a state. It was
considered man's duty to beget children so as to leave behind in his own
place another worshiper of the gods.[47] With such convictions how could
the Pythagoreans ever allow abortive remedies to be applied? How
could they fail to condemn practices of this kind, so common among
their compatriots?[48]

It stands to reason, then, that the Hippocratic Oath, in its abortion-
clause no less than in its prohibition of suicide, echoes Pythagorean doctrines. In no other stratum of Greek opinion were such views held or
proposed in the same spirit of uncompromising austerity.[49] When the
physician, after having forsworn ever to give poison or abortive remedies, adds: "In purity and holiness I will guard my life and my art," it
must be the purity and holiness of the "Pythagorean way of life"[50] to
which he dedicates himself.

B. The General Rules of the Ethical Code

The question now arises whether what is true of certain of the
ethical clauses of the Hippocratic Oath is true of all of them, in other
words, whether the whole medical code is in agreement with Pythagorean philosophy. By this latter term I mean Pythagoreanism as it was
understood in the fourth century B.C. It is to this form of the dogma
that the rules discussed so far were related, and it seems fair to assume
that the rest of the stipulations, if at all influenced by Pythagorean
thinking, correspond to the same concept of Pythagoreanism. At any
rate, wherever I shall speak of Pythagorean doctrines without qualifi-

cussion Plato's views certainly were more lax than those of the Pythagoreans, cf.
Laws, VIII, 841 d, and above, p. 18.

[47] Cf. 58 C 4, p. 465, 5 [Diels-Kranz]: . . . ὅτι δεῖ τεκνοποιεῖσθαι ἕνεκα τοῦ καταλιπεῖν
ἕτερον ἀνθ' ἑαυτοῦ θεῶν θεραπευτήν; cf. also *ibid.*, p. 464, 22. These statements are considered by Diels to be part of the old Pythagorean *Symbola*. Plato, *Laws*, VI, 773 e;
776 b, agrees with the point of view of the Pythagoreans, much as he deviates from
it in other passages.

[48] Reinach, *op. cit.*, p. 321, on the evidence of a very late Orphic fragment, claims
that it was the Orphics who favored rejection of abortion. But his argument is no
more cogent in this respect than it is in regard to suicide, cf. above, n. 38.

[49] It seems worth pointing out that both stipulations of the *Oath* show some
affinity with ideas credited especially to Philolaus, cf. above, n. 44, and below, p. 56.
This philosopher lived for some time in Thebes. It is therefore hardly by chance
that this city alone in late sources is said to have had laws against suicide, cf.
above, n. 29. It seems probable that the well-known theory of the famous philosopher
was projected into the legislation of Thebes.

[50] Cf. Plato, *Republic*, X, 600 b: . . . Πυθαγόρειον τρόπον . . . τοῦ βίου.

cation, it is neither the teachings of the "historical" Pythagoras, nor those of the later so-called Neo-Pythagoreans which I have in mind, but rather those theories and beliefs which writers of the fourth century B.C., men like Plato, Aristotle and their pupils, attributed to Pythagoras and his followers.[51]

To start, then, with the analysis of that section of the ethical code which deals with the treatment of diseases proper:[52] here mention is made of diet, drugs and cutting. In a more technical language, medicine is viewed as comprising dietetics, pharmacology and surgery. Consequently those matters are discussed which seem most important for the attitude of the physician within these three departments of his art.[53] Now a division of medicine into these branches is not unusual and in itself is not indicative of any particular medical or philosophical school. But, according to Aristoxenus, the Pythagoreans were among those who accepted this particular classification of medicine; moreover, the sequence of the various parts of the healing art in the Pythagorean doctrine is the same as it is in the Hippocratic Oath, dietetics coming first, pharmacology next, surgery last.[54]

[51] For the very complex Pythagoras problem, cf. e.g., F. Ueberweg- K. Praechter, *Die Philosophie des Altertums*[12], 1926, pp. 61 ff. That the various forms of Pythagoreanism, especially the earliest doctrine and that of the fourth century B.C., must be sharply distinguished admits of no doubt after the studies of E. Frank, *Plato u. d. sogenannten Pythagoreer*, 1923. To him I am also indebted for his advice in many a controversial matter discussed in this paper.

[52] The ethical code can be divided into two parts of which the first (cf. above, p. 5, 12–18) outlines rules for the healing of diseases, whereas the second (cf. above, p. 5, 19–23) regulates the physician's behavior in all matters indirectly connected with the treatment, such as his relations to the patient, to the patient's family, and so forth.

[53] Cf. e.g., Münzer, *Münchener Medizinische Wochenschrift*, 1919, p. 309; Körner, *op. cit.*, p. 7. Concerning poison and abortive remedies as drugs, cf. above, p. 9. The οὐ τεμέω-clause, whatever its meaning (cf. below, pp. 26 ff.), certainly refers to surgical procedure. Deichgräber, *op. cit.*, p. 31, translates διαιτήματα with "Verordnungen" and adds, n. 24: ". . . eigentlich handelt es sich . . . um diätetische Verordnungen." There is no reason for taking the word to mean anything but "diätetische Verordnungen"; moreover, whatever may be understood by this term, the application of drugs cannot be covered by it, cf. below, p. 25. Therefore Körner, *op. cit.*, p. 11, is not right in saying: ". . . Diät . . . es ist also das gesamte Heilverfahren gemeint"; he himself admits that διαιτήματα does not include drugs.

[54] Littré, *op. cit.*, IV, p. 622, says that such a division is known only since the time of Herophilus, cf. Celsus, I, 1; cf. also below, p. 30. As a matter of fact, it is attributed to the Pythagoreans by Aristoxenus, cf. 58 D 1, p. 467, 5 ff. [Diels-Kranz]. Since this passage is fundamental for the interpretation of Pythagorean medicine, and the most extensive one preserved, I shall give it here in full: τῆς δὲ ἰατρικῆς μάλιστα μὲν ἀποδέχεσθαι τὸ διαιτητικὸν εἶδος καὶ εἶναι ἀκριβεστάτους ἐν τούτῳ · καὶ πειρᾶσθαι πρῶτον

21

In detail, the physician is asked to use dietetic means to the advantage of his patients as his judgment and capacity permit; moreover he is enjoined to keep them from mischief and injustice.[55] That the doctor's dietetic prescriptions should be given to help the patient is an obvious truth. It is the goal of all good craftsmanship to seek the best for the object with which the craftsman is concerned. Every ancient physician would have subscribed to such a formulation.[56] It suffices to say that the Pythagorean physicians did not feel differently, for this school acknowledged the useful and the advantageous as second among the aims of human endeavor.[57]

But what exactly is meant by the promise to keep the patient from mischief and injustice? Can this really imply, as some scholars have suggested, that the physician shall enforce his treatment even against the resistance or indifference of his patient's family?[58] It is true, interference of others may occur and the physician may have to contend with it, but this happens rarely, too seldom indeed to have been con-

μὲν καταμανθάνειν σημεῖα συμμετρίας ποτῶν τε καὶ σίτων καὶ ἀναπαύσεως. ἔπειτα περὶ αὐτῆς τῆς κατασκευῆς τῶν προσφερομένων σχεδὸν πρώτους ἐπιχειρῆσαί τε πραγματεύεσθαι καὶ διορίζειν. ἄψασθαι δὲ [χρὴ] καὶ καταπλασμάτων ἐπὶ πλείω τοὺς Πυθαγορείους τῶν ἔμπροσθεν, τὰ δὲ περὶ τὰς φαρμακείας ἧττον δοκιμάζειν, αὐτῶν δὲ τούτων τοῖς πρὸς τὰς ἑλκώσεις μάλιστα χρῆσθαι, ⟨τὰ δὲ⟩ περὶ τὰς τομάς τε καὶ καύσεις ἥκιστα πάντων ἀποδέχεσθαι.

[55] Cf. above, p. 5, 12–13. Littré, *op. cit.*, IV, p. 631, says: "Je m'abstiendrai de tout mal et de toute injustice"; the same meaning is given by F. Adams, *The Genuine Works of Hippocrates*, II, 1886, p. 279, and also by Jones, *op. cit.*, p. 9. But εἴρξειν is transitive; it cannot possibly refer to the physician himself, cf. Daremberg, *op. cit.*, p. 8, n. 6, with regard to Littré's translation: "Le text se refuse absolument à ce sens." With Daremberg agree Deichgräber, *op. cit.*, p. 31, and Körner, *op. cit.*, p. 11. The latter quite rightly points out that in Littré's interpretation the words are a mere duplication of what is said later on, cf. below, p. 33.

[56] Cf. e.g., Ps. Hippocrates, *Epidemiae*, I, 11, quoted above, n. 23, where the aim of medicine is defined as "to help or not to harm."

[57] For the Pythagoreans, cf. p. 474, 36 ff. [Diels-Kranz] (Aristoxenus). The συμφέρον and ὠφέλιμον were second in rank to the καλόν and εὔσχημον. It is worth noting that in later Pythagorean tradition Pythagoras himself is said to have come into this world for the benefit (εἰς ὠφέλειαν) of mankind, and to have philosophized and acted to this end (ἐπ᾽ ὠφελείᾳ), cf. Iamblichus, *De Vita Pythagorica*, 30; 162; 222.

[58] Cf. Körner, *op. cit.*, p. 11: "Der Arzt soll es (sc. the treatment) auch durchsetzen gegenüber Gleichgültigkeit oder Widerspenstigkeit der Umgebung des Kranken. Nur so kann es verstanden werden, .wenn der Schwörende im Anschluss an die Anordnung des Heilverfahrens verspricht, Gefährdung und Schädigung vom Kranken abzuwehren." Daremberg, *op. cit.*, p. 8, n. 6, compares the statement with the Hippocratic ὠφελεῖν ἢ μὴ βλάπτειν (cf. above, n. 56), but here it is certainly the physician himself who is supposed not to do any harm, and yet, as Daremberg has shown (cf. above, n. 55), this is not what is meant in the *Oath*. The other interpreters are silent about the implications of the words in question.

sidered in the medical code. Moreover, while mischief may be done to the sick by his friends, why should he suffer injustice from those who wish him well?[59] And why should this danger be any greater in regard to the dietetic treatment of diseases for which case alone mention is made of it, than it would be in regard to everything else the physician may prescribe or do? No, it can scarcely be protection from the wrong done by others that the physician vows to give to his patients. But since it can neither be protection from the wrong which he himself may do,[60] one must conclude that he promises to guard his patients against the evil which they may suffer through themselves. That men by nature are liable to inflict upon themselves injustice and mischief, and that this tendency becomes apparent in all matters concerned with their regimen, this is indeed an axiom of Pythagorean dietetics.[61]

The Pythagoreans defined all bodily appetites as propensities of the soul, as a craving for the presence or absence of certain things. Most of these appetites they considered as acquired or created by men themselves, and therefore they thought human desires were to be watched closely and to be scrutinized severely. As a natural process they acknowledged only that the body should take in an appropriate amount of food and should be cleansed again appropriately after it had been filled. To overload oneself with superfluous food and drink was regarded as an acquired inclination of the soul.[62]

But unfortunately all bodily passions have the tendency to increase indefinitely. Of themselves they become "idle, irreverent, harmful and licentious,"[63] as one can readily see in those who are in the position to live according to their wishes. In order to live right from early youth on, one must learn to hold in contempt those things that are "idle and

---

[59] Körner, *loc. cit.*, very significantly translates δήλησις and ἀδικίη with "Gefähr-dung und Schädigung," terms which do not bring out the full impact of the Greek words.

[60] Cf. above, n. 55.

[61] In order to gain a picture of Pythagorean medicine the evidence must be put together bit by bit. Modern literature on the subject is scarce. The outline given by I. Schumacher, *Antike Medizin*, I, 1940, pp. 34 ff., proves unsatisfactory because here the sources are not properly evaluated. Of great importance are the study of the doctrine of κάθαρσις by E. Howald, *Hermes*, LIV, 1919, pp. 203 ff., and the discussion of some of the fragments by A. E. Taylor, *A Commentary on Plato's Timaeus*, 1928, pp. 629 ff.

[62] Cf. 58 D 8, p. 474, 40–p. 475, 8 [Diels-Kranz] (from Aristoxenus).

[63] *Ibid.*, p. 475, 14–17: μάλιστα δ' εἶναι κατανοῆσαι τάς τε ματαίους καὶ τὰς βλαβερὰς καὶ τὰς περιέργους καὶ τὰς ὑβριστικὰς τῶν ἐπιθυμιῶν παρὰ τῶν ἐν ἐξουσίαις ἀναστρεφομένων γινομένας.

superfluous."[64] It is necessary, therefore, to select the nourishment of the body with great caution, to determine its quality and quantity most carefully, a supreme wisdom entrusted to the physicians.[65]

This is the Pythagorean doctrine concerning the regimen of the healthy. It is clear, I think, that in such a theory bodily and psychic factors are blended in a peculiar way. At the same time there is a moral element involved: unhealthy desire is uncontrolled desire; a decision is to be made between those appetites which ought to be satisfied and those which ought to be disregarded. Moreover, the Pythagorean teaching, in a strange manner, insists on negative instances. Not that alone which one does is important; that which one does not do, or is not allowed to do, carries just as much consequence. Right living is brought about not only, not even primarily, through positive actions, but rather through avoidance of those steps that are dangerous, through the repression of insatiable desires which if left to themselves would cause damage.[66]

The same consideration for body and soul, the same combination of precepts and prohibitions seems to be characteristic of the Pythagorean treatment of diseases. Most illnesses, in the opinion of these philosophers, are due to opulent living; too much food is consumed which cannot be digested properly, and thus extravagance destroys the body, just as it destroys wealth.[67] If health, the retention of the form, changes into disease, the destruction of the form, the body needs purification through medicine, just as the sick soul needs purification through music.[68] The physician in such a case must give assistance by changing

[64] *Ibid.*, p. 475, 11: . . . ἀφέξονται δὲ τῶν ματαίων τε καὶ περιέργων ἐπιθυμιῶν . . . .

[65] Cf. *ibid.*, p. 475, 20–33; for ancient theories concerning the dietetics of the healthy in general, cf. L. Edelstein, *Die Antike*, VII, 1931, pp. 255 ff. [303* ff.].

[66] A late Pythagorean poem still defines the right measure to be applied in matters concerning health, the μέτρον, as ὅ-μή σ' ἀνιήσει, that which will not harm you (*Carmen Aureum*, l. 34); for the date of this poem, cf. below, n 110.

[67] Cf. Diodorus, X, 7, 1: ὅτι παρεκάλει τὴν λιτότητα ζηλοῦν· τὴν γὰρ πολυτέλειαν ἅμα τάς τε οὐσίας τῶν ἀνθρώπων διαφθείρειν καὶ τὰ σώματα. Aristoxenus expresses the same idea by speaking of human beings as a ποικιλώτατον . . . γένος κατὰ τὸ τῶν ἐπιθυμιῶν πλῆθος (p. 475, 18–19 [Diels-Kranz]). A similar view is ascribed to Pythagoras himself by Apollonius, cf. Iamblichus, *De Vita Pythagorica*, 218; cf. also Rohde, *op. cit.*, p. 164. I owe this reference to Schumacher, *op. cit.*, p. 56.

[68] Cf. 58 C 3, p. 463, 26 [Diels-Kranz]: ὑγίειαν τὴν τοῦ εἴδους διαμονήν, νόσον τὴν τούτου φθοράν (from Aristotle). This concept can be elaborated by comparing the definition of health as harmony, the proper attunement of the body, *ibid.*, p. 451, 11 (early Peripatetic tradition), and by referring to Alcmaeon's definition of health as ἰσονομία of the qualities, and of disease as μοναρχία of one quality (24 B 4 [Diels-Kranz]; note also the expression φθοροποιόν). For medicine as κάθαρσις cf. *ibid.*, 58 D

the patient's regimen. He must use dietetical means, as the Hippocratic Oath says.[69] In choosing them he will be intent on his patient's benefit according to the best of his judgment and ability. Whatever he prescribes, as a true follower of Pythagoras he will remember one fundamental truth: everything that is given to the body creates a certain disposition of the soul. Men in general, though they are aware of the fact that some things, such as wine, may suddenly bring about a striking change in a person's behavior, do not apprehend that every kind of food or drink causes a certain mental habit, slight as the variations may be. But the physician knows that—his art primarily consists in this knowledge.[70] Consequently, he must see to it that the soul of the sick, through a wrong diet, does not fall into "idle, irreverent, harmful and licentious passions." Since he acts according to this principle when assisting the healthy,[71] he must certainly do likewise when treating the sick. Or in the words of the Hippocratic Oath: the physician must protect his patient from the mischief and injustice which he may inflict upon himself if his diet is not properly chosen.[72] He must be a physician of the soul no less than of the body; he must not overlook the moral implications of his actions, nor even the negative indices to be watched; for the regimen followed by a person concerns both his bodily and his psychic constitution.[73]

1, p. 468, 19 ff.: ὅτι οἱ Πυθαγορικοί, ὡς ἔφη Ἀριστόξενος, καθάρσει ἐχρῶντο τοῦ μὲν σώματος διὰ τῆς ἰατρικῆς, τῆς δὲ ψυχῆς διὰ τῆς μουσικῆς; cf. Howald, op. cit., p. 203.

[69] That in these instances the prescription of diet is the correct way of treatment follows from the alleged cause of the diseases, cf. above, pp. 23 f. This is also confirmed by the fact that dietetics was the principal treatment given by the Pythagoreans, as Aristoxenus says, cf. below, p. 30. The methods outlined in the Platonic *Timaeus*, a Pythagorean dialogue if there is any, are identical. Plato uses almost the same words: διὸ παιδαγωγεῖν δεῖ διαίταις . . . (89 c); Littré, op. cit., IV, p. 622, also referred to this passage in explanation of the Hippocratic δίαιται; cf. Körner, op. cit., p. 11.

[70] Cf. p. 475, 25–33 [Diels-Kranz]: διὸ δὴ καὶ μεγάλης σοφίας ⟨δεῖσθαι⟩ τὸ κατανοῆσαί τε καὶ συνιδεῖν, ποίοις τε καὶ πόσοις δεῖ χρῆσθαι πρὸς τὴν τροφήν. εἶναι δὲ ταύτην τὴν ἐπιστήμην τὸ μὲν ἐξ ἀρχῆς Ἀπόλλωνός τε καὶ Παιῶνος, ὕστερον δὲ τῶν περὶ τὸν Ἀσκληπιόν (from Aristoxenus).

[71] Cf. above, pp. 23 f.

[72] Mischief (δήλησις) obviously is identical with what Aristoxenus calls βλαβεραὶ ἐπιθυμίαι; injustice (ἀδικία) is a concept that is implied by ὑβριστικαὶ ἐπιθυμίαι; cf. above, p. 23.

[73] Note that Plato in the *Timaeus*, 87 d, says that nothing is more dangerous than the ἀμετρία . . . ψυχῆς . . . πρὸς σῶμα; later on he states that most of the so-called physicians are deceived in their treatment because they seek the cause of the disease in the body, whereas in reality it is to be found in the soul (88 a).

The rules concerning dietetics, then, agree with Pythagoreanism, in fact they acquire meaning only if seen in the light of Pythagorean teaching. That the pharmacological precepts, the stipulations concerning poison and abortion, are Pythagorean in origin has already been demonstrated.[74] It remains to be shown that the laws laid down for surgery, too, are most easily understandable on the theory that they are founded on Pythagorean doctrine.

The physician vows: "I will not use the knife either on sufferers from stone, but I will give place to such as are craftsmen therein"; this at least is the most common rendering of the words in question.[75] Supposing that it be correct, what should be the reason for the prohibition here pronounced? The treatment of stone-diseases by operation, in Greek medicine, seems to have been an old-established procedure; at any rate, since the rise of Alexandrian medicine, such an operation was performed throughout the centuries.[76] Why then is it forbidden in the Oath?

From the Renaissance down to the nineteenth century there was only one answer to this question: the Oath in the clause concerning lithotomy intends to draw a line between the practice of internal medicine and that of surgery. This separation, it was added, is introduced because surgery was held to be beneath the dignity of the physician.[77] With finer historical judgment, Littré rejected this generally accepted

[74] Cf. above, p. 20. What the Pythagoreans understood by pharmacology and how they made use of it can be concluded from Aristoxenus' statement, quoted above, n. 54. For more details cf. below, pp. 30 f.

[75] For the text, cf. above, p. 5, 17–18; for the translation, cf. Jones, *op. cit.*, p. 11 (but cf. below, n. 89); Littré, *op. cit.*, IV, p. 631; Daremberg, *op. cit.*, p. 5; Pétrequin, *op. cit.*, I, p. 187; J. Hirschberg, *Vorlesungen über hippokratische Heilkunde*, 1922, p. 27; Körner, *op. cit.*, p. 12.

[76] Littré, *op. cit.*, IV, pp. 615 ff., has argued very convincingly that the operation must have been known since an early period because in Ps. Hippocrates, *De Morbis*, I, 6, diagnosis of the disease by means of a catheter is referred to as part of good craftsmanship. From Celsus, VII, 26, it follows that in his time great improvements in technique were made. Meges and Ammonius, whom he mentions, probably lived in the first century A.D.; cf. Hirschberg, *op. cit.*, p. 31; but the operation was certainly performed before; cf. Littré's interpretation of the passage, *op. cit.*, I, p. 342. For lithotomy in late centuries, cf. Ps. Galen, *Introductio* (Galen, XIV, p. 787 K.). Hirschberg, *op. cit.*, p. 32, believes that the Alexandrian physicians were the first to practice lithotomy, but this assumption he derives from the interdiction of this operation in the Hippocratic *Oath* which he considers a very old document (cf. *ibid.* p. 27). Such an argumentation, of course, is not cogent, since it is precisely the date of the *Oath* which has not been established so far.

[77] Cf. e.g., Th. Zwinger, *Hippocratis Opera*, 1579, p. 59. Cf. also I. Cornarius, *Hippocratis Opera*, 1558, p. 8; P. Memmius and J. Fabricius in their commentaries

view. He pointed out that the ancient practitioner was a surgeon as well as a physician and considered the interpretation current before his time to be influenced by modern prejudices; but he had to admit that if this were so the statement seemed to defy explanation.[78] Indeed if the words in question do not have the meaning usually presumed, what else could they signify?

Littré with great hesitation and caution intimated that the stumbling block could perhaps be removed by the assumption that the Oath does not refer to lithotomy at all, but to castration. Some modern scholars have accepted this suggestion. For moral reasons they have said the physician abhorred such a treatment.[79] I shall not repeat the argument that has been brought forward before: to reject castration on moral grounds and yet to leave it to others would be "like compounding a felony, if not something worse."[80] Although from a linguistic point of view it is not impossible to understand the text as referring to castration, such a rendering is not consistent with the subject matter. For it is not attested that the ancients ever thought of applying castration as treatment of stone-diseases.[81] The sentence under discussion, therefore, must concern lithotomy, not castration.

Now some scholars, recognizing the fact that the Oath refers to

on the *Oath*, published in 1577 and 1614 respectively. Cf. in general Körner, *op. cit.*, pp. 14 ff.; but cf. also below, n. 85.

[78] Cf. Littré, *op. cit.*, IV, pp. 616–17.

[79] Cf. Littré, *op, cit.*, IV, p. 620 (with reference to R. Moreau, a physician of the seventeenth century; cf. *ibid.*, p. 618); Th. Gomperz, *Griechische Denker*, I⁴, 1922, p. 231; in general S. Nittis, The Hippocratic Oath in reference to lithotomy, A new interpretation with historical notes on castration, *Bulletin of the History of Medicine*, VII, 1939, pp. 719 ff.

[80] Cf. Jones, *op. cit.*, p. 48; cf. also Körner, *op. cit.*, pp. 12 ff. Nittis being aware of the difficulties pointed out by Jones and Körner tries to evade them by translating ἐκχωρήσω etc. by "I will keep apart from men engaging in this deed" (*op. cit.*, p. 721). He thinks that this might be the meaning of the verb ἐκχωρήσω, but he is unable to adduce any evidence for such a usage: the meaning of χωρέω of course does not prove anything in regard to that of ἐκχωρέω, and ἀποστήσομαι to which Nittis refers as a parallel has exactly the sense of ἐκχωρέω as it is usually taken. How inappropriate Nittis' rendering is, one can easily conclude from an old variant of the *Oath*: οὔτ' ἐμοῖσι δὲ οὔτ' ἄλλοισι ἐκχωρήσω . . . (Jones, *op. cit.*, p. 19).

[81] Nittis, who has carefully investigated the history of castration, comes to the following conclusion (*op. cit.*, p. 728): "Castration . . . was . . . probably practiced for the cure and prevention of diseases. Lithiasis is not mentioned directly by any writer as one of the diseases preventable by castration . . . ." In view of the fact that castration cannot be meant here, it is unnecessary to discuss the many emendations proposed to facilitate this interpretation, cf. Hirschberg, *op. cit.*, p. 29. To rectify an assertion which has frequently been made, I wish to mention at least that ancient

lithotomy, contend that impotence was likely to result from the operation and that the physician recoiled from this risk—"it was against his liking"; "a higher concept of his profession" is supposed to have determined his renunciation of operative treatment by which he lost a good source of making money.[82] But such an interpretation can hardly be correct. To emphasize it once more: if the physician for moral reasons refuses to undertake the operation, he cannot possibly say in the same breath that he "will give place to such as are craftsmen therein."[83] The author of the Oath in other instances does not shrink from forbidding unconditionally what is held immoral or objectionable: when prohibiting the use of poison and of abortive remedies he does not say that the application of these drugs should be left to somebody else. The concession made in regard to lithotomy proves beyond doubt that the operation as such is not condemned: the performance of lithotomy, though not considered the business of the physician, is left to others for whom apparently it is judged legitimate.[84]

If this is true it seems to follow that lithotomy was to be given into the hands of specialists who were better able to do the job, that the Oath requires the physician to keep strictly within the limits of his own knowledge and recognize the superior skill of others who in some instances could be of greater help to his patients.[85] Such an explanation again leads into great difficulties. To be sure, specialization in certain operations or diseases of certain organs was known in antiquity. The stone-disease may have been one of these illnesses; lithotomy may have been practiced by craftsmen who were experts in this specific operation.[86]

---

physicians are known to have practiced castration for purposes other than medical, cf. Littré, *op. cit.*, IV, pp. 618 ff.

[82] Cf. Hirschberg, *op. cit.*, p. 30: "Eine solche Operation ging der Gilde gegen den Strich." As he says, Wilamowitz and Diels accepted his view. So does Deichgräber, *op. cit.*, p. 37, who writes: "Auch hier erhebt sich der Eid über die Sphäre der gewöhnlichen Handelsweise zu einer höheren Auffassung und wieder wird dem praktischen Arzte eine Erwerbsquelle verschlossen."

[83] Cf. above, p. 26.

[84] Incidentally, it is not attested that in the opinion of the ancients lithotomy could injure the procreative faculty, cf. Hirschberg's discussion of the medical aspect of the problem, *op. cit.*, pp. 30 ff., especially the passages from Celsus and Paulus of Aegina, *ibid.*, p. 32.

[85] Cf. Körner, *op. cit.*, pp. 15 ff. A very similar interpretation has been proposed by J. H. Meibom, *Hippocratis Jus Jurandum*, 1643, p. 163.

[86] The question of specialists in antiquity has been widely discussed. That from Alexandrian times on medicine became specialized can hardly be doubted. In Rome specialization in certain diseases reached a climax. Nothing definite is known about

But lithotomy as performed in antiquity was not a more daring operation than many another which the general practitioner undertook without hesitation. Why then should the physician acknowledge his own
limitations in this particular case?[87] If moderation on his part is the
general issue, why is he not asked to forego the treatment of all diseases
for which the ancients had specialists? It is true, a distinction is made
in the Oath between that which the physician should do and that which
he should leave to others. But this division is recommended only in regard to lithotomy, and it has to be understood with reference to this
particular instance.

There is no way out of the dilemma! The words must mean what
in the opinion of all early interpreters they seemed to mean: lithotomy
is here excluded because the performance of operations is held to be
incompatible with the physician's craft, and by the one example given
the Oath intends to exclude surgery in general from the field of the
physician. It is possible that originally more operations were named as
forbidden, that these references are missing only in the preserved text.
But such a hypothesis cannot be verified.[88] It is more probable, however, that the statement as it stands is intact but in itself carries broader
implications. For instead of translating "I will not use the knife either
on sufferers from stone," it is equally well possible to translate "I will
not use the knife, not even on sufferers from stone."[89] This would signify

the classical period. In spite of Cicero's emphatic statement that Hippocrates still
mastered the whole range of medical knowledge (*De Oratore*, III, 33) it is hard to believe that in the Hippocratic period specialization was unknown (contrary to Littré,
op. cit., IV, p. 615, n. 1, who follows A. Andreae, *Zur ältesten Geschichte der Augen-
heilkunde*, 1841); the material is too scanty to admit a decision of the issue.

[87] For operations performed by general practitioners, cf. Littré, *op. cit.*, IV, p.
617. That other operations made were more dangerous than lithotomy (contrary to
Körner, *op. cit.*, p. 15) has been emphasized by Hirschberg, *op. cit.*, p. 30, who also
stresses the fact that the ancient writers do not speak of an especially high mortality
rate in this instance.

[88] Körner, *op. cit.*, n. 16, mentions the possibility of a lacuna after οὐ τεμέω δὲ;
cf. also *C. M. G.*, I, 1, p. 4, 19: post δὲ lacunam statuit Diels (though for other reasons; cf. Hirschberg, *op. cit.*, p. 30). Deichgräber, *op. cit.*, n. 11, considers such an
assumption unnecessary.

[89] Jones is the only one who has strongly emphasized the possibility of such a
rendering. Moreover he has stressed the great difference in meaning that the two
translations involve (*op. cit.*, pp. 46–47; cf. also *ibid.*, p. 11, n. 1, and Hippocrates,
I, pp. 293 ff. [Loeb]); cf. also Nittis, *op. cit.*, p. 720, who goes so far as to say that
the usual translation of the words is grammatically incorrect. I am not sure that in
this respect he is right, but I do prefer the other rendering. Deichgräber, *op. cit.*,
n. 11, says of the crucial words: "οὐδὲ verstärkt die Negation wie Z. 15 (*sc.* after οὐ

that the physician directly renounces operative surgery altogether. He will not resort to it even in the case of that disease which more than any other, according to the testimony of the ancients, drove men to suicide.[90] The prohibition could not be formulated in more emphatic and solemn words.

Whatever rendering is chosen, the statement under discussion enjoins a separation of medicine and surgery. Driven back to this interpretation which no doubt is drastically at variance with reality, one feels almost inclined to say with Littré that such an explanation must be rejected, and that consequently the motive for the interdiction of lithotomy in the Oath remains obscure.[91] Yet this seems to be too rash a conclusion. It is true that the depreciation of surgery was foreign to ancient physicians in general.[92] It is likewise true, however, that one medical sect valued surgery less highly than dietetics and pharmacology, I mean the Pythagorean physicians. As Aristoxenus says, they believed "most of all" in dietetics; they applied poultices more liberally than did their predecessors, but "thought less" of the efficacy of drugs; "they believed least of all in using the knife and in cauterizing."[93] In other words, according to Aristoxenus, the Pythagoreans attributed different values to the various branches of medicine, and in their classification operative surgery together with cauterization was ranked lowest. If one remembers that in Aristoxenus' opinion the Pythagoreans explained

---

δώσω δέ); μήν beteuert, wie oft gerade in Eidschwüren und Versprechen." But in the passage quoted by Deichgräber, οὐδέ is used, not οὐδὲ μήν; this fact is indicative of a difference in meaning. For οὐδὲ μήν in the sense of intensification (not even), cf. Kühner-Gerth, *Griechische Grammatik*, II, 2, § 502, 4 b, p. 137. Cf. also the old Latin translation (Jones, *op. cit.*, p. 37): non incidam autem neque lapiditatem patientes; another translation (*op. cit.*, p. 35) corresponds to the rendering of most modern interpreters.

[90] Cf. above, n. 14, finis.

[91] Cf. Littré, *op. cit.*, p. 617. It is of course impossible to say with Jones, *op. cit.*, p. 48, or K. Sprengel, *Apologie des Hippokrates*, I, p. 77 (cf. Littré, *op. cit.*, I, p. 342), that the words in question are a later addition. If this statement were missing, surgery would not be referred to at all in the *Oath*.

[92] Cf. e.g., Littré, *op. cit.*, IV, p. 617. A separation of surgery from internal medicine can be traced at best to Galen's time (cf. Galen, X, pp. 454–55 K.; Jones, *op. cit.*, p. 48), that is, in the sense that physicians refused to practice surgery because they held it beneath their dignity. The study and teaching of the various branches of medicine had become specialized long before, cf. Celsus, *Introductio*, 9; cf. also above, n. 86.

[93] Cf. 58 D 1 [Diels-Kranz] (quoted above, n. 54); cf. Porphyry, *Vita Pythagorae*, 22: φυγαδευτέον πάσῃ μηχανῇ καὶ περικοπτέον πυρὶ καὶ σιδήρῳ καὶ μηχαναῖς παντοίαις ἀπὸ μὲν σώματος νόσον . . . (Aristoxenus = *Fr.* 8 [Müller]).

most diseases as the result of unreasonable living,[94] one is at first inclined to conclude that they were mainly interested in dietetics and pharmacology, because these were the more appropriate means of treatment. Still this can hardly be the whole truth. For Plato in the *Timaeus*, when outlining the Pythagorean treatment of diseases, does not mention cutting or cauterizing at all, though he agrees with Aristoxenus in placing the importance of pharmacology after that of dietetics.[95] Evidently, then, there must have been Pythagoreans who refused to apply any surgical means of treatment which were otherwise so universally used in Greek medicine. This inference from the Platonic *Timaeus* seems quite certain though no express statement to this effect is preserved.[96]

It is most likely that Aristoxenus' report is one of his typical attempts to reconcile the rigorous Pythagorean attitude with the demands of common sense and the exigencies of daily life: such compromises he introduces in many instances where other sources attest the uncompromising attitude of the Pythagoreans.[97] Seen from this angle, the

[94] Cf. above, pp. 22 ff.

[95] Cf. *Timaeus*, 87 c ff.; esp. 89 d.

[96] Note how in contrast to the passage in the *Timaeus*, Plato in the *Republic*, III, 405 c ff., defines medicine as the art which should deal with drugs or cauterization and cutting, whereas the pedagogics of dietetic medicine is rejected (406 d). It can hardly be by chance that Plato omits a reference to cutting and cauterization in the *Timaeus*. In K. Sprengel– I. Rosenbaum, *Versuch einer pragmatischen Geschichte der Arzneikunde*, I, 1846, p. 251, it is said: "Der schneidenden und brennenden Werkzeuge enthielt er (*sc.* Pythagoras) sich gänzlich," but the only testimony adduced is the fragment of Aristoxenus (cf. above, n. 54). J. F. K. Hecker, *Geschichte der Heilkunde*, I, 1822, p. 77, claims that: ". . . die Pythagorische Arzneikunst sich viel mit äusseren Mitteln beschäftigte, von der kühnern Chirurgie aber ganz entfernt blieb." He does not give any proof for this assertion. The more recent books on Pythagorean medicine do not discuss the problem at all. For the modern it may be difficult to imagine a medical art without surgery in the strict sense of the word (the treatment of fractures and so forth is of course not curtailed by the prohibition of operative surgery). Yet in antiquity popular opposition to "cutting and cauterization" was strong indeed. Cf. e.g., Plato, *Gorgias*, 456 b, and the parallels collected in Stallbaum's commentary *ad locum*. The attitude of the ancients never changed in this respect; cf. the most impressive statement of Scribonius Largus, *Compositiones*, p. 2, ll. 3 ff. [Helmreich]: ". . . siquidem verum est antiquos herbis ac radicibus earum corporis vitia curasse, quia timidum genus mortalium inter initia non facile se ferro ignique committebat. quod etiam nunc plerique faciunt, ne dicam omnes, et nisi magna conpulsi necessitate speque ipsius salutis non patiuntur sibi fieri, quae sane vix sunt toleranda."

[97] Note e.g., Aristoxenus' denial of the contention that Pythagoras refrained from all bloody sacrifices, p. 101, 13 ff. [Diels-Kranz], or his claim that he did not reject beans as nourishment, *ibid.*, p. 101, 19 ff., whereas others see in this prohibition a means of purification, *ibid.*, p. 463, 10 (Aristotle), p. 451, 15 ff. (early Peripatos).

stipulation of the Oath appears as another compromise, more lenient and at the same time more rigid than that reported by Aristoxenus: the use of cauterization obviously is allowed, operative surgery is completely eliminated. On the other hand, the Pythagorean physician will allow others to help his patient in his extremity. The stipulation against operating is valid only for him who has dedicated himself to a holy life. The Pythagoreans recognized that men in general could not observe any elaborate rules of purity; in this fact they saw no argument against that which they considered right for themselves. To give place to another craftsman, especially in such instances where the patient might fall prey to a sinful temptation,[98] certainly was a duty demanded by philanthropy, by commiseration with those who suffered.[99]

But why should the Pythagorean have avoided the use of the knife? The answer can only be a conjecture: he who believed that bloody sacrifices should not be offered to the gods and saw in them a defilement of divine purity could well believe that he himself would be defiled in his purity and holiness by using the knife in bloody operations.[100] However that may be, it is only in connection with Pythagorean medicine that the injunction of the Hippocratic Oath, according to which operative surgery was forbidden to the physician, acquires any meaning and

---

P. Corssen, *Rheinisches Museum*, LXVII, 1912, p. 258, intimated that Aristoxenus in his interpretation of Pythagorean philosophy is inclined to make the doctrine appear less rigid than it is portrayed by others. Cf. moreover Ueberweg-Praechter, *op. cit.*, p. 64.

[98] Cf. above, n. 14; p. 17.

[99] Already in Peripatetic attacks on the Pythagorean way of life the question was raised how a state could be governed in which everybody followed the Pythagorean taboos. The answer was that these purity-observances were not meant to be valid for everybody; cf. Porphyry, *De Abstinentia*, I, and J. Bernays, *Theophrastos' Schrift über Frömmigkeit*, 1866, p. 13. Moreover, the Pythagorean ideal of government is that of an aristocracy with proportionally divided rights and duties, cf. M. Pohlenz, *Aus Platos Werdezeit*, 1913, p. 154, n. 1 (Dicaearchus).

[100] There is no need for an elaborate discussion of the Pythagorean rejection of bloody sacrifices in which their insistence on purity manifested itself most clearly, cf. e.g., Diogenes Laertius, VIII, 13, and in general Bernays, who quite rightly speaks of the "Pythagoreische Blutscheu" (*op. cit.*, p. 33); cf. also the Pythagorean objections to the drinking of wine "the blood of the earth," Corssen, *op. cit.*, pp. 246 ff. (Androcydes). For the concept of defilement, cf. such expressions as Plato, *Laws*, VI, 782 c: τοὺς τῶν θεῶν βωμοὺς αἵματι μιαίνειν; cf. also Bernays, *op. cit.*, p. 130. For purification rites in regard to the knife that is used in bloody sacrifices, cf. Bernays, *op. cit.*, p. 91. Note that Aristoxenus, according to whom surgery, though valued least, was nevertheless practiced by the Pythagoreans, denies that they offered only bloodless gifts to the gods; cf. above, n. 97.

plausibility at all. The rules given in regard to surgery no less than those concerning dietetics and pharmacology are Pythagorean in character.[101]

Those stipulations of the Oath which deal with the medical treatment proper are finally followed by two more general provisions bearing on medical ethics in the strict sense of the word. The behavior of the physician toward his patient and the patient's family is regulated; reticence is imposed upon him in regard to whatever he may see or hear. Is it really true that in non-medical literature no parallels can be found to these postulates?[102] In my opinion these ethical rules, too, in their specific wording are understandable only in connection with Pythagorean doctrine.

As for the first vow, he who swears the Oath promises to come, into whatever house he enters, to help the sick, refraining from injustice and mischief, especially from all sexual incontinence.[103] That the physician should act for the sole purpose of assisting his patient, is a demand that seems self-evident. It certainly is as compatible with any ethical standard to which a doctor may subscribe, as it is with Pythagorean ethics.[104] It may seem equally natural that the physician is bidden to refrain from all injustice and mischief. Yet, the appropriateness of the statement does not imply that it is not in need of further explanation, be it in regard to its meaning or its motivation.[105]

Those who believe that only medical parallels can be adduced for the stipulations of the Oath point to seemingly similar utterances in one of the so-called Hippocratic writings, the book "On the Physician."[106] Here it is stated that in his relations with the sick the doctor ought to be just, for the patients have no small dealings with their physician.

---

[101] Cf. above, pp. 21 f., where it is shown that even the sequence of dietetics, pharmacology and surgery, as given in the *Oath*, corresponds to the sequence of these branches of medicine in the report of Aristoxenus.

[102] Cf. Deichgräber, *op. cit.*, p. 37: "Während sich die drei ersten Bestimmungen (*sc.* concerning dietetics, pharmacology, and surgery) mit ausserhalb der medizinischen Kreise und des medizinischen Bereiches geltenden Maximen vergleichen lassen, ist für diese Beschränkungen eine derartige Gegenüberstellung nicht möglich. Nur ein Vergleich mit den sonst in der hippokratischen Pflichtenlehre geltenden Anschauungen lässt sich durchführen . . ." (cf. however below, n. 109). The other interpreters do not attempt at all to give an explanation of these rules.

[103] Cf. above, p. 5, 19–21.

[104] For the ὠφέλιμον and its rôle in Pythagoreanism, cf. above, n. 57.

[105] Cf. Körner, *op. cit.*, p. 16, who in his interpretation of the *Oath* simply says: "Das nun folgende Gelöbnis bedarf keiner Erklärung."

[106] Cf. Deichgräber, *op. cit.*, p. 38; but cf. also Daremberg, *op. cit.*, p. 57.

They put themselves into his hands, and the physician comes in contact with women and maidens and with very precious possessions indeed; so toward all these self-control should be used.[107] I do not wish to raise the issue, whether justice is here commended for utilitarian rather than moral reasons. Nor do I emphasize the fact that only if it had a moral bent could this assertion be likened to the Oath.[108] In refutation of the argument of modern interpreters it is enough to say that the parallel referred to is by far less comprehensive and less rigorous than the statement which it is supposed to explain. The Oath, unlike the Hippocratic treatise "On the Physician," does not speak only of the avoidance of injustice, it also excludes mischief. Moreover, the Oath enjoins continence in regard to women and men alike; it stresses that the same continence must be observed toward free-born people and slaves, features that are entirely missing in the other passage.[109] A more satisfactory interpretation of the words in question, therefore, must be sought.

Now a plea for justice and continence may of course be derived from many ancient philosophical systems. As for justice, the Platonists and the Aristotelians praised its dignity no less than did the Pythagoreans.[110] But so much it is safe to claim: that the physician is required to abstain from all intentional injustice and mischief—such a formulation

---

[107] Cf. *C. M. G.*, I, 1, p. 20, 18 ff. In my paraphrase of the very difficult passage I have partly followed Jones' translation, *Hippocrates*, II, p. 313 [Loeb].

[108] For the idealistic point of view consistently observed in the *Oath*, cf. above, p. 28, and below, p. 50. As a matter of fact the author of Περὶ ἰητροῦ is a utilitarian, cf. below, n. 124.

[109] That this is so, is also admitted by Deichgräber, *op. cit.*, p. 38, who adds that the attitude taken in the *Oath* is in agreement with that taken by certain philosophers, but he does not say who they are.

[110] For Plato and Aristotle, cf. below, n. 117, for the Pythagoreans in general, cf. Zeller, *op. cit.*, I, 1, p. 390. I admit that the ultimate principles of Pythagorean ethics are not well known, but this much one may venture to say: justice played an important rôle in their system. Otherwise, why should justice determine men's relation to the gods and to all other creatures in the world (cf. 58 C 4, p. 464, 8 [Diels-Kranz]; Diogenes Laertius, VIII, 23; Iamblichus, *De Vita Pythagorica*, 168)? Why should Pythagoras have said of salt that it should be brought to table to remind us of what is just—for salt preserves whatever it seasons, and it arises from the purest sources, sun and sea (cf. 58 C 3, p. 463, 27 [Diels-Kranz])? Cf. also *Carmen Aureum*, ll. 13–16. But I do not wish to lay too much emphasis on this source, since it is of relatively late date (usually ascribed to the first century B.C. or A.D., cf. Ueberweg-Prächter, *op. cit.*, p. 518). Hierocles in his commentary on the *Carmen Aureum*, *Fragmenta Philosophorum Graecorum*, ed. F. G. A. Mullach, I, 1883, p. 433, goes so far as to claim that justice was the principal virtue of the Pythagoreans. But this is a late Neo-Platonic re-interpretation.

savors of the famous Pythagorean sayings by which injustice and mischief are proscribed, even if committed against animals and plants.[111] And indeed, to blend the concept of justice with that of forbearance is characteristic of the Pythagoreans. They abhorred violence; only if provoked by injustice would they resort to force. In this recoiling from aggression the asceticism of Pythagorean ethics culminated.[112] Moreover, the consequences drawn in the Oath from the ethical standards there imposed are in strict keeping with those principles which the Pythagoreans enforced upon their followers. Their views on sexual matters were severer than those of all other ancient philosophers. They alone judged sexual relations in terms of justice, meaning thereby not that which is forbidden or allowed by law: for the husband to be unfaithful to his wife was considered to be unjust toward her.[113] The Pythagoreans upheld the equality of men and women. They alone condemned sodomy.[114] Besides, in the performance of moral duties, they did not discriminate between social ranks. In that respect free-born people and slaves, for the Pythagoreans, were on equal footing.[115] Everything, then, that the Oath stipulates in regard to sexual continence agrees with the tenets of Pythagorean ethics, in fact with the ideals of these philosophers alone.

[111] Cf. Diogenes Laertius, VIII, 23 (from Androcydes, cf. Corssen, *op. cit.* p. 258): φυτὸν ἥμερον μήτε φθίνειν μήτε σίνεσθαι, ἀλλὰ μηδὲ ζῷον ὃ μὴ βλάπτει ἀνθρώπους In other passages the words used are even more reminiscent of the phraseology of the *Oath*, cf. Iamblichus, *De Vita Pythagorica*, 168: μήτε ἀδικεῖν . . . μήτε φονεύειν; *ibid.*, 99: μήτε βλάπτειν μήτε φθείρειν.

[112] The renunciation of violence is a natural consequence of the Pythagorean concept of purity and holiness. I do not think that such an ideal is to be found in any other ethical system of the ancients. Zeller rightly ascribes to the Pythagoreans "Gerechtigkeit und Sanftmut gegen alle Menschen," *op. cit.*, I, 1, p. 462.

[113] Cf. Ps. Aristotle, *Oeconomica*, I, 4: . . . ὑφηγεῖται δὲ [ὃ] καὶ ὁ κοινὸς νόμος, καθάπερ οἱ Πυθαγόρειοι λέγουσιν, ὥσπερ ἱκέτιν καὶ ἀφ᾽ ἑστίας ἠγμένην ὡς ἥκιστα δεῖν [δοκεῖν] ἀδικεῖν· ἀδικία δὲ ἀνδρὸς αἱ θύραζε συνουσίαι γιγνόμεναι. Cf. also Diodorus, X, 9, 3; 4; Iamblichus, *De Vita Pythagorica*, 132, and in general, above, pp. 19 f.; cf. also Zeller, *op. cit.*, I, 1, p. 462, n. 2. How foreign such reflections are to common Greek thought becomes apparent from Aristotle, who considers adultery unjust if committed for gain's sake; otherwise he calls it self-indulgence, *N. E.*, 1130 a 24 ff.

[114] Concerning women in the Pythagorean school, cf. Iamblichus, *De Vita Pythagorica*, 267; cf. Zeller, *op. cit.*, I, 1, p. 314, n. 4. As for the γεννήσεις παρὰ φύσιν, rejected by the Pythagoreans, cf. p. 476, 4–5 [Diels-Kranz], quoted above, n. 46. Even Plato, *Laws*, VII, 841 d, does not go as far as the Pythagoreans. For the usual Greek point of view, cf. Aristotle, *N. E.*, 1148 b 29 ff.

[115] For the Pythagorean attitude toward slaves, cf. E. Zeller–W. Nestle, *Grundriss d. Geschichte d. griech. Philosophie*[13], 1928, p. 40; but they speak only of "humane Behandlung." It would be more adequate, however, to speak of equality,

Finally, as a Pythagorean postulate the clause takes on a peculiar significance for the physician. It is justice first of all that is required from him. This virtue, to the average people, meant to live in accordance with the laws of the state.[116] To Plato, wherever he does not speak of justice in his own peculiar usage as the perfect working of the human soul in all its functions, justice was mainly a civic virtue. Aristotle tried to establish justice as a political virtue, and as one that applies to contracts and dealings in the law-courts.[117] All these aspects are also inherent in the Pythagorean concept of justice, and they certainly are of some concern for the physician. While in his direct dealings with men, in his personal contact with them and their households, it may be of less importance whether generally speaking he is a law-abiding citizen, it makes a great difference indeed, whether he is an honest man or not. It is in this sense that even the author of the Hippocratic book "On the Physician" counsels the doctor not to infringe upon the possessions of others with whom he is doing business.[118] But such justice, essential as it may be for good morals, is not all that the Pythagorean ideal of justice implies. To the adherents of this dogma, justice was the social virtue par excellence. As Aristoxenus reports,[119] they believed that "in

though there is no express statement to this effect among the Pythagorean testimonies, cf. J. Burckhardt, *Vorträge*, 1919, p. 193. As Aristoxenus says, p. 471, 8 f. [Diels-Kranz], the true Pythagorean will not punish anybody in anger, be he slave or free. Moreover, according to Aristotle, *N. E.*, 1132 b 22, the Pythagoreans define justice as reciprocity without qualification; cf. Zeller, *op. cit.*, I, 1, p. 390, n. 1. Aristotle adds that reciprocity fits neither distributive nor rectificatory justice, meaning thereby that punishment must differ in regard to the official status of the offender. In the *Magna Moralia*, 1194 a 28, the Pythagorean definition of justice is rejected because it cannot hold good in relation to all persons, "for the same thing is not just for a domestic as for a freeman." Obviously, then, the Pythagoreans did not believe that justice should be administered differently in the case of slaves. They believed in the equality of all human beings.

[116] Cf. Aristotle, *N. E.*, V, ch. 1, where also the proverbial saying is quoted: "In justice is every virtue comprehended," 1129 b 29–30.

[117] For Plato, cf. especially *Republic*, IV, 441 c ff., and *Laws*, VI, 757 a ff.; in general cf. Zeller, *op. cit.*, II, 1⁴, pp. 884–86. For Aristotle, cf. *N. E.*, V, chs. 2 ff.

[118] Cf. above, p. 34.

[119] 58 D 5, p. 470, 1 ff. [Diels-Kranz]: ἐπεὶ δὲ καὶ ἐν τῇ πρὸς ἕτερον χρείᾳ ἐστί τις δικαιοσύνη, καὶ ταύτης τοιοῦτόν τινα τρόπον λέγεται ὑπὸ τῶν Πυθαγορείων παραδίδοσθαι. εἶναι γὰρ κατὰ τὰς ὁμιλίας τὸν μὲν εὔκαιρον, τὸν δὲ ἄκαιρον, . . . ἔστι γάρ τι ὁμιλίας εἶδος, ὃ φαίνεται νεωτέρῳ μὲν πρὸς νεώτερον οὐκ ἄκαιρον εἶναι, πρὸς δὲ τὸν πρεσβύτερον ἄκαιρον. . . . τὸν αὐτὸν δ' εἶναι λόγον καὶ περὶ τῶν ἄλλων παθῶν τε καὶ πράξεων καὶ διαθέσεων καὶ ὁμιλιῶν καὶ ἐντεύξεων. . . . ἀκόλουθα δὲ εἶναι καὶ σχεδὸν τοιαῦτα, οἷα συμπαρέπεσθαι τῇ τοῦ καιροῦ φύσει τήν τε ὀνομαζομένην ὥραν καὶ τὸ πρέπον καὶ τὸ ἁρμόττον, καὶ εἴ τι ἄλλο τυγχάνει τούτοις ὁμοιογενὲς ὄν.

any relation with others" some kind of justice is involved. "In all inter-course" it is possible to take "a well-timed and an ill-timed attitude." In order to do what is proper, one must differentiate according to cir-cumstances. Speech and actions necessarily vary depending on the particular situation and the persons concerned. From the right decision result timeliness, appropriateness, and fitness of behavior, and it is justice that reveals itself in good manners.[120] Interpreted in the light of Pythagorean teaching, then, the recommendation of justice epitomizes all duties of the physician toward his patient in the contacts of daily life, all he should do or say in the course of his practice; it gives the rules of medical deportment in a nutshell.[121]

Last but not least: the promise of silence. The physician accepts the obligation to keep to himself all that he sees or hears during the treatment; he also swears not to divulge whatever comes to his knowl-edge outside of his medical activity in the life of men.[122] The latter phrase in particular has always seemed strange. It is so far-reaching in scope that it can hardly be explained by professional considerations alone.[123] To be sure, other medical writings also advise the physician to be reticent. The motive in doing so is the concern for the physician's renommée which might suffer if he is a prattler.[124] But the Oath de-mands silence in regard to that "which on no account one must spread abroad." It insists on secrecy not as a precaution but as a duty.[125] In

[120] Such a concept of justice seems entirely different from what Greek philoso-phers in general understand by justice. Aristotle, *N. E.*, 1126 b 36 ff., for instance discusses under temperance that which the Pythagoreans call justice. On the other hand, the Pythagorean definition of justice in part overlaps with the common one in so far as the law also touches upon conduct, cf. Aristotle, *N. E.*, V, ch. 1, and above, p. 36. In Aristoxenus' representation Pythagorean ethics often approximates the tenets of popular reflection, cf. Zeller, *op. cit.*, I, 1, p. 460, and above, n. 97.

[121] Deichgräber, who was the first to emphasize the importance which the con-cept of justice has in the *Oath* (*op. cit.*, pp. 37; 41 ff.), goes so far as to say that the *Oath* embodies the ideal of the just physician (cf. above, n. 10). This in my opinion is an exaggeration because the *Oath* combines the ideal of justice with that of for-bearance (cf. above, p. 35); moreover, holiness and purity are also insisted upon (cf. above, p. 20). Justice then, important as it is, is not the only standard which is here applied to human actions. Cf. also below, n. 128.

[122] Cf. above, p. 5, 22–23.

[123] Cf. Jones, *op. cit.*, p. 50.

[124] Cf. Hippocrates, Περὶ ἰητροῦ, *C. M. G.*, I, 1, p. 20, 9: τὰ δὲ περὶ τὴν ψυχὴν σώφρονα, μὴ μόνον τῷ σιγᾶν . . . μέγιστα γὰρ ἔχει πρὸς δόξαν ἀγαθά. Deichgräber, *op. cit.*, p. 37, refers to this passage; he himself admits that the statement serves merely utilitarian purposes.

[125] Incidentally, Körner, *op. cit.*, p. 6, translates ἃ μὴ χρή ποτε ἐκλαλέεσθαι ἔξω by "wenn es nicht in die Öffentlichkeit gebracht werden muss," and in his interpreta-

the same way silence about things which are not to be communicated to others was considered a moral obligation by the Pythagoreans. They did not tell everything to everybody. They did not indiscriminately impart their knowledge to others. They expected the scientist to be reticent and ready to listen.[126] They observed silence even in daily life. That they were taciturn beyond all other men no less than the fact that they were frugal in their habits made them the object of ridicule in ancient comedy.[127] Certainly if the doctor who promises not to talk about anything that he may see or hear is to be placed in any philosophical school, it must be the Pythagorean.

To sum up the results of the analysis of the ethical code: the provisions concerning the application of poison and of abortive remedies, in their inflexibility, intimated that the second part of the Oath is influenced by Pythagorean ideas. The interpretation of the other medical and ethical stipulations showed that they, too, are tinged by Pythagorean theories.[128] All statements can be understood only, or at any rate

---

tion, *ibid.*, p. 17, states that this clause means that the physician should keep to himself everything except that which it is his duty to bring to public attention. In other words, Körner finds in the *Oath* a distinction between that which the physician owes to his patient and that which he owes to the community. Apart from the fact that the physician's obligations toward the state are nowhere mentioned in the document, such an interpretation is not warranted by the words. ἔξω is not "Öffentlichkeit" but simply "outside." Moreover, the text gives no indication as to what the physician should say, but only as to what he should keep to himself. Cf. also next note.

[126] Cf. Diogenes Laertius, VIII, 15 (Aristoxenus): μὴ εἶναι πρὸς πάντας πάντα ῥητά. Cf. 58 D 1, p. 467, 4 [Diels-Kranz]: σιωπηλοὺς δὲ εἶναι καὶ ἀκουστικοὺς . . . (from Aristoxenus after introductory remarks about the sciences accepted by the Pythagoreans [music, medicine, mantics]); cf. also below, pp. 47 f., concerning the transmission of knowledge in the Pythagorean school. Later, the ability to be reticent, in Pythagorean education, was considered the strongest proof of self-continence, the sign by which to distinguish good from bad pupils. Compare ἃ μὴ χρή in the *Oath* with Iamblichus, *De Vita Pythagorica*, 71: καὶ τὴν σιωπὴν καὶ τὴν λαλιὰν παρὰ τὸ δέον (from Apollonius [?]; cf. Rohde, *op. cit.*, p. 137).

[127] Cf. the fragment from Alexis, p. 479, 36 [Diels-Kranz]; cf. also, *ibid.*, p. 466, 20: γλώσσης πρὸ τῶν ἄλλων κράτει θεοῖς ἑπόμενος (old *Symbolon*), and *ibid.*, p. 97, 33 (Isocrates, *Busiris*, 29); in general cf. Zeller, *op. cit.*, III, 2, p. 80, n. 1. I need hardly refer to the proverbial *Silentium Pythagoricum*.

[128] Deichgräber, taking Apollo as the symbol of purity and justice, has characterized the morality advocated in the *Oath* as Apolline ethics, but this term as he uses it, is an invention *ad hoc* (*op. cit.*, p. 42: . . . "wenn man so will, die Idee des apollinischen Arztes"). To be sure, the Delphic religion promoted a certain ethical attitude, but the little that is known about it concerns men's relation to God and Fate rather than to his fellow men, cf. E. Howald, *Ethik des Altertums, Handbuch der Philosophie*, 1926, p. 11. An ethics as it is found in the Hippocratic *Oath* was a historical reality only in Pythagoreanism. That in some respects this philosophical

they can be understood best, as adaptations of Pythagorean teaching to the specific task of the physician. Even from a formal point of view, these rules are reminiscent of Pythagoreanism: just as in the Oath the doctor is told what to do and what not to do, so the Pythagorean oral instruction indicated what to do and what not to do.[129] Far from being the expression of the common Greek attitude toward medicine or of the natural duties of the physician, the ethical code rather reflects opinions which were peculiarly those of a small and isolated group.

system itself was influenced by Delphic concepts is possible; the ancients thought so themselves, cf. Diogenes Laertius, VIII, 8 (Aristoxenus). But such an agreement between Delphi and Pythagorean philosophy does not cover all those detailed injunctions in which the Oath coincides with the Pythagorean system.

[129] Cf. p. 464, 4 [Diels-Kranz]: Ἀκούσματα . . . τρία εἴδη . . . τὰ δὲ τί δεῖ πράττειν ἢ μὴ πράττειν. Deichgräber, op. cit., p. 41, contends that the Oath "nur negative Bestimmungen enthält." Although the negative formulations are more numerous in the Oath, one cannot overlook the most emphatic positive statements concerning the physician's purity and holiness (cf. above, p. 5, 15–16), and concerning his promise to bring help to his patient (cf. above, p. 5, 12; 19).

II. THE COVENANT

The ethical code by the acceptance of which the physician gives a higher sanction to his practical endeavor is preceded by a solemn agreement concerning medical education. The pupil promises to regard his teacher as equal to his parents, to share his life with him, to support him with money if he should be in need of it. Next he vows to hold his teacher's children as equals to his brothers and to teach them the art without fee and covenant if they should wish to learn it. Finally he takes upon himself the obligation to impart precepts, oral instruction and all the other learning to his own sons, to those of his teacher and to pupils who have signed the covenant and have taken an oath according to the medical law, to all these, but to no one else.[130]

Whatever the precise purport of the single terms and phrases used in this covenant, so much is immediately clear in regard to its general meaning and is commonly admitted: the teacher here is made the adopted father of the pupil, the teacher's family becomes the pupil's adopted family. In other words, the covenant establishes between teacher and pupil the closest and most sacred relationship that can be imagined between men, and it does so for no other apparent reason than that the pupil is being instructed in the art.

In explaining this stipulation modern interpreters usually allege that in Greece, in early centuries, medicine like all the other arts was passed on from father to son in closed family guilds. When at a certain time these organizations began to receive outsiders into their midst, they are said to have demanded from them full participation in the responsibilities of the "real" children. Consequently those who wished to be admitted to all the privileges and rights of the family had to become its members through adoption. The Hippocratic covenant, then, it is claimed, is an engagement which was signed by newcomers joining one of the medical artisan families, and it was probably the family of the Asclepiads in which this formula held good.[131]

The evidence for such a theory, in my opinion, is insufficient. Galen is the only ancient author who asserts that the Asclepiads, after having been for generations the sole possessors of medicine, later shared their knowledge with people not belonging to their clan. And even he says

[130] Cf. above, p. 5, 5–11.
[131] Cf. e.g., Littré, *op. cit.*, IV, pp. 611 ff.; I, pp. 341 ff.; Daremberg, *op. cit.*, p. 2; for later proponents of this view, cf. Jones, *op. cit.*, p. 44.

that these outsiders were men whom the family esteemed "on account of their virtue"; he does not contend that they were made members of the family or forced to accept any obligations.[132] It is hardly by chance, therefore, that Galen himself does not refer to the Hippocratic Oath as bearing out the truth of his story. In any case, his words cannot be adduced as corroborative proof for the assumptions of modern scholars. Nor does it increase the strength of the modern argument if Galen's testimony is combined with that of Plato, according to whom "physicians taught their sons medicine and . . . Hippocrates taught outside pupils for a fee."[133] Though Plato says this, it still does not follow that the outsiders became the adopted children of their masters. On the contrary, who will believe that the young Athenian aristocrat Hippocrates of whom Plato speaks would have considered paying a fee to the great Hippocrates for instruction, had that meant that he should enter the family of the Coan physician![134]

If thus the usual interpretation of the Hippocratic covenant is unsupported by external testimony, it is equally unfounded as far as the wording of the text is concerned. For the covenant itself does not refer to a family guild of physicians. It speaks only of the pupil and the teacher, leaving open the question whether the latter is the son of a physician, the member of a clan of doctors, or not.[135] In view of this fact it does not help to concede, as some scholars have done, that adoptions of outsiders into artisan families are hardly known from any other source, and yet to maintain that the Hippocratic covenant only con-

---

[132] Cf. Galen, *Opera*, II, pp. 280 ff. K. The most important words are: . . . καὶ τοῖς ἔξω τοῦ γένους ἔδοξε καλὸν (!) εἶναι μεταδιδόναι τῆς τέχνης . . . ἤδη γὰρ τελέοις ἀνδράσιν, οὓς ἐτίμησαν ἀρετῆς ἕνεκα, ἐκοινώνουν τῆς τέχνης.

[133] Cf. Jones, *op. cit.*, p. 56; the Platonic passages referred to are *Laws*, IV, 720 b; *Protagoras*, 311 b. Substantially the same considerations are to be found in Littré, *op. cit.*, IV, pp. 611 ff., and in most authors who take the covenant as a document indicative of the state of family organizations.

[134] Cf. *Protagoras*, 311 b. Hirschberg, *op. cit.*, p. 28, seems the only one to admit that Plato does not give evidence for the *Oath*. For he emphasizes that in Plato's time the regulations found in the Hippocratic covenant—which he considers early— did no longer exist.

[135] As far as I know Jones has been the first to stress this fact. Cf. Jones, *Hippocrates*, I, p. 293: "Some scholars regard the *Oath* as the test required by the Asclepiad Guild. The document, however, does not contain a single word which supports this contention. It binds the student to his master and his master's family, not to a guild or corporation." Cf. also *The Doctor's Oath*, p. 56: "a private agreement between master and apprentice." Nevertheless Jones accepts the general view (*ibid.*, p. 44) that the covenant has something to do with the Asclepiad guild; but cf. also below, n. 157.

firms what must be presumed anyhow on the basis of generally valid laws of economic development. In all civilizations, it is stated, crafts were first restricted to family guilds; eventually these organizations became mere trade unions accessible to all; in a transitory period between these two stages the families adopted outsiders as "quasi-children."[136] I am not prepared to discuss the correctness of these so-called economic laws, nor do I wish to judge whether they are applicable to the Greek situation. The Hippocratic covenant at all events neither confirms such a theory, nor can it be explained by it; for there is no indication in the text that the document is concerned with family interests or family politics.[137]

Yet, if through the covenant the pupil is not received into a family guild, if he is made rather the adopted son of his teacher—was such a relationship common among the Greeks of any period? Some scholars answer this question in the affirmative. In the time preceding that of the Sophists, they say, the teacher generally was esteemed as the "spiritual father" of his pupil.[138] But this assertion can be made only if the Hippocratic covenant is taken as the basis for speculations and generalizations which are not warranted by any additional evidence. Granted that the covenant is determined by a concept of spiritual kinship between teacher and pupil, it is nowhere attested that the same idea prevailed in all schools and guilds of the pre-classical era, or in any of them for that matter.[139] Surely, it is not permissible to conclude from

[136] Cf. Deichgräber, *op. cit.*, pp. 32 ff. He says, p. 32: ". . . eine Idee, wie wir sie vielleicht im griechischen Vereinswesen hier und dort voraussetzen dürfen, aus antiken Nachrichten aber kaum kennen." As a matter of fact, even E. Ziebarth, *Das griechische Vereinswesen*, 1896, p. 96, to whom Deichgräber refers, apparently in explanation of his "vielleicht" and "kaum" (n. 18), knows of no other testimony than the Hippocratic *Oath*. Concerning Galen, II, p. 280, cf. above, p. 40. Plato, *Republic*, X, 599 c and *Fragmenta Historicorum Graecorum*, ed. G. Müller, II, 1848, p. 263, passages which Ziebarth quotes in addition, do not yield anything concerning the problem of adoption.

[137] I should mention that in consequence of the usual interpretation of the covenant different ethical standards have to be presupposed for the two sections of the *Oath* (cf. above, p. 7). To use the characterization of Deichgräber who has most strongly brought out this discrepancy (*op. cit.*, p. 38; p. 42): the first part shows a business point of view, whereas the second is determined by Apolline concepts of purity. Concerning this problem, cf. also above, n. 128, and below, pp. 50 ff.

[138] Cf. E. Hoffmann, Kulturphilosophisches bei den Vorsokratikern, *Neue Jahrbücher f. Wissenschaft u. Jugendbildung*, V, 1929, pp. 19–20. This article, in spite of its importance, is strangely neglected in the literature on the *Oath*.

[139] Hoffmann, *loc. cit.*, says: "Über andere als ärztliche Schulen haben wir aus jener Zeit leider nur Legenden, aber diese Legenden sagen uns ganz Ähnliches. In

the covenant that the lack of such evidence in regard to other than medical teaching in the sixth and early fifth centuries is merely fortuitous. For it is uncertain when the Hippocratic Oath was composed, and the document which itself needs explanation and identification cannot possibly serve as the starting point for theorizing about otherwise unknown circumstances.[140] There is no reason, then, to assume that the adoption of the pupil by the teacher was a common characteristic of archaic education. Nor is such a practice known to have been customary in ancient scientific or practical training at any other time.[141]

There is one particular historical setting, however, one particular province of Greek pedagogics where a counterpart of the Hippocratic covenant can be found: the Pythagoreans of the fourth century apparently were wont to honor those by whom they had been instructed as their fathers by adoption. So Epaminondas is said to have done; and in Epaminondas' time it was told of Pythagoras himself that he had revered his teacher as a son reveres his father.[142] If the Hippocratic

---

dem Bunde der Pythagoreer z. B. war die Treue unter den Schülern des Meisters wie die Treue zwischen Brüdern: Damon und Phintias. Die geistigen Söhne des Meisters sind eben Brüder." Hoffmann himself, then, admits that these stories portray situations only distantly related to those of the *Oath*, for he speaks only of "similarity." Note, moreover, that the legend of Damon and Phintias, to which alone Hoffmann refers in proof of his statement, concerns events taking place in the fourth century B.C., in the time of Dionysius of Syracuse; cf. p. 472, 1 ff. [Diels-Kranz]. In view of the uncertainty in regard to the history of the old Pythagorean school (cf. above, pp. 20 f.), it is impossible simply to reconstruct conditions of the sixth century on the evidence of the fourth century. Finally, even if the old Pythagorean society was a fraternity and was based on a spiritual kinship with the master, Pythagoras would not necessarily be the direct teacher of his pupils as is the master of the covenant; he would be the teacher and father of all Pythagoreans, even of those who lived long after him, because he was the founder of the school. In how far the covenant is determined also by a concept of spiritual kinship between teacher and pupil will be discussed below, n. 191.

[140] For the divergent assumptions concerning the date of the *Oath*, cf. below, pp. 55 ff. Hoffmann's thesis which presupposes the pre-Sophistic origin of the *Oath* without adducing any proof can be characterized only as *ignotum per ignotius*.

[141] S. Nittis, The Authorship and Probable Date of the Hippocratic Oath, *Bulletin of the History of Medicine*, VIII, 1940, pp. 1012 ff., who takes the covenant as the statute of a medical fraternity around 420 B.C., comparable to that of other fraternal societies of this time and later centuries, has not succeeded in finding one instance where in such organizations the pupil was adopted by the teacher.

[142] Cf. Diodorus, X, 11, 2: καὶ πατὴρ αὐτοῦ (sc. of Epaminondas) θετὸς ἐγένετο δι' εὔνοιαν (sc. his teacher Lysis); cf. Plutarch, *De Genio Socratis*, ch. 13, 583 C: . . . πατὴρ . . . ἐπιγραφείς. That the expression does not indicate a particular attachment of Epaminondas to Lysis is evident from what Diodorus, X, 3, 4, says about Pythagoras' relation to his teacher, Pherecydes: ὡσανεί τις υἱὸς πατέρα (Aristoxenus, cf. p. 44, 34

covenant is viewed against the background of such testimony, the specific form in which the pupil is here bound to his teacher is no longer an unexplainable and isolated phenomenon. Compared with Pythagorean concepts of teaching and learning as they were evolved in the fourth century B.C., the vow of the medical student assumes definite historical meaning.[143]

This result seems to imply that the covenant as a whole must be influenced by Pythagorean philosophy. The agreement between the Hippocratic treatise and the Pythagorean reports concerns so unusual a circumstance that they are most unlikely to be independent of each other. Nor is it probable that the Pythagoreans derived their pattern of instruction from a medical manifesto that in the range of medical education and indeed of general education is without parallel.[144] Nevertheless one should hesitate to claim Pythagorean origin for the covenant by reason of one feature only, even if it be the main feature of this document.[145] But as matters stand, all the other demands enjoined upon the pupil may likewise be explained only in connection with Pythagorean views and customs, or at least they are compatible with them.

To take those duties first which the pupil acknowledges in regard to his mentor: he is asked to share his life with his teacher and to support him with money if need be.[146] This statement usually is considered an extravagant exaggeration that cannot be taken at its face value. Or, to avoid the stumbling block of excessive and improbable magnanimity, the words are said really to signify that the pupil should share with his master his livelihood, not his life, and if need be support him with money. Such an interpretation, however, itself falls prey to the objection that it gives to certain terms an unusual sense and makes the two stipulations of which the sentence consists meaningless repetitions.[147] In the light of what is known about the Pythagoreans the words

[Diels-Kranz]). Aristoxenus, too, relates of Epaminondas, p. 104, 3 [Diels-Kranz]: καὶ πατέρα τὸν Λῦσιν ἐκάλεσεν (for the source of this passage, cf. ibid., p. 103, n. 13). In these passages, which Hoffmann apparently overlooked, the father-son relation is expressly attested, and it is supposed to exist between the pupil and his teacher, just as in the Hippocratic Oath.

[143] Hoffmann, then, was fundamentally right in his suggestion that the Hippocratic Oath and Pythagorean doctrine are related, though the details of his argument are erroneous.

[144] Cf. above, pp. 42 f.   [145] Cf. above, p. 40.
[146] Cf. above, p. 5, 5-6.
[147] For the former view, cf. e.g., Jones, Hippocrates, I, p, 292: "Indeed, such

chosen ring true. That the Pythagorean pupil shared his money with his teacher if necessary, one may readily believe. To support his father was the son's duty, even according to common law. This obligation was the more binding for the Pythagorean, who was taught to honor his parents above all others.[148] But the Pythagorean also came to his teacher's assistance in all the vicissitudes of life, wherever and whenever he was needed: he tended him in illness; he procured burial for him. All this is admiringly reported of Pythagoras himself.[149] The Pythagorean pupil was indeed supposed to share his life with his master, as the son does with his father. He did much more than advance money to him in case of an emergency.[150]

Next, the Hippocratic covenant admonishes the pupil to regard his teacher's offspring as his brothers, and without fee and covenant to teach them his art if they wish to learn it.[151] That the teacher's children

---

clauses could never be enforced; if they could have been, and if a physician had one or two rich pupils, his financial position would have been enviable." *Ibid.*, p. 295: "These (*sc.* clauses) might well contain promises to the teacher couched in extravagant language if taken literally, but which were intended to be interpreted in the spirit rather than in the letter." For the reinterpretation of the text, cf. e.g., Jones, *The Doctor's Oath*, p. 9: "To make him partner in my livelihood, and when he is in need of money to share mine with him"; Deichgräber, *op. cit.*, p. 31: "Mit ihm den Unterhalt zu teilen und ihn mitzuversorgen, falls er Not leidet." If pupil and teacher share their livelihood, how can the one be in need without the other being in need also? Or how could the one support the other in such a case? For βίος in the sense in which I have translated it, cf. the *Oath* itself, above, p. 5, 16; 25. Incidentally, Deichgräber, *op. cit.*, n. 7, rightly rejects as unwarranted Ziebarth's interpretation, *op. cit.*, p. 97, according to which the second part of the sentence is supposed to mean that if need be the pupil has to pay the teacher's debts.

[148] For the Pythagorean insistence on the reverence to be paid to parents, cf. Diogenes Laertius, VIII, 23: ἀνθρώπων δὲ μάλιστα τοὺς γονέας (*sc.* τιμᾶν); cf. p. 460, 12 ff. [Diels-Kranz] (Aristoxenus). In addition, one must remember that, according to Pythagorean doctrine, even friends shared everything, if one of them had lost his property, cf. below, n. 154.

[149] Cf. Diodorus, X, 3, 4, and above, n. 142. The same story is told by Iamblichus, *De Vita Pythagorica*, 183-84, who concludes with the following words: οὕτω περὶ πολλοῦ τὴν περὶ τὸν διδάσκαλον ἐποιεῖτο σπουδήν. This statement is perhaps taken from Nicomachus, cf. Rohde, *op. cit.*, p. 159, but the story itself is older, as is clear from Diodorus and also from Aristoxenus, cf. above, n. 142. For the Pythagorean emphasis on the importance of an appropriate burial, cf. Plutarch, *De Genio Socratis*, 585 E.

[150] The importance which such a life companionship had for the Pythagoreans in general is evident also from the name later given to them: κοινόβιοι, Iamblichus, *De Vita Pythagorica*, 29; cf. also the term συμβίωσις as characteristic of the relationship between the brothers, *ibid.*, 81.

[151] Cf. above, p. 5, 7-8. Concerning the exact meaning of the term "covenant," συγγραφή, cf. below, n. 158. Deichgräber, *op. cit.*, n. 9, is certainly right in rejecting

should be the pupil's brothers naturally follows from the fact that the disciple acknowledges his master as his father. Thus the teacher's sons and his pupils become one flesh and blood.[152] But the preference shown for the interest of the members of the family, the unselfishness commended in the relationship to them, the confidence put in their reliability without any insistence on formal guarantees—all these features are characteristic of Pythagorean ethics.[153] The Pythagoreans were admonished to turn to their brothers first, and to make friends with them before all others outside the family. Moreover, all Pythagoreans considered themselves brothers and were believed, like brothers, to have divided their earthly goods among themselves. Their unquestioned belief in their brothers' trustworthiness did not falter even in the face of death.[154]

---

the interpretation "Schuldschein" as opposed to "barer Lohn" (μισθός) proposed by Th. Meyer-Steineg–W. Schonack, *Hippokrates, Über Aufgaben u. Pflichten d. Arztes, Kleine Texte*, 1913, nr. 120. Such a meaning of the word is not attested.

[152] Note that the pupil is asked to consider his teacher's children (γένος τὸ ἐξ αὐτοῦ) as his "male brothers" (ἀδελφοὶ ἄρρενες). Jones, *op. cit.*, p. 9, translates "brothers"; he thinks that the word ἄρρενες is "quite otiose" (*ibid.*, p. 43, n. 1). Deichgräber, *op. cit.*, p. 31, translates "männliche Geschwister." Earlier interpretations are collected and rejected by Daremberg, *op. cit.*, p. 6, n. 3. Daremberg himself translates "propres frères," *ibid.*, p. 5. Yet in Greek law the rights of kin differ as to male and female lineage, the former preceding the latter; cf. W. Erdmann, *Die Ehe im alten Griechenland*, 1934, pp. 117 ff.; pp. 125–6. ἀδελφοὶ ἄρρενες therefore probably means "brothers of male lineage" (for ἄρρενες in this sense, cf. e.g., Isaeus, VII, 20). Thus the relationship between adopted and real children is made as close as possible. Note that in *Carmen Aureum*, l. 4 (quoted below, n. 154) the ἄγχιστ᾽ ἐγγεγαῶτες are mentioned after the parents. They constitute the so-called ἀγχιστεία which is contrasted with the relatives of female lineage even in the late laws of Charondas, cf. Diodorus, XII, 15, 2, and Erdmann, *op. cit.*, p. 134, n. 62.

[153] That the form of a "Hausgemeinschaft" which is envisaged in the Hippocratic covenant is also typically Pythagorean will be shown below, pp. 57 f.

[154] For the seeking of their brothers' friendship, cf. Sotion, *Fragmenta Philosophorum Graecorum*, II, p. 47 [Mullach]: οἱ ἀδελφοὺς παρέντες καὶ ἄλλους φίλους ζητοῦντες παραπλήσιοι τοῖς τὴν ἑαυτῶν γῆν ἐῶσι, τὴν δὲ ἀλλοτρίαν γεωργοῦσιν (Sotion is a Neo-Pythagorean of the first century A.D.; cf. F. Susemihl, *Geschichte der Griechischen Literatur*, II, 1892, p. 332, n. 459); cf. *Carmen Aureum*, l. 4: σούς τε γονεῖς τίμα, τούς τ᾽ ἄγχιστ᾽ ἐγγεγαῶτας; but the statements seem to echo old tradition, cf. the insistence on family relations, Diogenes Laertius, VIII, 23, quoted above, n. 148; cf. also below, pp. 57 f. For the Pythagorean communism, cf. Diodorus, X, 3, 5: ὅτι ἐπειδάν τινες τῶν συνήθων ἐκ τῆς οὐσίας ἐκπέσοιεν, διῃροῦντο τὰ χρήματα αὐτῶν ὡς πρὸς ἀδελφούς. Cf. also Aristoxenus, p. 472, 16 ff. [Diels-Kranz], and Diogenes Laertius, VIII, 10; Gellius, *Noctes Atticae*, I, 9, 12. For the Pythagorean willingness to respond unhesitatingly to every demand made by one of their brothers, cf. the famous story of Phintias and Damon, Aristoxenus, p. 472, 1 ff. [Diels-Kranz]. Note especially ἡ προσποίητος πίστις (*ibid.*, p. 472, 7), and ἔφη οὖν ὁ Διονύσιος θαυμάσαι τε καὶ ἐρωτῆσαι, εἰ ἔστιν ὁ ἄνθρωπος οὗτος, ὅστις ὑπομενεῖ θανάτου γενέσθαι ἐγγυητής (*ibid.*, p. 472, 19).

Under these circumstances, how could the Pythagorean do other than teach his adopted brothers without fee the knowledge which he had acquired? What assurances could he expect or ask of them before he instructed them in the art that he had learned from their father?

Finally, the fact that in the Hippocratic covenant teaching is divided into precepts, oral instruction and the other learning,[155] is best understood as a Pythagorean classification. The precepts of Pythagoras, handed down from one generation to the other, were greatly renowned throughout the centuries. "Oral instruction" and "learning" were the two categories under which Aristoxenus listed all that was "taught and said" in Pythagorean circles, and all that the members of the school tried "to learn and remember."[156] That knowledge, according to the covenant, is to be imparted to a closed circle of selected people alone, most assuredly is in agreement with those principles on which the transmission of Pythagorean doctrine was based. The Pythagoreans differed from all other philosophical sects in that they did not divulge their teaching to everybody.[157] They carefully examined those who wished to join them. It is attested even that they exacted an oath from the pupil who was to be admitted, just as the Hippocratic treatise speaks of out-

---

[155] Cf. above, p. 5, 8–11.

[156] The terms used in the covenant are: παραγγελίη, ἀκρόησις, ἡ λοιπή μάθησις. For the first of these, cf. Aristoxenus, p. 477, 13 [Diels-Kranz]: παραγγέλματα (sc. of Pythagoras). For the second and third, cf. μαθήσεις καὶ ἀκροάσεις, Aristoxenus, ibid., p. 467, 18. The exact meaning of these words is difficult to ascertain. Παραγγέλματα are maxims, perhaps similar to what in other reports are called ἀκούσματα, short practical rules without rational explanation, cf. p. 463, 33 [Diels-Kranz]; ἀκροάσεις probably are lectures; and μάθησις should comprise all other studies, whether theoretical or practical. Similarly the terms may also be used in the Hippocratic covenant. Cf. also next note. Whatever the correct explanation may be, one need not agree with Jones' statement, op. cit., p. 43, n. 1: ". . . I feel sure that all scholars will consider the division of instruction into παραγγελίη, ἀκρόησις, and ἡ λοιπή μάθησις curious and unusual."

[157] Cf. Diogenes Laertius, VIII, 15, quoted above, n. 126 (Aristoxenus), and in general Zeller, op. cit., I, 1, pp. 315 ff. On account of the restriction of teaching demanded in the covenant one cannot explain παραγγελίη, ἀκρόησις, μάθησις (cf. preceding note) by parallels taken from non-Pythagorean schools of philosophy, or from other Hippocratic writings (cf. e.g., Daremberg, op. cit., p. 7, n. 5; Jones, op. cit., p. 9, n. 2). For these schools were open to everybody, and ἀκρόησις in Ps. Hippocrates, Παραγγελίαι, ch. XII, means "lecture before a crowd," just as the Παραγγελίαι themselves with which Jones compares the παραγγελίη of the covenant (op. cit., p. 9, n. 2) formed a published book available to every reader. Incidentally, Jones, op. cit., p. 45, refers to the Pythagoreans who, he says, perhaps held meetings from which outsiders were excluded. But he does not make use of this parallel for the interpretation of the Oath.

siders who sign the covenant and take an oath before they are allowed to participate in the course of studies.[158]

To sum up: not only the main feature of the covenant, the father-son relationship between teacher and pupil, but also all the detailed stipulations concerning the duties of the pupil can be paralleled by doctrines peculiar to the followers of Pythagoras.[159] If related to Pythagoreanism, the specific formulas used in the covenant acquire meaning and definiteness. What otherwise appears exaggerated, or strange, or even fictitious, thus becomes the adequate expression of a real situation. Since the rules proposed show no affinity with any other Greek educational theory or practice, it seems permissible to claim that the Hippocratic covenant is inspired by Pythagorean doctrine.

[158] For the Pythagorean Oath, cf. below, pp. 53 f. The covenant refers to pupils who are συγγεγραμμένοι τε καὶ ὡρκισμένοι νόμῳ ἰητρικῷ; Jones, *op. cit.*, p. 9, translates: "who have signed the indenture and sworn obedience to the physician's Law." But Deichgräber's rendering, *op. cit.*, p. 31: "vertraglich verpflichtet und vereidigt nach ärztlichem Brauch" seems more correct. The ξυγγραφή referred to here obviously is the same from which the teacher's children are exempted, cf. above, p. 45; but it is hardly identical with the covenant which the *Oath* contains, cf. below, p. 49. Nittis, *op. cit.*, p. 1019, says that the phrase implies that "others (*sc.* those who were not sons of physicians) had to qualify by a test, enrollment in the society, which naturally meant meeting the financial obligations of the association, taking the *Oath* and the payment of tuition." Not only does the covenant not concern societies, but as far as I can see, ξυγγραφή never has the meaning given to it by Nittis.

[159] As far as I am aware, my interpretation has covered all the points mentioned in the covenant, except the payment of a teaching-fee by the outside student, a regulation to be inferred from the fact that fees are remitted to the children of the master (cf. above, p. 45). The evidence available does not indicate whether the Pythagoreans took money for instruction. But even Hippocrates taught medicine for a fee (cf. Plato, *Protagoras*, 311 b), and many philosophers charged money for their courses.

III. The Unity of the Document

Covenant and ethical code, the two parts of which the so-called Hippocratic Oath consists, in the preserved text form a unity. Without any marked transition the first section is followed by the second.[160] Is there any reason for believing that the two have not always belonged together?

It seems certain that the obligations laid down in the covenant and in the ethical code are assumed by the physician simultaneously, that is, at the moment of his entering the medical profession as a practitioner in his own right. The promise to help the teacher and the stipulation concerning the teaching to be given to others point to the fact that he who takes the Oath has become an independent craftsman.[161] In the same way the rules regarding the practitioner's behavior are best understandable if imposed upon the doctor who is now starting out on his career. For as long as the pupil is still under the supervision of his teacher, his actions of necessity are regulated by his master's orders. In short, covenant and ethical code are signed together, not by the beginner but rather by the student who has completed his course.[162]

[160] It should be noted, however, that the covenant is given in infinitives, whereas the code is given in the first person. That this difference in style is an indication of archaic speech Deichgräber, *op. cit.*, p. 30, n. 3, has assumed but has not proved; that it is indicative of an original independence of the two sections is quite possible. Perhaps the covenant originally was used in various fields of instruction and was only taken over into the medical manifesto; if that were so, it would be easier to understand why the covenant refers to "the art" instead of to medicine. This, no doubt, would be a better explanation of this strange fact than the one given by Jones, *op. cit.*, pp. 50–51, who says that the physician "here called his profession, with glorious arrogance, 'the art'." Incidentally, the juxtaposition of aorist and future tenses which Jones blames as incorrect, *op. cit.*, p. 7; p. 43, n. 1, is not an uncommon usage, cf. Kühner-Gerth, *Griechische Grammatik*, II, 1, § 389, p. 195 A 7, esp. p. 197 *finis*.

[161] Moreover, as Deichgräber has rightly pointed out, *op. cit.*, p. 32, the covenant mentions another oath, apparently sworn before instruction begins.

[162] Cf. Deichgräber, *op. cit.*, p. 32: ". . . der Schwörende, offenbar ein Schüler, der nach Abschluss der Ausbildung in die Praxis geht, ..." Jones, *op. cit.*, p. 44; pp. 56 ff., seems to be of the same opinion, but he characterizes the covenant as an agreement between pupil and teacher, while he calls the ethical code an obligation toward the society of physicians. There is no reason for such a distinction, cf. below, pp. 60–61. It is true, as O. Temkin suggests, that because in ancient medicine the apprentice assisted his master in his practice (cf. e.g., Ps. Hippocrates, *Prorrhetikon*, II, IX, p. 20 L.), the ethical rules might apply to the student. Cf. also C. Singer, *A Short History of Medicine*, 1928, p. 17. Yet for the reasons just given it seems more likely that the *Oath* was administered after the teaching had ended and the pupil became responsible for his own actions.

Moreover the two parts are a spiritual unity. For it is not true, contrary to what is sometimes claimed, that the covenant exhibits a realistic business attitude, whereas the ethical code is determined by a lofty and exalted standard of conduct.[163] The agreement concerning teaching and the rules of professional behavior both reflect the same idealistic outlook on human affairs, they are steeped in Pythagorean doctrine. The same can be said of the preamble and the peroration by which the document is introduced and concluded as one coherent formula.

In the invocation, Apollo the physician, Asclepius and his children, and all the gods and goddesses are made witnesses of the vow to be taken.[164] That all the divine powers are called upon is the usual form in which an ancient oath, at least an oath of some importance, is pronounced, for this makes the protestation all the more solemn.[165] That Apollo the physician and his son Asclepius are named in particular is quite appropriate for a medical oath. It is also in agreement with Pythagorean views that a member of the medical profession should invoke these deities. According to Aristoxenus, the art of selecting the right food and drink for the human regimen, in the belief of the Pythagoreans, had first been practiced by Apollo and Paeon, while later it was taken over by the physicians, the sons of Asclepius. The Pythagorean doctor, the healer of diseases by diet, then, must have revered precisely the gods whom the Oath addresses.[166] That Asclepius' divine children, Panaceia and Hygieia, are called upon in addition is not astounding. The names of all the members of the divine medical family come naturally to the

[163] Cf. Deichgräber, *op. cit.*, p. 34; p. 38. Deichgräber fails to explain how statements of so different an ethos should ever have become a unity. Jones, who also sharply distinguishes the two parts, seems not to find any difference in regard to the ethical standards though in his opinion the covenant is somewhat at variance with the code, cf. especially, *op. cit.*, p. 43.

[164] Cf. above, p. 5, 2–4.

[165] Cf. E. Ziebarth, *De iure iurando*, 1892, pp. 17 ff.; Deichgräber, *op. cit.*, n. 13.

[166] Cf. p. 475, 32 f. [Diels-Kranz] (quoted above, n. 70). Apollo the physician, as the *Oath* has it, obviously is Apollo and Paeon of whom Aristoxenus speaks; the two were often merged into one deity of medicine; cf. H. Usener, *Götternamen*, 1896, pp. 153 ff. Note that contrary to Deichgräber, *op. cit.*, p. 42, Apollo here is not necessarily the Delphic god, the god of purity. The Delphic Apollo renounces medicine in favor of his son Asclepius, cf. Wilamowitz, *Der Glaube der Hellenen*, II, 1932, p. 35. Nor is he commonly regarded as patron of the physicians (Deichgräber, *ibid.*); statements to this effect, such as Callimachus, *Hymnus in Apollinem*, II, 45–6, are very rare. But for the Pythagoreans, who reformed medicine according to their concept of purity and who introduced music into medicine (cf. p. 467, 13–15 [Diels-Kranz]), the Delphic Apollo may indeed have been identical with the god of medicine.

mind of the believer in Apollo and Asclepius when he takes upon himself those obligations that will guide his future life as a physician.[167]

Having invoked the gods as witnesses and having bound himself to live in purity and holiness, justice and forbearance, he who swears asks that he may enjoy his life and art in fame if the vow is kept inviolate; if it is not carried out, the opposite shall befall him.[168] Does this peroration indicate that in his very heart the physician is motivated not by ethical standards but rather by the wish to attain success? Is it his reputation that he wants to see enhanced by all his actions and that he forswears in case of his failure to fulfil his obligations?[169] This can hardly be the meaning of the words in question. For it is not fame or a good name among his clients for which the juror prays, it is fame for all time among all men, it is immortal fame that is here implored or renounced.[170] Such a wish one cannot reasonably call aspiring to a good reputation in the interest of business, though a good reputation was of great practical importance for the ancient doctor.[171] Rather is this prayer characteristic of the Greek love for glory, of the ancient belief in eternal fame on this earth as a stimulus to all good deeds. No less a man than Solon, in exactly the words of the Oath, asks for renown among all future generations in recompense for what he has done and written. In the same vein Plato acknowledges that the craving for undying fame is the real motive of all great achievements.[172]

[167] For Hygieia and Panaceia as daughters of Asclepius, cf. e.g., *Paean Erythraeus in Aesculapium*, ed. I. U. Powell, *Collectanea Alexandrina*, 1925, p. 136.

[168] Cf. above, p. 5, 24–26. That the prayer for divine blessing is coupled with an execration is typical for a solemn oath; cf. R. Hirzel, *Der Eid*, 1902, p. 138; cf. also H. Schöne, *Sokrates*, I, 1913, p. 127; Deichgräber, *op. cit.*, n. 14. It should also be emphasized that it is usual to invoke the gods at the beginning, while at the end only the consequences that will ensue in this world are mentioned; cf. Hirzel, *op. cit.*, p. 69.

[169] Cf. Deichgräber, *op. cit.*, pp. 35–36, who sees in the wish for fame the confirmation of his opinion that even here the utilitarian point of view is not set aside. The physician's regard for his reputation, he thinks, is only tempered by his concern for what is right, *ibid.*, p. 41.

[170] Cf. above, p. 5, 25–26: δοξαζομένῳ παρὰ πᾶσιν ἀνθρώποις ἐς τὸν ἀεὶ χρόνον. The expression is as tautological as the words of Plato, *Symposium*, 298 c: κλέος ἐς τὸν ἀεὶ χρόνον ἀθάνατον καταθέσθαι.

[171] I am the last to deny the significance which the physician's regard for reputation had in ancient medicine; cf. L. Edelstein, *Problemata*, IV, 1931, chap. III [87*]. But the attitude outlined in the *Oath* is enjoined in opposition to the realities and exigencies of daily life; here an attempt is made to better existing conditions, to remedy the rather deplorable state of affairs, cf. below, p. 59.

[172] Cf. Solon, I, 3–4: ὄλβον μοι πρὸς θεῶν μακάρων δότε καὶ πρὸς ἀπάντων/ ἀνθρώπων αἰεὶ δόξαν ἔχειν ἀγαθήν. Plato, *Symposium*, 298 c ff.; cf. also Pindar, *Isthmiae*, IV, 12;

That such an insistence on glory is in the opinion of the Greeks entirely compatible with an idealistic attitude can be proved by many instances. Even the earliest philosopher who upheld a philanthropic and moral belief against the philosophy of success saw in glory the righteous aim of human actions.[173] Nor did the Pythagoreans shun this goal. Aristoxenus reports that they were opposed only to such glory as consists in the approbation of the many, but thought it foolish to despise all fame.[174] It is for this reason that glory, though sometimes deprecated by the Pythagoreans and grouped together with the vices, in other instances is extolled as praiseworthy.[175] Most important: the Pythagoreans, too, were striving for that glory which makes a man's name live for all time to come. Pythagoras himself was said to have exhorted his pupils to philosophical endeavor by stating that "education stays with men unto death, and for some it brings immortal fame even after death."[176] No doubt, the Pythagoreans approved of the desire for fame. The physician who prays for glory does not violate the code of Pythagorean ethics.[177]

---

and in general J. Burckhardt, *Griechische Kulturgeschichte*, ed. J. Oeri, IV³, pp. 233 ff. (for the heroic time, *ibid.*, p. 17).

[173] I am thinking of the so-called *Anonymus Iamblichi*, 80 [Diels-Kranz]; cf. especially II, p. 402, 19–20 [Diels-Kranz]; cf. in general W. Capelle, *Die Griechische Philosophie*, II, 1, p. 24 (Göschen nr. 858) and also R. Roller, *Untersuchungen zum Anonymus Iamblichi*, Diss. Tübingen, 1931. Cf. below, n. 177.

[174] Cf. p. 473, 32 ff. [Diels-Kranz]: ἀνόητον μὲν εἶναι καὶ τὸ πάσῃ καὶ παντὸς δόξῃ προσέχειν . . . ἀνόητον δ' εἶναι καὶ πάσης ὑπολήψεώς τε καὶ δόξης καταφρονεῖν. (In the index of Kranz this passage is said to deal with δόξα in the sense of "opinion"; but δόξα παρὰ τῶν πολλῶν, lines 33–4, clearly is "fame"; note also the connection in which the passage is quoted by Iamblichus). A very similar statement is found in Iamblichus, *Protrepticus*, ch. 6, p. 40, 7 [Pistelli]; cf. also Iamblichus, *De Vita Pythagorica*, 72 (Apollonius), cf. Rohde, *op. cit.*, p. 137.

[175] Cf. such passages as p. 471, 23 [Diels-Kranz] (φιλοτιμία, ἐπιθυμία, ὀργή), or Iamblichus, *De Vita Pythagorica*, 69 (δόξα, πλοῦτος); cf. also *ibid.*, 188; 226. On the other hand, cf. *ibid.*, 223: . . . τὴν σωτηρίαν τῆς ἐννόμου δόξης, δι' ἣν αὐτός τε μόνα τὰ δοκοῦντα ἑαυτῷ ἔπραττε . . . .

[176] Cf. Iamblichus, *De Vita Pythagorica*, 42: . . . τῆς δὲ παιδείας καθάπερ οἱ καλοὶ κἀγαθοὶ τῶν ἀνδρῶν μέχρι θανάτου παραμενούσης, ἐνίοις δὲ καὶ μετὰ τὴν τελευτὴν ἀθάνατον δόξαν περιποιούσης (from Timaeus through Apollonius [cf. Rohde, *op. cit.*, p. 134; P. Corssen, *Sokrates*, I, 1913, pp. 199 ff.]; "aus . . . Bruchstücken ächter Tradition" [Rohde, *ibid.*]).

[177] Burckhardt, *Griechische Kulturgeschichte*, IV, p. 166; *Vorträge*, p. 198, holds that Pythagoras was the only philosopher who opposed the Greek craving for glory. But Porphyry, *Vita Pythagorae*, 32: φιλοτιμίαν φεύγειν καὶ φιλοδοξίαν (from Diogenes), the only passage quoted by Burckhardt, must be interpreted in the light of the testimony of Aristoxenus referred to above, n. 174. In addition it should be noted that

Yet one may object: even granted that the content of the invocation and the peroration seems to be Pythagorean, were the followers of
Pythagoras allowed to take an oath, to swear in the names of the gods?
Certainly some Pythagorean sources stipulate that one should not
swear by the gods, but should rather make oneself the witness of one's
own words.[178] Still this hardly means that the Pythagoreans intended
to ban all oaths and all invocations of divine witnesses. No Greek could
ever have gone that far.[179] It is true, "Pythagoras" tried to remedy the
notorious Greek predilection for making oaths. Yet the aim of the
Pythagoreans was the restriction, not the abolition of vows. As Diodorus
expressly states, in the opinion of the school, an oath should be sworn
only on rare occasions.[180] Even the late Pythagoreans, though they seem
to have been stricter in this respect, did not renounce vows altogether.
Just as the physician is supposed to take an oath when he settles down
to practice, so those who intended to become members of the Pythagorean society took an oath of allegiance.[181]

At this point, I think, I can say without hesitation that the so-called
Oath of Hippocrates is a document, uniformly conceived and thoroughly
saturated with Pythagorean philosophy. In spirit and in letter, in form
and content, it is a Pythagorean manifesto. The main features of the
Oath are understandable only in connection with Pythagoreanism; all
its details are in complete agreement with this system of thought. If only

---

the idealistic ethical system to which I have alluded (cf. above, n. 173) is known only
from Iamblichus, who integrates these passages into his *Protrepticus* as the final
incentive to the study of philosophy. The name of the author whom he follows is
unknown (cf. II, p. 400, n. 1 [Diels-Kranz]). Could he have been a Pythagorean?

[178] Cf. Diogenes Laertius, VIII, 22: μηδ᾽ ὀμνύναι θεούς· ἀσκεῖν γὰρ αὐτὸν δεῖν ἀξιόπιστον
παρέχειν (from Androcydes, thus Corssen, *Rh. M.*, LXVII, 1912, p. 258).

[179] Cf. Hirzel, *op. cit.*, p. 112, who points out the difference between this attitude
and that of the Jews and Christians.

[180] Diodorus, X, 9, 2: ὅτι Πυθαγόρας παρήγγελε τοῖς μανθάνουσι σπανίως μὲν ὀμνύναι,
. . . ; cf. Hirzel, *op. cit.*, pp. 98 ff.; Burckhardt, *Griechische Kulturgeschichte*, III, p.
320. H. Diels, *Archiv f. Geschichte d. Philosophie*, III, 1890, p. 457, does not do justice to this divergence of the tradition. Diodorus' statement most probably goes
back to Aristoxenus, on whom he largely depends, cf. E. Schwartz, *s. v.* Diodorus,
Pauly-Wissowa, V, p. 679, for it is in perfect agreement with Aristoxenus' compro-
mising attitude, cf. above, n. 97.

[181] For the Neo-Pythagoreans in general, cf. Zeller, *op. cit.*, III, 2, p. 146 (I, 1,
p. 462, n. 7), and again for the similarity of the Pythagorean attitude with that of
the Essenians, *ibid.*, III, 2, p. 284, n. 5; cf. also Hirzel, *op. cit.*, pp. 99–100. Julian,
VII, 236 D, probably in opposition to the Christians, says: . . . οὔτε τὸ ὅρκῳ χρῆσθαι
προπετῶς τοῖς τῶν θεῶν ὀνόμασιν [sc. ἐπέτρεπεν]. Pétrequin, *op. cit.*, p. 173, was the first
to compare the Hippocratic *Oath* with Pythagorean fidelity to a vow.

one or another characteristic had been uncovered, one might consider the coincidence fortuitous. Since the concord is complete, and since there is no counterinstance of any other influence, all indications point to the conclusion that the Oath is a Pythagorean document.

IV. DATE AND PURPOSE OF THE OATH

The origin of the Hippocratic Oath having been established, it should now be possible to determine the time when the Oath was written and the purpose for which it was intended. What answers regarding these questions are to be deduced from the analysis of the document?

As for the date, it seems one must conclude that the Oath was not composed before the fourth century B.C. All the doctrines followed in the treatise are characteristic of Pythagoreanism as it was envisaged in the fourth century B.C.[182] It is most probable even that the Oath was outlined only in the second half or toward the end of the fourth century, for the greater part of the parallels adduced are taken from the works of pupils of Aristotle.

Yet is such an assumption not irreconcilable with certain external data? Aristophanes, it is said, in one of his comedies performed in 411 B.C. makes mention of the Hippocratic Oath.[183] Not even the ancient commentators dared to claim that the Hippocrates referred to here was the physician of Cos. Eager as they were to find allusions to great historical names wherever that was possible, and even where it was most unlikely, in the case in question they expressly stated that the Hippocrates whom Aristophanes names was an Athenian general.[184] Nor can one infer from linguistic considerations that the Oath was written in the

---

[182] The only exceptions to this statement are the references to Sotion and to the *Carmen Aureum* (cf. above, n. 154). I think it permissible to say that, the whole argument taken into consideration, these two instances do not invalidate the claim that the interpretation given rests on the testimony of fourth century authors.

[183] D. Triller in the eighteenth century seems to have been the originator of this claim. Littré first followed him, *op. cit.*, I, p. 31, but later rejected the theory, cf. *ibid.*, II, p. xlviii; IV, p. 610. Pétrequin, however, repeated Triller's argument, *op. cit.*, p. 172, n. 1, and it has again been brought forward by Jones, *op. cit.*, p. 40.

[184] Cf. Aristophanes, *Scholia in Thesmophoriazusas*, v. 273; in *Nubes*, v. 1001; and Daremberg, *op. cit.*, p. 1, n. 1. I must confess that I fail to discover any reference to an Oath of Hippocrates in the lines in question. Euripides swears by Aether, the abode of Zeus (272). The interlocutor asks why he does so instead of swearing τὴν Ἱπποκράτους ξυνοικίαν. This, Jones, *op. cit.*, p. 40, takes to mean: "by the community of Hippocrates." But ξυνοικία is a tenement house in which many families live, and it is apparently the joke of the whole statement that the interlocutor does not understand why the oath should be made by the house of Zeus rather than by the house of Hippocrates. That by ξυνοικία "Aristophanes probably had in mind the opening words of Oath, with their comprehensive ξυνοικία of divinities" (Jones, *ibid.*), I cannot believe, the less so, since ξυνοικία is never used in the sense required by Jones' interpretation. It should also be noted that Athenaeus, III, 96 e–f, says that "the sons of Hippocrates were ridiculed in comedy for swinishness," a statement which certainly refers to the Aristophanes passages under discussion.

fifth century. Granted for the sake of argument that the great Hippocrates was the author of the Oath; that he was in Athens in the year 421 B.C.; that the words "covenant" and "law" in Athens between March and October, 421, were used interchangeably to cover the same meaning, just as they are supposedly used in the Oath—all this would have no bearing on the date of this document, for it is written in the Ionic, not in the Attic dialect.[185] There is, then, no reason for rejecting the date that seems to follow from the internal evidence on the basis of external data.[186]

On the other hand, one may argue: it is true, the Oath agrees with reports of fourth century writers on Pythagoreanism; yet these accounts, though they stem from the fourth century, must not necessarily describe the Pythagorean system as it was evolved or understood at that time; the passages may in part at least reflect older conditions or reproduce more ancient traditions; the composition of the Hippocratic Oath, therefore, could well fall into an earlier period. However, such reasoning is not probable. I shall not dwell on the fact that the Pythagorean system of the fifth or even of the sixth century is practically unknown, that whatever is reported about the old Pythagorean teaching as a whole is, if not the invention, at least the interpretation of authors of the fourth century.[187] Two of the main provisions of the Oath are connected with theories that are attributed either directly or indirectly to Philolaus, a contemporary of Plato. This makes the turn of the fifth to the fourth century the *terminus post quem* for the composition of the Oath.[188] Moreover, even if one or another ethical precept ascribed to the Pythagoreans

---

[185] Cf. Nittis, *Bulletin of the History of Medicine*, 1940, p. 1020. I am far from admitting that Nittis' statements concerning the terms νόμος and ξυγγραφή are convincing, but for the reason given above I see no need to go into the details of his theory. In regard to the external evidence, I should mention at least that the Hippocratic *Oath* in reality is first mentioned by Erotianus and by Scribonius Largus in the first century A.D. Erotianus' list of Hippocratic writings probably goes back to Hellenistic sources, but even so the *Oath* would not be attested before the third century B.C. (cf. Deichgräber, *op. cit.*, n. 1).

[186] That the fifth century origin of the *Oath* cannot be proved by reference to general sociological laws has been shown above, pp. 41 f.

[187] Cf. above, pp. 20 f.; in general Ueberweg-Praechter, *op. cit.*, pp. 67 ff.; cf. also *ibid.*, p. 66: "Im allgemeinen gilt, abgesehen von jener Lehre (*sc.* that of metempsychosis), jedenfalls der Satz, dass wir nur von einer Philosophie der Pythagoreer, nicht des Pythagoras sprechen können, wie dies in der Tat auch schon bei Aristoteles geschieht." And these Pythagoreans, as far as their names are known, are Philolaus and his contemporaries or successors, cf. *ibid.*, p. 61.

[188] For Philolaus and his relation to Plato, cf. e.g., Ueberweg-Praechter, *op. cit.*, p. 65 (44 A 5 [Diels-Kranz]); cf. above, p. 17 and p. 19.

by Aristoxenus and accepted in the Hippocratic Oath was held also by older Pythagoreans, the whole program of instruction envisaged in the Oath in conformity with the Pythagorean model is characteristic of fourth century Pythagoreanism; for it presupposes the destruction of the Pythagorean society in the last decades of the fifth century.[189] As Aristoxenus relates, it was after the uprising in Italy that Lysis went to Thebes where he taught Epaminondas and was revered by him as his adopted father. In a letter ascribed to him, Lysis protests against those who after the dissolution of the society made the Pythagorean dogma available to everybody. Pythagoras himself, Lysis asserts, had charged his daughter never to give his writings to those "outside of the house."[190] Whether this letter is genuine or not, it must have been for some such reasons that Lysis bound Epaminondas to himself as his adopted son. This afforded the only solution which made it possible to initiate outsiders into the Pythagorean doctrine, and yet to keep it a secret, a "family secret," as is also the intention of the Oath.[191] But such a rela-

[189] For the time of the dissolution of the Pythagorean society through which the members of the school were brought from Italy to Greece, cf. Zeller, *op. cit.*, I, 1, pp. 332 ff.; Ueberweg-Praechter, *op. cit.*, p. 65; K. v. Fritz, Pythagorean Politics in Southern Italy, 1940, p. 92.

[190] Cf. p. 104, 1 ff. [Diels-Kranz], and Diogenes Laertius, VIII, 42; Hercher, *Epistolographi Graeci*, p. 603, 5. For the authenticity of the letter, cf. p. 421, 12 ff. [Diels-Kranz]. The situation is viewed in the same manner by Aristoxenus, cf. Diogenes Laertius, VIII, 15, and Timaeus, cf. *ibid.*, 54. Nicomachus also summarizes the situation by asserting that the Pythagoreans restricted their teaching to the members of their own families, cf. Iamblichus, *De Vita Pythagorica*, 253; 251; Porphyry, *Vita Pythagorae*, 58. Nicomachus uses the same words ἔξω τῆς οἰκίας which appear in the letter of Lysis.

[191] Cf. above, p. 45. The belief in a spiritual kinship between teacher and pupil (cf. above, p. 42) may also have been influential in the founding of this system of education, for even in their ethical behavior the Pythagoreans were bidden to take toward each other the attitude of the good father toward his children, cf. p. 471, 24 [Diels-Kranz]; *ibid.*, 477, 15 (Aristoxenus), where again this fatherly love is compared with that of the benefactor; both must be free from envy. If men owe to nature their lives, but to education their knowledge of the right life (Diodorus, XII, 13, 3 [Charondas]; cf. Rohde, *op. cit.*, p. 168), the teacher can well be called the spiritual father of the pupil. But basically the insistence on an adoption of the pupil is determined by external factors, by the new situation in which the Pythagoreans found themselves in the fourth century B.C. In this connection it seems worth pointing out that in the Platonic *Phaedo*, which is strongly influenced by Pythagorean concepts, Socrates is once referred to as the father of his pupils (116 a), just as late Neo-Platonists, for whom the Platonic and Pythagorean dogmas coincide, again speak of their teacher as their father and even of the teacher's teacher as their grandfather, cf. Marinus, *Vita Procli*, 29. For the importance of the father-son relation in later mystery cults, cf. R. Reitzenstein, *Die hellenistischen Mysterienreligionen*³, 1927, p. 20 (cf. also first edition, 1910, p. 27).

tionship between teacher and pupil could be instituted only after the disappearance of the great fraternity that had existed before. Only at that moment did the transmission of the Pythagorean doctrine become the concern of the individual Pythagorean; in earlier times it had been promoted by the society itself. The Hippocratic Oath, which calls the teacher the adopted father of the pupil, can hardly have been composed, therefore, before the fourth century B.C.[192]

Nor is it likely that the document is of later origin. In the fourth century B.C. Pythagoreanism reached the peak of its importance. Its influence gradually began to wane from the beginning of the Hellenistic period. When in the first century B.C. the Pythagorean system was revived and again became a potent factor in philosophical speculation, it took on traits very different from those which are characteristic of the earlier dogma and the prescripts of the Oath.[193] Moreover, in Alexandria medical ethics was integrated into the teaching of the medical sects. Closely connected as these newly established schools were with philosophy, Pythagoreanism played no part in their teaching. A direct influence of Pythagorean philosophy on medicine, however, is not probable.[194]

Yet in the fourth century B.C. the Hippocratic Oath in every respect

[192] That the *Oath* cannot be traced to pre-Sophistic times for the reasons adduced by Hoffmann, has been shown above, p. 42. Meyer-Steineg–Schonack, *op. cit.*, p. 4, assume the date of the sixth century without even attempting to give a proof for their assertion; cf. also Deichgräber, *op. cit.*, n. 24.

[193] For the general development of Pythagoreanism, cf. Ueberweg-Prächter, *op. cit.*, p. 65; pp. 513 ff.; esp. p. 516. Even if the Pythagorean school was not entirely in eclipse in Hellenistic centuries, it certainly had lost its strong hold over the philosophical mind. Yet in the fourth century B.C. Pythagoreanism through Plato, Aristotle and their schools had become a subject of general interest for the educated. As the references in the Middle Comedy prove, the followers of Pythagoras were also figures familiar to everyone. The Neo-Pythagorean movement of the first century B.C. is influenced by mystic tendencies; the ascetic features are overstressed; the practical interest in human affairs which the *Oath* presupposes, cf. below, p. 59, is almost entirely lacking. That is why I cannot believe that the *Oath* is in any way connected with this late teaching.

[194] It has sometimes been claimed that the Hippocratic *Oath* was written in Hellenistic times. The proof offered is the fact that medicine is here divided into dietetics, pharmacology and surgery, cf. Münzer, *Münchener medizinische Wochenschrift*, 1919, p. 309; cf. Körner, *op. cit.*, p. 7. That this division is not typical of Alexandrian medicine has been shown above, n. 54. C. Singer, *From Magic to Science*, 1928, p. 18, goes so far as to say: "Despite the Ionic Greek dress in which this formula is known to us, there is evidence that it is of Imperial date, and of Roman rather than of Greek origin"; cf. the same, *A Short History of Medicine*, 1928, pp. 16 ff.: parts earlier than Hippocrates, the *Oath* as such very much later. Singer does not make explicit why he holds this belief.

was a timely manifesto. In that period many individual attempts were made to improve medical conditions. Abuses, to be sure, had been criticized even before.[195] But it is in those Hippocratic treatises that were written in the second half of the fourth century or even later, that one finds the first outlines of a system of medical deontology. Moreover, these endeavors at reform were instigated by the reflection on ethical problems as it developed in the rising philosophical schools.[196] Thus a medical ethics devised in accordance with Pythagoreanism is well in agreement with the general trend of thought in that period. On the other hand, from the point of view of fourth century Pythagoreanism it was quite justifiable that those concepts which underlay philosophical instruction were applied also to the teaching of the healing art, and that Pythagorean ethics was infused into the practice of medicine. The school ranked medicine together with music and mantic as the supreme sciences. Medical skill, to its members, was the greatest wisdom attainable by men.[197] The standards of medical education, therefore, could not be set too high. Moreover, the Pythagoreans thought that "love for what is truly noble" manifests itself in practical pursuits and in the sciences— for here the love for good habits and the devotion to them become apparent—and consequently they called the fair and dignified sciences "full of love for the noble." To imbue medicine with the spirit of Pythagorean holiness and purity was a task enjoined by the Pythagorean dogma itself.[198]

[195] Cf. especially the surgical books of the *Corpus Hippocraticum* which are usually ascribed to the fifth century; cf. e.g., K. Deichgräber, Die Epidemien und das Corpus Hippocraticum, *Abh. Berl. Akad.*, 1933, nr. 3, p. 98. In general L. Edelstein, *Problemata*, IV, pp. 100 ff. [96* ff.].

[196] I am referring to the books *Decorum*, *Physician* and *Precepts*. For their late date and for the Epicurean or Stoic influence on them, cf. Jones in his introduction to these treatises, Loeb vols. I and II; cf. also the chapter "Ancient medical etiquette," *ibid.*, II, pp. xxxiii ff. The Ps. Hippocratic *Law*, another book of this type, has been connected with the Democritean school by Wilamowitz, *Hermes*, LIV, 1919, pp. 46 ff.; cf. however, F. Müller, *Hermes*, LXXV, 1940, pp. 39 ff., who dates the treatise in the fifth century. I was unable to secure this article which is abstracted in *Classical Weekly*, XXXVI, 1942, p. 84.

[197] Cf. 58 D 1, p. 467, 3 [Diels-Kranz]: τῶν δ' ἐπιστημῶν οὐχ ἥκιστά φασιν τοὺς Πυθαγορείους τιμᾶν μουσικήν τε καὶ ἰατρικὴν καὶ μαντικήν (Aristoxenus); cf. *ibid.*, p. 464, 9: τί σοφώτατον τῶν παρ' ἡμῖν; ἰατρική (old Ἄκουσμα).

[198] Cf. p. 478, 17 ff. [Diels-Kranz]: τὴν ἀληθῆ φιλοκαλίαν ἐν τοῖς ἐπιτηδεύμασι καὶ ἐν ταῖς ἐπιστήμαις ἔλεγεν εἶναι· . . . ὡσαύτως δὲ καὶ τῶν ἐπιστημῶν τε καὶ ἐμπειριῶν τὰς καλὰς καὶ εὐσχήμονας ἀληθῶς εἶναι φιλοκάλους . . . (Aristoxenus). What men gain in the usual pursuits of life only is λάφυρά που τῆς ἀληθινῆς . . . φιλοκαλίας. The term φιλοκαλία itself seems to be preeminently a Peripatetic concept, cf. *N. E.*, 1125 b 12; 1179 b 9; cf.

It stands to reason, then, that it was in the fourth century B.C. that Pythagorean philosophy led to the formulation of the Hippocratic Oath. Does this imply that the document must have been outlined by a philosopher rather than by a physician? Not at all. The Hippocratic Oath is a program of medical ethics, and there is no reason to question that it was composed by a doctor. But ancient physicians often belonged to philosophical schools or studied with philosophers. The Pythagorean teaching aroused considerable interest among the physicians of the fourth century.[199] It is quite possible that a physician, strongly impressed by what he had learned from the Pythagoreans either through personal contact or through books, conceived this medical code in conformity with Pythagorean ideals.[200]

One last question remains: what is the purpose of the Oath? Is this document an ideal program with no direct bearing on reality? Or was the Oath actually administered?[201] In my opinion one need not doubt that this vow was made by many an ancient physician, that it was sworn to and regarded by them as their "Golden Rule" of conduct. If it is true that Epaminondas considered his teacher his adopted father, a physician could honor his master in the same way. If it is true that Epaminondas, the great statesman, in his life strove to practice Pythagorean virtue, a physician could do so as well.[202]

---

also *E. E.*, 1250 b 34; 1251 b 36. It almost approaches the meaning of "love of honor," cf. Xenophon, *Symposium*, IV, 15. Zeller's interpretation of the fragment ("Die Wissenschaft . . . kann nur da gedeihen, wo sie mit Lust und Liebe betrieben wird," *op. cit.*, I, 1, p. 462) does not do justice to the words.

[199] Thus Philolaus is mentioned in Meno's history of medicine, 44 A 27 [Diels-Kranz]. Androcydes, a physician, wrote on Pythagorean symbols, cf. C. Hölk, *De acusmatis sive symbolis Pythagoricis*, Diss. Kiel, 1894, pp. 40 ff.; Corssen, *Rh. M.*, LXVII, 1912, pp. 240 ff. Another Pythagorean physician of that time (Phaon) is perhaps referred to in a fragment preserved from the Middle Comedy, p. 479, 26 [Diels-Kranz].

[200] That the covenant is probably modeled according to a general pattern of Pythagorean training has been suggested above, n. 160. Nevertheless the work as a whole could be that of a physician, and the rules concerning medical conduct could hardly have been drawn by anybody except a practitioner.

[201] Cf. Jones, *op. cit.*, p. 57: "We must clearly understand, however, that the extant evidence does not prove conclusively that the *Oath* was ever actually administered. It is conceivable that it was a mere ideal, a counsel of perfection expressed in the form of an oath . . . ." Cf. also Deichgräber, *op. cit.*, p. 32 (before he uses the *Oath* as the basis for his reconstruction of the early history of Greek crafts!): "Für die sichere Beantwortung dieser Fragen (*sc.* when and where the *Oath* was sworn) fehlt es an näheren Nachrichten und übertragbaren Analogien."

[202] For the exemplary character of Epaminondas' life, cf. e.g., Nepos, *Epaminondas*, ch. 3.

To be sure, no special societies of Pythagorean physicians are attested, no guilds are known for which Pythagorean philosophy was the statute of organization. But the covenant is a private agreement between pupil and teacher.[203] The Oath as a whole is hardly an obligation enforced upon the physician by any authority but rather one which he accepted of his own free will. It is not a legal engagement; as the wording indicates, it is a solemn promise given and vouchsafed only by the conscience of him who swears.[204] This again is in keeping with Pythagorean ethics. For the school insisted that all instruction must be based on the willingness of teacher and pupil, on voluntary rule as well as on voluntary obedience.[205] And was not the whole reform which Pythagoras instituted a reform of the life of the individual, an appeal to man, not as a citizen, but as a private person, to lead a better, a purer, a holier existence? As Plato saw it, the Pythagorean "way of life" meant not a political or a group movement; Pythagoras wanted to stir up the conscience of the individual.[206] Throughout antiquity many responded to this summons. Certainly, in its application to the task of the physician it also found its devotees.

[203] Cf. above, p. 41.

[204] Hirzel, *op. cit.*, p. 140, has shown that those oaths which in the end ask for reward or punishment (cf. above, p. 51) are indicative of a transition from the legal to the merely ethical sphere.

[205] Cf. p. 470, 35 [Diels-Kranz] (Aristoxenus): . . . καὶ τὰς μαθήσεις τὰς ὀρθῶς γινομένας ἑκουσίως δεῖν ἔφασαν γίνεσθαι, ἀμφοτέρων βουλομένων, τοῦ τε διδάσκοντος καὶ τοῦ μανθάνοντος· ἀντιτείνοντος γὰρ ὁποτέρου δήποτε τῶν εἰρημένων οὐκ ἂν ἐπιτελεσθῆναι κατὰ τρόπον τὸ προκείμενον ἔργον.

[206] Cf. Plato, *Republic*, X, 600 a ff.; Burckhardt, *Griechische Kulturgeschichte*, III, p. 320; *Vorträge*, pp. 199 ff. It is Burckhardt who has brought out this essential point, proving it from the fact that Plato contrasted Pythagoras and Orpheus with men like Charondas and Solon. In accepting Burckhardt's characterization of the intent of Pythagorean philosophy, I do not wish to pass judgment on the controversy whether the Pythagorean movement in Italy actually was a political movement or not, cf. v. Fritz, *op. cit.*, *passim*. Within the limits of this investigation it is not the early Pythagorean school, but Pythagoreanism as represented in the fourth century B.C. that has to be considered, cf. above, p. 20, and for this form of the Pythagorean dogma Burckhardt's interpretation is undoubtedly correct and in agreement also with the reports of Aristoxenus. Cf. also J. Burnet, *Early Greek Philosophy*[4], 1930, p. 89 (cf. also E. Frank's review of v. Fritz' book, *American Journal of Philology*, LXIV, 1943, pp. 220 ff., which appeared when this study was already in print).

V. CONCLUSION

The so-called Hippocratic Oath has always been regarded as a message of timeless validity. From the interpretation given it follows that the document originated in a group representing a small segment of Greek opinion. That the Oath at first was not accepted by all ancient physicians is certain. Medical writings, from the time of Hippocrates down to that of Galen, give evidence of the violation of almost every one of its injunctions. This is true not only in regard to the general rules concerning helpfulness, continence and secrecy. Such deviations one would naturally expect. But for centuries ancient physicians, in opposition to the demands made in the Oath, put poison in the hands of those among their patients who intended to commit suicide; they administered abortive remedies; they practiced surgery.

At the end of antiquity a decided change took place. Medical practice began to conform to that state of affairs which the Oath had envisaged. Surgery was separated from general practice. Resistance against suicide, against abortion, became common. Now the Oath began to be popular. It circulated in various forms adapted to the varying circumstances and purposes of the centuries.[207] Generally considered the work of the great Hippocrates, its study became part of the medical curriculum. The commentators supposed that the master had written the Oath as the first of all his books and made it incumbent on the beginner to read this treatise first.[208]

Small wonder! A new religion arose that changed the very foundations of ancient civilization. Yet, Pythagoreanism seemed to bridge the gulf between heathendom and the new belief. Christianity found itself in agreement with the principles of Pythagorean ethics, its concepts of holiness and purity, justice and forbearance.[209] The Pythagorean god

[207] For the manuscript tradition in general, cf. Jones, *op. cit.*, pp. 2 ff.; 12 ff.; cf. also J. H. Oliver–P. Maas, *Bulletin of the History of Medicine*, VII, 1939, pp. 315 ff. (a medical Paean); and for the *Oath* in non-medical ancient literature, cf. E. Nachmanson, *Symbolae Philologicae, O. A. Danielsson dedicatae*, Upsala, 1932, pp. 185 ff.

[208] Cf. Ps. Oribasius, *Commentarius in Aphorismos Hippocratis*, Basileae, 1535, p. 7. I need not deal here with the historical process by which ancient medical works came to be ascribed to Hippocrates, cf. L. Edelstein, The Genuine Works of Hippocrates, *Bulletin of the History of Medicine*, VII, 1939, pp. 236 ff. [133* ff.]; cf. the same, *Problemata*, IV, ch. IV.

[209] Cf. above, n. 45; n. 181, where the coincidence of certain Pythagorean doctrines with Jewish (Essenian) and Christian teachings was noted. Cf. also the material collected by Meibom, *op. cit.* pp. 131 ff., who speaks of "Hippocratis religiositas."

who forbade suicide to men, his creatures, was also the God of the Jews and the Christians. As early as in the "Teaching of the Twelve Apostles" the command was given: "Thou shalt not use philtres; thou shalt not procure abortion; nor commit infanticide." Even the Church Fathers abounded in praise of the high-mindedness of Hippocrates and his regulations for the practice of medicine.[210]

As time went on, the Hippocratic Oath became the nucleus of all medical ethics. In all countries, in all epochs in which monotheism, in its purely religious or in its more secularized form, was the accepted creed, the Hippocratic Oath was applauded as the embodiment of truth. Not only Jews and Christians, but the Arabs, the mediaeval doctors, men of the Renaissance, scientists of the Enlightenment, and scholars of the nineteenth century embraced the ideals of the Oath.[211] I am not qualified to outline the successive stages of this historical process. But I venture to suggest that he who undertakes to study this development will find it better understandable if he realizes that the Hippocratic Oath is a Pythagorean manifesto and not the expression of an absolute standard of medical conduct.

[210] Cf. the so-called Διαδοχὴ τῶν δώδεκα ᾿Αποστόλων, The Apostolic Fathers, with an English translation by Kirsopp Lake, I, 1925, pp. 310–312 [Loeb]; cf. also Gregory of Nazianzus, XXXV, col. 767 A [Migne]; Hieronymus, Epist., 52, 15 (XXII, col. 539 [Migne]).

[211] It would be difficult here to substantiate this general statement; a few references to the pertinent literature must suffice. For the Jews and Arabs, cf. H. Frieden-wald-G. Sarton, with reference to M. Meyerhof, Isis, XXII, 1934, pp. 222–23; cf. also Jones, op. cit., pp. 29 ff.; Deichgräber, op. cit., pp. 38 f. Some mediaeval references are collected ibid., pp. 39–40, cf. also E. Hirschfeld, Deontologische Texte des frühen Mittelalters, Archiv f. Geschichte d. Medizin, XX, 1928, p. 369. For the Renaissance and later centuries the commentaries on the Oath quoted above, n. 77, furnish some evidence of the importance of the document; cf. besides S. V. Larkey, The Hippocratic Oath in Elizabethan England, Bulletin of the History of Medicine, IV, 1936, pp. 201 ff. Cf. also Erasmus, Methodus ad Veram Theologiam, ed. H. Holborn, 1933, p. 151; p. 180. For the eighteenth century, cf. e.g., J. P. Frank, The People's Misery: Mother of Diseases, H. E. Sigerist, Bulletin of the History of Medicine, IX, 1941, p. 100. Goethe, too, took over the principles of the Oath in his Wilhelm Meister, cf. Hoffmann, op. cit., pp. 18 ff.

HIPPOCRATIC PROGNOSIS*

E ver since the work of Ermerins, modern scholars have interpreted prognosis as the objectively significant knowledge of what the outcome of sickness would be; moreover, Littré and Daremberg formulated the still accepted judgment that prognosis constitutes the scientific achievement of ancient medicine.[1] The knowledge expressed in ancient prognosis seems scientific to the modern physician because it resembles modern knowledge. It is for this reason that prognosis is deemed a scientific achievement, and that the physician who practiced it is considered a good, scientific physician. Yet, even though the extant prognostic writings reveal amazing knowledge, this fact does not yet tell us anything about the significance and practice of prognosis in ancient medicine. Such considerations alone, however, can determine how prognosis is to be evaluated.

Moreover, it has been claimed that in prognosis the ancient physician, starting out from the patient's behavior during sickness, succeeded in interpreting disease as a process independent of the affected organ.[2] And in this sense, too, prognosis is called the scientific achievement and discovery of ancient medicine, in which prognosis took the place of the true insight into natural phenomena which it still lacked.

But it must be said in objection to this that ancient medicine held substantial theories about diseases and was not persuaded that it lacked the necessary insight into the course of disease—as is claimed today

---

* From Chapter II, *Peri aerōn und die Sammlung der hippokratischen Schriften.* Berlin: Weidmannsche Buchhandlung, 1931 (Problemata, Heft 4), see above, p. ix.

[1] F. Ermerins, *De Hippocratis doctrina a prognostice oriunda,* 1832. Littré, "Introduction," to his edition, I, 451 ff. Daremberg, *Oeuvres choisies d'Hippocrate,* Paris, 1855, pp. 121–22. Further, M. Neuburger, "Zur Entwicklungsgeschichte der Prognostik," *Wiener medizinische Presse,* 48, 1907, p. 1 ff. Th. Meyer-Steineg, "Die Bedeutung der Prognose in den hippokratischen Schriften," *Arch. f. d. Gesch. d. Naturwiss.* 6, 1913. According to K. Sudhoff, *Kurzes Handbuch der Geschichte der Medizin,* Berlin, 1922, p. 74, the two last mentioned works are the medically authoritative ones. Also the handbooks: Haeser, *Geschichte der Medizin,* and R. Fuchs, in Puschmann, *Handbuch der Geschichte der Medizin,* I, 242 ff.

[2] First by Littré, "Introduction," I, 453 ff.

simply because medicine has advanced. And, above all, there is in ancient medicine no such theory of a disease *per se*, independent of the
affected organ. For *Prognostikon*, the interpretation of which forms the
sole basis for this assumption, is concerned with the prognosis of acute
diseases, not with that of disease *per se*.

Prognostikon begins by pointing out the importance of prognosis
in general (Khlw. I 78,2–8). Then its significance for treatment is indicated (τὴν δὲ θεραπείην 78,9 ff.), and the benefit to be derived from it
(79,3–8). It would be better if the physician were able to cure all his
patients, better than merely being able to foresee what the outcome
of the sickness will be (78,10–13). But that is not possible. Patients
cannot always be saved, but sometimes die—and, indeed, some die
from the severity of their illness before they can even call the doctor
(78,14–16), others soon, a day or so, after the doctor arrives (78,16–17).
For this reason the physician, before he takes up the fight against all
diseases with his art, must know the nature of the diseases that run a
rapid course (τῶν τοιούτων νοσημάτων), how superior they are to the
strength of the body, and whether there is something divine (θεῖον) in
them (–79,3).[3] For such a prognosis will help him to protect himself
against the charge that he is responsible for a patient's death and to
give medical aid more easily (79,3–8). The significance of prognosis for
treatment is thus exemplified in the diseases that rapidly lead to death—
an exception, for not all diseases are so rapidly fatal; and in the eventu-

---

[3] Following Kuehlewein's punctuation, the passage is translated as follows:
"It would be better to cure everyone. But that is impossible. And since not everyone can be saved, but men die—some before they can call the doctor, others shortly
after his arrival, before the physician is able to fight the disease with his skill." The
clause, πρὶν ἢ τὸν ἰητρὸν πρὸς ἕκαστον νόσημα ἀνταγωνίσασθαι (78,17–18) is thus referred
to this, and not to what follows, as in my interpretation. But the sick do not die in
one or two days, before the physician, in those one or two days, can begin to fight
the disease with his art (ἀνταγωνίσασθαι). He can begin to fight the disease in the
one or two days when people are still alive, though perhaps the time is not sufficient
for conquering it. If the concept, ἀνταγωνίσασθαι, then, is meaningless when the sentence is construed in this way, the words "fight against every disease" (πρὸς ἕκαστον
νόσημα) are equally incomprehensible. It makes sense to say, "people die before the
physician can overcome their disease" (πρὸς τὰ νοσήματα); it makes no sense to say
people die before the physician can fight every single one of the many diseases that
they have, or before he can fight every conceivable disease. On the other hand, the
expression πρὸς ἕκαστον νόσημα becomes meaningful if understood in the sense that
the physician, in order to protect himself, should first determine prognostically the
serious and rapidly fatal diseases, before starting to fight every disease he encounters.
Only if the πρίν clause is taken to refer to what follows does the meaning of prognosis
emerge, the foreknowledge before treatment, which is absolutely essential.

ality of these serious diseases that come so quickly to a crisis, the physician is advised to make a prognosis.

The development of the theme, beginning at this point, shows how prognoses should be made; that is, how they should be made in acute diseases (σκέπτεσθαι δὲ χρὴ ὧδε ἐν τοῖσιν ὀξέσι νοσήμασιν 79,9), namely, in certain diseases which are called acute because the crisis is reached rapidly and because death usually ensues very quickly. In this way, the entire subsequent doctrine of prognosis is referred expressly to acute diseases and is expressly limited to such diseases, as indeed was to be expected from the explanation, in the introduction, of the importance of prognosis. For the introduction derived the very necessity for prognosis from the example of certain rapidly fatal diseases. It is, thus, only for these diseases that the main body of the writing gives prognoses.

The writing closes with sentences which delimit once more both the meaning and the reach of the prognoses given (ch. 25). Much can be done (108,4 ff.), it is contended, if the symptoms noted in the book are learnt, and if one knows how to interpret them correctly. Moreover, one should not be confused by the absence (ποθέειν) of any disease from the foregoing list of names, for all diseases whose outcome is decided within the time specified (ὁκόσα ἐν τοῖσι χρόνοισι τοῖσι προειρημένοισι κρίνεται) are characterized by the same symptoms (108,9–11).[4] One should, therefore, not be disturbed by the absence of certain diseases, whose course, of like duration, runs through the same stages, i.e., by the absence of any *acute* disease. This conforms to the introduction, which drew its conclusion as to the importance of prognosis from certain rapidly fatal diseases; it conforms also to the development of the theme, which started out (78,9) with express reference to these acute diseases, which lead so quickly to death.

The formulation of the conclusion (that one should not be bothered by the absence of any disease from the foregoing list) becomes understandable when one realizes that "acute diseases" (ὀξέα νοσήματα) is a comprehensive term. In *On regimen in acute diseases* (Khlw. I 111,4 ff.), one reads that by "acute diseases" those diseases are meant which

---

[4] Wilamowitz, *Hermes*, 64, 1929, pp. 483–84, believes the words 108,4 ff. have been added. His only argument is that the form of direct speech is used (γνώσηι 10). But it cannot be proved that this form could not be used here; it is found in *Prognostikon* itself, as Wilamowitz himself says. One cannot simply ignore this coincidence of forms in the tradition. The objective correctness of the words and the way in which they further the logical argument—for they are not without meaning—are shown in the interpretation given here.

the ancients called "pleurisy and pneumonia and phrenitis and *kausos* and the others of this sort where the fever generally is continuous" [transl. Ed.] (πλευρῖτιν καὶ περιπνευμονίην καὶ φρενῖτιν καὶ καῦσον καὶ τἄλλα ὅσα τούτων ἐχόμενα, ὧν οἱ πυρετοὶ τὸ ἐπίπαν συνεχέες). At some definite point in the development, therefore, single diseases with individual names were grouped together under one name which emphasized the rapid course common to them all. Thus, even though an author, whose intention it is to deal with all similar diseases, mentions only the comprehensive term at the beginning of his discussion, and in developing his theme gives individual names as occasion arises, he can very well say in conclusion that his reader should not be disturbed by the absence of single names or single diseases that happen not to be mentioned.[5] For since they are all alike, what is said under one name is valid for each of them, no matter how varied the individual names. When one realizes that it is the acute diseases from which most people die, that they are the most dangerous of all sporadic diseases (as one reads in *On regimen in acute diseases* [Khlw. I 111,7 ff.]), and when one sees how, in the majority of the passages in the Hippocratic writings that deal with acute diseases, the phenomenon of sudden death astonishes people and makes them aware of their helplessness, the significance of prognosis for just these diseases becomes apparent. And it does not seem strange that a whole investigation should be devoted to them alone.[6]

The prognosis of the *Prognostikon* refers to a special case, that of the acute diseases. It is concerned with the patient's behavior when ill, but it knows nothing of the concept of a disease *per se* in the acute illnesses. It is, therefore, not possible to infer from this writing and its teachings any generally applicable prognosis based on the idea of a disease *per se* considered apart from the organ affected by it and determining the course and development of the illness.

---

[5] It was on this ending that Littré based his interpretation of prognosis as a theory of disease *per se*, interpreting the words οὐδενὸς νοσήματος ὄνομα theoretically, rather than historically, as I attempt to (cf. L. I 453; II 95). In the concluding clause he thought he saw the rejection of a point of view which was concerned with single, acute diseases instead of with acute disease itself; and he inferred further a corresponding general theory of disease as such. He overlooked the fact that in the *Prognostikon* itself individual diseases are mentioned (98,13; 97,17; 92,1; 99,10).

[6] The mere comparison of the various descriptions of acute diseases in the *Corpus* is sufficient support for this statement. It is not by chance that in *On affections* (ch. 13 VI 220 L.), it is in connection with these diseases that the question of responsibility is discussed, and that *On diseases, III* (VII 140 L.), prognosis is advised in only one definite case of the disease in question.

The meaning of prognosis in Hippocratic medicine can only be demonstrated by assembling all the writings and all the isolated utterances about it and by attempting in this way to gain an insight into its nature.

In Hippocratic medicine as in every kind of medicine, prognosis is, first of all, the prediction of the outcome of a disease, as well as its fluctuations and transmutations. In this sense, prognostication is an anticipation of the future.

But in ancient medicine, prognosis also includes a knowledge of the patient's present condition and of his earlier symptoms, of what, in fact, already exists and has already existed. In this sense, prognostication is the anticipation of statements that the patient or a third party might make about the present or the past.

Finally, prognosis includes the physician's determination of whether the patient has followed his directions or not, and in what way he has transgressed. Here, too, prognostication is an anticipation of facts which, in themselves, could as well be learnt from a third party.

When prognosis is not concerned with the future, but with the present and the past, it serves to make the physician independent of the utterances of others. His ability to determine the present and past condition of the patient without recourse to others prevents his being deceived by incomplete statements. His knowledge of what is happening and of what has been going on beforehand, without having to ask, inspires astonishment and admiration, and he immediately wins people's confidence. He avoids being deceived by patients who conceal the fact that they have disobeyed his orders, and, by the same token, when the outcome is bad, he avoids the reproaches heaped upon him by patients—although the failure is their own fault—and those which others could make to him.

And if the physician knows what course the disease will take, he is also better able to prepare for what is to come. But what preparations he should make, what he should do, indeed, the most important thing, medical intervention itself, these are influenced only in so far as sure knowledge of a successful outcome enables the physician to act with greater confidence and calm, while his foreknowledge of the stages through which a disease will go prevents his being suddenly and unexpectedly confronted by new facts—which is important for the physician's personal dignity. Once the patient has gained confidence in the physician because of what the latter says about his past and present condition, a prediction of the successful outcome of the disease will calm him and increase his confidence still more. If, on the other hand, when the physician takes over the care of the patient, he predicts a fatal outcome, this exonerates him from all blame for what happens.

Prognosis and prediction are, consequently, of significance for *people*, for the physician and for the patient, and only thereby for the curing of the disease itself. In the therapeutic procedure prognosis is, therefore, important not as knowledge from which to derive other knowledge; its importance is psychological.

A prognosis is made either semeiotically, by taking the way the organs are functioning and the whole constitution of the body as signs, or mantically, by divination, without paying attention to the patient's physical condition. But it is also possible to start out from general circumstances which determine man's condition, from the season, the winds, etc., and to draw from them inferences regarding the disease.

Besides this prognosis referring to diseases and the diseased, ancient medicine possessed also a prognostic doctrine of the healthy. For, to many physicians, health was synonymous with balance, whether of the fluids of the body, of material taken into the body, of human activities, or a balance of the last two. Disease, on the other hand, was synonymous with a disturbance of that balance, i.e., with a disproportion of the parts. The balance of health could necessarily never be permanently sustained, but attained only for the moment. For the relationship between the various parts is continually subject to change because of the constant intake of fresh nourishment, because of constantly new activities, and because of automatic seasonal increase and decrease in the body fluids or in their circulation under the influence of heat and cold. For this reason, everyone must try at all times to correct the imbalance as it arises. Thus dietetics is of great importance and the healthy man is as much under the control of the physician as the unhealthy. It is just as possible to set up prognoses for the healthy person as in the treatment of disease. The body is altered by the general conditions of the seasons and the winds, indeed, by the particular ways of life. But it is only through prognosis that preventive measures become possible and help can be given.

I shall try to substantiate this general picture of prognosis by detailed interpretation of the various prognostic writings.

The *Prognostikon* teaches semeiotic prognosis. Man and his behavior in sickness are observed, and the statements are then differentiated according to age and sex. From the symptoms one concludes what is going to happen. But no symptom should be taken singly; the important thing is the combination of all relevant circumstances; this aspect is repeatedly stressed in the body of the writing (e.g., 94,15 ff.) and expressly underlined in the conclusion. Significant in this is the comparison of the diseased condition with the healthy (79,11), as well as a consideration of the particular traits which characterize the patient (79,12; 82,5). These characteristics can, presumably, be established by asking questions, such as one asks in establishing the truth of certain statements (79,21). The favorable or unfavorable outcome of a disease depends on the stage that has been reached in its course (e.g., 79,19) and on the crises. The possible turning of the present condition into other forms of disease is taken into consideration; indeed, there is even the prediction of a deformed limb as the result of illness (99,2).

Yet even though such prognosis is based on the interpretation of symptoms, general data must nevertheless be utilized, at least as correctives. Diseases which are endemic in single localities must be taken into account, and the physician's statements must be modified accordingly (ch. 25), for they supplement the phenomena already described (107,20–21). The characteristics of the season must be considered, for they are generally believed capable of provoking certain diseases and, thus, of causing a deterioration of the patient's condition (107,22). Nevertheless, the necessary inclusion of these general factors of endemic diseases and seasonal influences does not mean that the interpretation of symptoms should vary, relative to the different countries in which physicians practice. Symptoms have the same meaning in Libya, in Delos, and in Scythia (107,22–108,7). The over-refined kind of prognosis, therefore, which takes geographical data into account and thereby splits medicine into numerous splinter medicines, is rejected. Indeed, the writing tends altogether to a generalized point of view.

The *Prognostikon*, then, is concerned with the prognosis of acute diseases. The individuality of its author can be grasped. The *Coan Prognoses*, semeiotic in character like the *Prognostikon*, is a miscellany without individual character that gathers together existing prognoses and classifies them systematically under large subdivisions.[7] There is, in addition, a collection of single predictions, *Prorrhetikon I*, also *Prorrhe-*

[7] [Pp. 68–73 of the German text, which the author omitted but summarized in the next sentence, contain analyses of *Coan Prognoses* and of *Prorrhetikon I* and *II*, as well as comments on the interdependence of these works.—Ed.]

tikon II, in form an independent book meant for publication, that gives prognoses for the entire gamut of diseases.

In these semeiotic books, prognosis is based on experience and observation of the human body. But in the writing *On the nature of man*, an attempt is made to start out from external circumstances and reach conclusions concerning the course the disease is likely to take.

This book contends that diseases that begin in winter end in summer, while those that begin in summer end in winter, unless they terminate after a definite number of days of crisis (ch. 8 VI 50–52 L.). On the other hand, diseases that come in spring end in autumn, just as autumn diseases disappear in spring, unless they persist beyond term and become chronic (ἐνιαύσιον 52,1). This general prognosis, greatly narrowed down by the added limitations,[8] is a consequence of the theory of the four humors, according to which disease arises from a disturbance of the balance of the humors. Disturbance occurs when one of the humors predominates, and every season automatically provokes such predominance of one of the humors. When it results in sickness it is automatically canceled out again by the opposite season. In this prognostic doctrine, the individuality of the patient is completely neglected. In no other writing in the Corpus, to the best of my knowledge, is prognosis expressed in so dogmatic a form; and indeed such dogmatism is only possible within strict four-humoral theory.

Even the writing, *On the number seven* (π. ἑβδομάδων), combines the influence of the season with bodily symptoms when the outcome of fever and other diseases is to be determined prognostically. The disease will end well if the season is not on its side, fighting along with it; for generally speaking, man's nature cannot overcome the nature of the universe.[9] In both the semeiotic prognoses and the conclusions based

[8] Fredrich, *Hippokratische Untersuchungen*, Berlin, 1899, pp. 15–16 (Philologische Untersuchungen, 15) athetizes these limiting sentences, considering them alien in content and objectionable in form. But they are, precisely, intended to limit the theory, whose generality is too unrealistic (cf. also Schöne, *Göttingische gelehrte Anzeigen*, 1900, 658). For the meaning of ἐνιαύσιον, cf. VII 66 L.

[9] VIII 663,14–15 L. Compare the description of the unfavorable outcome (667,1). The corresponding prognostic passage in *On critical days* (ch. 2 IX 298 L.) is actually excerpted from *On the number seven*. In the *Aphorisms* (IV 486 ff. L., part III) only the origin of disease and its aggravation are discussed in relation to the seasons, not the outcome of the disease (cf. Nos. 1 and 19). In the same way, it is the origin of disease that is of concern when age and diseases are related to each other, except in pronouncement No. 28, which speaks of crises. The statements (11–14), which agree with *On airs, waters, places*, abandon that writing's general pronouncements about the termination of diseases. They designate the outcome only in No. 12 in τίκτουσι

on general conditions, it is unreservedly taken for granted that it is possible to make prognoses; it is not asked whether there may not be certain limits to that possibility. It is true, pronouncements are made relative to sex and age, but even these more specialized groups still presuppose that people of a certain age or sex are alike and that the same thing is valid for them all, just as the disease of one of them seems comparable to that of another. In the final analysis, all such theorizing is still dogmatic and standardizing.

The book, *On diseases I*, attempts to determine the extent to which one can predict the outcome of a disease. In the following cases, the disease runs an unconditionally inevitable course, and the outcome (ἀνάγκαι) is, therefore, unconditionally predictable (ch. 3 VI 142–46 L.): Wounds in certain cases lead to mutilation, in certain cases to death, in certain cases to recovery; some diseases are lethal, others of doubtful outcome; finally, a number of diseases are not fatal unless complicated by an additional malady. Some diseases are of long, others of short, duration, while in some this or that change is to be expected. In this survey of wounds and diseases, the facts are the starting point from which it is determined when anything at all can be said about the future, and how much can be said about it.

In other diseases, however, there is no prognostic knowledge. The elucidation of lung and chest suppurations, for instance, is followed by the statement that people who suffer from such diseases die soon (that is, if the disease has a fatal outcome, which is not necessarily the case: the right treatment may be helpful, e.g., 162,13–14), yet they may live long. This cannot be determined with certainty because one man's body differs from another's, one man's suffering from another's, as do the times when the individuals are sick (διαφέρει γὰρ σῶμα σώματος καὶ πάθημα παθήματος καὶ ὥρη ὥρης ἐν ἧι ἂν νοσέωσιν);[10] it is not possible to predict any point precisely (τὸ ἀκριβές). For even the assertion that the outcome of a disease is related to the time of year, which some people consider definite, is not unconditionally true, because the years and the seasons

---

ὥστε ἢ . . . ἀπόλλυσθαι and κατάρροοι ξυντόμως ἀπολλύντες, that is, in a quite different sense. *On humours*, too, only deals with the origin of diseases (V 496 No. 15 L.).

[10] My reading here differs from that of Littré. In omitting καὶ ἡλικίη ἡλικίης after σώματος, I follow θ (cf. note 19, p. 169). Littré deleted the words καὶ ὥρη ὥρης ἐν ἧι ἂν νοσέωσιν without the slightest justification in the manuscript (cf. note 1, p. 170). The words make good sense and correspond to the formulation in the development of the second prognosis, 184,1. The time of year in which a man is sick is important.

are not always alike; instead, one year differs from another, as does season from season (διαφέρει γὰρ καὶ ἔτος ἔτεος καὶ ὥρη ὥρης).[11] Men may die of their illnesses at any time of the year, and in every season they may survive them (ch. 16, 168–70).

And at the end of the second section concerned with the etiology of individual diseases (chs. 17–21, 170–82), it is said that as to the question of a good or an incomplete recovery from a disease, it makes a difference whether the patient is a man or a woman, young or old, at what time of year he becomes sick, and whether he has had some other disease beforehand, or not. And again, one man's suffering differs from another's, one man's body from another's, the treatment of one physician from that of another. For these reasons, too, the course of the disease will necessarily vary as far as duration is concerned (ἀνάγκη διαφέρειν καὶ τὸν χρόνον), and sometimes it will end in death, and sometimes in a cure; sometimes it will last a long time and sometimes be over quickly (ch. 22, 182–84,9). Finally, it is shown how the patient's age determines the appearance of the disease (184,9 ff.).

It is in view of this possibility to differentiate in making the prognosis—i.e., according to the patient's individuality—that, at the end of the account of the acute diseases, the discussion is restricted to the manner in which death will occur if the disease ends unfavorably (chs. 32–34, 202–4). Up to this point, only the general possibilities for the actual termination of the disease have been given (e.g., 196,1–5).

Generally speaking, the ideas expressed in the writing *On diseases I*, and the theory resulting from them, eliminate the possibility of predicting the course of a disease. All events and all persons are unique phenomena, and their nature and definition can be experienced, but not known beforehand. What will be cannot be concluded from what was, for nothing repeats itself. Only very rarely can the future be judged with certainty. Almost always the physician faces the future just as uncertainly as do the patient and those who love him.

The *Prognostikon* made firm prognoses for the acute diseases; it classifies phenomena; patients of a type are considered alike; diseases of a type always run the same course. Compared to the teachings of *On diseases I*, the *Prognostikon* is more rigid, less receptive to experience, less responsive to the constant variations of reality. It is of the opinion

[11] Here, in conformity with the textual sequence in footnote 10, above, I delete the words ἐν ἧι ἂν νοσέωσιν, which Littré added after ὥρης (note 6, p. 170), after having previously deleted them (cf. note 1, p. 170).

that it can teach medicine, and that whoever learns the doctrine is a physician. With this point of view, it contradicts profound and basic ideas of other physicians. At the same time, it becomes evident that belief in foreknowledge of the future is not accepted by all physicians nor in all writings. The practice of prognosis requires a particular doctrine, particular views of man and disease. The physician's art and prognostic acumen do not necessarily go together; on the contrary, profound medical learning may even be the basis for rejecting prognosis. It is possible to be a physician without practicing prognosis.[12] And if prognosis is practiced at all, there are various motives for it and various ways of using it. A physician may seek and use knowledge of the future in the interest of others; he may also seek it for his own advantage. It is by these criteria that the meaning of prognosis must be judged.

Prognostikon bases the importance of prognosis for therapy on the contention that the physician who has foreknowledge of the future, being prepared far in advance for coming developments (79,4–6), can give his patients better care. The physician is spared sudden decisions in difficult situations. Thus far, only the advantages of prognosis in treating the disease have been considered; but, in addition, his prediction of the favorable or unfavorable outcome of his patient's illness relieves him of all responsibility (79,6–8), and he is justifiably admired, for he is a good physician (79,3–4). Prognosis, therefore, gives the physician a method of demonstrating his superiority, of protecting himself from accusations, of avoiding the mistakes he might make, not because he knows too little, but because he might be confused by the necessity of acting suddenly. *Prognostikon* teaches that a prognosis should be made for every case. In other writings, it is only in specially difficult cases that the physician is advised to undertake and carry out the treatment only after predicting the outcome or, at least, any great, imminent danger (e.g., Khlw. II 25,10; 100,8; 219,8; VII 140 L.). Any

---

[12] Not only *On diseases I*, but *On flesh* also finds prognosis possible only in certain cases, i.e., in the most acute diseases, at least in the sense that there are dates on which the outcome is decided (VIII 612,10 L.). Apart from this, there is no reasonable way to forecast the course of illnesses, except in the case of wounds (614,2–3). The surgical books, too, deny the possibility of exact prediction (Khlw. II 57,3 ff.; 97,19 ff.; 223,11). The reasons for denying such possibility vary in the various writings. In therapeutic writings, isolated passages reject the prognosis of a date, e.g., VII 118,10 L.; VIII 86,16 L. But all writings which neglect to mention prognosis in cases where other writings advocate it in so doing implicitly reject prognosis as such.

physician, however, whose judgment rejects prognostic knowledge and who is unable to say what will happen, foregoes a means of protecting himself from attack or of gaining respect and admiration.

The question arises: To whom should the prognosis be communicated? The physician will be eager to prophesy a favorable outcome to the patient himself; he will also tell the people around him. But supposing he foresees death? *Prorrhetikon II* instructs the physician to tell a third party that such and such will ensue (ἄλλωι προσημαίνειν IX 22 L.). In *On decorum*, it is absolutely forbidden to tell the patient what lies in store for him, for this has often had "other" (unexpected, evil) consequences (CMG I₁ 29,17). *Prognostikon* does not discuss this problem. One may be sure that patients were often told the worst, without any consideration: that *Prorrhetikon II* advises the physician to tell his prognosis to a third party suggests that such was the case. The numerous statements in the Hippocratic writings, that the physician's words at the bedside should be cautious, give one an inkling of how often other physicians disapproved of both the form and content of what patients were told.[13]

When the physician, in making a prognosis, is mindful of not becoming culpable in the eyes of others and of gaining their admiration, these others are not limited to the patient, his family, and perhaps his friends; the physician thinks, beyond these people, of the general public. Ancient life lacked the rigid distinction between public and private life of modern times. Besides, men lived in relatively small communities and therefore knew more about each other than they do today. Thus the physician's prognoses were talked about, and he won respect not only in one house, or in one family, but in a city or even cities. This added to the importance of prognostic knowledge and to the temptation to use it.

At the beginning of *Prorrhetikon II* one reads that people talk of many excellent and astonishing prognoses that physicians have made (IX 6 L. τῶν ἰητρῶν προρήσιες ἀπαγγέλλονται συχναί τε καὶ καλαὶ καὶ θαυμασταί). And people make even greater wonders of them than they, in fact, were (IX 10 ἅμα δὲ καὶ τοὺς ἀπαγγέλλοντας τερατωδεστέρως διηγεῖσθαι

---

[13] E.g., *Epidemics 6* (V 290; 308 L.). Galen, in his *Commentary on Epidemics 6* (V 308), tells (XVII B 145 K.) of a physician who answered his patient's question whether he would die: "If you are not the child of Leto, who is blessed with fair children, you will die." Another patient who asked the same question received the reply: "Patroclus, too, died, and he was a better man than you." These utterances are typical of what may be said.

ἢ ὡς ἐγένετο). Thus prognosis became a weapon in the struggle for public recognition, which in those centuries played a much greater rôle in defining a physician's reputation than today. At the same time, it fitted in with the spirit of the *agon*. The amazing prognoses of certain physicians were not too difficult for anyone to imitate who wished to engage in such contests (τῶι βουλομένωι τὰ τοιάδε διαγωνίζεσθαι *Prorrh.* IX 8). Anyone who took pleasure in competition, then, might make such predictions (ἀλλὰ χρὴ προλέγειν καταμανθάνοντα πάντα ταῦτα ὅστις τῶν τοιούτων ἐπιθυμεῖ ἀγωνισμάτων IX 10). This is corroborated by *On joints*: τὰ δὲ προρήματα λαμπρὰ καὶ ἀγωνιστικά (Khlw. II 205,20). And this same spirit of competition must be implied when the *Epidemics* record: This was the disease in question. It was predicted that the patient would die, and such and such would be the circumstances of his death. He died as predicted (*Epidemics 5* V 248; 256 L.).

When the Greek physician makes prognoses of the outcome of diseases, it is only the human element—not medical considerations—which concerns him. Of all the Hippocratic writings, only *Epidemics I* and *III* use prognosis in a wider sense.

In *Epidemics III*, according to the κατάστασις given before the second series of descriptions of individual diseases, one reads (Khlw. I 231,19):

For all the diseases which follow, spring was the most dangerous time and killed most people; summer, on the other hand, was the best time with the smallest number of deaths. In autumn and during the season of the Pleiades, deaths occurred again, usually after four days of sickness. According to this, the coming of summer seems to me to be helpful, for summer diseases are dispelled by the ensuing winter, and the ensuing summer alters the diseases of winter. And yet, the summer itself was not a favorable one . . . I believe (232,7) that it is an important part of the art to be able to judge correctly what is written down. For he who understands it and knows how to make use of it cannot make many mistakes. But the exact character of the seasons must be learnt, and the disease; the good that is common in the season or disease, and the bad also; then, which disease lasts long and is fatal, or lasts long but is not fatal, which ends quickly in death, and which is short and ends in recovery. In this way, it becomes possible to recognize the order of the crises, and this in turn makes it possible to predict. He who is versed in these matters knows who must adjust his way of life, and when and how this must be done (–232,19).

Thus, the physician should compare the disease he is treating and the nature of the seasons at the time of the sickness he is observing with the statements in the books of *Epidemics*. By comparing, he acquires the ability to recognize and predict the critical days and to determine the way of life to be followed. That such a comparison of the cases treated with the cases described makes prognosis possible is understandable, if one presupposes—as does *Prognostikon*[14]—that there are classes of people who react alike and classes of diseases which are of the same nature. It is more difficult to understand why the comparison should lead not only to prediction of the outcome, but also to prescribing the regimen the patient should follow, for in listing the cases the patient's way of life is not mentioned.

In *On regimen in acute diseases*, one sees that the questions whether medication should be given to the patient at the very beginning of treatment or not (Khlw. I 122,3 ff.) and whether it should be given uniformly throughout the illness or should be changed on certain days, the days of crisis (e.g., 115,7 ff.), constituted grave problems for medical treatment. With this in mind, the passages in the *Epidemics* which include specific reference to the days of crisis may be understood as meaning that comparison of the cases to be treated with those in the literature yields just such knowledge of the important days on which the regimen should be changed, however its content may have been envisaged. In this context, the content of the regimen is a matter of indifference and it is, therefore, possible for it to be entirely absent from the books on *Epidemics*. It is mentioned in a different context, not in the books on prognosis. In any case, prognosis hereby attains a degree of importance for treatment itself, at least inasmuch as it is considered correct to change the patient's regimen on specific days in the course of the disease.

Chapters 15–16 of the third book of *Epidemics* correspond to chapters 23–25 of the first book. In the latter, it is at first only a question of the prognosis of the outcome of the disease. Then, in the twenty-fifth chapter, after general considerations about fevers and their crises, one reads that, taking these considerations as a starting point, the physisician must also regulate his patient's regimen (δεῖ δὲ καὶ τὰ διαιτήματα σκοπεύμενον ἐκ τούτων προσφέρειν 201,9). These signs and others must be

---

[14] In *Epidemics*, fatal and favorable terminations of illnesses are recorded in the same way, descriptions of fatal cases being, in fact, more numerous. This "honesty," about which so much has been said (cf. Littré II 588), hinges upon the circumstance that prognosis of a bad outcome is more important for the physician than that of a good outcome, because a bad outcome counts more heavily against him than a good outcome does for him.

considered if he is to know whether a disease will be short and fatal, or not fatal; which patient should be given medication, and which not; when medication should be given, and what, and how much (καὶ τίνι προσαρτέον ἢ οὐ καὶ πότε καὶ πόσον καὶ τί τὸ προσφερόμενον ἔσται 201,15–17). This is what is said, though nowhere in all the descriptions of cases is there any mention of the patient's regimen. The regimen, then, cannot be learnt from the books on *Epidemics;* there remains only the reference to the critical days and to a change of regimen at those times. The nature of the change is known to the physician.

The books on *Epidemics* are the only writings to use prognosis in treating the sick.[15] Elsewhere the setting up of prognoses in treating a patient always hinges on psychological considerations.

The modern physician, too, gives his opinion of what the outcome of an illness will be, because people ask him. He, too, feels obliged to tell at least those close to the patient that he can no longer save him. But he will not use prognosis for the purpose of attracting patients and impressing people. For him, at least ideally, prognostic knowledge is nothing more than the consequence of his insight into the course the disease will run. In Hippocratic medicine, prognosis gives the physician who practices it a means of avoiding sudden decisions and, above all, of impressing people and influencing them.

In the historical interpretation of this prognosis of the outcome of diseases—at least insofar as the prognostic knowledge is based on symptoms in the human body—misunderstanding was bound to arise when, in periods characterized by quite different knowledge and methods, the physicians studied the writings of the fifth and fourth centuries in the spirit of scholasticism. The descriptions of symptoms appeared to be material to be used in diagnosing the disease. It was believed that all this infinitely detailed observation of diseases was made so that the physician might *know* what was wrong with the patient, in order to proceed from the diagnosis of the disease to the correct treatment.[16]

[15] The observations of crisis in various other passages (e.g., VII 144; 148) are also to be explained in accordance with the interpretation of the *Epidemics* books. I shall not cite these passages individually.

[16] If such were the case, however, the Herophilean distinction between preknowledge (πρόγνωσις) and prediction (πρόρρησις) would be meaningful, not merely subtle, as Galen says (CMG V₉, 203,19–20). An interesting early testimony for this objective interpretation of the prognostic material is, in my opinion, seen in the *characteres* added to the single descriptions of diseases, if they really are abbreviated forms of the names of diseases.

No attention was paid to the motivations and purposes which determined prognostic knowledge according to the writings themselves, nor to the fact that all these judgments existed only that they might be communicated to others. All utterances alien to this point of view were forgotten or ignored, and *Prognostikon*, the writing which could most easily be so interpreted, if the brief introduction and the conclusion were taken as mere embellishments, became the most important prognostic book. The same procedure was followed by the interpreters who, as an ultimate exaggeration, declared that in *Prognostikon* diagnosis of disease *per se* had been achieved.

Hippocratic and modern prognosis of the outcome of disease are comparable; but prognostic cognition is much more widespread in ancient medicine than in modern, for it was also supposed to embrace the patient's present condition, the pre-history of his illness, and his behavior in the absence of the physician. And just as prognosis of the outcome of disease does not help in understanding the nature of the disease, so in these areas of prognosis so far removed from modern medicine, it is the desire to protect the physician and to influence people which constitutes the motive and aim of the physician.

Only in expressions which read like formulae is there any question in the Hippocratic writings of the physician's obligation to tell the patient what is happening to him, what has already happened, and what the future will bring. The physician had to know from experience what he should say in individual cases.[17] And, at any rate, by making prognoses, he profits, in that he is credited with real knowledge of diseases, so that people dare to let him treat them (*Prognostikon*, Khlw. I 78,3–8).

What allows the physician to gain people's confidence, however, at the same time allows the patient to test the physician and to give his confidence only to the one who deserves it. The physician can tell a man who knows nothing of medicine anything he wants about the origin and treatment of disease. But if the physician tells him what is happening to him and what has already happened, this gives every patient the certainty that the physician to whom he is about to entrust himself understands his business, because he is able to judge the physician's words.

[17] Such formula-like phrases are found in Khlw. I 78,4–5; 189,24–190,2 (in a slightly different phrasing). The idea expressed in them is presupposed in the objective discussions of this theme with which I shall be concerned below.

This idea of the protection of the patient through prediction can be inferred from the words of the *Prognostikon;* in another passage, it is openly expressed. In the writing *On the physician* (CMG I₁ 24,21 ff.), one reads that, when wounds are present, the identification of the responsible weapons is a very important part of war surgery. For then the wounded man knows if he is being wrongly treated, and, by rights, only the physician who knows the signs (σημεῖα) will handle the treatment.[18]

The writing *On wounds in the head* discusses which kinds of missiles produce torn flesh or broken bones, whether in this wound or that the missile came from above or from the side, and so on (Khlw. II 12,6 ff.). It is taken for granted that the physician asks the patient how and in what way he was wounded (11,14; 14,16), in order, before examining him, to ascertain what kind of wound he has received (11,19). But once the inference is made that a certain kind of wound corresponds to a certain kind of missile, it is easy to conclude that a certain kind of missile corresponds to a certain kind of wound. Indeed, the strong insistence on interrogating the patient as to the circumstances of his injury suggests that the physician all too often determined these circumstances in prognosis in order to impress. Even the book on head wounds contains an exhortation, in the case of certain injuries, when certain conditions around the wounded part can be seen from a distance, to declare, without touching the patient, that the bone has been injured (ἀπόπροσθεν σκεψάμενον [λέξαι] μὴ ἀπτόμενον τοῦ ἀνθρώπου 11,2–3). In this way the physician impresses people before examining the patient and ascertaining whether the bone is really injured, and in what way (ἀπτόμενον τοῦ ἀνθρώπου πειρᾶται εἰδέναι σάφα 11,3–5), and before interrogating him (11,11).

Prognosis of past events, present condition, and future developments was intended to win the patient's confidence and patronage. But the physician must also try to maintain the patient's confidence in him while he is in his care, and this he can achieve by his ability to tell the patient to his face whether he is following orders or not. Many think they can discover all the patient's transgressions and everything in which he has been remiss; at least, such is the impression they try to

---

[18] τῶν ὅπλων ἐνόντων καὶ σημεῖα πεπορίσθαι τέχνης ἐστι πλεῖστον μέρος καὶ τῆς πρὸς ταῦτα χειρουργίης. τούτου γὰρ ὑπάρξαντος οὐκ ἂν παραλίποιτο τρωματίας ἀγνοηθείς, ὅταν (!) χειρουργῆται μὴ προσηκόντως· μόνος δ'ἂν ὁ τῶν σημείων ἔμπειρος εἰκότως ἐπιχειροίη. On the interpretation of these symptoms, cf. Khlw. II 12,6–14,13.

produce. *Prorrhetikon II* gives directions for determining certain errors on the part of the patients (IX 12,2; 14,4; 18,5; v.u. L.). More than this, it believes, the physician cannot achieve (14,8 ff.). *Prognostikon* speaks only of the impression such prognoses make, without going further into the matter (Khlw. I 78,5). The writing *On decorum*, however, shows that the physician is interested in such prognoses not only because they impress people but also because they enable him to escape responsibility for the harm caused by disobeying his orders.[19]

These are the delineations of prognosis in diseases, whether it is concerned with the outcome of the disease, with its history, or with the patient's following the physician's instructions. Since it is a means to influencing people, there is always the danger that it will be misused. This misuse consists not only in saying things of which one is not sure, or of which one has no knowledge at all. It consists, above all, in the attempt on the part of many physicians to create the impression that they owe their knowledge to superhuman powers of divination. Mantic prognosis attempts to make a statement without looking for evidence in the patient or in things; or at least it encourages people to believe that the physician arrives at his verdict in such a manner. Naturally, this mantic prognosis could not be recorded and can be grasped only as reflected in the books that have been preserved. Thus, *Prorrhetikon II* shows a physician coming to a patient whom everyone thinks lost, including the attending physician and the man's own friends. The stranger enters and declares that the man will not die, but will go blind (IX 6,5 L.). The author of *Prorrhetikon* does not pretend to make such prognoses by divination; his intention is to supply signs to guide the physician in arriving at a decision (ἐγὼ δὲ τοιαῦτα μὲν οὐ μαντεύσομαι, σημεῖα δὲ γράφω 8,2). For even this apparently superhuman knowledge—this knowledge that others, at least, consider superhuman—was in reality discovered in a very human way by means of certain clues, by signs, which the physician has obtained; one must simply know how such things are done (8,7 ff.). But the men who practice prognosis in this way are, after all, physicians, and the significance of prognosis manifests itself most clearly in this final, inflated form of practice.

The practicing physician is always faced with the question of what

---

[19] Cf. CMG I₁ 29,3 ff.; 29,20 ff. A pupil should supervise the patients or protect the physician from blame (ψόγος); beforehand, responsibility (αἰτία) is stressed. It follows that this prognosis of errors, too, is not universally practiced by physicians but can be replaced by other measures.

the future will bring. People want to know whether they will get well. The patient's feelings are dominated by this desire, and he continually asks the physician what is in store for him. Thus the physician is pressed to make prognoses. The decision not to answer such questions is not an easy one to make, and the more a physician is dependent on his patients, the less can he afford not to comply with their wishes. There is, therefore, a strong temptation to make prognoses, for they are the easiest way of gaining people's confidence. They increase the respect men feel for the physician, particularly if they are Greeks; for knowledge of the future is, for the Greek, really reserved to the gods; for modern man, on the other hand, it is self-evident that the control of the future through science lies within human power.[20]

In addition to prognosis of diseases and of human behavior during sickness, there is prognosis for the healthy. The writing *On regimen and health* (VI 72 ff. L.) gives one an idea of what such prognosis was like. It first (ch. I) determines the general manner of life for winter, spring, summer, and fall. Then the general statements are subjected to correction in accordance with age and constitutional makeup (ch. 2.)[21] Then come directions about walks, baths, and clothing (ch. 3), theories about alterations in the constitution (ch. 4), orders concerning the use of purgatives (ch. 5), special rules for women and children (ch. 6), and finally rules of conduct for people in training (ch. 7 οἱ γυμναζόμενοι).

The physician who takes this view proceeds on the basis of a definite concept of the human body. With the changing seasons, the basic materials comprising the body are subject to certain alterations deter-

---

[20] For this attitude of the Greeks, cf. e.g., Isocrates κατὰ τ. σοφιστῶν XIII § 7–8· A late commentary on the *Prognostikon* still pays special attention to the significance of prognosis which has just been described (*Scholia in Hippocratem et Galenum*, ed. Dietz, 1834, I, 55).

[21] Only the seasons and the patient's constitution and age are important. A reads the ending correctly according to the sense, as follows: δεῖ οὖν πρὸς τὴν ἡλικίην καὶ τὴν ὥρην καὶ τὰ εἴδεα διαιτήματα ποιεῖσθαι ἐναντιούμενον κτλ. 76,2–3. Littré and Villaret (*Hippocratis de nat. hominis liber*, Diss. Berlin, 1911, 45, 12), in accordance with the other manuscripts, read: πρὸς τὴν ἡλικίην καὶ τὴν ὥρην καὶ τὸ ἔθος καὶ τὴν χώρην καὶ τὰ εἴδεα διαιτήματα ποιεῖσθαι. But more is involved in the concepts χώρη and ἔθος than has been said in the preceding sentences, and a summons to be guided by custom in setting up a regimen is impossible, since it is custom which is about to be determined. Reference to the χώρη would, in principle, be feasible. But it seems unthinkable that in this writing a factor is called important in determining a regimen without the consequences being drawn when dietetic doctrine is concerned. The addition of the two concepts makes the statement parallel to enumerations occurring elsewhere of the things to which attention must be paid in medicine. Cf. the listing in Fredrich, *op. cit.*, p. 6, 2.

mined by nourishment and activity, and these alterations must immediately be counterbalanced if they are not to lead to sickness. For this
reason, everyone must regulate his life by taking certain measures.
And these interventions can be foreseen and predetermined because
they are related to general conditions. Of course, only the rich can really
do all they should for their health; the poor lack time for it. The writing
On diet pays keenest attention to this social distinction. It first determines the way of life of people in general, who eat and drink what they
happen to have, who have to tax their energies and do such work as
happens to be necessary. The writing gives them rules, insofar as this
is possible (ch. 68 VI 594 L.). But the author's real discovery, which
makes it possible, on the basis of a way of life, to avoid disease by means
of a prediagnosis (προδιάγνωσις 472,5), is valid only for people who can
devote themselves completely to their health and neglect everything
else for its sake (ch. 69,604). For both categories of people instructions
are given, invading the most intimate aspects of the life of the individual.[22]

This kind of prognosis has medical significance, for the physician
intervenes on the basis of it. In it a pessimism concerning the body is
expressed that is alien to modern views of sickness and health. In ancient medicine, wherever human health is understood as a balance of
certain elements, or where certain elements are thought to course, constantly changing, through the body, there is neither in theory nor in
practice a healthy man. For health has no being but is a continuous
becoming. The result is a nervosity in daily life and the use of medicines
even when one is healthy, a practice foreign to modern man. Even
though to modern thinking too, man, theoretically speaking, is not
completely healthy, in practice a differentiation is made between a state
of health and a state of disease, so that the life of the healthy is not
under the control of the physician. To be healthy means, simply, not to
be sick.

---

[22] There is no point in enumerating the details. The important thing is the
clarity with which the idea of the influence of the social order on the way of life is
grasped and the complete frankness with which it is expressed; cf. Plato, *The republic*, III, 406a ff., the argument against Herodicus. Incidentally, one must not be deceived by the small number of writings in the *Corpus* concerned with the healthy
man's life; this literature was really very extensive. The beginning of *On diet* shows
this in its arguments with its predecessors and in defining its position in relation to
them. Nevertheless, this is, of course, only a peripheral part of medicine; writings
by physicians must always be primarily concerned with diseases and their cure.

Just as one finds together with the prognosis of the outcome of sickness the attempt at a prognostic determination of the errors the patient may make during treatment, so prognosis for the healthy is accompanied by a prognosis of the errors they are likely to make, for instance in the exercises that belong to their regimen. This kind of prognosis also concerns athletes (*Prorrhetikon II*, IX 6,14; 14,10 ff. L.). Finally, healthy people can be told what diseases they will at some time encounter, a feat performed especially in the case of persons who lead an active life (6,11). Anyone who enjoys such things may make such prognoses; but he should do so with caution, for if the prognosis is correct he will be an object of awe, but if it is false, he will lose favor and suddenly seem to be out of his mind (10,8 ff.).

Such is the whole compass of prognosis in Hippocratic medicine in all its details. The Greek physician, starting by determining what course the disease will run, seeks to broaden the prognosis into a determination of the present condition and what preceded it. He is desirous of demonstrating his superiority; he wants to dominate over others, to be independent of what they might be able to tell him, though perhaps they might not express it correctly. And when the physician does not have to ask questions but already knows what he needs to know, he is admired by the public.

THE HIPPOCRATIC PHYSICIAN*

The Hippocratic physician is a craftsman. As a craftsman, he practices either as a resident or as an itinerant; he may also settle for a while in some town, leave again, work in another town, or wander all over the country. When he is in a town, he works in his shop or in his patient's home. The shop is a place in which today one person, tomorrow another, plies his trade—not a hospital, not a consulting room in the physician's house. Sick people come to the shop for examination and treatment, or the physician goes to his patient's home. An itinerant physician works in the patient's house or has a booth set up in the marketplace of the town, or elsewhere, and practices there.[1]

The medical craft is not under any restrictions. Anyone can practice it without having to pass an examination and without being accredited by any authority. As a craftsman, the physician of antiquity is classified socially as a businessman. While the modern doctor, in spite of the payment he receives, is not on the same social level as the other craftsmen who, like him, are paid for their services, the ancient physician is the equal of the other craftsmen and thereby occupies a low position in society.[2]

These circumstances determine the attitude of the patient to the physician and, consequently, the attitude of the physician to the patient. For the patient, the physician is not the doctor, the educated man to

---

* From Chapter III, *Peri aerōn und die Sammlung der hippokratischen Schriften.* Berlin: Weidmannsche Buchhandlung, 1931 (Problemata, Heft 4), see above, p. ix.

[1] For the data on which these general statements are based, cf. Daremberg-Saglio *s.v. medicus* III₂ 1669 ff. Aischines, *Contra Timarchum*, § 124, describes the workshop as a store.

[2] Everything I say about the status of the physician applies to the average physician. A famous physician naturally has a higher position although he can no more escape a lowering of his social status than can the great sophists. Since, in addition, most physicians are strangers, they are also excluded from the city community and from communal life. Today, there may still be individuals who consider the medical profession not suitable to their rank, but no entire social class is of this opinion, as is the class representative of ancient society. On the independence of crafts, cf. Daremberg, *op. cit.*, 1676.

whose knowledge he defers and whom he recognizes as an authority in his field; on the contrary, the physician is a craftsman who must prove that he knows his business and that he is just as eager to do his work well as to earn money. The patient, therefore, tries to reach an objective judgment of the physician's qualities in order to distinguish the charlatan from the true physician. In his actions, the physician must take this into consideration; he must give people an opportunity to reach a decision about him and his ability. The authority that is essential in every treatment must first be established, and this means that the physician's behavior is dictated by non-medical considerations to a much greater extent than are the actions of today's physician in his relations with his patient.[3]

The physician has many opportunities to show his worth. Into his workshop there come not only people who have some business there, i.e., not only sick people, but others who come to meet acquaintances, to converse, and to watch the physician. In the physician's workshop, then, there is an audience which discusses what the physician does, while the physician explains his treatment and attempts to persuade not only his patient, but also the bystanders, that he is a good physician and knows his business.[4]

When the physician goes to the patient's home, he is accompanied by his pupils and others, and there he meets the sick man's friends and relatives. The more communal character of life in antiquity permits an audience even during treatment, which lacks the intimacy that modern man takes for granted.[5]

It is essential for the physician to prove himself and important for the layman as a future patient to know physicians and to understand something about medicine, and the form of life furnishes possibilities for the physician to make himself known beyond the individual case, to make a reputation for himself which frees him from the necessity of convincing people anew with each treatment. But when the physician

[3] My purpose is to show that the personal element in the Greek physician's attitude toward his patient, which is so highly praised in today's discussions, was conditioned by the circumstances of ancient medicine; and that, at the same time, it has overtones which made of it something quite different from what is now understood by the physician's relation to his patient, which, it is generally claimed, is to be found already in Greek medicine.

[4] Cf. the interpretation of some of the relevant passages, p. 99 f. below.

[5] This follows, for instance, from Plato, *Gorgias* 456 b. Cf. also (as elsewhere when no particular reference is given) the handbooks and, in addition, Becker, *Charikles*, Leipzig, 1854, I, 231 ff.; Welcker, *Kleine Schriften*, III, especially 226 ff.

is a stranger and unknown to the people, the impression he makes at the moment is all-important.[6]

If he begins as an itinerant, the physician, like all other artisans, has to knock on people's doors and ask whether they can use his services. Since there are not resident physicians everywhere—they are always to be found in big cities and never in the countryside—people cannot run to the doctor with every illness. So that when one passes through, he can be sure that there will be work for him. But it can also happen that he asks about work in a house where another physician is just treating a patient. Nevertheless, he is admitted, for perhaps he knows his craft better than the doctor who is already there. He enters the room and tells the patient, "You will get well! There will only be a crippling of a finger of the left hand." If the other physician, who has been treating the sick man up to this point, has considered the case hopeless and has given everyone to understand that he no longer believes in the possibility of a cure, or if the new physician merely makes a better impression than the old one, the new physician will be retained and the old sent away.[7]

If a physician sets up his booth in a town, he has to recommend himself and his work to those who pass by, just as any artisan praises his wares; or he may have a crier proclaim his services. If someone then lets himself be persuaded to come to him, the physician treats him, and a marvelous treatment that proves successful with one patient will recruit new ones.

If the physician settles in one place and rents a shop, as long as he is still a stranger he will inquire of people whether he can be of service to them. He will put in an appearance in the workshops of other physicians and have his say, just like the people sitting around. Wherever possible, he will show that what his colleague proposes to do is wrong, that the case must be handled differently, that he understands the matter better, and that the patient should therefore put himself under his care. But he can also have others take him to a sick man, prove his superiority at

<hr />

[6] The medical man has only one possible career, that of becoming a city-appointed physician, and this position is rare, for only large cities can afford to engage a physician. It is, however, only with such an appointment that the physician no longer needs to establish his authority himself.

[7] For an example of the way in which work was solicited, see Xenophon, *Symp.* I § 11. What is here related about one craftsman is, of course, valid for all, as in every period of primitive craftsmanship. For the ἰατρὸς εἰσελθών, cf. Khlw. I 131,10 ff.; IX 6,5 L.

the patient's bedside by means of clever explanations and refutation of what the physician in charge proposes to do, and so make it clear that people must come to him when they are sick and anxious to receive proper treatment.[8]

Once the physician has acquired a certain reputation, or even become famous, people send for him; he is called from one town to another, and when he travels across the country he has friends everywhere. He can stay with them, and people come to be treated by him, or merely to see him and hear him speak.

This is how the physician practices. If he is properly trained, he has gained his knowledge as the pupil of another physician. It is a craftsman's knowledge, like any other, simple and secure in its grasp of the subject matter. It may be broadened, new medicaments may be discovered like new techniques in an art, but by and large medical knowledge is a known quantity.[9] The difference between individual craftsmen lies not in their knowledge but in their skill.[10]

The Hippocratic writings, oriented toward practice as they are, reflect real life so precisely that one can attempt to reconstruct a picture of the physician's activities from scattered statements in them, and thus it should be possible to add some individual characteristics to the general description I have already given.[11] I shall first deal with the physician as surgeon, as seen in the individual surgical writings.

[8] For this point, too, cf. the interpretation on p. 99 f. below.

[9] One must not assume that the ancient physician experienced the restlessness of the modern scientist, who sees medicine as science in a perpetual process of change through one discovery after another. In modern medicine, the emphasis rests, in principle, on knowledge—and my comparison of ancient and modern medicine is necessarily confined to their principles. The practicing physician stands on the lowest rung in the medical hierarchy, even though the individual may have felt differently about the value of what the practitioner does. And, above all, the physician's practical occupation appears to be the application of insight scientifically discovered; it is this which renders it superior to the occupation of the shoemaker or tailor. In principle, the doctor is forbidden to consider his education finished; he is duty bound to keep abreast of the advances in medical science. Clearly, then, the concepts of knowledge in ancient and modern medicine are poles apart. For details of the concept of *technē*, cf. below, p. 106.

[10] My portrait of the Hippocratic physician is necessarily confined to the typical; it describes the general situation, in contrast with which one must see individual achievement. One must start from this typical picture, which, as such, does not give the most favorable impression of the physician, in order to obtain a true measure of the greatness of an individual's accomplishment.

[11] In the following exposition of the physician's stance, I have taken account of the modern discussion of medical ethics, so lively at the moment, though I have taken no position in regard to detailed issues. My task is merely to interpret the

The writing *In the surgery* discusses everything that is of importance to surgery. It teaches how the room in which treatment is given should be equipped, how the light should enter it, how the patient and the physician should be seated, what clothing is appropriate for the surgeon, how he must hold his hands and take care of them. The surgeon must be able to perform every manipulation with the right and the left hand, striving to accomplish his purpose correctly, well, quickly, effortlessly, in good posture, and without embarrassment (ἀγαθῶς καλῶς ταχέως ἀπόνως εὐρύθμως ἀπόρως Khlw. II 33,9). And when bandages are described, one reads again that the physician should work fast, effortlessly, with skill and good posture (ταχέως ἀπόνως εὐπόρως εὐρύθμως 34,2). These terms are defined as follows: fast (ταχέως) means finishing the business expeditiously; effortlessly (ἀπόνως) means doing it with a light touch; skillfully (εὐπόρως) means showing oneself equal to the task; with good posture (εὐρύθμως) means proceeding in such a way that it is pleasant to watch.

For the way in which the dressing is applied, there are two categories: "well and neatly" (ἀγαθῶς; καλῶς 34,6). By "neatly" (καλῶς) is meant here that the dressing is simple, tidy, applied evenly and alike on even and similar parts, and unevenly and unlike on parts that are unlike and uneven (34,6 ff.). A "well"-made dressing (ἀγαθῶς) is achieved by pressure, or by a multitude of bandages, and by applying the dressing so that it cannot slip (34,12 ff.).

These statements on the method of treatment take into consideration the impression the surgeon makes when practicing. In this respect, the writing *In the surgery* differs from the teachings of other writings.

The point of departure in the writing *On fractures* is the question of the position in which the injured limbs should heal. Then signs are enumerated by which to tell whether a dressing fits correctly (καλῶς καὶ ὀρθῶς Khlw. II 53,12). Yet "neat" does not designate the external form of the dressing, as in the writing *In the surgery*, but the objective correctness of the whole, and there is no consideration at all of the question of good deportment (εὐρύθμως) during the application of the dressing,

---

ancient material. Yet, I have tried to learn from the present debate what must be considered as material. I should mention specifically one earlier study because it has helped me in the interpretation of general questions by providing detailed material: G. Weiss, "Die ethischen Anschauungen im Corpus Hippocraticum," *Arch. f. Gesch. d. Mediz.* 4, 1911; Weiss appends a comprehensive collection of references to his interpretation of the physician's attitude.

nor of the procedure's being pleasant to watch, and the like. This is an essential difference.

The surgeon needs instruments for his work, and if he practices in a large city he should have instruments made for all necessary operations (68,19). But they should be used only when human strength does not suffice. A good surgeon would not stoop to (σολοικότερον 72,7) using instruments except when necessary. Of course, good and bad surgery are both possible with, and without, instruments (καλῶς καὶ αἰσχρῶς 73,19); and, clearly, people find it more convincing (πιθανώτερον) if the physician uses an instrument; it also makes him more readily appear blameless (ἀναμαρτητότερον). Nevertheless, as a feat it must be valued less highly (ἀτεχνότερον 74,1). In these words there is no decision as to which course should be taken; it is left to the individual to choose what makes him appear efficient and blameless in the eyes of the people. Whereas just now, in the discussion of dressings, the doctor's actions were restricted to the essential, here judgment is suspended. Still, the physician who defers to the judgment of the crowd seems less capable because the kind of treatment he uses is simpler, although good results may be obtained from both methods. Besides the opinion of others, there is, therefore, also the matter of the quality of his work for the physician to consider, and this consciousness of his own expertise is the determining factor. Thus he will try as far as possible to avoid the physical damage which can arise from an operation. Predictable occurrence of such mutilation argues for the use of special caution and special means. Regard for his clients and regard for himself and his work are constantly intermingled: it is extremely distressing and deleterious when a leg is shortened (μεγάλη ἡ αἰσχύνη [subjectively] καὶ βλάβη [objectively] βραχύτερον τὸν μηρὸν ἀποδεῖξαι 77,3–4). And, in the same way, in the following phrase, the desire to perform an operation correctly combines with the realization of how harmful it is to one's reputation to treat a patient poorly, or not as well as others: ". . . if one wishes to work correctly and with a light touch" (εἰ δέ τις μέλλοι καλῶς καὶ εὐχερῶς ἐργάζεσθαι 90,13); or again, in the words: ". . . it is unpleasant and inefficient . . ." (αἰσχρὸν καὶ ἄτεχνον 93,6), or in the advice to use an instrument only when one can confidently expect to achieve one's goal (96,22).

The physician's art is limited by the impossibility of restoring everyone to health. One should not blind oneself to this impossibility but should predict what is pending (100,6). Indeed, the physician should try to refuse treatment that has little hope of success and involves many dangers, if he can do so without reprobation (ἤν τις καλὴν φυγὴν ἔχηι 101,9 ff.). In other words, he should refrain from treating such a case, not simply because he knows help is not possible, but also because treating a hopeless and dangerous case will harm him. Hope is slight, the difficulties great; if he does not intervene, people think he is not knowledgeable; if he does intervene, he hastens death (αἴ τε γὰρ ἐλπίδες ὀλίγαι καὶ οἱ κίνδυνοι πολλοί · καὶ μὴ ἐμβάλλων ἄτεχνος ἂν δοκέοι εἶναι, καὶ ἐμβαλὼν ἂν ἐγγυτέρω θανάτου ἀγάγοι . . .). Then it is better for the physician's prestige to have nothing to do with the case.

In sum, the attitude of the author of *On fractures* is that of conscious mediation between the practically necessary and what is dictated by a consideration of public opinion.

In the instructions in the writing *On joints* importance is again attributed to the physician's ambition and determination to perform his duties well. For it is said that the physician should see to it that a situation does not arise which objectively has perhaps no particularly harmful significance but gives evidence of improper treatment (καὶ κάκιον μὲν ἂν οὐδὲν εἴη, αἴσχιον δὲ καὶ ἀτεχνότερον Khlw. II 128,19). The physician should know when a proposed operation will be successful but will result in crippling, and he should predict this if he considers it proper to do so (εἰ ἄλλως ἐθέλοις 134,1). The physician does not wish to be suspected of having caused a physical deformity through his lack of skill. Sometimes, at the beginning of their illness, patients insist on being treated; the doctors do everything they can, but after a while the patients no longer bother to take good care of their wounds, for they experience little pain. The physicians run away and discontinue treatment, quite glad about their patients' unconcern, because they would have been unable to prevent crippling anyway (οὐ δυνάμενοι καλὰ τὰ χωρία ἀποδεικνύναι 135,18 ff.). Their personal interest then is more important to them than the patient's. The author relates the occurrence without any criticism, but he does not necessarily condone it, for he himself has advised the physician to predict an impending deformity.

Some physicians consider in their treatment only the good impression they can make. They apply a magnificent nose bandage; for two or three days the patient rejoices over his wonderful bandage, and the physician is proud of his skill. On the third day, the patient is in great pain. The physician is satisfied with the fact that he has shown his mastery in the art of bandaging (155,8). He happens to be one of those very skillful but very stupid doctors (ἰητροὶ μὴ σὺν νόωι εὔχειρες 152,16), one of those with a light touch but weak intelligence (οἱ τὴν ἀνόητον εὐχειρίην ἐπιτηδεύοντες 155,3) who rejoice over a beautiful bandage without giving the matter further thought (οἱ χαίροντες τῆισι καλῆισιν ἐπιδέσεσιν ἄνευ νόου 154,16). They are, nevertheless, physicians.

In this case, the physician thinks only of the impression his treatment is making on others, not at all of the fact that it harms the patient. Many a physician, to be sure, refrains from a therapeutic course which in itself is not harmful and, if properly followed, has good results, even though he knows that it is very impressive and makes people everywhere praise the physician. He chooses a different, less pretentious course as long as it is just as effective. The author of the writing *On joints* says that he would be ashamed to make use of succussions on a ladder (κατασείσιες ἐν τῆι κλίμακι), with which physicians work who are eager to amaze the populace. For the populace ask only for the wondrous, not whether the treatment is beneficial or injurious (167,10 ff.). Although he has as yet seen no success from such treatment, he considers it completely within the realm of possibility that it could succeed, provided the procedure is correct (168,1–2). Nevertheless, he rejects this kind of treatment as more befitting the charlatan than the true physician. Yet his personal rejection of it does not prevent his showing exactly how the method must be used if the physician wants to use it correctly (168,13 ff.).[12]

The question may be asked, how far the physician should extend his knowledge. Should he limit it to the curable and know of the incurable only that it is incurable? Or is he also interested in the course of a disease which he cannot cure? The author of *On joints* decides, in opposition to the opinion of others (205,11 ff.), to extend his knowledge to the course of incurable cases also: first of all, so that the physician may not cause people unnecessary pain, and then because predicting what will happen is impressive and demonstrates the superiority of the physician (τὰ δὲ προρήματα λαμπρὰ καὶ ἀγωνιστικά). However much he himself refuses to make an impression with display and unworthy methods, the desire to make an impression and to set off his own ability against that of others does, nevertheless, motivate his actions and thoughts even when he is concerned with advancing the formulation of a problem; he does not desire increased knowledge merely for the sake of knowing

---

[12] This shaking of patients on ladders fastened to gables and walls (169,12–13) is one of the many methods used in ancient surgery which, by their very nature, are bound to be public exhibitions and tempt the physician to dazzle the populace.

more. And it remains uncertain whether personal motives could not also induce him to prefer a particular form of treatment. For he says, in describing a case, that a certain operation is good and correct and suitable to the matter in hand, and, at the same time, a good advertisement if the physician is pleased by such things and would like to boast of them (ἀγαθὴ μὲν ἤδε καὶ δικαίη καὶ κατὰ φύσιν ἡ ἐμβολὴ καὶ δή τι καὶ ἀγωνιστικὸν ἔχουσα, ὅστις γε καὶ τοῖσι τοιούτοισιν ἤδεται κομψευόμενος 224,19 ff.). He only goes as far as to say that, of many therapeutic possibilities, the physician should choose the one that attains its object with the least display (236,16 ff.). This is the seemly course for a respectable physician (ἀνδραγαθικώτερον; τεχνικώτερον), and any other amounts to deceiving the populace (δημοειδὴς κιβδηλίη). Yet he knows that there are cases in which the physician is forced to employ a treatment that is bound to be harmful, simply because people demand it, and because they are suspicious of the physician if he does not employ it (220,14 ff.).

Men's ignorance of medical matters is very dangerous. Sometimes physicians persuade themselves and their patients that they can heal an injury although it is incurable; they deceive themselves about the nature of the malady. They may do it without evil intent and believe it themselves. In any case, it causes much difficulty for the physician who knows, and speaks, the unpleasant truth. For people naturally listen to the physicians who assure them that all is well. It is they who have the advantage; the other physician will not be listened to. A physician needs courage to see not only the momentary condition of his patient and the confirmation of his treatment which this condition represents, but to go on observing to the end and perhaps to admit that, seen in retrospect, his treatment was bad. Still more courage is required to write down the bad result of the treatment employed and publish it; but such action combats ignorance and is more correct than that of physicians who are content with momentary success (182,3).[13]

The writing On joints, then, is more indulgent toward the physician's wish to make an impression on people than is that On fractures.[14]

The writing On the physician presents a completely objective view. It rejects all bandaging that is done only to make a good impression and that allows certain techniques because they please people (ἐπιδέσιες

[13] This honesty, more than the honesty shown in Epidemics, could be called intellectual honesty (cf. "Prognosis," p. 78 above, ftn. 14).

[14] On the relationship of these two writings, see Edelstein, Peri aerōn und die Sammlung der hippokratischen Schriften, Berlin, 1931, p. 168 ff.

εὔρυθμοι καὶ θεητρικαί CMG I₁ 21, 32 ff.). That is senseless ostentation, not becoming to the true physician.

In the remaining surgical writings, there are no statements about the physician's deportment.[15] Of the general medical books, only *On diseases I* also discusses surgical activities (ch. 10 VI 158 L.). The dexterity (εὐχειρίη) that is demanded is merely correct and appropriate action. A particularly graceful finger position, beautiful to look upon (τὸ δὲ τοῖσι δακτύλοισιν εὐσχημόνως λαμβάνειν), or any embellishment of the bandages constitutes a dexterity which has nothing to do with medical ability but is a thing apart and must be judged as such (οὐ πρὸς τῆι τέχνηι κρίνεται, ἀλλὰ χωρίς).

The surgical practice of the Hippocratic physician can be reconstructed down to the last detail because the polemical character of the great surgical books has preserved it with clarity. So complete a picture of the practice of dietetics cannot be put together, in spite of the much greater number of dietetic writings in the *Corpus*, for the dietetic writings are much more sober and not polemical.[16] It is only possible to combine isolated passages from different books to reconstruct the image of the dietetic physician. Even so, the surgical writings, which are more detailed, must be used to interpret adequately the occasional utterances of the therapeutic writings.

I start with the question of the physician's attitude toward undertaking the care of a patient. If the case is not serious, he naturally does not hesitate to treat it, but if the disease is serious and if there is little likelihood of a cure, various procedures are possible.

The physician may undertake treatment of the serious case, declaring right away that there are only slight prospects of a cure: he takes the case, but he declines responsibility by predicting the outcome (Khlw. I 79,8).

But the physician can also deliberate whether he should undertake to treat a difficult case at all, and whether he wants to do so or not is

[15] The writing *On wounds in the head* touches upon the physician's behavior only once: he should announce what kind of injury he believes to be present before making an examination (Khlw. II 11,2; cf. p. 81 above, where the difference between this writing and *On the physician* is discussed also). Other statements in writings of the *Corpus*, which could be added, tell nothing new. A passage of interest from the point of view of war surgery is to be found, V 254 L.

[16] Only the books on the diseases of women are polemical. Occasional polemics occur in *Epidemics* and elsewhere, but they are restricted to refutations of specific views and are not written in a novelistic style. Incidentally, some polemical remarks are directed not against abstract ideas, but against the actions and opinions of cer-

his decision. Thus, in the therapeutic writings a case is described; it is stated that it is a serious case such as usually ends fatally; the necessary treatment is given, but this treatment is introduced by the words, "If you so desire, treat it thus" (e.g., VII 126,7; 194,13 L. ἢν θεραπεύῃς; ἢν δὲ βούλῃι). It is left, then, to the physician's discretion to undertake, or to decline, to treat a case, and that the question is left open can only be because of the desire not to have a bad outcome charged to the physician. For he has drugs at his disposal which, although not specifically helpful, could nevertheless be tried. In other passages, one reads that the physician should take a case if there is some prospect of success; but he should know which cases are without hope of success and why, and if he treats them his administrations should be as helpful as is still possible (τὰ μὲν ἀνυστὰ ἐκθεραπεύειν τὰ δὲ μὴ ἀνυστὰ εἰδέναι διότι οὐκ ἀνυστὰ καὶ θεραπεύοντα τοὺς τὰ τοιαῦτα ἔχοντας ὠφελέειν ἀπὸ τῆς θεραπείης ἐς τὸ ἀνυστόν VI 150–52 L.).

This possibility of declining to treat a particular disease must be distinguished from the advice to abstain from intervening in certain instances. The physician is forbidden to give treatment when the disease is in a critical stage because, according to theory, intervention at that time is injurious (VII 148,7 L.). Moreover, there are certain situations in which a fatal outcome of the disease seems so sure that intervention is prohibited (VII 72,6 v. u. L.). The reason for this is the impossibility of being helpful and probably—though this can only be proved by analogy with the surgical books—the intention not to harass the sick person unnecessarily. And in such cases, of course, it is also desirable, in the physician's interest, that he refrain from treating them.

Nevertheless, it must be borne in mind that this concerns only certain very serious cases, that only an occasional writing expresses such a prohibition, that on the basis of other theories the possibility of any prognostic knowledge of the outcome of a disease can be contested, or limited to so few complications in the course of the disease that, relatively speaking, they do not count at all (cf. p. 73 ff. above). Finally, in a great many descriptions of disease, in spite of the statement that the illness ends in death, at least in most cases, medicaments that should be employed are nevertheless named (e.g., VII 84,8 ff. L.), and

---

tain people (οἱ ἰητροί . . . e.g., V, 78 L.). In other words, one learned of the views of one's colleagues not just from books, but much more often from personal observation of what they were doing and saying.

this is done without urging a prognosis and without making treatment optional or advocating rejection of the case. This means that one cannot speak of a general rule that incurable cases should not be treated.[17]

The physician strives to be cautious in accepting patients so that no blame may be attached to him, not to torment the sick unnecessarily in carrying out his treatment, and also not to involve himself unnecessarily in hopeless cases. In his final decision he does not think only of himself; he also takes other factors into account. He may refuse a case only if he can do so without reprobation, as the surgical writings have it (cf. p. 92 f. above), and as the writing *On diseases of women* indicates with the words: "It is best not to treat this woman, but if he must, then only after making a prognosis" (ταύτην μάλιστα μὲν μὴ ἰῆσθαι, εἰ δὲ μὴ προειπόντα ἰῆσθαι VIII 150,12 L.).

The surgeon must pay attention to the manner and posture in which he operates and applies dressings. In dietetics, it is important for the physician—who can do nothing but give drugs—to show himself to advantage by proper procedure and correct behavior. Thus many passages speak of the physician's behavior, of his clothes, the way to enter the sickroom, how to take a seat, to speak, and to act. When this is discussed in the writings on ethics, the solutions to the problem are at variance; but the contradictory solutions do not affect the importance physicians consciously attach to behavior and appearance, which to them are a matter of courtesy toward the patient (αἱ τοῖσι κάμνουσι χάριτες V 308 L.).[18]

The importance of paying attention to what one says is constantly emphasized (e.g., V 308 L.). The physician should not alarm the patient, but comfort and encourage him. At the same time, the physician's words are the best means of obtaining obedience. If the physician is to help, his relationship to his patient must be that of the person in command to the one who obeys. The patient must be in the physician's hands (ὑποχείριος CMG I₁ 20,21), though such a relationship is difficult to attain.

The physician cannot presume that his orders will be obeyed, so

[17] It is true, in *On the physician* (CMG I₁ 10,21; 14,1) the principle is defended that the physician should not treat hopeless cases because he should not undertake what he cannot accomplish. But as the evidence quoted in the text shows, this is only one point of view.
[18] *On decorum, On the physician*, ch. I, and *Precepts*, together with scattered passages in the *Epidemics* provide the material relevant for the topic to be discussed (e.g., V 290, 308 L.).

he should visit his patient frequently to make sure that he is following orders. He should leave one of his pupils behind to watch over the patient (CMG I₁ 29,30). If the physician is unable to prevent mistakes (ἁμαρτίαι) on the part of his patient, he will suffer for it himself, for the physician will be taxed with the unfavorable result of the treatment, even though the patient himself is to blame (29,3 ff.). The patient is believed to be credulous, devoid of real judgment, and a liar (29,4), opinions which are indicative of the opposition on which the physician must count.

Frequently the physician is unable to stay as long as the treatment would demand, perhaps because he is called away to another city, perhaps because, where he is, he has too few patients or too poor ones to be able to remain. The physician's fee is, therefore, a source of worry for the patient, because he may leave if he does not receive sufficient remuneration. The physician should learn not to charge very much when the patient is unable to pay; he should see his reward in his patient's gratitude and in the reputation he gains for also treating the poor (CMG I₁ 32,4 ff.). In any case, it is important whether the physician states at the beginning of the treatment how much he will demand in payment, or whether he waits until the end (31,16 ff.). On the other hand, the patient is free to leave one doctor and go to another. Moreover, it is not unethical for a physician to treat a colleague's patient: people run after every new doctor who promises new, unheard-of things (31,26), and one should not interfere with this.

What I have said also describes the attitude of the physician who practices dietetics; it is shaped, as is that of the surgeon, by conscious consideration of the person of the patient. But it is possible for the physician to influence people not only by what he does; his words too help him to attain his goal in surgery as in dietetics.

The physician has to tell the patient what to do, and in certain cases the patient must also be told why he has to follow this or that instruction. Besides, when another doctor or other persons are present while the treatment is given, and they enter into the conversation and say what they think should be done, the physician will also have to enter into a discussion with them. It is essential to attack opposite opinions and to explain and justify what one personally considers right.

One physician gives orders during treatment of an injured hand. He points out that the hand must be bandaged in the position he has chosen because it is held in the same position in archery. And everyone is amazed at his cleverness (Khlw. II 47,6–16). Another physician proceeds differently but makes just as clever a speech, advances just as wonderful arguments, and makes an equally great impression on people (49,8–16). On one occasion, a physician claims that the injury with which the patient has come to him can only be explained in a certain way; and all the physicians and laymen present agree with him. Only one physician disagrees. A discussion arises and the dissenting physician persuades the others, with some difficulty, that he is right, not the physician in charge (Khlw. II 111,12–112,4). Where diseases are concerned, there can be a discussion of the cause of the illness from which someone is suffering, and of the way it should be treated. In this discussion (ἀντιλογίη), the physician must pay attention to whether his opponent makes untenable statements, and at such points he must interfere and prove him wrong (*On diseases I*, ch. 1 *finis* VI 142 L.).[19]

Thus the physician in his practical activity is daily in need of oratorical skill, and it is not astonishing that he should train as a speaker. But wherever people come together medical questions are brought up, and one talks about the nature of medicine and its possibilities, just as one discusses any other questions. In such conversations, physicians present their medical theories and opinions; man's nature and the structure and composition of his body are discussed. Some maintain that he is composed of four elements, others that he is made of earth and water, and whatever other theories may be propounded (*On the nature of man*, ch. I VI 32 L.). Laymen have to inform themselves about medicine and correct treatment; otherwise, when they are sick, they are unable to distinguish the true physician from the false. It is for this reason that people listen to such discourses, and it is for this reason that physicians deliver them.[20]

[19] The book *On diseases I*, is an introduction to the art of debating written for physicians (cf. ch. 1). All essential problems of the medical art and the etiologies of diseases are expounded with the object of showing which statements are admissible and which not. Similarly, one must understand the appendices to various writings about general medical questions as lessons in debating addressed to physicians (e.g., π. τόπων τ. κατ' ἄνθρωπον ch. 41 ff. VI 330 L.).

[20] Another way of informing the public is to publish books meant for the laity, giving instruction in medical matters. The writing *On affections* (VI 208 L.) is a book of this kind. The beginning stresses expressly the importance for the layman of understanding something of medical questions, as far as he can as a layman (ch. I). The writing is by no means a manual for self-treatment, enabling one to dispense with the need for a doctor when one is ill; rather, it is a book from which the layman can learn how to judge a physician. In the centuries of rhetoric, however, the spoken word was still fully the equal of the book as a source of enlightenment. Under these

But the physician must speak up not only to inform people about the nature of medicine and tell them which is the right treatment. Like every other *technē*, the medical *technē*, too, is the object of attacks; and indeed the very existence of a *technē* is disputed. This question is of great importance to the physician, for if there is really no such thing as a *technē*, then medicine is useless. Men will regain their health without its help and the physician is superfluous. Against this danger the physician must defend himself. He must take a stand in the art's fight for existence. How he does this is seen in the writing *On the art*.

This writing is believed to be the work of a sophist.[21] But, as the words used in the writing show, it is the work of a physician, and it is of significance as the treatise which documents the physician's rhetorical stance and his rhetorical battle detached from all specifically medical objectives.

The speaker begins with a description of the people who try to discredit the *technai*. Those who thus attack the other *technai* should be curbed by the people concerned, in the field they are concerned with, and, moreover, by people capable of it (τοὺς μὲν οὖν ἐς τὰς ἄλλας τέχνας τούτωι τῶι τρόπωι ἐμπίπτοντας οἷσι μέλει τε καὶ ὧν μέλει οἱ δυνάμενοι κωλυόντων CMG I₁ 9,14). This speech will be directed against those who try to take advantage of medicine; it is full of courage in the face of the pettiness of the people it accuses; it is equipped for battle in behalf of the *technē* it seeks to succor, and, finally, equal to the task, thanks to the sagacity and education of its author (δυνάμενος δὲ διὰ σοφίην ἧι πεπαίδευται 9,18). When the author says that attacks against other *technai* must be answered by those concerned and, indeed, in the fields that concern them, he must be a physician, who now speaks for medicine. If this were not

conditions, the physician understandably did not always rely only on his natural gift of speech in order to gain the upper hand in the debates in which he had to engage; as a physician, he often studied and practiced the art of rhetoric. It would be meaningless to call such a physician an *iatro* sophist, for, in the centuries in which the Hippocratic writings were written, the connection between rhetoric and medicine was still natural, just as rhetoric was an intrinsic part of the daily life of the whole population, especially the life of politics; it was not merely the empty talk which it became at a much later period. That there may have been individual physicians in the fifth and fourth centuries for whom rhetoric was only an external show does not take away the significance which rhetoric itself had for medicine.

[21] Th. Gomperz, *Die Apologie der Heilkunst*, Wien, 1890, laid the basis for this interpretation. Although his attribution of the writing to a particular sophist has not been accepted, the speech is at least regarded as the exhibition of a sophist in all the books and manuals I have seen.

so, it would be in medicine alone that it is not the expert who speaks, and the author would be the only one to ignore the principle he has himself just set up. It is, then, a physician who speaks, anxious to defend his own *technē* in the general attack on the *technai*, and knowing that he does battle at only one point—at the point where he stands as a physician. It is under this assumption that one must try to understand what follows.

After the introduction, there first comes a brief epistemological reflection on the problem of existence (ch. 2). The author connects the problem of the existence of a medical *technē* with the problem of existence as such, as fits a man of culture. There is, to be sure, no real discussion of the problem of existence, and the author is under no illusion that he has adequately expounded the subject. And so in conclusion he says: "Anyone who is not content with what is said here and does not quite comprehend it can obtain instruction from other speeches (περὶ μὲν οὖν τούτων, εἰ γέ τις μὴ ἱκανῶς ἐκ τῶν εἰρημένων ξυνίησιν, ἐν ἄλλοισιν ἂν λόγοισι σαφέστερον διδαχθείη 10,15–16). The orator himself has learnt his epistemology from others and emphasized his good education at the very beginning. Therefore, he refers his audience to another authority which will teach in detail, if they so wish, what he only hints at. Medicine is his field and his theme, and he turns to it after this general preamble.

His discourse is to have two parts. First, he intends to set forth what medicine is and what it can, and should, do (10,19). In the second part, his intention is to show how medicine achieves its goals (11,1). In the first part, (11,5 ff.), he goes through individual questions and objections concerning the problem of chance and comes finally to the question (14,1) whether physicians may justly be blamed if they refuse to treat a disease that is too far advanced. He does not blame them, basing his judgment on general arguments.

The *technē* cannot attack everything in the same way, and only the mad can demand that it be capable of things for which it was not made. The same is true of nature. The aim should be to attain only the attainable (–14,10). Thus it is impossible (14,11) to treat a malady which is stronger than the remedies at medicine's disposal (–14,21). The demand to treat everyone carries conviction only for those physicians who are such in name only (–14,24). This discussion of treatment under all circumstances concludes the first part; it is itself concluded with the statement that the true physician does not bow to the opinion of the inexpert but counts on those who, through exact deliberation (14,26 λελογισμένοι), know just what the *technē* can do, and what it cannot do, what the physician must be blamed for, and what the patient. The whole first part deals with general questions, with objections that can, in fact, be leveled against every *technē;* they are fought in their guise as attacks on medicine, simply because it is medicine that is being defended and the orator is a physician.

"As far as the other *technai* are concerned, another speech at another time will say what must be said. As for medicine, what it can perform, how it is to be judged, these things have been discussed and will be discussed further" (τὰ μὲν οὖν κατὰ τὰς ἄλλας τέχνας ἄλλος χρόνος μετ' ἄλλου λόγου δείξει, τὰ δὲ κατὰ τὴν ἰητρικὴν οἷά τέ ἐστιν ὥς τε κριτέα, τὰ μὲν ὁ παροιχόμενος, τὰ δὲ ὁ παρεὼν διδάξει λόγος 15,3–5). With these words the speaker goes over to the second part, in which he discusses the existence of the medical *technē* from the standpoint of bodily conditions and the resources of medicine, instead of on the basis of general problems, as in the first part. At the start, the speaker designated the answering of attacks made on each individual *technē* as the duty of the experts (δυνάμενοι) of each *technē*. In placing his own task beside those of others at the beginning of the oration, and also at the transition from the first part to the second, he designates it as a part of a large interconnected struggle. When he mentions other speeches to be made at some other time in defense of the other *technai*, he cannot be thinking of a speech he intends to make himself but, in accordance with the introductory chapter, of speeches that experts will make for their specialties, as he now speaks for medicine.

The conclusion, too, demonstrates that here a physician is speaking. The author ends with the statement that medicine can defend itself against the attacks made upon it, that it is justified in refusing to treat too difficult cases, and that, if it does give treatment, it has no share in the unfavorable outcome (19,3–5). This is demonstrated by what was just said; but it is also demonstrated by the proofs the experts prefer to give through their deeds, rather than in words (19,5–6). And, indeed, physicians rely on the proof of their deeds rather than on proofs in argument. Of course, the speaker is just such a physician; he does not wish to make a speech, but he is obliged to do so because medicine is so fiercely attacked in the general discussion. Physicians prefer the testimony of their deeds because the crowd is more readily, and more suitably, persuaded by what it sees than by intellectual discussion; and it is not a question of the physicians' neglecting oratory and not troubling themselves with it (οὐ τὸ λέγειν καταμελήσαντες,[22] ἀλλὰ τὴν πίστιν τῶι πλήθει, ἐξ ὧν ἂν ἴδωσιν, οἰκειοτέρην ἡγεύμενοι, ἢ ἐξ ὧν ἂν ἀκούσωσιν 19,7–9). The explanation—that in general the experts refrain from making speeches because a speech does not convince the crowd—makes sense only if the speaker is addressing a cultured audience and paying them a tribute, and making an excuse to people who are fond of speeches; that is, when a physician speaks to interested, cultured people.[23]

The assertion that *On the art* is the work of a sophist is based primarily on the two passages that mention another speech (λόγος), which is to be given. The first passage is concerned with the discourse on epistemological questions (10,15), which was referred to before in the discussion of the transition from the introduction to the main body of the writing. The second passage is the transition from the first to the second part (15,3 ff.), to which reference has just been made. And because it is claimed that at one point the author declares it to be his duty to discuss epistemological problems and, at another, to speak of the attacks made on the *technai* in general, he is supposed to be a sophist who must have his say on all subjects. But in neither passage does the author speak of himself, and it is, therefore, not possible to deduce from the words alone what kind of speaker he has in mind. This can only be discovered by interpretation. In accordance with the over-all sense, it is out of the question that the author, who is a physician, could be the speaker on these two occasions.

Although the writing *On the art* is the composition of a physician, he has, in the battle he wages, distanced himself to the utmost from his activity as a physician, however much he may have to fight this fight in his very capacity as a physician. But in these general discussions, he can still utilize the same dialectic training which he must normally apply in the sickroom and in public.[24]

---

[22] I read καταμελήσαντες contrary to Heiberg, who reads καταμελετήσαντες (Samb. et Fevr., cf. Gomperz, *Apologie der Heilkunst*, 1910² p. 58 *ad* l. 13). Only this reading, I believe, gives the full contrast to the following ἡγεύμενοι.

[23] It is thus that I think the words must be interpreted, Gomperz' views notwithstanding. He sees the ending as a compliment on the part of a sophist to his audience of physicians, whom he wishes to defend against the reproach (his own or whose?) that they set no store by speeches.

[24] The writing *On the art* shows how important it is to make distinctions in judging ancient medicine. Its dialectic training and argumentation can, of course, only be put to use before certain audiences. With unsophisticated people the argu-

The importance of the physician's training in dialectics, however, is not exhausted by its usefulness as a means for handling people. Schooling in rhetoric, at the same time, furnishes the means of proving medical theories. While a modern theory of diseases can only be based on experiments and observations, a theory which presents heat and cold, the air, or the four fluids as the causes of diseases can only be proved by dialectics, by logical argumentation. It is not possible to demonstrate experimentally how the balance of fluids in the human body is disturbed, nor how this imbalance evokes diseases. But it is possible to claim that a disturbance of the balance of the fluids determines diseases, and it is possible to attempt verification of the claim by means of arguments, analogies, sophistry. In its purely theoretical aspect, this medicine by hypothesis[25] is the real achievement of ancient medicine. And it is of necessity logical; it is, therefore, accessible only to men educated in philosophy and rhetoric and can only be represented by such men in public discussions.

The necessity of justifying itself before men and the logical penetration, generally, of the physician's activity and knowledge have resulted in the completely clear expression in the medical writings of the

---

ment would be simpler and more concrete. (The great difference between city and country in these centuries must also have resulted in great differences in treatment.) Littré has assembled details of the oratorical activities of the physician (IV 613). Diels maintains (*Hermes* 46, 1911, p. 273,2) that these activities included inaugural addresses of state physicians and designates some speeches in the *Corpus* as such. But the passage (Xenophon, *Mem.* IV 2,5), to which Diels simply refers by name in evidence of his opinion, says only that the physician, at the time of his appointment, has to furnish information concerning his teachers and his activity. This cannot be called an inaugural address. Plato, *Gorgias* 456b, furnishes an imaginary situation.

[25] The concept "hypothesis" I have borrowed from the writing *On breaths* (CMG I₁ 36,6; 37,19). The polemic of this speech, which attacks "hypothetical" medicine, should not be allowed to obscure the importance of the theories it opposes. *On ancient medicine* gives just one view of the matter. At the end of the writing *On breaths*, it is claimed (CMG I₁ 101,21) that the speech has proved the hypothesis to be true (ἀληθὴς ἡ ὑπόθεσις ἐφάνη), as one must read "hypothesis" in accordance with M, rather than "promise," as Heiberg conjectures. For how could a "promise" to demonstrate the cause of the disease (111,18) be "proved true" by the speech? The speaker demonstrated the power of the *pneuma* in all things, then took up the more important diseases in which the hypothesis he has proposed, viz., that the *pneuma* is the cause, had proved correct. And as proofs of a hypothetical theory, *On breaths* and similar writings must be valuated positively and not dismissed merely as the "miserable fabrications of sophists."

fundamental concepts and ideas of the ancient healing art. One need only assemble them to understand medicine as it understood itself.[26]

Medicine is a *technē*. Every *technē* implies doing, and, in doing, one is bound just as much by the potentialities of the object as by those of the *technē* itself. Success can be achieved only within the limits of the given possibilities, and in principle one should only seek success within these limits (CMG I₁ 14,7).

This idea of the limits of medicine, however, also be expressed in the following way: the medical *technē* is linked to three conditions: the disease, the patient, the physician. The physician is the servant of the *technē*. The patient, together with the physician, must fight the disease (Khlw. I 190,3 ff.).

Or one can say: men are mortal, and it is impossible to cure them all (Khlw. I 78,10).

Implicit in the realization of the limits of medicine is the consequence that the physician cannot be made responsible for everything that happens. But even if it is conceded that medicine, being a human activity, is restricted by certain limits, the existence of *tychē* (chance) appears to forbid attributing success to any action of the *technē*. If *tychē* exists at all, everything may be *tychē*.

The answer is: *tychē* does exist. But *atychia* (ill-luck) usually accompanies bad treatment; *eutychia* (good luck) usually goes with good treatment. And in spite of the fact that people claim that *tychē* and not *technē* saves men, they entrust themselves to the *technē* and not to *tychē*. Consequently, it can be asserted that *technē* exists (CMG I₁ 11,10 ff.).

Or one says: chance exists, but medicine is independent of it. For the physician can treat correctly if chance is on his side, but he can do the same if it is against him, because knowledge, unlike chance, can be mastered and is always accessible. And all that counts is correct action.

Medical action, then, is independent of chance. Nor does it leave room for chance. Medicaments cure without *tychē*. For if, in truth,

[26] I have assembled only those passages which seem to me most essential in this connection. [In the original German I translate the Greek terms in the ensuing discussions of individual concepts only occasionally, since, in translation, these discussions appear affected and merely captious and therefore pointless, while they elucidate the terms used if one has their Greek counterparts before one. Here, however, I have made an attempt to translate the words in question and have transliterated such well-known terms as *tychē* and *technē*. *Technē*, I am well aware, is usually translated as "art"; but this rendering easily conveys the idea that the art of the ancient physician is like the art of the modern physician, while in reality, the ancient art is a craft, just like the "art" of the ancient painter and sculptor.—Author].

medicaments had to be administered with the help of *tychē* in order to be of use, non-drugs would be equally helpful if only they were given with the help of *tychē*. But this no one will admit. Medicine, then, does not need chance.

Nevertheless, those people are in error who would exclude chance entirely from medicine, or from any other field, on the grounds that it has nothing to do with expertise. For it is only with reference to those who know—the experts—that one can talk of having *tychē* or not having *tychē*, because having *tychē* is equivalent to doing the right thing, and not having *tychē* is equivalent to not doing the right thing out of ignorance. (The last three discussions, *On places in man*, ch. 46 VI 342–44 L.).

Or, one can say that there are certain cases in which the physician and medicine are dependent on chance, good and bad. These cases can be defined and, when they are defined, the physician forfeits the right to ascribe certain successes to his own prowess; but others also forfeit the right, on the basis of chance, to deny the reality of the *technē* (*On diseases I*, ch. 8 VI 154 L.).

Chance, then, does not do away with the reality and existence of medicine. But the object of medicine is man, and in man certain processes are carried out automatically, further limiting the medical possibilities.

Through the *automaton* (spontaneously), favorable and unfavorable phenomena arise in every disease. They are nevertheless predictable (*On diseases I*, ch. 7 VI 152–54 L.).

Through the *automaton*, there arise not only individual changes for the better or for the worse, but also the favorable or unfavorable outcome of the disease may be determined by it. Indeed, it may effect a favorable outcome which could not have been achieved by human means, or an unfavorable outcome which human means could not have prevented (*Prorrhetikon II* ch. 8 IX 26; end of ch. 9 28 L.).

Every process arising from the *automaton* is an event of unknown cause. Something whose cause men do not know they call *theion* (divine) (VI 352 L.; CMG I₁ 74,12 ff.). Therefore, instead of saying that the physician should have knowledge, and foreknowledge, of the *automaton*, as one reads in *On diseases I* (cf. above), we can say he must have foreknowledge of the *theion* in diseases (Khlw. I 79,1).[27]

[27] When the concept of the divine is interpreted in this way, its use at the beginning of the *Prognostikon* is understandable (Khlw. I 79,1), for throughout, the book

And instead of saying these people will get well through the *automaton*, and human help can accomplish nothing, one can say that medicine knows what it owes to the gods; it honors them in sickness and suffering. Physicians yield to the gods, for the power of medicine is not absolute (οὐ γὰρ ἔνι περιττὸν ἐν αὐτέηι τὸ δυναστεῦον). Physicians attempt much and accomplish much, but many things cure themselves (CMG I₁ 27,13 ff.).

Some people say that even if medicine has to acknowledge the *automaton*, it does not itself belong to the realm of the *automaton*. For everything that comes into existence comes into existence through a cause (*dia ti*), and if there is a cause, the *automaton* disappears. Medicine belongs to the realm of things caused and therefore not to the realm of the *automaton* (CMG I₁ 13,1 ff.).[28]

Thus are the limits of medicine defined. What law governs its behavior within these limits?

Medical activity is action on the basis of knowledge. But medical knowledge cannot be acquired quickly because, in medicine, there can be no fixed dogma (*On places in man*, ch. 41 VI 330 L.). For medicine is not like the art of writing (*graphikē technē*). A man who knows his letters can write everything, and all who know the letters write in the same way, now and always. In medicine, anything can mean anything. Pains come from the most diverse and contradictory causes (ch. 42). Likewise, anything may constitute a medication if only it changes the existing condition (ch. 45).

But it is also impossible for medicine to have a fixed dogma because the people to be treated are all different. There is no "man" as such. All the general pronouncements concerning man, such as the philosophers make, correspond in their lack of individualization rather to principles of the art of writing than to principles of medicine (*On ancient medicine*, CMG I₁ 51,13).[29] Medicine, and medicine alone, comprehends

---

speaks of diseases that supervene (i.e., which come "spontaneously") and cause favorable or unfavorable changes (the same thought as in *On diseases I; On diseases I* also documents the possibility of foreseeing such phenomena). Wilamowitz, *Hermes*, 64, 1929, p. 482, gives a different interpretation.

[28] In the same way, the divine character of diseases is disproved in both *On airs, waters, places* (74,12 ff.) and *On the sacred disease* (VI 352 L.), by establishing the cause. Obviously these are merely two ways of expressing the same thing.

[29] ἧσσον νομίζω τῆι ἰητρικῆι τέχνηι προσήκειν ἢ τῆι γραφικῆι. That the comparison refers to the art of writing and its unindividualized rigidity, better suited to philosophical dogmas than to medicine, follows from the passage just cited, VI 330 L.

man's individual nature in its relations to all things—which is admittedly no simple matter.

Because of this individuality of each case, it is not possible, or seldom possible, to hit upon precisely the right thing (*to akribes*). Bodily sensations are the sole measure of medicine (CMG I₁ 41,22).

But for this reason it is also impossible to predict what will happen, although within certain limits there is *anankē* (necessity) (*On diseases I* ch. 3 VI 142–46 L.).

Prediction is also impossible because one treatment differs from another (Khlw. II 97,20; 223,2 ff.).

In a positive sense, this individualization of medicine—through the variations among the physicians who treat and among the patients who are treated—means that the physician must know when the right moment (*kairos*) has come to act (e.g., *On places in man*, ch. 44 VI 338 L.).

Beside the difficulty of learning and practicing medicine, there is the difficulty of teaching it. One pronounces a certain name, but this name does not correspond exactly to the phenomenon it designates (Khlw. II 125,12).[30] Thus it is difficult and again a matter of art to interpret correctly what is written, if indeed the theory is written down or can be put in writing at all (Khlw. II 151,2).

Finally, medical teaching is subject to the difficulty which besets all doctrine, that it is indeed possible to say what should be done in a particular case when one is confronted with it, but that one cannot give general advice about what should be done without seeing the particular case (end of *On regimen*, VI 470 L.).

One can say how medical instruction should begin (VI 278 L.), but one cannot say how treatment should begin (VI 156 L.).

Medicine already exists and does not have to be discovered (CMG I₁ 37,1; VI 342 L.). What remains is only the discovery of new ways and means along the old path. No new theories are required about the origin of diseases.

The old ways are clung to not only as regards new theories but in relation also to new ways of treatment. The physician, like all crafts-

---

The use of *graphikē* in this sense is usual in comparisons. Cf. Isocrates κατὰ τῶν σοφιστῶν XIII § 10.

[30] In the context in which they occur, these words refer to surgery, and it is certainly most difficult to represent surgery in a book, but I apply the passage to every kind of medical representation because the doctrine of *kairos* which it enunciates is important in the whole of medicine.

men, is conservative, but the public runs after the outlandish, the uncustomary (e.g., Khlw. II 46,17 ff.).

Thus does Hippocratic medicine see itself. Its own words testify to the fact that ancient and modern medicine are far removed from one another. And the difference is one not only of detail, but of fundamental outlook.

REVIEW*

M. Pohlenz, *Hippokrates und die Begründung der wissenschaftlichen Medizin.*

Berlin, de Gruyter, 1938, pp. 120.

This book is a new vindication of the doctrine of Hippocrates and his work in opposition to recent and earlier skepticism. The system of the founder of scientific medicine is reconstructed from the two Pre-Alexandrian testimonies still available (pp. 63–79) and then identified with theories of a few of the so-called Hippocratic writings (pp. 79–80), especially with those of *Airs Waters Places* and *Sacred Disease;* the latter treatises are analyzed at great length in the first part of Pohlenz' book (pp. 3–62). Finally Hippocrates' importance for later generations and his influence on them are evaluated (pp. 81–96). An appendix containing the footnotes and a short survey of recent literature (pp. 97–120) complete the work.[1]

Pohlenz' main problem is the determination of Hippocrates' system; all the other inquiries made are either supplementary to this or based on its solution. The question as to how the testimonies of Plato (*Phaedrus* 270 C) and of Aristotle's pupil Meno (V, 35 ff.)[2] are to be interpreted, therefore, must be the chief topic of this review also. Like Pohlenz, I shall deal first with the later testimony of Meno, who relates the Hippocratic explanation of diseases, and then consider that of Plato, the earlier witness, who describes the Hippocratic method only (cf. Pohlenz, p. 75).

Pohlenz claims that the account given in the Meno-Papyrus has never been analyzed before as it should have been; for the original words of Meno have not been clearly distinguished from later additions on the part of the doxographer who made the excerpts from Meno's history of medicine (p. 65). The text, as it stands, so Pohlenz says himself, unmistakably attributes to Hippocrates an explanation of diseases

---

* *American Journal of Philology*, 1940, vol. 61, pp. 221–29.
[1] In the meantime Pohlenz has given a summary of his views in *Die Antike*, XV (1939), pp. 1 ff.
[2] *Anonymi Londinensis ex Aristotelis Iatricis Menoniis et aliis Medicis Eclogae,* ed. H. Diels, *Supplementum Aristotelicum*, III, 1 (1893).

by the φῦσαι ἐκ τῶν περιττωμάτων, "Gase, die sich aus den Perittomata entwickeln" (p. 66). Yet, according to Meno, Pohlenz maintains, Hippocrates spoke of φῦσαι alone (p. 67) and explained diseases through the air taken into the body with nutrition (p. 68). The concept of the air excreted from the remnants of food is an interpolation of the doxographer (p. 67) which must be eliminated so as to make the text intelligible and consistent (p. 68).

It seems strange that Pohlenz should charge the doxographer with having altered Meno's words. For the report in question, at the beginning (V, 36–37) and at the end (VI, 42), is expressly characterized as the opinion of Aristotle, i.e., of Meno. The doxographer disagrees with this opinion, so much so that he adds his own views concerning Hippocrates' doctrine, which he outlines in accordance with some of the so-called Hippocratic writings (VI, 43 ff.). Why, then, should he have changed Meno's account? And if he did, why has he interpolated a concept which he himself later on does not ascribe to Hippocrates? Or has the later description of the Hippocratic theory, so utterly at variance with the previous one, been added by somebody else? Pohlenz, who does not enter into these questions at all, seems to believe that not only the doxographer but also a third person may have participated in the preparation of the excerpts as they are preserved (p. 65).

However these difficulties may be accounted for, Pohlenz thinks that he can prove the probability of the assumed alteration by two facts: the doxographer, he says, has classified all the theories with which the Hippocratic doctrine is grouped under a term originally foreign to them, namely that of περιττώματα (p. 65); besides, he has introduced into the summary of the Platonic theories a concept which is not to be found in the Platonic text (p. 66). I am not prepared to decide whether Hippocrates himself could use the word περιττώματα. That, in the sense of remnants of food, it occurs for the first time in Diocles' fragments does not prove that it was not used before (contrary to Pohlenz, pp. 65–66); the material preserved from earlier writings is too scanty to allow such a conclusion.[3] It is, however, the less necessary to discuss this question since Pohlenz himself in his argumentation puts all em-

---

[3] I note that Ilberg, in his copy of Diels' edition of the Meno-Papyrus, now in the Institute of the History of Medicine at the Johns Hopkins University, refers (Index s. v. περισσώματα) to E. Howald, *Hermes*, LIV (1919), pp. 187 ff. and G. Méautis, *Philologische Wochenschrift*, XLV (1925), pp. 184 ff.; both authors endeavor to prove the early occurrence of κάθαρσις and περιττώματα.

phasis on the alleged misrepresentation of Plato's views: "... wie unbekümmert ... der Doxograph nicht nur formal umstilisiert, sondern auch sachlich umgestaltet, können wir in einem Fall (*scil.* in the Plato-report) noch mit Händen greifen," he says (p. 66).[4]

I shall not insist that the doxographer, if he is not correct in his description of the Platonic doctrine, need not necessarily be incorrect in his representation of the Hippocratic dogma. I rather ask whether he really misrepresents Plato's theory. Pohlenz claims that the doxographer ascribes to Plato, as he does to Hippocrates, an explanation of diseases by the φῦσαι ἐκ τῶν περιττωμάτων (XVII, 46–47); this term, however, does not occur in the *Timaeus* on which the résumé is obviously based; the doxographer, then, has falsified his source (cf. Pohlenz, p. 66). But the text of the Plato-report reads thus (XVII, 44–47):

$$\pi\alpha\rho\grave{\alpha}\ [\delta\grave{\epsilon}]$$
$$\tau\grave{\alpha}\ \pi\epsilon\rho\iota\tau\tau\acute{\omega}\mu\alpha\tau\alpha\ \sigma\upsilon\nu\acute{\iota}\sigma\tau\alpha[\nu\tau\alpha\iota\ \tau\rho\iota\chi\tilde{\omega}\varsigma]$$
$$\alpha\grave{\iota}\ \nu\acute{o}\sigma\upsilon\iota,\ \mathring{\eta}\ \pi[\alpha]\rho[\grave{\alpha}\ \tau\grave{\alpha}\varsigma]\ \phi\acute{\upsilon}\sigma\alpha\varsigma\ [\tau\grave{\alpha}\varsigma\ \grave{\epsilon}\kappa\ \tau(\tilde{\omega}\nu)]\ \tau\epsilon\text{-}$$
$$\rho\iota\tau\tau\omega\mu[\acute{\alpha}\tau(\omega\nu)\ \mathring{\eta}\ \pi\alpha\rho\grave{\alpha}]\ \chi\omega\lambda\grave{\eta}\nu\ \mathring{\eta}\ \phi\lambda\acute{\epsilon}\gamma\mu\alpha\ \cdot$$

It is then, first of all, not the doxographer who, as Pohlenz says, speaks of air excreted from the περιττώματα. The concept of the φῦσαι ἐκ τῶν περιττωμάτων is a conjecture of the editor of the papyrus. If the words, as restored, do not correspond to the Platonic text, the editor has erred, not the doxographer.[5]

But one may object: even if φῦσαι ἐκ τῶν περιττωμάτων is a conjecture, the words φῦσαι and περιττώματα (cf. also XVII, 14) are preserved in the papyrus, and yet neither of them is to be found in the *Timaeus* (cf. Pohlenz, p. 66). Does this difference not suffice to prove a misunderstanding of Plato's views and, consequently, to cast suspicion upon the correctness of the representation of Hippocrates' views? To be sure, Meno speaks of φῦσαι, whereas Plato speaks of πνεῦμα (*Timaeus* 84 D).

---

[4] K. Deichgräber (*Abhandlungen der Preussischen Akademie der Wissenschaften*, Phil.-Hist. Klasse [1933], Nr. 3, p. 153) was the first to assume this inaccuracy of the report on Plato. Diels (*Hermes*, XXVIII [1893], p. 425), however, had already asserted the methodological value of the Plato-account, because it affords a check on Meno's reliability. For other minor divergencies cf. A. Rivaud, *Platon, Œuvres Complètes*, X (1925), p. 115, n. 4. Cf. note 13 *infra*.

[5] It is misleading, it seems to me, for Pohlenz in quoting the papyrus (p. 66, n. 2) not to indicate the lacunae and emendations. Especially if an argument is based on such a text, the reader is entitled to be informed about what is preserved in the original and what is modern conjecture.

But it is the air that has entered the human body with which Plato is concerned, and this air is commonly called φῦσα or φῦσαι by physicians.[6] Plato himself was aware that the term which he uses was antiquated and that, already in his time, φῦσα was the more common medical expression (cf. *Republic* 405 D).[7] The change in terminology made by the doxographer is, then, certainly no falsification of Plato's opinion. Moreover, it is true that Plato does not use the expression περιττώματα. Yet the second cause of illness which he mentions is phlegm, the third bile (Meno, XVII, 47; *Timaeus* 85 A ff.). These qualities, in Aristotelian language, are named περιττώματα.[8] The third class of diseases (*Timaeus* 84 C) which Meno is paraphrasing comprises then two species which are correctly referred to by the term which Meno introduces.

But what about the φῦσαι ἐκ τῶν περιττωμάτων, if this is the correct restoration of the lacuna? Pohlenz is right in pointing out that in *Timaeus* 84 D Plato is discussing the air which the human being breathes (p. 66). Yet, in *Timaeus* 84 E, a passage which, strangely enough, is not quoted by Diels, who in his notes refers only to *Timaeus* 84 C–D, the first way in which illness arises is characterized thus: πολλάκις δ' ἐν τῷ σώματι διακριθείσης σαρκὸς πνεῦμα ἐγγενόμενον καὶ ἀδυνατοῦν ἔξω πορευθῆναι . . . . This Martin takes to mean: "Souvent aussi, la chair se trouvant raréfiée dans quelque partie du corps, il s'y engendre de l'air, qui, n'en pouvant sortir . . ."[9] Such a sense, however, could well be epitomized by φῦσαι ἐκ τῶν περιττωμάτων. For disintegrated flesh is the material from which, according to Plato, bile, phlegm, etc. are produced.[10] Moreover, Meno, in consequence of the importance of the περιττώματα in all three cases,

[6] Cf. *Breaths*, ch. 3 (*Hippokrates*, ed. J. L. Heiberg, *Corpus Medicorum Graecorum*, I, 1 [1927], pp. 92, 20; 95, 15, etc.); cf. Pohlenz, p. 67, n. 2, and p. 67 where he himself understands φῦσα as air breathed in by the human being.

[7] I was reminded of this passage by H. Cherniss.

[8] Cf. Aristotle, *Historia Animalium* 511 b 9; Pohlenz (p. 66, n. 2) also refers to this passage, yet, in his interpretation of the Plato passage, takes the word to mean remnants of food, a meaning which it cannot have either here (XVII, 45) or before (XVII, 14), although in the Hippocrates-account it is used in the limited sense of remnants of food (cf. Aristotle, *De Generatione Animalium* 724 b 26; Pohlenz, p. 65, n. 3).

[9] Th. H. Martin, *Études sur le Timée de Platon*, I (1841), p. 225. Already Marsilius Ficinus translates: Saepe etiam intra corpus discreta et rarefacta carne innascitur spiritus: qui cum foras egredi nequeat . . . (quoted from Plato, ed. I. Bekker, III, 2 [1817], p. 126). With Martin's translation agree R. D. Archer-Hind, *The Timaeus of Plato* (1888), and F. M. Cornford, *Plato's Cosmology* (1937).

[10] Cf. *Timaeus* 82 C, and A. E. Taylor, *A Commentary on Plato's Timaeus* (1928), p. 591.

would with some justification have subordinated them to the general heading νόσοι παρὰ τὰ περιττώματα (XVII, 45).

Of course, one cannot decide whether Meno understood the Plato passage as do Martin and others. It is also possible to translate the words in question differently: "And often, when the flesh is disintegrated, air which is enclosed in the body and is unable to pass out. . . ."[11] Such an interpretation is suggested as the right one by the fact that in 84 D, too, it is not air alone which, according to Plato, brings about illness; it is air combined with some other substance, with ῥεύματα which are produced from phlegm (cf. *Timaeus* 85 B, and for the expression ῥεύματα again *Republic* 405 D). If the lungs are filled with these rheums, the usual passage of the air is hindered, and it is for that reason that diseases are caused. If in 84 E Plato is also referring to the air coming from outside, the discussion of air as cause of diseases would be uniform. In both cases, as distinguished by Plato, air would be harmful only together with some other substance, with rheums or with disintegrated flesh in Platonic terms, with phlegm or bile, or in Aristotelian categories with περιττώματα. Meno, then, may have spoken of φῦσαι μετὰ περιττωμάτων[12] and he would have been equally justified in calling the third class of diseases νόσοι παρὰ τὰ περιττώματα. The advantage of such an emendation is that in his summary, then, he does not omit the explanation of diseases brought about by air from outside (84 D), although one must not forget that his résumé as a whole is not exhaustive and that he leaves out other points also.

At any rate, whatever restoration is adopted, the trustworthiness of the Hippocrates report cannot be disproved on the evidence adduced by Pohlenz. Many other instances, moreover, confirm the correctness of the data given in the papyrus (cf. Deichgräber, *op. cit.*. p. 159). It is

[11] Plato, *Timaeus etc., with an English translation* by R. G. Bury (The Loeb Classical Library), p. 229; cf. Taylor (*op. cit.*, p. 601) who interprets: ". . . whenever an abnormal 'division' or cavity is formed within the flesh, wind collects to fill it, and is unable to find a proper outlet." Cf. also A. Rivaud, *op. cit.*, p. 217: "Souvent aussi, la chair se disjoint à l'intérieur du corps; de l'air s'y enferme et, ne pouvant pas en sortir. . . ."

[12] Cf. *Timaeus* 83 E μετὰ πνεύματος αἷμα; 83 B ξανθὸν χρῶμα μετὰ τῆς πικρότητος. According to the above interpretation I propose to read in the papyrus:

παρὰ [δὲ]
τὰ περιττώματα συνίστα[νται τριχῶς]
αἱ νόσοι, ἢ π[α]ρ[ὰ τὰς] φύσας [τὰς μετὰ] τε-
ριττωμ[άτ(ων) ἢ μαρὰ] χολὴν ἢ φλέγμα·

true that sometimes the account is enlarged by the addition of similes[13] and that the language is colored by later terminology, but the basic facts, it seems, are authentic. What Meno relates about Hippocrates, therefore, has to be accepted as it stands; it cannot be reinterpreted as Pohlenz proposes to do. Hippocrates, according to Meno at least, has explained diseases by the air excreted from the remnants of food, and well he may; there is no reason either to assume that Meno was mistaken in his description of the Hippocratic dogma.[14] For similar theories are known from other great physicians of Hippocrates' time; the importance of food for the development of diseases, the influence of digestion is stressed over and over again in the *Corpus Hippocraticum*. The doctrine that it is air, not a liquid, which is excreted from the remnants of food (cf. e.g., Meno, V, 12 ff.) would be the specifically Hippocratic modification of a more common dogma.

As I cannot agree, then, with Pohlenz' interpretation of the Meno-Papyrus, I cannot follow him in his interpretation of the *Phaedrus* either. This second and most important testimony on Hippocrates Pohlenz takes to mean that, according to Plato, Hippocrates found it impossible to understand the nature of the body without the nature of the cosmos (ἄνευ τῆς τοῦ ὅλου φύσεως 270 C), and, consequently, he ascribes to Hippocrates a thorough observation of the seasons, of the air, etc. (p. 78; cf. pp. 4–5). That in Plato as well as in other writers τὸ ὅλον may mean "cosmos" is certain; Pohlenz (p. 75, n. 1) gives additional proof for such a sense. It is equally certain, however, that the word, especially in the Platonic dialogues, signifies the whole, the logical or organic unity, a usage for which Pohlenz does not cite any parallel. The problem is not whether τὸ ὅλον can be understood only in the one way or in the other, it is rather which of the two meanings of the word is implied in the passage in question.[15]

[13] For instance in the Plato report (XVI, 24 ff.); cf. Diels, *Hermes, loc. cit.*, and note 4 *supra*. That the simile given in the Hippocrates passage can be original (Pohlenz, p. 67) I do not deny (cf. *R.-E.*, Supplement VI [1936], 1323). The probability, however, is not increased by the observation that similes are added in other places.

[14] This was, for instance, the belief of Diels, *loc. cit.*, pp. 424–434; cf. the introduction to the edition of Meno, p. xvi. That Meno had an adequate knowledge of ancient medicine seems now generally assumed. That his account of Hippocratic views is consistent (contrary to Pohlenz, p. 68) has been shown *R.-E., loc. cit.*

[15] Already in antiquity the opinion of the interpreters was apparently divided; Galen (*Corpus Medicorum Graecorum*, V, 9, 1 [1914], p. 55, 16; cf. p. 53, 26) understands τὸ ὅλον as cosmos; Hermias (*In Platonis Phaedrum Scholia*, ed. P. Couvreur [1901], p. 245, 5) takes it to mean the whole body (cf. *R.-E., loc. cit.*, 1319). Of mod-

Socrates claims that the procedure of medicine and that of rhetoric are identical; in both arts it is necessary to give a diaeresis of the object concerned (διελέσθαι φύσιν 270 B).[16] He, then, asks whether it is possible to understand the nature of the soul, the object of rhetoric, without the nature of the whole (270 C). Phaedrus answers with a reference to Hippocrates, who holds it impossible to acquire even medical knowledge without such a method (ἄνευ τῆς μεθόδου ταύτης ibid.). Whereupon Socrates, who is not satisfied with Hippocrates' authority before inquiring into the validity of the argument, tries to explain what kind of investigation Hippocrates and right reason demand concerning nature (περὶ φύσεως ibid.). They demand, he says, for the understanding of every nature (περὶ ὁτουοῦν φύσεως 270 D) two things: first an investigation as to whether the object is simple or multiform, and then a division of the object into its parts together with a determination of the relation of these parts to each other and to the factors influencing them (ibid.). In other words, they demand definition and diaeresis; that these two processes are inseparable has been stressed even before (e.g., 265 D–226 B); each diaeresis involves a conception of the whole which is to be divided into its parts. The nature of the whole, then, which, as Socrates says, is presupposed by every right understanding, must be the comprehension of the particulars into one idea;[17] the method which Hippocrates follows

---

ern interpreters L. Robin (*Platon, Œuvres Complètes* [Collection Budé], IV, 3 [1933]) sides with Galen; cf. also Wilamowitz, *Platon* (1929),[3] p. 462, and W. H. S. Jones, *Hippocrates with an English Translation* (The Loeb Classical Library), I, p. xxxiii. Hermias' interpretation is upheld by B. Jowett, *The Dialogues of Plato translated into English*, I[3] (1892), p. 479, but already proposed as the only satisfactory solution by W. H. Thompson, *The Phaedrus of Plato* (1868), p. 124. Cf. L. Edelstein, Περὶ ἀέρων *und die Sammlung der Hippokratischen Schriften*, Problemata, IV (1931), pp. 129–135; G. M. A. Grube, *Plato's Thought* (1935), p. 213, n. 1. P. Shorey (*What Plato said* [1933], p. 205) refers to *Lysis* 214 B and *Charmides* 156 B ff.; he seems to understand τὸ ὅλον as cosmos and as the whole of the body; so does W. Nestle, *Hermes*, LXXIII (1938), p. 18.

[16] I doubt that *Laws* 946 B κλήρῳ διελόντας τὸν νικῶντα, the passage to which Pohlenz refers (p. 75, n. 1) has the same meaning as διελέσθαι in the *Phaedrus*. At any rate, the division of the soul has its analogy in medicine as Pohlenz himself, in spite of his qualifying interpretation of διελέσθαι in the notes (p. 75, n. 1), admits in his text (p. 76). For the identity of the dialectical procedure of the *Phaedrus* with that of the late dialogues, the *Sophist* and the *Politicus* cf. J. Stenzel, *Studien zur Entwicklung der platonischen Dialektik von Sokrates zu Aristoteles* (1907), p. 62.

[17] For this use of τὸ ὅλον cf. e.g., Stenzel, *op. cit.*, p. 66 and R.-E., *loc. cit.*, 1318–1320. *Symposium* 205 B and D give a particularly good example of this sense of τὸ ὅλον and εἴδη (the whole and the parts of a concept) even in a context which is not strictly dialectical.

also in medicine must be the general definition of its object, the human body.

Socrates discusses the identity of the methods used in rhetoric and medicine so as to explain what he said before and what Phaedrus did not understand. Πᾶσαι ὅσαι μεγάλαι τῶν τεχνῶν προσδέονται ἀδολεσχίας καὶ μετεωρολογίας φύσεως πέρι· τὸ γὰρ ὑψηλόνουν τοῦτο καὶ πάντῃ τελεσιουργὸν ἔοικεν ἐντεῦθέν ποθεν εἰσιέναι (269 E–270 A), Socrates claimed and then exemplified his statement by the relation of Pericles to Anaxagoras. Does Socrates, by speaking of μετεωρολογία φύσεως πέρι, refer to "Meteorologie" or "Himmelsspekulation," that is astronomy and mathematics, and is the word chosen by Plato in order to indicate his agreement with Hippocrates, who by the same term expressed the belief that astronomy is necessary for medicine (Pohlenz, p. 78)? In the *Republic* (529 A) Glaucon praises the study of astronomy because "it compels the soul to look upward (εἰς τὰ ἄνω ὁρᾶν) and leads it away from the things here to those higher things," but Socrates answers (529 A–530 C): "You seem to me in your thought to put a most liberal interpretation on the study of higher things (τὴν περὶ τὰ ἄνω μάθησιν); for apparently, if anyone with back-thrown head should learn something by staring at decorations on a ceiling, you would regard him as contemplating them with the higher reason (νοήσει) and not with the eyes. Perhaps you are right, and I am a simpleton. For I, for my part, am unable to suppose that any other study turns the soul's gaze upward (ἄνω ποιοῦν ψυχὴν βλέπειν) than that which deals with being and the invisible . . . It is by means of problems, then, . . . as in the study of geometry, that we will pursue astronomy, too, and we will let be the things in the heavens, if we are to have a part in the true science of astronomy and so convert to right use from uselessness that natural indwelling intelligence of the soul."[18] It is, then, certainly not observation of the heavens, not even the usual form of astronomy which Socrates acknowledges as propaedeutics to higher knowledge. What he alludes to in demanding for all great arts ἀδολεσχία καὶ μετεωρολογία φύσεως πέρι can only be a study detached from the visible world, "discussion and high speculation about

---

[18] Plato, *The Republic with an English Translation* by P. Shorey (The Loeb Classical Library), II, pp. 181–183; 187–189. For a more detailed interpretation of the passage cf. E. Hoffman, *Vorträge der Bibliothek Warburg* (1923–24), pp. 34 ff., and Shorey in the notes to his edition.

the truth of nature,"[19] of the nature of the object (cf. περὶ φύσεως 270 C; φύσις 270 B–D), as he says here, of generalization and diaeresis, as he states later on (270 B ff.). One can hardly conclude from this passage that Plato agreed with Hippocrates, who held it necessary that the physician know the influence of the seasons on the development of diseases. The words, understood in their Platonic sense, only confirm that Hippocrates recommended definition and division of the object of medicine, of the human body.

Finally, Plato always regards it as the task of the good craftsman to apprehend the whole of his object, and in particular, as that of the physician, to study the whole of the body and not only its parts. So he says in the *Charmides* (156 C) as well as in the *Laws* (902 D–E; 903 C). Should the great Hippocrates, whom Plato admires, not fulfill the conditions set up by Plato for good craftsmanship? Should he, on the contrary, be inclined to speculations or studies of which Plato himself does not approve? Neither the procedure of diaeresis nor the terminology used in it are inventions of Plato; they are known to earlier generations. There are no valid historical objections, then, to the assumption that Hippocrates actually demanded definition and division; because he did so, he need not be a Platonist, nor a believer in the Platonic idea (contrary to Pohlenz, p. 75, n. 1). On the other hand, Diocles, the follower of Hippocrates, maintained that it is the whole nature of the body which is responsible for diseases. Moreover the method of diaeresis, Galen says, was an integral part of later medical theories which depended on Hippocrates' system.[20]

To be sure, if the testimonies of Meno and Plato are interpreted as I think they have to be, Hippocrates is not the founder of the πνεῦμα theory (cf. Pohlenz, pp. 73 ff.; 92 ff.) but of scientific medicine in the Platonic sense of the word science (cf. *Philebus* 16 C). Moreover, there is no book among the so-called Hippocratic writings which can be

---

[19] I am using Jowett's translation (*loc. cit.*, p. 478). That μετεωρολογία may have such a meaning is shown by Edelstein, *loc. cit.* The Platonic doctrine of the ἄνω and κάτω is outlined by G. Teichmüller, *Studien zur Geschichte der Begriffe* (1874), p. 391.

[20] Concerning the diaeresis before Plato cf. A. E. Taylor, *Varia Socratica* (1911), pp. 212–246; E. Hoffman, *Anhang zu Zeller, Philosophie der Griechen*, II, 1 (1922), p. 1073. For Diocles (ἡ ὅλη φύσις) cf. Fragment 112 (p. 163, line 2 Wellmann and W. Jaeger, *Diokles von Karystos* [1938], p. 29). The Hippocratic diaeresis was taken over by Mnesitheus and Diocles, cf. Galen XI, p. 3 (Kühn) = Mnesitheus, Fragment 3 (H. Hohenstein, *Der Arzt Mnesitheos aus Athen*, Diss. Berlin [1935]).

ascribed to Hippocrates himself. That even from Pohlenz' point of view this could not be done, I believe, is certain.[21] But I do not discuss the question, since I think that the interpretation on which Pohlenz relies in his attempt to establish the authenticity of certain books is not convincing. It is true that after a hundred years of research it is still impossible to claim that the genuine works of Hippocrates have been ascertained.[22] But Hippocrates' method, his doctrine are known, though his books are lost. The writings of many great scientists and philosophers have been destroyed, only testimonies concerning their achievements are left. To acknowledge that is no verdict, no negativism; it is a statement of fact.

[21] Cf. L. Edelstein, "The Genuine Works of Hippocrates," *Bulletin of the History of Medicine*, VII (1939), pp. 236 ff. [133* ff.].
[22] Cf. W. Jaeger, *op. cit.*, p. vi.

REVIEW*

WILLIAM F. PETERSEN, *Hippocratic Wisdom. A Modern Appreciation of Ancient Scientific Achievement.*

Springfield, Illinois: Charles C Thomas, 1946, xix + 263 pp.

This book presents a cross section of the whole content of the so-called works of Hippocrates. In the first part (pp. 1–151), excerpts from the philosophical, physiological, therapeutic and surgical writings are conveniently grouped in twelve chapters dealing with the main aspects of Hippocratic medicine; an intermediary text, or commentary, provides an evaluation of the passages selected, and points to the relation of ancient and modern medical thought. In a short résumé, a general appreciation of the Greek merit is added (pp. 152–162; cf. also Introduction, pp. ix–xix). The second part, the "Appendix," supplies the references and the notes which discuss in greater detail the scientific problems at issue (pp. 165–242). Finally, there follows a glossary, an index of illustrations and of contents (pp. 243–263). To my knowledge, this collection of "Hippocratic Wisdom" is the most comprehensive survey of the doctrines proposed in the *Corpus Hippocraticum* that is available in English.

With such a short characterization of the book under review I should perhaps consider my task done. For, as Dr. Petersen says in his introduction, "this is not a book for Greek scholars—it is written for young physicians and for medical students" (p. xi). And later on he adds: "The interpretation is thus physiological and medical, not philological and historical" (p. 165). Being but a philologist and an historian I am not in a position to praise or criticize a physiological and medical analysis. Yet, Dr. Petersen has interpreted translations selected and in part corrected by him; he has defined the meaning of terms used by Greek writers; he has outlined a picture of Greek medicine as he supposes it to have been. Thus, although preoccupied with scientific questions, he has also been concerned with the solution of linguistic and historical problems. To this extent at least, I think, it is not improper for the philologist and historian to judge Dr. Petersen's results and to

* *Bulletin of the History of Medicine*, 1946, Vol. 20, pp. 475–82.

this extent I consequently feel allowed to scrutinize his book and to evaluate it.

For the rendering of the texts on which his argument rests, the author has relied on standard translations (p. xiv), that is, he has accepted by preference the translation of Jones; Sticker, Littré and Kuehlewein have been used for comparison (the last apparently in regard to variant readings); Kapferer's notes have also been considered (p. 165). Yet this short summary does not give an adequate impression of the range of the work done by Dr. Petersen. Jones' translation, as well as that of Adams—I wonder why the latter was not consulted, it is quite worthy of being taken into account, and after all it was made by a physician—both these translations include only a small part of the *Corpus Hippocraticum*. Since Dr. Petersen draws material from almost all the Hippocratic writings, his contribution to the Englishing of Hippocrates passages is quite considerable. And if I may express an opinion in the matter, his renderings read well. They are usually phrased in a clear and vivid language; the content is expressed with simplicity and brevity.

As for the correctness of those translations which Dr. Petersen reproduces *verbatim*, I do not intend to offer any criticism. One might, of course, argue about many points. Even Jones' excellent rendering can sometimes be questioned. On p. 67, for instance, I should say with Littré: "She did not eat anything the whole time" instead of "No appetite for any food the whole time"; or on p. 34: ". . . it [Asia] is not oppressed with cold either, yet it is damp and wet by excess of rains and snow" instead of ". . . it is not oppressed with cold, nor yet damp and wet with excessive rains and snow." I mention these two examples only in order to impress upon the reader the fact that throughout Dr. Petersen's book he is faced with translations, that is, with interpretations, that divergence of opinion may exist among the translators even concerning the meaning of passages as simple and factual as the ones referred to, that if he wishes to evaluate the correctness of a translation, he should not fail to differentiate between the various translators— Jones, Kapferer, Littré, Sticker are not on the same level. I wish Dr. Petersen had always indicated not only the Greek source but also the source of his translation; this would have greatly facilitated the critical study of his book. In many cases, I also wish that he had accepted one translator rather than the other. But Dr. Petersen has given those renderings which he has judged best, and in general he has given them with fidelity and accuracy. In checking a fair number of his selections—

I have naturally not compared all of them with the original—I have noted only two major defects. First the omission of whole sentences within a given context has not been marked; there ought to be some indication of a lacuna—for instance, on p. 33 after *those of the other*, or on p. 48 after *at all ages*—for one expects to become acquainted with Hippocrates' thought and for this purpose one should be told whether one is reading his words in their entirety or not. Second, relatively often a few words of the Greek text have dropped out in the translation. Thus on p. 61 one must add after *lung abscesses:* especially those from pleurisy or pneumonia; after *phlyctenae may occur about the body:* the patients repudiate food; after *the very beginning:* from the above mentioned signs which will appear and from the pain in the beginning; after *fortieth day:* and sixtieth day; after *about the twentieth day:* for those whose suffering is easier it will be retarded in proportion.

To turn now to Dr. Petersen's corrections of the standard translations, they consist mainly in the introduction of modern scientific terms. In a few cases, the elimination of the ancient concepts takes place before the very eyes of the reader. Thus Dr. Petersen writes on p. 26: "Male seed (*semen*) passes into the uterus and there commingles with the female seed (*egg*)." Hippocrates' obsolete theory of generation here is parenthetically identified with the modern one. But in the next sentence it is said: "While both semen and egg are necessary . . ." The Greek, of course, again has male and female seed (and even Kapferer, in his translation, has kept the terms of the original and in a footnote has stressed the difference of Hippocrates' views from those of later times). Having once adopted the words semen and egg, Dr. Petersen employs them throughout the next two sentences until the translation must return to the old concepts in order to make the statement meaningful at all, and suddenly one reads: "The same male may produce seed of different potentials . . ., and so, too, may the female. . . ." But it is only rarely that one can follow up the process of change in such a way. In the great majority of the passages, one is confronted with modern terminology pure and simple. One finds: "The growing organism is organized by the warm air. Like goes to like; all material goes to its predestined related tissue from which too it has originated" (p. 29). Or one hears of gastrointestinal activity and of metabolism (p 73). Instances of this kind are very numerous; I need not collect them; everybody will find them for himself.

Now in my opinion, such translations impute to Hippocrates doctrines that doubtless were unknown to him. The impression is given that the Hippocratic physicians were scientists in the modern sense, which they certainly were not. The statement, for instance, in which Hippocrates, according to Dr. Petersen, speaks of organism, organize, predestined tissues, this statement, to the best of my knowledge, actually reads: "The flesh [of the embryo] having been increased through [the influence of] the air is divided into members, and of it like goes to like, the solid to the solid, the loose to the loose, the moist to the moist, and each goes to its proper place according to the kinship [homogeneity] from which it originated." This, to be sure, sounds less modern, but I think it is a more adequate translation of the Greek (and by the way almost identical with Littré's translation). Yet Dr. Petersen would probably counter my assertion with the claim that by expressing the views of Hippocrates in the medical terminology of today he has succeeded in bringing out what the physician Hippocrates meant to say, while my rendering simply shows that I rely on dictionaries and that I do not know medicine. I have advisedly said that Dr. Petersen would probably make this objection, for so much, it seems, was the application of modern terms to Greek medicine a foregone conclusion to him, that he does not even mention or justify his procedure in his introduction, or in any other place of his discussion proper, as far as I am aware. I have gathered his arguments from the introduction to a new translation of Hippocrates which he contemplated undertaking with the late E. Andrews. (Since the programmatic remarks outlined by the latter have been printed by Dr. Petersen [pp. 167 f.], I trust I am not doing an injustice to him by assuming that they have determined his own course.) Here it is said that "in the past Hippocrates was utterly unreadable" and that this was often "due to the fact that the English translator, being hopelessly ignorant of modern medicine, often looked up his words in Greek dictionaries published half a century or more ago, as many of the best were" (p. 168). It is true, I am hopelessly ignorant of modern medicine, and I have consulted a dictionary. Yet I have not used one published in the nineteenth century, but rather Liddell and Scott, *A Greek-English Lexicon*, re-published in 1925 and the following years, an edition for which Dr. E. T. Withington, physician, translator of Hippocrates and historian of medicine, read "the whole of the extant remains of Greek medical literature, and there is scarcely a page in the Lexicon which does not bear traces of his handiwork" (L. & S., p. vii). Dr. Withington certainly was not hopelessly ignorant of modern medicine, and yet I cannot find any of the terms employed by Dr. Petersen in Liddell and Scott. The reason is, I think, that Dr. Withington tried to understand the Greek words, as the Greeks intended them to be taken, regardless of the progress of modern medicine. And thus indeed they must be understood, they must be interpreted in their historical connotations. Otherwise an entirely distorted picture of the past obtains. By introducing modern terminology Dr. Petersen has seriously invalidated the correctness of the translations which he presents, and I cannot agree with him when he expresses the belief that "the use of standard translations" has protected him from the charge of "reading something into the text" (p. xiv).

The unhistoricity which the passages quoted have taken on through Dr. Petersen's corrections, moreover, is heightened by the setting into which he has fitted most of his material. I have no quarrel with those who think that they will get ancient medicine across, as the phrase goes, by dramatizing it. But it is a definitely inappropriate framework that is here chosen. Hippocrates is made to lecture to his students (pp. 87–125); patients are presented (p. 107); the reader is asked to imagine that he has taken a seat "in the white marble amphitheatre that was attached to the surgical dispensary of Hippocrates" (p. 86). The Greek students of the fifth and fourth centuries were not lectured to. There was no marble amphitheatre attached to a surgical dispensary in which the pupils came together. There was no presentation of cases similar to that in modern hospitals. Dr. Petersen, I am sure, would object even to a movie that in representing the history of Henry V would introduce as stage accessories a jeep and an airplane. That Shakespeare gave the Tudor rapier to the quarrelsome gentlemen of the time of Henry V he would at best excuse as poetical license. The anachronistic manner in which he himself proceeds in a scientific book seems the more objectionable to me, since it serves to confirm the impression, already aroused by the text proper, that Greek medicine and modern medicine after all are not so different.

But Dr. Petersen has not only corrected passages and placed them against an imaginary background, he has also arranged the material in a manner of his own. Rarely does one read two or three pages which are taken from the same book. While page 63 is made up of eight quotations from the *Coan Prenotions*, p. 64 consists of excerpts from *Places in the Body*, *Coan Prenotions*, *Epidemics VII*, *Diseases II*, and p. 52—half a page really—is made up of selections from *Humours*, *Ancient Medicine* and *Breaths*. Nevertheless the reader is asked to take all these statements as a unity. In the introduction of E. Andrews to which I referred before I find the admission that "such a method at once lays one open to the charge of indirect misquotation by changes in context. This may be a very serious charge." Yet Andrews adds: "I can only say that we have tried desperately to avoid such pitfalls and have always been acutely conscious of the inherent faults of the method and its possibilities for leading one astray" (p. 168). I consequently presume that Dr. Petersen has acted in the same spirit, although I admit that I am doubtful of the possibility of remedying "the inherent faults of the method." And the fact remains that all these excerpts taken together are supposed to represent the views of Hippocrates, not the "historical" Hippocrates to be sure—for Dr. Petersen is not concerned with the question whether the Hippocratic books are genuine or which are the authentic ones, he grants that they were written by various people, that "they cover a longer time period than that of the life span of one individual" (p. 165). Still, the quotations embody the "Hippocratic thesis"; Dr. Petersen has followed "an apparently original line of thought that binds the whole," and the thesis which he defends "is foreshadowed in *Ancient Medicine;* is basic (but overgrown with weeds) in *Breaths;* carries through in *Sacred Disease* and *Regimen;* and finds its clearest expression in *Airs, Waters, Places*" (p. 169). Even the most ardent "unitarian" of the nineteenth century, or of antiquity for that matter, would have found it difficult to defend the compatibility of these books. To make his assumption convincing Dr. Petersen envisages an Hippocrates who in his youth was imbued with the doctrines of Anaximenes and Anaxagoras, then after long travels came also under the influence of Democritus, and still later adopted in addition certain views of Heraclitus (pp. 172–173). Were such a man known to have lived, I would grudgingly admit his existence. To postulate his reality I should not dare. That supposing he ever did live, he was "the physician who had an understanding of the body and its dysfunctions unsurpassed for twenty-three centuries" (p. 153), I cannot believe.

Thus far I have dealt only with Dr. Petersen's presentation of the material. It is time for me to consider the more interpretative parts of the book under review. Here I notice first of all that, according to Dr. Petersen, Hippocrates "wrote for the many. That the many might understand, he used the current word symbols. He accepted the prejudices of the time" (p. xiv). To say: "Prayer indeed is good, but while calling

126

on the gods a man should himself lend a hand" is common sense in a social milieu where superstition and religion still held sway among the multitude, and the author considers it legitimate "to interpret some statements of the texts in the light of such asides" (p. xv). In other words, Hippocrates did not write down everything he knew; there is a kind of hidden truth in his utterances. Or as the programmatic remarks formulate it: Hippocrates "was a philosopher. He was hence well versed in that peculiarly abrupt telegraphic lingo whose solution has been the cause of untold heartaches until modern Greek scholars guessed the correct answer: that is, that it was intentionally misleading—a sort of secret code by which members of the initiated pass on cosmic thought to others of the favored few" (p. 168). I do not know who the scholars are who are here referred to, or who those are on whose authority Dr. Petersen bases his verdict. Whoever they may be, I dare say they are mistaken. No Greek philosopher or physician of the classical period was intent on hiding the truth which he had found. Nobody hesitated to write about the genesis of the cosmos, or of man, or about the nature of diseases, as he saw fit. The greatest heresies were discussed and defended openly, as the preserved documents attest; even the existence of the gods was openly challenged. If a philosopher or a physician wished to use the current word symbols in a different sense because otherwise they would not conform to the peculiar bent of his thought, he said so. Dr. Petersen himself prints the statement of Hippocrates which is evidence of this fact: "When I speak of 'becoming' or 'perishing,' I am merely using popular expressions; what I really mean is 'mingling' and 'separating'" (p. 131). In some notes of E. Andrews, in which he opposes Jones' translation of two fragments of Heraclitus, I find that he objects to Jones' rendering of *logos* by *Word* because "it's positively Biblical and smacks of a bewhiskered Jehovah, whom the Greeks were spared for five more centuries" (p. 167).[1] To my mind, the

---

[1] Incidentally, the criticism of Jones' translation is quite unwarranted. Although *Word* for *logos* sounds Biblical and although *logos* is also defined "in dictionaries as 'reason,'" *Word* is the meaning here required. Historians of Greek philosophy are agreed in this respect (cf. e.g., J. Burnet, *Early Greek Philosophy*, 1930, p. 133, n. 1). Nor are the new renderings of the two fragments that are proposed an improvement. As for the first, *all things* for *panta* is a perfect translation, and it is not true that *panta* is "the ordinary Greek word for Nature" (again Jones agrees with Burnet, *op. cit.*, p. 132). The word *essential* which Andrews has is not indicated in the text at all. Jones' translation seems in every respect superior to that of Andrews and the correctness of the latter does not become more convincing by such statements as: "Now how could it have meant anything but this? After all a man whom Aristotle

assumption of a hidden meaning of the Hippocratic writings, or of any philosophical statements of the fifth and fourth centuries, is much more "Biblical," and smacks of those who believed to serve the cause of their Master by speaking of a double truth hidden in divine revelation, or by writing themselves in the language of double truth. Such men the contemporaries of Hippocrates indeed were spared, and theories similar to theirs have no place in the interpretation of the Greek material with which Dr. Petersen is dealing.

I must confess that I am skeptical also of the appropriateness of the author's second principle of interpretation, that of symbolic interpretation. As. Dr. Petersen phrases it, reliance on the work of others has not deterred him "from substituting certain modern equivalents for words used in a symbolic sense by the Greek physician." And he continues: "The strangely sounding '*Fire and Water*' is, for example, simple enough when we realize that these terms symbolized our catabolism and anabolism, our energy and matter" (p. xiv). I am not aware of any testimony that would justify the claim of a symbolic use of words on the part of Hippocrates, nor does Dr. Petersen explain what is the basis of his supposition of such a usage, or under what conditions he feels free to interpret a concept as symbolic. From the passage just quoted and from a further discussion of the same example given later on in the book (pp. 128 f.), I can only infer that the author's view is the following: whenever a Greek term sounds strange—because it is utterly irreconcilable with modern scientific opinion, I suppose—the interpreter asks himself whether this term may not have symbolic implications. He then ferrets out whether if taken symbolically it might not coincide with the results of the most recent investigations. Thus the concept of the "hottest and strongest ethereal fire" becomes "to all intents and purposes, the formulation of a modern energy concept, namely, the transmission of energy in wave motion. Until recently considered as immaterial, it is now accepted as involving the transmission of matter, in a form that has weight" (p. 128). Or to put it differently: "We accept energy as wave

---

revered and annotated couldn't have written as Jones would have it" (p. 166). I do not feel impressed either by the fact that in the rendering of the second fragment of Heraclitus not a single word is translated "in terms that cannot be found as definitions even in a small Greek dictionary," or that some renderings "are quite in accord with ordinary Greek usage" (p. 167). What would scientists say, were a philologist to write on medicine on the basis of small dictionaries and ordinary usage of words? Jones is again correct and in agreement with Burnet (*op. cit.*, p. 133).

motion that transmits matter—Hippocrates said fire (*energy*) imperceptible to sight or touch, that contains water (*matter*)" (p. 129). And the terms fire and water are then used by the interpreter "with acceptance of the implication that Hippocrates had anticipated our modern observations, achieved by the most delicate of instruments" (ibid). Granted for argument's sake that Hippocrates—or rather Heraclitus (cf. notes on p. 231), but Dr. Petersen considers Hippocratic the treatise on *Regimen* which reproduces Heraclitus' philosophy—granted that Hippocrates, when he spoke of imperceptible fire, mixed with water, was interested in the explanation of the same phenomena in which those are interested who speak of matter and energy, it would still make all the difference in the world that to Hippocrates, or Heraclitus, both fire and water were qualities or substances. For fire, though not perceptible to sight or touch, exists in some material form just as does water; it must be nourished by water, and so forth (cf. J. Burnet, *Greek Philosophy*, I, 1928, pp. 59 ff.). In my opinion, nobody who wrote before Plato and Aristotle—and most of the Hippocratic books were written before their time; certainly that on *Regimen*—could have understood a discussion about matter and energy as such. Simple historical considerations make it impossible to link the Hippocratic theory with the modern theory—even if the presupposition of symbolic meaning were acceptable at all. And I wonder whether even in cases in which ancient and modern thought can be linked together, the scientist will find in the Greek texts more than a weak glimmering, a dim foreshadowing of his own doctrines, whether he will ever find what one might really call an anticipation of his theories (it may be otherwise with facts). For scientific thought develops and changes, and "one cannot enter the same river twice," as Heraclitus says.

But at this point I strike my colors and lay down my arms. For if I went any further, I might become involved with Dr. Petersen's third principle of interpretation, that of medical interpretation. His own findings have provided "a modern verification of the ancient clinical observations, by answering the hows and the whys." And he has decided to write his commentary because he "found it fascinating to piece together some of the basic observations and clinical deductions and make coherent pictures from apparent jig-saw puzzles" (p. xiii). I have admitted from the beginning that I am not competent to follow him in this undertaking, and all objections made from my point of view do not, of course, imply that his book is without value in regard to those questions which he has at heart. Only this much I venture to say: that his commentary contributes to the "knowledge of the historical continuity of the tradition" which is indispensable today (p. xv) seems doubtful to me. For the picture of "Hippocratic wisdom" which he presents to the student and to the young physician contains a great number of details which are unhistorical. Nor can I succeed in persuading myself that the picture as a whole nevertheless is a more or less adequate likeness, as it sometimes happens that in spite of the incorrect drawing of details the face or figure of a person emerges lifelike in a portrait.

In offering my criticism it has certainly not been my intention to reopen the time-honored debate as to whether the physician or the philologist is the better qualified interpreter of Greek medicine, a debate to which Dr. Petersen himself alludes, quoting Pitschaft's opinion, according to which "only a physician should interpret the Hippocratic texts, for the opinions of the school man can, have little usefulness in so practical a field as medicine," and that of Much, according to which "only a physician is justified in interpreting the physician Hippocrates . . . others . . . should confine themselves to the religiophilosophic or purely humanistic phases" (pp. 165 f.). I for one do not believe in the mutual exclusion of the two approaches, and I plead for cooperation between the scientific and the philological interpreter. Obviously, it is the task of the physician to judge about the diseases described, about the treatment followed, to appreciate the value of Greek medicine. This is not the business of the philologist, and here he must be guided by the physician. But if the scientist takes upon himself the responsibility of interpreting the Greek texts, if he is to establish their medical significance, he must start from the groundword laid by the philologist, he must inquire about certain facts that can be established through philological and historical research.

For in history no less than in science, there are facts which one cannot afford to overlook; new discoveries are made which one must take into account, and doubtful instances ought not to be considered certain. The scientist will not allow himself the slightest deviation from the evidence while he is experimenting or describing natural phenomena. Being a stickler for facts, for precision, in his own field, he should not adopt a different attitude when turning to the interpretation of past phenomena. In a biography of Hippocrates it is no longer possible to speak of Cos as "Temple site of Asklepios" (p. 171). The Coan temple, as the excavations have shown, was founded around 300 B.C., that is, decades after the death of Hippocrates. Nor did Hippocrates write "for the group of properly trained and accepted physicians of the guild of Asclepios" (p. 47, n. 1). The Hippocratic books were available to everybody, and the "guild" of physicians was not interested in the training of its members; no medical examinations were given. One cannot quote an Hippocrates letter as Hippocrates' work, *On mental disease* (p. 48, cf. 199); all these letters were composed in the first century B.C. (Hippocrates therefore cannot be credited with knowing of contagion.). Simply to maintain that the name Asclepius signifies "clear bright air after a storm" (p. 46) is unwarranted after the admission of eminent Greek scholars that they are unable to give any etymology whatsoever. Again, that Hippocrates met with Democritus (p. 172) is at best doubtful and attested only by late sources, among them the spurious Hippocratic letters. That Hippocrates practiced human anatomy (p. xiv) is, to say the least, uncertain and the reader should be informed of arguments that speak against this assumption. Whether Hippocrates had "an excellent understanding of the anatomy of the circulation (heart, lungs and vessels)," this issue depends on the minute interpretation of texts and it cannot be solved by reference to one article that is in favor of a positive answer (p. 22).

To repeat it once more, it is certainly the province of the physician to interpret Hippocratic medicine so that the presentation of its wisdom can "develop a point of view—a wide horizon" (p. xix). I cannot believe, however, that he will achieve this aim—the highest aim indeed which can be set for an interpretation of Greek medicine—unless he is willing to learn from others, just as others must be willing to learn from him, unless in fine he proceeds as did his master Hippocrates of whom the ancients said that "he knew neither to deceive nor to be deceived."

THE GENUINE WORKS OF HIPPOCRATES*

During the last few decades the belief has been current that none of the so-called Hippocratic writings could be ascribed with any certainty to Hippocrates himself. Philologists used to frown at those who did not share this skepticism, especially at physicians who still claimed authenticity for some of the Hippocratic books.[1] In recent years a decided reversal of this attitude has taken place. After Wellmann had dared again to assume the genuineness of some Hippocratic treatises and had been acclaimed by Wilamowitz,[2] various new lists of the genuine works of Hippocrates have been proposed within a rather short period of time by K. Deichgräber, Die Epidemien und das Corpus Hippocraticum, *Abhandlungen der Preussischen Akademie der Wissenschaften*, 1933, *Phil.-Hist. Klasse*, Nr. 3; M. Pohlenz, *Hippokrates und die Begründung der wissenschaftlichen Medizin*, Berlin, 1938; and W. Nestle in an article with the title "Hippocratica," *Hermes*, 73, 1938,

* Bulletin of the History of Medicine, 1939, vol. 7, pp. 236–48.

[1] W. Schonack, *Janus*, 14, 1909, 664: "In dieser Hinsicht besteht ein scharfer Gegensatz zwischen Medizinern und Philologen. Die Mediziner, für die das Hippokratische Corpus über zwei Jahrtausende ein Wissensschatz von unnennbarem Werte gewesen ist, . . . wollen mit Gewalt wenigstens einige Schriften als echt festhalten, während die bösen Philologen in ihrem Skeptizismus so weit gehen, dass in ihren Kreisen, soweit sie sich mit medizin-historischer Forschung beschäftigen, eine Meinung herrschend geworden ist, die sich kurz und bündig so ausdrücken lässt: 'Nichts von allem, was uns erhalten ist, ist eignes Werk des Hippokrates.' "

[2] M. Wellmann, *Hermes*, 64, 1929, 16 ff.; U. v. Wilamowitz, *ibid.*, 480 ff. Wellmann's theory was refuted by O. Regenbogen, *Quellen und Studien zur Geschichte der Mathematik*, Abt. B, 1930, 132, 1. Before Wellmann an attempt at determining genuine works of Hippocrates was made by H. Schöne, *Deutsche Medizinische Wochenschrift*, 1910, 418; 466. Schöne, however, considered as truly Hippocratic not a book of the *Corpus Hippocraticum*, but a treatise which does not belong to it. His view was opposed by H. Diels, *Sitzungsberichte der Preussischen Akademie der Wissenschaften*, *Phil.-Hist. Klasse* 1910, 1140 ff.; 1148. Hippocrates-criticism up to the time of Littré is summarized in his edition of the works of Hippocrates (*Oeuvres Complètes d'Hippocrate*, I, 1839, 154–199).

1 ff. Now those philologists or historians of medicine or physicians who do not admit the authenticity of at least a few of the so-called Hippocratic writings are frowned at and reprimanded because of their exaggerated and unfounded skepticism.[3]

As regards the methods used as well as the results attained by these recent inquiries, their similarity to those of Littré is striking. For it is in accordance with Littré's procedure that Deichgräber, Pohlenz, and Nestle discard the evidence of tradition transmitting a great number of books as the works of Hippocrates and aim at establishing the authenticity of Hippocratic books only through Pre-Alexandrian testimonies about his doctrine.[4] Moreover, while Littré took as genuine: *Ancient Medicine, Prognostic, Aphorisms, Epidemics I* and *III, Regimen in Acute Diseases, Airs Waters Places, Joints, Fractures, Instruments of Reduction, Wounds in the Head, Oath, Law*,[5] Deichgräber counts among the genuine works: *Epidemics I* and *III, Epidemics II, IV,* and *VI, Humours, Surgery, Instruments of Reduction,* and finds a close relation

[3] Deichgräber, 7: "Und doch ist diese Skepsis, so behaupte ich, im Grunde nicht berechtigt. Wenn die Philologie den Masstab anlegt, nach dem sich ihr Urteil zu richten hat, dann muss sie zugeben, dass ihre Skepsis unberechtigt oder doch voreilig ist." Pohlenz, 1: " 'Hippokrates ist zur Zeit ein berühmter Name ohne den Hintergrund irgend einer Schrift,' stellte Wilamowitz 1901 fest. 'Wir wissen von Hippokrates nichts, als dass er gelebt hat,' schreibt Henry E. Sigerist 1932 in dem Buche, in dem er Leben und Werk der 'Grossen Ärzte' schildern will. Und solche Urteile können wir heute allenthalben von Philologen wie von Medizinern vernehmen. Lähmend hat sich diese Skepsis auf die Forschung gelegt . . . Ist diese Bankrotterklärung der Forschung berechtigt?—" Nestle, 35: ". . . nach der lange herrschenden absoluten Skepsis . . . ⟨werden⟩ wir als echt anerkennen . . ." It is then appropriate that the latest publication of an English translation of Hippocratic treatises comprises as genuine the works which were attributed to Hippocrates by Adams in his translation of the genuine works of Hippocrates (*Medical Classics*, III, 1938, I, V, referring to F. Adams' conclusion in *The Genuine Works of Hippocrates*, I, 1886, 105–106 [repeated from I, 1849, 129–30]).

[4] Cf., e.g., Pohlenz, 63: "Die antike Überlieferung entscheidet in diesem Falle (sc. in the question of authenticity) nicht." 79: "Plato und Aristoteles sind nicht nur die ältesten und sichersten, sondern sogar die einzigen Zeugen, auf die wir uns verlassen können, wenn wir über Hippokrates Authentisches feststellen wollen." Cf. Deichgräber, 7; 146; 162. As regards Littré cf. *l. c.* I, 292. Adams opposes Littré's claim that the Pre-Alexandrian testimonies are superior in value to any other principle of criticism; to him ancient evidence of the genuineness of books has to be accepted, if it cannot be disproved (*l. c.* I, 1849, 47; cf. the interesting argument, *l. c.* 29, referring to Littré, I, 171). But according to ancient tradition the authenticity of each book has been disputed, cf. *Realencyclopädie der Klassischen Altertumswissenschaft*, Supplement VI, 1936, 1315–1317.

[5] *L. c.* I, 293; cf. 434; the coincidence of Littré's results with those of the modern interpreters is stressed by Deichgräber, 169–170, and Nestle, 35, themselves.

between these books and *Prognostic, Fractures, Joints, Nature of Man,* finally *Airs Waters Places, Sacred Disease,* and even *Epidemics V* and *VII*.[6] Pohlenz holds to be authentic: *Sacred Disease, Airs Waters Places, Prognostic, Epidemics I* and *III;* he is still undecided as to the authenticity of *Fractures* and *Joints*.[7] Nestle asserts the genuineness of *Prognostic, Epidemics I* and *III; Airs Waters Places, Fractures, Joints, Instruments of Reduction,* parts of the *Aphorisms, Sacred Disease, Regimen in Health,* and *Epidemics II, IV,* and *VI*.[8] Scholarship, then, seems to have returned to where it stood a hundred years ago.

Yet have these new attempts to identify books of Hippocrates really led to results which are convincing? It is this question which I want to discuss. In doing so I have no intention of throwing doubt upon the correctness of the concept of Hippocratic medicine which Deichgräber, Pohlenz, and Nestle presuppose in the solution of their task. This concept is, in the main, derived from the interpretation of what Plato says about Hippocrates in the *Phaedrus* and of what Meno relates about him in his history of medicine.[9] The understanding of these passages is difficult indeed; I must confess that I do not agree with their explanation as proposed by the three scholars.[10] But for the moment I am not concerned with the interpretation of these testimonies. I only ask whether Deichgräber, Pohlenz, and Nestle, according to their own presuppositions, have succeeded in showing that certain books can be regarded as the genuine works of Hippocrates, either with likelihood or with a high degree of probability or with certainty.[11]

If Hippocratic medicine considers the human being in its depend-

---

[6] Deichgräber, 163; cf. 169–170.   [7] Pohlenz, 79–80.   [8] Nestle, 35.

[9] Plato, *Phaedrus,* 270 C–D; Meno's Iatrica, *Supplementum Aristotelicum* III, I, ed. H. Diels, 1893, V, 35 ff.; cf. Diels, *Hermes,* 28, 1893, 407 ff.; cf. Deichgräber 7; 149–160; Pohlenz 2; 65–79; Nestle 17; Nestle rather neglects the Meno passage.

[10] The reasons for a different interpretation of the passage in question are given by L. Edelstein, Περὶ ἀέρων *und die Sammlung der Hippokratischen Schriften, Problemata,* IV, 1931, 129–137, and *Realencyclopädie, l. c.,* 1318–1324.

[11] This distinction between likelihood, a high degree of probability, and certainty is to be found in the books under review. Deichgräber, 163, says: "Nur als *wahrscheinlich* möchte ich es bezeichnen, dass Hippokrates einen Teil dieser Werke selbst verfasst hat." Cf. 170: "Zwar bleibt auch jetzt noch unsicher, was wirklich Eigentum des Hippokrates ist"; Pohlenz, 79, calls the results of his studies: ". . . ⟨ein⟩ Ergebnis, das sich zwar auch nicht mit mathematischer Sicherheit erweisen lässt, aber bei dem Stande unsrer Überlieferung ein *Höchstmass von Wahrscheinlichkeit* beanspruchen darf." Nestle, 22, however, contends: "Denn der von Th. Gomperz noch vermisste Fall, dass ein 'zweifellos echter Grundstock hippokratischer Schriften *nachgewiesen* wäre . . .' ist jetzt, seit Deichgräbers Forschungen, eingetreten . . ."

ence on the universe, methodically divides the parts of the body as well as their faculties, and explains diseases by the influence of air[12]—from which books is it that Plato and Meno themselves, to whom this concept of Hippocratic medicine is to be traced, gathered their knowledge about Hippocrates? This, no doubt, must have been the first question for Deichgräber, Pohlenz, and Nestle, as it was for Littré. But whereas Littré held that Plato referred to *Ancient Medicine* and consequently used this treatise as the standard for determining other books as Hippocratic,[13] the recent interpreters fail to find the writings which Plato and Meno read as those of Hippocrates. According to Deichgräber and Nestle the book that was followed by Plato cannot be pointed to; it is apparently not extant.[14] Pohlenz hazards at least a guess as to which it is, but he himself admits that he is not able to prove his thesis.[15] As regards the treatise which Meno believed to be genuine and which he reproduced in his account, there is general agreement that it has not been preserved.[16]

This is indeed a strange situation. The attempt is made, and its realization is claimed, of recovering a few Hippocratic writings according to the testimony of some early witnesses, although the books which these same witnesses have considered as Hippocratic, it is stated, can

[12] Cf. Deichgräber, 151; 156; Pohlenz, 68; 76; Nestle, 18; my characterization of their concept of Hippocratic medicine, is, of course, very general and abbreviated; details will be discussed later. Cf. pp. 140 ff.

[13] Cf. Littré, I, 294 ff. Littré did not yet have the history of medicine written by Meno (cf. I, 165 ff.), which was not found until 1893; he therefore could not take into account this testimony. Schöne's procedure (cf. *l. c.*) was not different from that of Littré; he, however, believed that Plato's words were to be found in a treatise not preserved in the *Corpus Hippocraticum*. The statement of Meno he declared to be incorrect, *l. c.* 418.

[14] Cf. Nestle, 18: "Welche hippokratische Schrift Platon im Phaidros vorgeschwebt habe, lässt sich nicht bestimmen." Deichgräber nowhere names the book to which, in his opinion, Plato is referring. That he thinks it lost is clear from his other statements; cf. especially 165, 1 and below p. 140, 26.

[15] Pohlenz, 78–79: "Ist da die Vermutung zu kühn, dass er (sc. Plato) mit dem merkwürdigen Worte 'Meteorologie' auf den Eingang der vielgelesenen Schrift (sc. Airs Waters Places) anspielte . . . Und dass er dies deshalb tat, weil er diese Schrift für ein charakteristisches Werk des Arztes hielt, den er sofort als den Vertreter der wissenschaftlichen Medizin zitieren wollte? . . . ein zwingender Beweis, dass Plato gerade die Schrift über die Umwelt (sc. Airs Waters Places) zitieren wollte, lässt sich nicht führen."

[16] Deichgräber, 162: "Die Schrift, aus der das Hippokratesreferat des Menon stammt, befindet sich nicht unter den besprochenen Schriften, sie ist nicht erhalten." Pohlenz, 69: "Menon hält sich an eine uns verlorene Schrift . . ." Nestle does not deal with the Meno passage and the resulting problems; cf. p. 135, 9.

no longer be detected. Of course, it is possible that these treatises have been lost; it is certainly not very plausible that this is so. If the works of Hippocrates have been handed down, and if the *Corpus Hippocraticum* represents the collection of the Hippocratic works or of the works of his school, it is rather astonishing that just the books which Plato and Meno considered as genuine should not have been preserved in spite of the testimony of these two most important authors as to the value of the writings in question.[17]

But if it is impossible to determine the books which have been excerpted by Plato and Meno, nevertheless there are some writings, Deichgräber, Pohlenz, and Nestle claim, which reproduce Hippocratic ideas as represented by Plato and Meno as well as by others, and which fit the biographical data known about Hippocrates. These books then must needs be ascribed to Hippocrates. In this line of reasoning a few difficult problems are involved which should be made explicit before the success or failure of the argument as such can be judged. Scholars say: the *Epidemics* contain the Hippocratic doctrine that diseases are to be explained by air; furthermore they follow Hippocrates' scientific principles; the *Epidemics* therefore have been written by Hippocrates.[18] Granted that the premises of this statement are correct, is the conclusion drawn from them correct also? Is it not possible that other physicians held the same doctrines and methods, either independently or in dependence on Hippocrates, and that consequently the books in which they are to be found were composed by other physicians than Hippocrates? Fevers which recur every five, seven, or nine days are known to Hippocrates, as Diocles says, and they are mentioned in *Epidemics II*, *IV*, and *VI*.[19] To be sure they are known, not only to Hippocrates,

---

[17] Pohlenz, 69: "Dass die aristotelische Zeit noch in der Lage war, echte Schriften des Hippokrates, der ja bis tief ins vierte Jahrhundert gelebt hat, zu kennen und zu erkennen, müssen wir bis zum Beweise des Gegenteils glauben." This is certainly true, but the question as to why these writings have been lost remains unsolved.

[18] Deichgräber, 162: "Auch eins fehlte nicht ganz, was als Ergänzung so erwünscht wäre: die Pneumalehre." Deichgräber (*l. c.*) has before stated that this theory "offensichtlich naturphilosophisch beeinflusst ist und auch noch naturphilosophisch gefärbt ist" and "der naturphilosophischen Methode, wie sie der Phaidros als Lehre des Hippokrates überliefert, voll entspricht." Pohlenz, 79–80: ". . . die Krankenjournale der ältesten Epidemienbücher, die jedenfalls ganz nach seinen wissenschaftlichen Gesichtspunkten angelegt und verwertet sind."

[19] Deichgräber, 162: "In eben diesen Epidemienbüchern wird ein fünf- sieben- und neuntägig wiederkehrendes Fieber angenommen, wird das gelehrt, was Diokles an Hippokrates' Fieberlehre auszusetzen hatte. Diese Beziehung hat schon Wellmann in einer Anmerkung zu dem Dioklesfragment vermerkt." Deichgräber believes

but also to others; because they are referred to in some books, it does not follow that these books were written by Hippocrates. A certain method of setting a dislocation is described in *Fractures;* Diocles blamed Hippocrates because he used such a method.[20] Again, this method may have been adopted by many others. In short, medical practice and theory, the knowledge of material facts which can be shared by hundreds of physicians, cannot prove the individual authorship of any book.

But there are also biographical data which confirm the genuineness of certain writings, it is claimed. Hippocrates practiced in Larissa; the *Epidemics* relate some case histories from Larissa; Gorgias was Hippocrates' teacher in rhetoric, the *Epidemics* to a certain extent follow the stylistic rules of Gorgias; Hippocrates studied with Herodicus, the *Epidemics* are influenced by the dietetic doctrines of Herodicus.[21] I do not insist on the fact that even if these data are correct Hippocrates, certainly, was not the only physician who came to Larissa, not the only writer who imitated the style of Gorgias, not the only pupil of Herodicus. It is evident that the biographies were written at a very late date.[22] Their authors then already knew the *Corpus Hippocraticum*. Uncertain as they were about the genuineness of the Hippocratic books in particu-

---

that Diocles fr. 97 really is a verbal quotation in which the name of Hippocrates has been preserved. That this is hardly true has been shown *Realencyclopädie, l. c.* 1308–9. Cf. also W. Jaeger, *Diokles von Karystos*, 1938, 230. But again I am proceeding from the assumptions as made by Deichgräber.

[20] Deichgräber, 162–3: "Zuletzt findet sich die Theorie, dass der Oberschenkel wieder eingerenkt werden könnte, in II. ἄρθρων." It is again hardly true that this passage (Galen XVIII A 731) originally contained the name of Hippocrates, cf. *Realencyclopädie, l. c.* 1308. Pohlenz's judgment, 80, is more cautious: "Unter den sonstigen Schriften des Corpus sind es in erster Linie die chirurgischen Fachbücher, bei denen man an hippokratischen Ursprung denken kann. Denn an der Einrenkung des luxierten Oberschenkels, die dort gelehrt wird, hat nach Galen XVIII A 731 schon Ktesias Kritik geübt und dabei, wie es scheint, ausdrücklich Hippokrates genannt."

[21] Deichgräber, 162: "Hippokrates hat nach der sicheren Nachricht der Biographie in Larissa in Thessalien praktiziert im ersten Drittel des vierten Jahrhunderts; Epid. III, wovon mindestens ein Teil um 410 geschrieben ist, enthält einige Krankheitsgeschichten aus Larissa. In Larissa dürfte Hippokrates mit Gorgias zusammengetroffen sein; Epid. II, IV and VI zeigen eigentümliche Stilkennzeichen, die an gorgianische Figuren erinnern und von gorgianischem Einfluss her verstanden werden könnten. Einfluss der diätetischen Lehre des Herodikos lässt sich nachweisen, der nach der Biographie Lehrer des Hippokrates war." Cf. also Nestle 37, 3. The biography, by the way, only says that Hippocrates died in Larissa (Soranus ed. J. Ilberg, *Corpus Medicorum Graecorum* IV, 1927, 177, 4).

[22] Cf. *Realencyclopädie, l. c.*, 1295.

lar, they believed in the authenticity of some writings, above all in that of the *Epidemics*. It is a priori probable, and in accordance with the general habit of these writers, that they derived their account of Hippocrates' life mainly from those books which they considered as genuine, that they invented stories by analogy, as Deichgräber himself stresses.[23] None of the data given in the biographies then can be used as proof for the genuineness of Hippocratic books unless it is shown that such data are based on evidence outside the Hippocratic works. This, however, is hardly possible for such facts as the relation of Hippocrates to his teacher, his travels, and so forth; especially since the sources of these biographies, as far as they can be ascertained, are mostly Hellenistic.[24] If one concludes from the coincidence of the biographies and of certain books that these treatises are genuine, the argument runs in a vicious circle.

But to all that, one could reasonably object: even if it is true that a single medical doctrine, a single biographical fact does not demonstrate the genuineness of certain books, the case is different as soon as all or most of the theories ascribed to Hippocrates, all or most of the biographical data related about him are to be verified in some books. Faced with such overwhelming evidence, it is nonsensical to speak of mere chance, of eventualities which are not capable of proof either. This, I think, would be a justifiable objection. But the argument for the genuineness of some books, I repeat, is irrefutable only under the condition that nothing important is missing in these writings; the books to be ascribed to the author must at least express his doctrine in its entirety, not only in parts. Otherwise the proof will never be cogent.[25]

[23] In his discussion of the biographical data themselves, when not considering their value for the identification of books, Deichgräber, 148, says: "Auch die Nachricht, dass Hippokrates später bei Herodikos von Selymbria in die Lehre gegangen ist . . . mag noch zu Recht überliefert sein. Sie ist schwerlich aus der Erwähnung des Herodikos in Epid. VI nachträglich erschlossen. Wenn dann jedoch Gorgias und Demokrit als Lehrer der Rhetorik bzw. der Philosophie genannt werden, so wird man unsicher, da spätere Ausbildungsformen in die Vergangenheit zurückprojiziert zu sein scheinen."

[24] Cf. *Realencyclopädie, l. c.,* 1295.

[25] I agree with Deichgräber's methodical principle as it is formulated, 163, in his final conclusion: "Wenn jetzt die Lehren, die von den ältesten Zeugen und von der Doxographie dem Hippokrates beigelegt werden, mit denen der Epidemien und der mit den Epidemien zusammenhängenden Schriften übereinstimmen, *ohne dass man behaupten kann, dass etwas, was da sein müsste, fehlt,* glaube ich mit Recht, wenn auch wieder mit der nötigen Zurückhaltung, die aufgestellte Hypothese als verifiziert ansehen zu können."

If one examines the studies of Deichgräber, Pohlenz, and Nestle from this point of view one comes to the conclusion that they consider such books as genuine works of Hippocrates which contain only parts of that doctrine which these authors themselves consider as Hippocratic; other very important parts are not contained in these books and it is difficult to understand how they could be fitted into their content. For it is only the dependence of the human body on the cosmos which the so-called genuine works show. The division of the body and its faculties—that means the discussion whether the body is simple or multiform, and if simple what power of acting it has; if multiform, to number the forms—this discussion is not contained in any of the so-called genuine works.[26] Yet Plato, as Deichgräber, Pohlenz, and Nestle claim, ascribes to Hippocrates a doctrine which combines meteorological medicine with logical analysis.[27] Furthermore, it is the explanation of

[26] Deichgräber, 165, 1, says: "Ich weise noch darauf hin, dass die Verbindung der Diairesis und des ὅλον -Prinzips innerhalb des Corpus sich nur hier nachweisen lässt." Deichgräber is referring to *Nature of Man* which, according to tradition, he ascribes to Polybus. At any rate, this book cannot have been written by Hippocrates, in spite of its agreement with Plato in one point, because it explains diseases by changes of the four humors, not by means of air as did Hippocrates according to the given interpretation of Meno. That modern scholars reject this book, the authenticity of which was maintained by Galen (cf. Galen's commentary on *Nature of Man*, *Corpus Medicorum Graecorum*, V, 9, 1, 1914, especially 53, 17 ff.) who discarded the Meno testimony, is indicative of another difficulty which I want at least to mention. Granted that Hippocrates, as Plato says, understood the human body as part of the universe, in which way did he do so? Deichgräber, 165, 1, stresses that such a theory "dass die Erkenntnis der Natur des Alls Vorbedingung ist für die Erkenntnis des Körpers" may have two aspects: it may mean that the microcosm is a reproduction of the macrocosm, or it may mean "Der Körper ist von den μετέωρα und ἀστρονομικά abhängig." Deichgräber, Pohlenz, and Nestle, without giving any reasons, ascribe to Hippocrates the second theory. Nothing can be concluded from the Plato passage itself; for this passage describes only the method of approaching the problem and does not say anything about its solution. Since *Nature of Man* rather follows the macrocosm-microcosm theory this book, for the modern interpreters, cannot be genuine although it, and it alone, partly corresponds to their interpretation of Plato's testimony on Hippocrates.

[27] Deichgräber, 151: "Zuerst wird man feststellen dürfen, dass er (sc. Hippocrates) seiner Medizin einen naturphilosophischen Unterbau gegeben hat, der zugleich das Fundament einer Diairesis darstellte. Weiter kann man auf Grund der Angaben bei Platon sagen, dass Hippokrates gefragt hat, ob der Körper ein ἕν oder ein πολυειδές ist, und was aus dem Zusammenhang hervorgeht, dass er den Körper für ein πολυειδές erklärt hat, dass es für ihn εἴδη bzw. μέρη τοῦ σώματος gab. Er hat weiter die aktiven Kräfte und passiven Möglichkeiten jedes dieser εἴδη unterschieden und vielleicht auch dargelegt." Pohlenz, 76: "Aber diese Einsicht (sc. that neither body nor soul can be understood without the nature of the whole cosmos) bedarf beide Male noch einer Ergänzung. . . . so ist es eine selbstverständliche Parallele zur

diseases by air alone which is employed in the so-called genuine works of Hippocrates. The explanation of diseases by air secreted from the remnants of food or by the air taken in with food, is missing in these writings. Yet Deichgräber and Pohlenz themselves find such an explanation in Meno's account.[28] It is then necessary to maintain that what is called the genuine work of Hippocrates gives only a very fragmentary reproduction of Hippocratic medicine. Important and characteristic features of his doctrine, as attested by Plato and Meno and as represented by modern interpreters, do not recur in these writings.[29]

Erosrede, wenn Plato 270 d dazu übergeht, von den Teilen der Seele, ihren Funktionen, von ihrem Tun und Leiden, von der Art, wie man auf sie einwirken kann, zu reden. Denn über all dies muss der wissenschaftliche Psychagoge Klarheit haben, so gut wie der Arzt über die entsprechenden Organe und Vorgänge des Körpers. Deutlich ist auch hier das Vorbild der wissenschaftlichen Medizin (sc. Hippocrates), und ausdrücklich wird noch einmal auf ihre analoge Aufgabe hingewiesen." Nestle, 18, considers the division even as the foundation of meteorological medicine.

[28] Cf. Deichgräber, 156: "Es bleibt schon jetzt nichts anderes übrig, als anzunehmen, dass dem Hippokrates ursprünglich mindestens zwei Krankheitsursachen zugeschrieben wurden, das Pneuma, das eingeatmet wird, und die φῦσαι, die aus der unverdauten Speise entstehen." The latter theory, by the way, is not to be found in any of the Hippocratic writings. Pohlenz, 68: "Nach Hippokrates haben die Krankheiten ihre Ursache in einer falschen Ernährung, durch die mit den Speisen in unzweckmässiger Weise Pneuma in den Leib dringt. Diese Erklärung beruht auf Hippokrates' Grundanschauung, nach der das Pneuma entscheidende Bedeutung für den Menschen hat. Es ist für ihn lebensnotwendig, kann aber innerhalb des Leibes bei anormalem Zustande auch störend und lebenshemmend wirken." That the air taken in with food may cause diseases is claimed in *Breaths* (*Corpus Medicorum Graecorum*, I, 1927, 94, 9); it is one of the many possible causes of diseases mentioned in this treatise. Such a theory is not to be found in any other Hippocratic writing, neither in *Sacred Disease* nor in *Airs Waters Places*. Pohlenz, 74, says: "Eine einzige Schrift gibt es ausser der Epideixis περὶ φυσῶν, auf die Menons Charakteristik der hippokratischen Lehre haarscharf zutrifft. Das ist die Schrift über die Heilige Krankheit, mit der auch in dieser Hinsicht am engsten die Schrift über die Umwelt verbunden ist." But this he can say only because he is thinking not of air taken in with food, the Hippocratic theory on his reckoning, but of air breathed in by the body; his analysis, 71–73, makes this evident. Earlier, 71, he claims: "Und wenn nach der Schrift π. φυσῶν das Pneuma in allen Speisen, ja überhaupt in allen Dingen vorhanden ist, so entspricht das ganz dem Weltgefühl des Arztes, der zwar nur vom Feuchten ausdrücklich das Gleiche aussagt (gleichlautend Heil. Krankh. 13 und Umw. 8 S. 62, 16), aber auch lebendig schildert, wie beim Südwind das Pneuma die ganze Natur durchdringt und wandelt (Heil. Krankh. 13)"; this indicates the real situation. It is the book on *Breaths* alone which shows a similarity, at least in one respect, with the Menonian report on Hippocrates as interpreted by Pohlenz. But again this book which fulfills one condition cannot be regarded by him as genuine because it contradicts all the other assumptions made about Hippocrates' doctrine.

[29] In view of these fundamental omissions it is not necessary to dwell any further on the problems connected with the other testimonies and with the biographical data.

It would hardly do to claim that the books preserved by chance must not necessarily reproduce all the views of an author. There are many treatises which are said to be Hippocratic; not even all of them taken together contain the doctrine of Hippocrates. Or should one suppose that Hippocrates could not express in two or three books what Plato and Meno in a few words expressed as the essentials of his theory? But apart from the fact that the proof for the genuineness of the Hippocratic works is invalidated, at any rate, since these books, as they are, do not correspond to the entirety of the Hippocratic system—let one imagine that the author of the *Epidemics* asks, as did Hippocrates, according to Plato, "whether that which we wish to learn and to teach is a simple or multiform thing, and if simple, then to inquire what power it has of acting or being acted upon in relation to other things, and if multiform, then to number the forms; and see first in the case of one of them, and then in the case of all of them, what is that power of acting or being acted upon which makes each and all of them to be what they are."[30] The strict empirical observation of the *Epidemics*, the renunciation of every explanation, of every system, do they really go together with the scientific endeavor, the classification which Plato admires in Hippocrates?[31] I think to raise the question means to answer it in the negative. Or let one imagine that the author of *Sacred Disease* explains diseases by air excreted from the remnants of food or taken in with food. Does such an explanation really go together with the explanation of diseases by gall and phlegm as employed in this treatise? Again such a question must be answered in the negative.

The recent inquiries, then, have not succeeded in establishing with certainty, with a high degree of probability, or even with likelihood the genuineness of any of the so-called Hippocratic books. These writings cannot be called Hippocratic according to Deichgräber's, Pohlenz's, and Nestle's own presuppositions. They do not reproduce Hippocrates'

---

[30] *Phaedrus*, 270 D: ἁπλοῦν ἢ πολυειδές ἐστιν, οὗ πέρι βουλησόμεθα εἶναι αὐτοὶ τεχνικοὶ καὶ ἄλλον δυνατοὶ ποιεῖν, ἔπειτα δέ, ἂν μὲν ἁπλοῦν ᾖ, σκοπεῖν τὴν δύναμιν αὐτοῦ, τίνα πρὸς τί πέφυκεν εἰς τὸ δρᾶν ἔχον ἢ τίνα εἰς τὸ παθεῖν ὑπὸ τοῦ, ἐὰν δὲ πλείω εἴδη ἔχῃ, ταῦτα ἀριθμησά-μενον, ὅπερ ἐφ' ἑνός, τοῦτ' ἰδεῖν ἐφ' ἑκάστου, τῷ τί ποιεῖν αὐτὸ πέφυκεν ἢ τῷ τί παθεῖν ὑπὸ τοῦ. The translation is taken from *The Dialogues of Plato* translated into English by B. Jowett, I³, 1892, 479.

[31] It is interesting to compare the Hippocratic system with that of Mnesitheus, which according to Galen is the further explication of it; cf. the detailed division of medicine and diseases, fr. 3 and 4, Hohenstein (H. Hohenstein, *Der Arzt Mnesitheos aus Athen*, Diss. Berlin, 1935).

ideas. Small wonder then that they are not the books which Plato and Meno considered genuine.[32] I feel, however, that the failure of the recent interpreters as of all the previous ones is fundamentally due to the peculiar difficulties of the problem with which they are faced. For the task set for them is not to show the genuineness or spuriousness of some writings which can be compared with others whose genuineness is unquestioned. Rather is it demanded that without any possible comparison one of the books of Hippocrates be identified, one book which then in turn can be used as a standard for other identifications. In this respect the Hippocratic problem is entirely different from the inquiries about the genuineness of Platonic or Galenic books. Yet neither Plato nor Meno quotes verbally from Hippocrates' works; they seem not even to use the specific language of Hippocrates, but to write in their own terminology.[33] Littré, then, quite rightly claimed that the style of Hippocrates too had to be deduced from that writing which had been proved to be genuine. But if the style is unknown, if no verbal quotation is preserved, one is unable to recognize the hand of one specific author in scientific treatises which might have been composed by many different writers. Under these circumstances how can one ever hope to succeed in demonstrating the authenticity of Hippocratic books?

If, however, it is hard to give positive proof for the genuineness of any Hippocratic treatise, it is comparatively easy to ascertain their spuriousness. That they contradict the Platonic-Menonian conception of Hippocratic medicine or do not correspond to it, is sufficient reason for rejecting them. This conclusion is valid at least as long as the attempt to identify the genuine works of Hippocrates is based on external testimonies, not on the evidence of a tradition which has labeled some books Hippocratic. It may seem strange or astonishing that the writings of Hippocrates have been lost. But the works of many great scholars and philosophers of antiquity have been destroyed. The longing to read Hippocrates' own writings, the difficulty of becoming reconciled to the fact that they are not extant, should at any rate be no reason for setting up the methodological postulate that they must have been preserved.[34]

---

[32] Cf. pp. 135 ff.

[33] As far as the Plato passage is concerned, this has already been pointed out by Littré, *l. c.* I, 305; the report of Meno obviously is only a summarizing of Hippocratic doctrine.

[34] Pohlenz, 1–2: "Es wäre eine schier unbegreifliche Tücke des Schicksals, wenn gerade die Werke des anerkannten Meisters spurlos verschwunden sein sollten. Es ist also einfach ein methodisches Postulat, dass unter den uns erhaltenen Schriften

Whether or not some of the so-called Hippocratic books were written by Hippocrates certainly "is a matter of merely antiquarian interest";[35] the solution of this problem does neither enhance nor depreciate Hippocrates' greatness or importance. Moreover, Hippocrates deprived of the books of the *Corpus*, but invested with the doctrine which tradition ascribes to him, does not live a shadowy existence either.[36] Plato and Meno give enough details so as to make clear the outlines of Hippocratic medicine. His scientific method, his explanation of diseases are known; his specific accomplishments can be fully ascertained if contrasted with the doctrines contained in the so-called Hippocratic writings; his importance for Greek medicine is indicated by the history of his influence on later generations.

An appreciation of the historical Hippocrates within these limits is incontestable; more knowledge about him and his works cannot be claimed with certainty. If such a judgment is called skeptical, it cannot be helped. As concerns the solution of scholarly problems, I do not see any difference or merit in their being positive or negative or skeptical. Whatever they are in this respect, they are true only if and as far as they are founded on reasons.[37]

---

auch solche von Hippokrates selber sein müssen. Und damit ist der Forschung eine Aufgabe gewiesen, der sie sich nicht entziehen darf, mag auch die Lösung noch so schwierig erscheinen."

[35] W. H. S. Jones, *Hippocrates* with an English translation (*Loeb Classical Series*), I, 1923, xxi.

[36] Cf. Jones, *l. c.* "the shadowy 'Hippocrates' of ancient tradition." This is true also against H. E. Sigerist, *The Great Doctors*, 1933, 36: "All that we certainly know of Hippocrates is that he lived, . . ."

[37] I note my agreement with Pohlenz, 2: "Natürlich ist der Wissenschaft nicht damit gedient, wenn sich kritiklose Traditionsgläubigkeit und dichterische Phantasie zu einem Hippokratesroman verbinden. Ihr Gang ist mühsamer und weniger kurzweilig."

REVIEW*

W. JAEGER, *Diokles von Karystos. Die griechische Medizin und die Schule des Aristoteles.*

Berlin, 1938, pp. 244.

J aeger's book is the first modern monograph on Diocles, whose fame in antiquity almost equaled that of Hippocrates. That recent scholars have neglected him may partly be due to the fact that only fragments of his writings are preserved.[1]

Against the common belief Jaeger tries to demonstrate that Diocles did not live before Aristotle. Rose's opinion to the same effect did not carry any conviction, for it was made as an aperçu rather than elaborated as a doctrine. Maass' splendid observation that Diocles avoids hiatus elucidated a detail of his style, but did not prove that he lived in the last third of the fourth century B.C., as Maass suggested (cf. Jaeger, pp. 13 ff.). By placing the scattered references to Diocles into the framework of Greek philosophy Jaeger puts on a new basis the discussion of the problems involved, for he shows for the first time to what extent Diocles' language and thought coincide with Aristotelian formulations and ideas. Jaeger then concludes that Diocles must have been dependent on Aristotle and that he must have been at least his contemporary, for otherwise Aristotle would be dependent on Diocles, and that too in regard to important metaphysical and ethical concepts as well as characteristic scientific terms and stylistic devices.

Such a line of reasoning, no doubt, contains an *a priori* assumption which is not incontestable. Aristotle in many respects is dependent on his predecessors, and if it were certain that Diocles lived earlier, one would have to resign oneself to the fact that it is Diocles who taught Aristotle. Yet, whereas scholars so far had concluded from ancient testimony that Diocles died around 350 B.C., certainly before Aristotle formulated his own philosophical system, Jaeger infers from the fragments that he died after 300 B.C. and before 288/7 B.C. (p. 119). In an article, published shortly after his book had appeared, Jaeger goes even

---

* *American Journal of Philology*, 1940, vol. 61, pp. 483–89.
[1] M. Wellman, *Die Fragmente der Sikelischen Ärzte Akron, Philistion und des Diokles von Karystos* (Berlin, 1901).

farther and tries to prove that Diocles lived from 340–260 B.C.[2] In both cases Jaeger's thesis is based on the interpretation of the same two statements which alone, it seems, provide direct information about Diocles' lifetime, the one coming from Theophrastus (Περὶ λίθων, ch. 5 = frag. 166 Wellmann), the other from Athenaeus (II 59a = frag. 125 Wellmann).

Frag. 166, although of secondary importance for Jaeger, must be considered first, because of certain difficulties which it involves. It reads thus: ἕλκει γὰρ (scil. τὸ λυγγούριον) ὥσπερ τὸ ἤλεκτρον, οἱ δέ φασιν οὐ μόνον κάρφη καὶ ξύλον, ἀλλὰ καὶ χαλκὸν καὶ σίδηρον, ἐὰν ᾖ λεπτός, ὥσπερ καὶ Διοκλῆς ἔλεγεν. Originally Jaeger claimed that Diocles, who was still alive around 300 B.C., must have been dead at the time when these words were written (before 288/7 [I, p. 119]), since Theophrastus speaks of him in the imperfect. Later he maintains only, again on account of the use of the imperfect, that Diocles was not in Athens when Theophrastus wrote (II, p. 13), another possible explanation of the tense discussed by Jaeger in his book, but there rejected as unlikely (loc. cit.).

The possibility of such a flexible interpretation of the imperfect (cf. also I, p. 14), in my opinion, does not enhance confidence in the certainty of either the one or the other conclusion. Moreover, Pliny, in paraphrasing the passage, says (XXXVII, 53): quod Diocli cuidam Theophrastus quoque credit. Jaeger, referring to the somewhat deprecatory expression Diocli cuidam, says: "Dieser Unterschied in der Bewertung des Diokles bei Theophrast und Plinius würde allein schon fast genügen, um zu beweisen, dass es sich um den grossen peripatetischen Arzt handeln muss . . ." (I, p. 117); and he claims that Diocles "für ihn (scil. Pliny) keine greifbare Grösse mehr ist" (loc. cit.). Yet since Theophrastus does not pass any judgment on Diocles' achievements, it is impossible to speak of differences in the evaluations pronounced by Theophrastus and by Pliny. Besides, it is hardly justifiable to cavil at Pliny's appreciation of Diocles' importance, for Pliny, who in other places mentions Diocles either simply by name or as the physician Diocles, calls him "the second in glory to Hippocrates" (XXVI, 10 = frag. 5 Wellmann). Since Pliny understood Theophrastus' statement to refer to a certain Diocles, this Diocles for Pliny could not be

---

[2] Vergessene Fragmente des Peripatetikers Diokles von Karystos, Abhandlungen der Preussischen Akademie der Wissenschaften, 1938, Phil.-hist. Klasse, No. 3, p. 17. (This paper I shall quote as II, whereas the book will be quoted as I.)

identical with the famous Diocles. Therefore it is dangerous, I believe, to use the fragment at all for determining the lifetime of Diocles of Carystus.[3]

The chronological evidence thus seems restricted to frag. 125: Διοκλῆς δὲ κολοκύντας μὲν καλλίστας γίνεσθαι περὶ Μαγνησίαν, προσέτι τε γογγύλην ὑπερμεγέθη γλυκεῖαν καὶ εὐστόμαχον, ἐν Ἀντιοχείᾳ δὲ σικυόν, ἐν δὲ Σμύρνῃ καὶ Γαλατίᾳ θρίδακα, πήγανον δ' ἐν Μύροις. The mention of Antioch, Jaeger says—taking up an argument of Rose entirely overlooked and forgotten later on—proves that Diocles was still alive when that city was founded or even for some time thereafter; Diocles must have lived, therefore, until 300 B.C. (I, pp. 67 ff.). Yet, as Theiler pointed out to Jaeger, Galatia is mentioned in the same fragment, and the name Galatia cannot have been used earlier than 270 B.C. (cf. II, p. 16). Jaeger, therefore, finally assumed as Diocles' term of life the years 340 to 260 B.C. (II, pp. 17; 36), and he claims that Diocles must have lived long enough to polemize against Herophilus whose *floruit* lies between 270 and 260 B.C. (cf. II, pp. 15; 36 ff.).

How does such a hypothesis fit in with the indirect evidence? When in his book Jaeger discusses Vindicianus' (4/5th century A.D.) doxographical survey of medical problems in which certain theories of Diocles are formulated as answers to the doctrines of Herophilus, he writes: "Wir müssen also entweder Wellmanns Voraussetzung preisgeben, dass in dem Exzerpt wörtliche Zitate aus Diokles vorliegen, oder folgern, dass Diokles im 3. Jahrh. lange genug gelebt habe, um eine Schrift gegen Herophilos verfassen zu können, der von Galen und anderen antiken Zeugen ausdrücklich als jünger als Diokles bezeichnet wird und nach herrschender Annahme erst vom zweiten und dritten Jahrzehnt an 'geblüht' hat. Dieser Synchronismus hat naturlich etwas Verlockendes, wenn man schon einmal dabei ist, die ganze Chronologie und Entwicklungsgeschichte der griechischen Medizin von Hippokrates bis zum Beginn des hellenistischen Zeitalters umzustossen. Aber hier stehen wir im Begriff, den Boden sicherer Tatsachen zu verlassen und statt der überwundenen Schwierigkeiten neue zu schaffen" (I, p. 200).

---

[3] There is at least one other fragment the genuineness of which is doubtful (frag. 99 Wellmann), cf. J. Heeg, *Sitzungsberichte der Preussischen Akademie der Wissenschaften*, 1911, pp. 991 ff. Wellmann's revindication of the fragment (*Hermes*, XLVIII [1913], pp. 464 ff.) is not convincing. Another physician Diocles is known from Galen (XIII, p. 87 Kühn, and Wellmann, p. 65, n. 1), not to speak of all the others by that name referred to in ancient literature. Cf. also D'Arcy Wentworth Thompson, *The Philosophical Review*, XLVIII (1939), pp. 212–213.

Indeed, the assumption that Diocles could have opposed views held by Herophilus is inconsistent with the testimonies of Celsus and Galen (frags. 4; 16 Wellmann) who agree that Diocles wrote before Herophilus.

Why does Jaeger now (II, p. 15) consider as genuine the so-called answers of Diocles to Herophilus which he himself had shown to be arranged by Vindicianus, as is typical of this late compilatory literature (I, pp. 200 ff.)? His main reason for changing his mind is the reference to Galatia (II, p. 16); and yet, Kaibel, in his edition of Athenaeus, had already remarked: γαλατείᾳ C E, videtur corruptum; Kaibel's statement is probably due to stylistic considerations, as Jaeger explains (*loc. cit.*). Jacoby, too, regards καὶ Γαλατίᾳ as an obvious insertion which destroys the careful antithesis otherwise to be observed in these words (Jacoby *apud* Jaeger, *loc. cit.*, p. 16, n. 2). Moreover, since the statement apparently means to tell where the best kind of lettuce is grown, it would be hardly appropriate to name two places of production (Smyrna and Galatia); also in the words immediately preceding and following only one place is mentioned for the best kind of vegetables referred to there (cf. E. Kind, *Philologische Wochenschrift*, LIX [1939], p. 528). Finally, Diocles, in giving the places of origin, usually speaks of cities, not of countries (Jaeger, II, p. 16). One must conclude, I think, that καὶ Γαλατίᾳ is a later insertion; additions in statements of this kind are certainly nothing extraordinary.

At any rate, the contention that Diocles lived long enough to write against Herophilus—a claim which is refuted by all indirect testimony—cannot be established by the evidence adduced by Jaeger.[4] Besides, the content of Diocles' teaching is in no way linked to the work done by Herophilus and his associates; on the contrary, Diocles' doctrine and method are characteristic of the bent of the older generation. To give one striking example: Diocles' anatomy is animal anatomy, not human anatomy (cf. I, p. 165), which is a distinctive feature of Hellenistic medicine. It is safe to say that none of the new medical concepts, as conceived by the physicians of the first half of the third century B.C.,

---

[4] Consequently it seems impossible to accept either Jaeger's identification of Diocles of Carystus with the Diocles mentioned in the will of Strato (II, pp. 10 ff.), or his new dates for the physicians of the fourth century B.C., which he bases on his chronology of Diocles (II, pp. 36 ff.). Furthermore, if Jaeger's thesis as formulated in his article is adopted, it becomes even more doubtful that the so-called letter of Diocles to Antigonus is genuine (I, pp. 70 ff.), for Diocles could hardly write to the king on an equal footing around 305/4 (I, p. 79) if he was at that time thirty-five years old and at the beginning of his career.

is reechoed in the fragments preserved from Diocles' writings. Had he really lived and worked from 340–260 B.C. his system would be an outright anachronism. That it was is, of course, not impossible; yet this could be concluded only on the basis of irrefutable evidence.

If the chronological argument from the fragments allows of any conclusion at all, it proves that Diocles lived until 300 B.C., the time in which Antioch was founded, or shortly after, in other words perhaps from 375–295 B.C. Such a result is not incompatible with Pliny's and Galen's opinion that Diocles lived shortly after Hippocrates (frag. 5 Wellmann, *secundus aetate* (*scil.* Hippocratis); frag. 26 Wellmann, μικρὸν ὕστερον Ἱπποκράτους),[5] for Hippocrates probably died around 380 B.C. The new date for Diocles' lifetime can also be reconciled with Celsus' reckoning of generations (frag. 4, *post quem* (*scil.* Hippocratem) *Diocles Carystius, deinde Praxagoras et Chrysippus, tum Herophilus et Erasistratus*). Yet, I think one must admit that Diocles' lifetime then extends over a longer period or begins at a later date than one would have guessed from the indirect information.

Nevertheless, even if one is inclined to disregard the one direct testimony (frag. 125) entirely, since it certainly has been altered by addition, and since the foundation of Antioch seems a rather late *terminus post quem* for Diocles' death—even then it would be in accord with all the other ancient witnesses to assume that Diocles was a contemporary of Aristotle. Before Jaeger nobody ever seriously considered this possibility, for the close ideological and stylistic resemblance between the work of the two men had not been observed and the question of their mutual dependence consequently was no issue. Now that this observation has been made, one becomes aware that nothing prevents assuming Diocles to have been of the same age as Aristotle or somewhat younger.[6] On the contrary, the evidence points in this direction, for according to all sources Diocles was later than Hippocrates; there is no indication that the two were contemporaries, they are always distinguished as belonging to different generations. The chronological argument then, rightly considered, is in favor of Jaeger's first thesis of a

---

[5] I fail to understand Jaeger's statement that a *floruit* of Diocles shortly before or around 300 B.C. is in agreement with Pliny's expression: *Diocles secundus aetate famaque Hippocratis* (II, p. 12), nor can I see that Galen's μικρὸν ὕστερον Ἱπποκράτους is already a misrepresentation of the tradition, because it puts Diocles immediately after Hippocrates (II, p. 37).

[6] Cf. Jaeger, I, p. 12: "Einen durchschlagenden Grund für . . . frühe Datierung des Diokles gibt es in der Tat nicht."

close proximity of Diocles and Aristotle. This again makes it unnecessary to explain their agreement by presuming that Aristotle borrows from Diocles.

All these considerations do not, of course, indicate the extent of the reciprocal influence of the two men, or whose influence was the stronger and more important. It stands to reason that Diocles, in the methodological discussions in which he shares the views of Aristotle,[7] is dependent on him. Tradition does not suggest any philosophical originality of Diocles, and the fragments show a combination of different trends rather than a strongly personal point of view. Diocles may also have taken over the terminology, which in many respects closely resembles that of Aristotle (I, pp. 16 ff.).[8] Allowance must be made, however, for some exception to the contrary even in regard to this relation. Too little is known about Diocles to exclude the possibility of his having some philosophical ideas of his own or devising some stylistic novelty.[9] The statement of Diocles (II, pp. 5 ff.) in which he disagrees with Aristotle in the explanation of winds shows that, in spite of all his dependence on Aristotelian philosophy, Diocles was able to judge for himself even in questions of natural philosophy. Nor is there any reason why it should have been necessary for him to learn what he learned by a careful study of the published *Ethics* as well as from the oral lectures which he had heard.[10]

Yet, if it is reasonable to assume Diocles' dependence on Aristotle in these matters, a similar subordination of Diocles the zoologist and physician is not probable. It is hardly a "Skandalon der historischen Vernunft" (I, p. 177) that Diocles' work is represented as one of the sources of Aristotle's zoological writings. In the first place, Diocles discussed questions of zoology not only in his meager dietetical books, as Jaeger at one place says (I, p. 176), but also in his treatise on anatomy, the first ever written (Galen, II, p. 282 Kühn = frag. 23 Wellmann). This book, then, could have been a source of information for Aristotle,

---

[7] ποιότης (?), ὅμοιον, ἀρχαὶ ἀναπόδεικτοι, ἁρμόττον (I, pp. 25 ff.; 37 ff.); the concept of teleology (pp. 51 ff.).

[8] ἐνδέχεσθαι (I, p. 23); ποσαχῶς λέγεται (p. 24); συμβαίνειν εἴωθε (p. 31).

[9] Especially if he had been a ῥήτωρ (frag. 99 Wellmann, and Jaeger I, p. 2). But Wellmann's emendation was rejected and the genuineness of the fragment disputed by Heeg (cf. *supra* n. 3).

[10] I, p. 59: "Nun scheint mir aber aus unserer Untersuchung zugleich unwiderleglich hervorzugehen, dass Diokles die ethische Lehre des späten Aristoteles nicht *nur* aus mündlichem Vortrag, sondern in ihrer genauen schriftlichen Formulierung gekannt hat, wie sie in der Nikomachischen Ethik uns vorliegt."

as Jaeger elsewhere admits (I, pp. 183–4), and a source of special importance if Aristotle himself did not write on anatomy (I, p. 165, n. 1). Such a work presupposes systematic knowledge and most probably contained a description of animal parts (contrary to Jaeger, *loc. cit.*); there is certainly no proof that it was unsystematic or lacking in description. Moreover, even disregarding the problem of the Coan zoological system (I, pp. 167 ff.), Aristotle himself testifies to his knowledge of forerunners in the field; he cannot have been the first to establish a system of zoology.[11] This fact in no way detracts from the remarkable qualities of his work or from the incomparable greatness of his achievement. Even where he takes over his knowledge, he maintains his independent attitude. Jaeger was doubtless correct when in his book he interpreted *De Generatione Animalium* II 7, 745 b 33–746 a 28 as a polemic against Diocles' divergent opinions (I, p. 166) and suggested that there may be many other such polemics in the Aristotelian writings (I, p. 167).[12] Still, even controversy does not exclude dependence, in the case of Aristotle any more than in the case of Diocles, the natural scientist.

As for Diocles the physician—no general considerations make it probable or acceptable that he, the son of a physician, wherever his opinions coincide with those of Aristotle, even in medicine, must be borrowing from him, or that in these instances both go back to the same source (I, pp. 218–19). To be sure, it would be hopeless to collect all the cases of their agreement and to divine which one is following the other (Jaeger, *loc. cit.*). Yet there are also cases in which Diocles deviates from Aristotle (e.g., I, p. 166); and certainly, if Diocles even as a physician had nothing to offer Aristotle he could not have been "the second in glory to Hippocrates" and one of the doctors whom Aristotle praises by saying: "those physicians who have subtle and inquiring minds have something to say about natural science and claim to derive their principles therefrom."[13] Finally, Aristotle asserts that philosophers should discuss the causes of death and disease only up to a certain point (μέχρι

[11] Cf. I. V. Carus, *Geschichte der Zoologie* (1872), pp. 57 ff.; 77. If Buffon, Cuvier, and Alexander v. Humboldt are inclined to see in Aristotle the first whom tradition mentions, the originator of zoology and its system (I, pp. 167–8), Aristotle himself answers (*Poetics*, 1448 b 27–30): τῶν μὲν οὖν πρὸ Ὁμήρου οὐδενὸς ἔχομεν εἰπεῖν τοιοῦτον ποίημα, εἰκὸς δὲ εἶναι πολλούς.

[12] Attention must be called, however, to the fact that this interpretation of these passages cannot be reconciled with the chronology set up in Jaeger's later article.

[13] *De Respiratione* 480 b 22 ff., Hett's translation (Loeb Classical Library [1935], p. 479).

151

του); he does not say that they have to become physicians themselves (*ibid.*). Why, then, should he not have learned from Diocles?

To sum up: Jaeger has shown, I believe, that Diocles was a contemporary of Aristotle and deeply influenced by Aristotelian philosophy, the first physician of the "synthetic type" (I, pp. 5; 220), integrating, as a true Aristotelian, the achievements of the whole past (I, p. 224). These results of Jaeger's interpretation, results of the greatest importance, must be protected and upheld against certain exaggerations to which he himself is liable in determining the rôle of Aristotle as compared with that of Diocles; they must be kept safe against the new position which Jaeger has later taken in regard to the chronological questions. Only then will a more appropriate appreciation of Diocles' achievements be reached.[14]

[14] When this was already in page-proof there appeared (*Philos. Rev.*, XLIX [July, 1940], pp. 393 ff.) an article of Jaeger's summarizing the views expressed in his book and paper here reviewed.

THE ROLE OF ERYXIMACHUS IN PLATO'S *SYMPOSIUM*＊

The intention of this paper is to show that Plato's representation of Eryximachus is not a caricature of the physician; that Eryximachus plays an important rôle in the framework of the dialogue and that there is a relationship between the position given to him and the contents of the *Symposium*.

Among the speakers at the banquet that brought together Agathon, Socrates and Alcibiades (172A–B), Eryximachus is the representative of the medical art. There is almost general agreement among modern interpreters that Plato, in representing him, has drawn an ironical portrait of the pedantic expert and scientist. When once it was claimed that "nowhere in literature do we have such a charming picture illustrating the position of the cultivated physician in society as that given in Plato's Dialogues of Eryximachus," Gildersleeve retorted that Eryximachus was a pedant, a system-monger "who was only on sufferance in that brilliant company and whom Plato holds up to ridicule as incorporating the worst foibles of the professor of the healing art."[1] Most other criticisms have been in more or less the same vein.

This common verdict on Eryximachus is not restricted to details of Plato's portrayal. Wherever he appears on the stage, it is claimed, he is ridiculed as a pedant.[2] Even before he contributes his share to the contest of speeches on Eros, he is said to show his pedantry. Unable to forget his professional solemnity, he seizes every opportunity to display his medical knowledge: when he is first mentioned, he immediately delivers a lecture on μέθη (176C–D); later on he discourses on λύγξ (185D–E).[3]

＊ Transactions of the American Philological Association, 1945, vol. 76, pp. 85–103.

[1] *AJPh* 30 (1909) 109. The statement is made in answer to W. Osler, *Counsels and Ideals* (Boston and New York, 1905) 24.

[2] Cf. U. v. Wilamowitz-Moellendorff, *Platon* I (third edition [Berlin, 1929]) 367: "Der Sprecher . . . soll unfreiwillig komisch wirken, wo immer er auftritt . . ."; cf. *ibid.* 361: "Der Arzt hat hier die Rolle des Pedanten."

[3] Cf. R. G. Bury, *The Symposium of Plato* (Cambridge, 1909) xxviii; A. Hug and H. Schöne, *Symposion* (*Platons Ausgewählte Schriften* 5 [third edition, Leipzig and Berlin, 1909]) xxxviii and 61, note 3.

This censure is hardly justified. Eryximachus' first intervention is due to Pausanias' complaint that he is still weak from yesterday's bout and to his request that the company consider how one could make today's drinking easy (176A). After Aristophanes has supported this wish for ease in drinking (176B) Eryximachus takes the platform. He inquires whether Agathon too finds himself not exactly in "good condition," and since this is admitted, and the other guests are not great drinkers anyhow (176B–C), he proceeds to state that excess in drinking is harmful and that he would advise against it, especially for those who are still somewhat heavy-headed (176D).[4] Advice has been sought, and who should be better prepared to give counsel than the physician, who can rely on his medical experience? Does not the question asked clearly concern medicine?[5] Again, in proposing a cure for hiccoughs (185D–E), Eryximachus does not intrude on the company with his medical lore. It is not he who has brought up the subject. Aristophanes has turned to him because he thinks that the physician is the man to tell him how to stop his hiccoughs; Eryximachus only gives the advice for which he has been consulted. By making Eryximachus act as a physician whenever the occasion calls for medical opinion, Plato can hardly have intended to satirize him.

But even in his speech on Eros, Eryximachus talks as a physician. To this ancestor of Molière's Diafoirus, Robin claims,[6] everything in the world appears within the infinitely enlarged compass of his art. His oration is marred by pedantic mannerisms: "If Eryximachus is allowed to take up his parable," Gildersleeve contends,[7] "it is because Plato wished to let his humor play on the weak sides of the profession."

[4] Eryximachus is not cut short by Phaedrus, as Hug-Schöne (see note 3) 21, note 2, maintain. He gives his counsel and has said all that he intended to say when he has finished.

[5] This is acknowledged in Phaedrus' words: ἄττ' ἂν περὶ ἰατρικῆς λέγῃς (176D). Physicians of the fourth century, not only philosophers like Antisthenes and Aristotle (cf. Hug-Schöne [see note 3] xxxviii, note 8), wrote on drunkenness and symposia; e.g., Mnesitheus (Athenaeus 11, p. 483f = Fr. 45 [H. Hohenstein, Der Arzt Mnesitheus aus Athen, Diss. Berlin, 1935]) and, in later times, Heraclides of Tarentum, Fr. 24 (K. Deichgräber, Die griechische Empirikerschule [Berlin, 1930]). Discussions of the influence of wine on men's health are also to be found in Hippocrates and Diocles; cf. Diocles, Fr. 141 (M. Wellmann, Die Fragmente der sikelischen Ärzte [Berlin, 1901]), and the parallels there given. Diocles recommends drinking πρὸς ἡδονήν (182, 1.2). The same expression is used in the Symposium (176E).

[6] L. Robin, Le Banquet (Platon, Oeuvres Complètes, 4.2 [Paris, 1929] Collection Budé) LII.

[7] AJPh 30 (1909) 109.

There is no gainsaying the assertion that Eryximachus loves to speak of medicine. Indeed, he begins his discourse with a dissertation on the medical art in order to pay homage to his profession, as he himself adds (186B). This, however, is not a sign of conceit on the part of the artisan; it simply shows a natural respect for his calling. Agathon too puts his art first, and in honoring poetry in this way, he expressly refers to the example of Eryximachus (196D).[8] Nor does Eryximachus give undue attention to his specialty. His analysis of medicine (186B–E) is shorter than his analysis of music (187A–E). To be sure, after having proved that Eros holds sway over medicine, he comes back to his art twice in order to elucidate certain points by comparison (187C; E), and once he speaks of health and disease when discussing the influence of Eros on the seasons of the year (188A–B). Such references, like the diction of his speech, clearly denote him as a medical man.[9] But after all, Eryximachus is a physician, and Plato apparently is interested in bringing out the typical characteristics of each speaker as well as the individual features of their personalities. Thus, in the speeches of Aristophanes and Agathon he uses motifs and stylistic devices that indicate the vocation of the two poets.[10] Aristophanes is pictured as "the very genius of the old comedy." He is "ready to laugh and make laugh before he opens his mouth, just as Socrates, true to his character, is ready to argue before he begins to speak."[11] The fact that Eryximachus talks like a

[8] Robin (see note 6) 24, note 2, concludes from the fact that Eryximachus discusses medicine first that for him it is *the* art. This judgment, in my opinion, is not justified because it does not take account of the motivation adduced by Plato. For another statement of Eryximachus that might be construed in Robin's sense, cf. below p. 157.

[9] A. E. Taylor, *Plato* (New York, 1936) 217, rightly says: "The style of the speech is appropriately sober, free from the artifices of rhetoric and marked by a plentiful use of professional terminology." Bury (see note 3) xxix notes the plainness of the oration and its lack of ornament but adds that its monotony (the recurrence of the same formulae) "marks it as the product of a pedantic, would-be scientific mind in which literary taste is but slightly developed and the ruling interest is the schematization of physical doctrines." Were such an evaluation made universal, many a great scientist, I am afraid, and even many a Greek scientist, would have to be classified as a pedant. P. Friedländer, *Platon* 2 (Berlin and Leipzig, 1930) 304, suggests that by emphasizing the pedantry of the arrangement Plato satirizes the style of certain Hippocratic writings. Could he not simply have imitated this style in order to give to Eryximachus' words their native color?

[10] For Aristophanes, cf. Bury (see note 3) xxx; Friedländer (see note 9) 306 ff.; for Agathon, cf. Bury xxxvi; B. Jowett, *The Dialogues of Plato* 1 (third edition [New York and London, 1892]) 531.

[11] Jowett (see note 10) 530.

physician, therefore, does not yet make him a pedant, and to those who interpret his medical air as a caricature of the expert, Eryximachus might well answer, as Aristophanes answered the physician when he blamed the comic poet for his buffoonery: I am not afraid to speak in this manner, for this is "the custom of my Muse" (189B).

On the other hand, if Eryximachus is reproached for "the dogmatism of his profession in trying to make good his pedantic correction of his predecessors,"[12] one should point out that the other speakers are dogmatic too. All of them give their opinions for what they are worth.[13] Besides, he is not the only one to detect the shortcomings of his rivals. Pausanias is dissatisfied with the speech of Phaedrus (180c); Aristophanes criticizes Eryximachus and Pausanias (189c); Agathon believes that his method of praising Eros is the correct one, while that of all the previous speakers was bad (194E); and Socrates charges that nobody so far has told the truth (198D). Moreover, if Eryximachus' argumentation seems a nuance too pedantic, this didacticism may have been intentional and meant to amuse himself and the rest of the company. The banquet is not a solemn affair. Those who are present are determined to have their fun; they indulge in jests and merrymaking, Aristophanes no more than Socrates and all the others.[14] At any rate, Eryximachus is quite capable of rising to the occasion. He defines medicine as the knowledge of separating fair love from foul (186c); he holds that Eros is the god who guides the work of the farmer and of the trainer (186E). Such ideas are fanciful and whimsical. He would certainly not have chosen the same language when conversing with his patients or with a peasant or a trainer. But for a party dedicated to the celebration of Eros his words are quite appropriate and give to his performance the mixture of the playful and the serious of which Agathon boasts in regard to his own oration (197E) and which is characteristic of all the speeches that are delivered.[15] Finally, that Eryximachus' professional attitude and seriousness are tempered by a sense of humor is obvious also in his altercation with Aristophanes (189A–B). The poet is well

[12] Gildersleeve (see note 1) 109; Friedländer (see note 9) 304, speaks of "Eitelkeit des Fachmanns" and "unliebenswürdige Krittelsucht."

[13] Cf. below p. 169.

[14] Taylor (see note 9) 217, was the first to suggest that Eryximachus' pedantry is "part of the fun of the evening and is presumably intentional." The gay tone of certain sections of the *Symposium*, the interplay of humor and seriousness, hardly need elaboration. Whether it is appropriate to contrast the *Symposium* as a comedy with the *Phaedo* as a tragedy (cf. Wilamowitz [see note 2] 356), is quite a different problem.

[15] Cf. Jowett (see note 10) 526.

aware of the physician's sarcasm when he answers him laughingly, and it is not for nothing that in his speech he guards himself repeatedly against any mocking remarks of Eryximachus (193B; D). Nor could Eryximachus have enjoyed the comic masterpiece of Aristophanes as much as he did (193E), had he himself lacked a sense of humor.[16]

Yet at this point one might object: even granted that the speech of Eryximachus is to some extent shaped by Plato's wish to characterize him as a doctor, that Eryximachus is not altogether portrayed as a pedantic fool, why is he made to claim that all he knows and all he is going to propound he has learned from medicine (186A–B)? How can medicine have taught him that Eros rules not only men and animals and plants, but all things, human and divine alike?[17] This assertion, it seems, indicates a rather ludicrous pride in the importance of the medical art and stamps Eryximachus as the prototype of the arrogant doctor. The speech as a whole, if not every detail of it, appears to be a travesty of the narrow-mindedness and conceit of the physician.[18]

It is true that Eryximachus' contention, at first blush, sounds preposterous. Yet before condemning him altogether it is perhaps pertinent to ask what exactly he has learned from medicine, what his art has led him to observe in regard to all the subjects which he mentions.[19] To put it briefly, it is this: the principle of a double Eros is valid in medicine, husbandry, gymnastics, music, astronomy and divination. Eryxi-

---

[16] Hug-Schöne (see note 3) xxxviii and 61, note 3, seem the only ones to allow Eryximachus "einen gewissen trockenen ärztlichen Humor."

[17] F. A. Wolf proposed to change the usual punctuation and to take the words ὡς μέγας κτλ as an independent sentence: nam ad *omnia* pertinere amorem, ad divinas etiam res ex arte medica discere non potuit (cf. G. F. Rettig, *Platons Symposion* 2 [Halle, 1876] 164). But such a change would be of no avail since the preceding ὅτι clause makes the same sweeping assumption. For the grammatical structure of the sentence, cf. Hug-Schöne (see note 3) 63, note 8.

[18] The statement made in 186A has been taken by K. F. Hermann (*Geschichte u. System der platonischen Philosophie* 1 [Heidelberg, 1839] 215) to show the pedantic self-complacency and glibness of the sophist; cf. also A. Schwegler, *Über die Composition des Platonischen Symposions* (Tübingen, 1843) 33. More recent interpreters are usually satisfied with pointing out that to Eryximachus medicine is the source of all knowledge (Hug-Schöne [see note 3] 63, note 7), and they parallel the assertion made here with that made in 176D. But the assumption that Eryximachus should have acquired from medicine a knowledge of all things human and divine is certainly a more far-reaching proposition than that medicine should have taught him a cure for hiccoughs.

[19] Thus, I think, one should best translate καθεωρακέναι μοι δοκῶ ἐκ τῆς ἰατρικῆς. The expression seems singular. Usually Plato says καθορᾶν ἐν cf. F. Ast, *Lexicon Platonicum* 2 [Leipzig, 1836]) s.v. Such phrases as καθορῶντες ὑψόθεν (*Sophistes* 216C) perhaps suggest that the words in question mean: looking out from medicine I have observed. . . .

machus' speech displays a familiarity with the basic presuppositions of the various arts, crafts and sciences.[20] Such knowledge, in my opinion, one should expect of a physician of the fifth century B.C., and Eryximachus may easily have acquired it in his pursuit of medicine.

In Eryximachus' time the value and nature of the arts were widely disputed. Many people asserted that the artisan did not accomplish anything through his art, that his success or failure depended entirely on chance. They went even so far as to deny that there was such a thing as an art; the word, they claimed, was an empty phrase behind which to hide one's ignorance and incompetence. To these attacks the artisans were forced to reply. By a careful analysis of the rules of the various arts they tried to establish the reality of their achievements, which they contended were the results of insight and true understanding. Wherever men gathered to talk about problems important to them individually, or to the community as a whole, one professional after another would defend his art and define the nature of his technique. The physician naturally was among those who participated in these debates. The Hippocratic writing *On the Art* reflects the atmosphere in which such discussions took place.[21] Here a physician speaks in behalf of medicine. He quotes the objections of the adversaries and refutes them word by word. He points to the difficulties of the other arts, to the parallelism between the physician's procedure and that of other artisans. He is apparently well versed in their problems, and he also knows as much philosophy as is needed to provide a more general foundation for his statements.[22]

[20] It has often been noticed that Eryximachus is preoccupied with the τέχναι. Cf. especially L. v. Sybel, *Platon's Symposion* (Marburg, 1888) 26 ff.; Bury (see note 3) xxix: "definitions of a precisely parallel kind for each of these departments [*sc.* of science] are evolved." Since these arts are concerned with all things human and divine, Eryximachus' talk assumes a cosmological aspect, but this tinge of natural philosophy is only incidental. In my opinion, he does not talk as a "Naturforscher," as has sometimes been held (e.g., Friedländer [see note 9] 305). The evaluation of Robin (see note 6) LII, note 1, seems more appropriate: "La *technicité* le préoccupe beaucoup plus que la *cosmologie*." The peculiarity of Eryximachus' approach is the more noteworthy since he was versed in natural philosophy, cf. below p. 160 f.

[21] *Hippocratis Opera*, ed. J. L. Heiberg, *Corpus Medicorum Graecorum* 1.1 (Leipzig and Berlin, 1927) 9 ff. This treatise gives the most vivid and most comprehensive picture of the problems debated, which are referred to also in the fragments of the Pre-Socratics and in the Platonic dialogues. In general, cf. also P. Shorey, *TAPhA* 40 (1909) 185 ff.; J. Wild, *Plato's Theory of Man* (Cambridge, 1946) 45 ff.

[22] The essay *On the Art* is usually considered the work of a sophist; e.g., Robin (see note 6) 24, note 2. That it must have been composed by a physician I have tried to show in Περὶ ἀέρων *und die Sammlung der Hippokratischen Schriften, Problemata*

Eryximachus, then, must have been familiar with the methods and theories not only of medicine but also of the arts in general. The relationship of his profession to gymnastics and husbandry and music must have been a matter of interest to him. The subject which he chooses as his topic at the banquet, the way in which he approaches it, even his contention that medicine led him to observe the facts which he is about to recount, all these features characterize him as a physician of the classical period. The speech is not a caricature but rather an historically correct picture of a medical man of that time. It cannot have been Plato's intention to deride Eryximachus as a pedant, a system-monger, unduly fond of medicine.

Of course, this does not imply that Plato may not in some respects have made light of Eryximachus, just as he lets his humor play on Aristophanes and even on Socrates. Perhaps it is true that the physician "by his fine phrases works himself up to the belief in his own triumphant cleverness."[23] The words with which his encomium of Eros ends (188E) betray belief in his own wisdom and superiority, though it is fair to add that every one of the guests seems well content with his own contribution and that Eryximachus is at least aware of the possibility that involuntarily he may have omitted certain points or that Aristophanes might find a different manner of glorifying the god. This much, however, I venture to affirm: there is no reason to believe that Plato had only ridicule for Eryximachus' medical theories, or that he scoffed at his opinions in general and made him perform his assignment badly.[24]

As far as it is possible to infer his doctrine from his brief résumé of medicine, Eryximachus seems to have demanded that the physician do justice to the good desire of the body and restrain its bad desire, that he produce the one where it is missing, and alter the other where it is prevalent, distinguishing right and wrong in regard to repletion and evacuation (186B–D). Apparently the doctor can reach this goal only

---

IV (Berlin, 1931) 105 ff. [101* ff.]. (I should have known then that Wilamowitz, *Platon* 2 [Berlin, 1919] 253, has maintained the same view without, however, giving any further proof.) Even if the author were not a physician, no educated artisan of Eryximachus' time could be unaware of the issue; the exigencies of the situation in which he found himself demanded that he be concerned with it.

[23] Gildersleeve (see note 1) 109; cf. also Robin (see note 6) LVI.

[24] Cf. Wilamowitz (see note 2) 367: ". . . und für seine Medizin hatte Platon im Grunde nur Spott, denn sie war keine Wissenschaft"; also *ibid.* 362. Among the detractors of Eryximachus' entire performance, F. G. Rettig, *Platons Symposion* 1 (Halle, 1876) 13 ff., is one of the most outspoken representatives. But cf. also Hug-Schöne (see note 3) xxxix.

by prescribing an adequate regimen for the patient.[25] Now the "states-man" Plato rejects dietetic medicine: for the elaborate rules of diet, as he says in his criticism of the medical science proffered with so much severity in the *Republic*, are detrimental to the fulfilment of civic duties. Surgery and the application of drugs alone can therefore be considered legitimate means of treatment (405A–408B). Yet the "scientist" Plato judges dietetics as the only adequate control of sickness, while he con-demns drugging as dangerous (*Timaeus* 89B–C).[26] Plato therefore must have felt some sympathy for Eryximachus' teaching. That he esteemed him and his father, that he respected their medical skill, is evident also from the *Phaedrus*. There the two are called upon as authorities (268A) together with other great artisans, Sophocles and Euripides (268C), and Hippocrates (270C), when the right procedure of any technique is ex-amined.[27] Moreover in the *Protagoras*, Eryximachus' interest in ques-tions of natural philosophy and astronomy is attested (315C). This too, in Plato's opinion, will have stood him in good stead.[28]

[25] Eryximachus expressly acknowledges that his art must take account of man's desires for the pleasure of eating (187E). The sources of his doctrine have been widely discussed. Taylor (see note 9) 218 holds that Pythagorean, Heraclitean and Empedoc-lean ideas are here amalgamated and that the theory as a whole is reminiscent of Sicilian medicine, to which Plato was greatly indebted (*ibid.* 217). I hesitate to attach a label to Eryximachus' views; they are so vague that they seem compatible with the teaching of many schools. The closest parallel to Eryximachus' speech of which I am aware is to be found in the Hippocratic writing *On Ancient Medicine* where πλήρωσις and κένωσις are named as the tendencies to be considered in the healthy and in the sick (*CMG* 1.1 [see note 21] 42, lines 11–12; cf. 41, line 18, and *Symposium* 186C) and where the art of the physician is summarized as knowledge of the right kind of regi-men. The passages adduced by Bury and Hug-Schöne (see note 3) *ad loc.* do not seem comparable; for in the Hippocratic books which they quote, πλήρωσις and κένωσις are not understood as tendencies of the body, as they are by Eryximachus, but rather as means of treatment on which the physician must rely.

[26] Note that Plato is aware of the seeming contradiction between his statements in the *Republic* and those in the *Timaeus*. For he recommends dietetics καθ' ὅσον ἂν ᾖ τῷ σχολή (*Timaeus* 89C). That most people have no leisure for the application of com-plicated dietetic rules was the decisive objection raised in the *Republic* (406C). Cf. also A. E. Taylor, *A Commentary on Plato's Timaeus* (Oxford, 1928) 628 [89C8].

[27] It is perhaps not amiss to point out that Eryximachus, "the noble son of a noble and sober father" (214B), attacks the bad habit of intoxication, and that Plato forbids the guardian of the *Republic* to indulge in μέθη (403E; cf. however *Laws* 637D ff.). Moreover, Acumenus, the father of Eryximachus, was fond of prescribing walks (*Phaedrus* 227A). Simple kinds of gymnastics are advocated in the *Republic* (404B; E; 407B), and even in the *Timaeus* (89A), gymnastic exercises are defended as a method of purging and renewing the body. For Acumenus, cf. also Xenophon, *Memo-rabilia*, 3.13.2.

[28] Wilamowitz (see note 2) 361 infers even from the *Protagoras* that Plato dislikes Eryximachus, for he appears "im Gefolge des Allerweltsweisen Hippias, den Platon

In his non-medical views Eryximachus is doubtless hinting at certain doctrines that are more fully developed in other Platonic writings. The sequence of arts which he advocates, the ascent from the bodily world through music and astronomy to the realm of the divine is the ascent which the *Republic* establishes in education and the *Timaeus* in the understanding of the cosmos. His definition of mantic foreshadows that given by Diotima.[29] The relative importance of his speech within the contest of orations is likewise obvious. It is his task to show the power of Eros in all departments of human activity. Phaedrus and Pausanias know only of Eros' significance for virtue, for morality. Aristophanes praises Eros as the aspiration of the soul that transcends itself and seeks its original unity. Agathon celebrates Eros as the possessor and dispenser of everything good. Eryximachus discusses one pertinent aspect of the subject that must be elaborated before Socrates can reveal the whole truth; and like all the other arguments, that of Eryximachus reappears in Socrates' encomium.[30]

Some interpreters charge Eryximachus with sophistry, obscurity and arbitrariness in dealing with his theme. They criticize the dogmatic manner in which he treats the views of Heraclitus (187A).[31] Yet the arguments he advances are certainly not worse, they rather seem better

---

besonders gering schätzt." But Eryximachus does no more than ask Hippias "some questions"; this can hardly have been a crime in Plato's eyes. Eryximachus' philosophical knowledge is apparent also in his speech; he quotes Heraclitus (187A), and his theory of the double Eros of the body may reflect the teaching of Empedocles; cf. Hug-Schöne (see note 3) xxxix.

[29] I have followed almost literally formulations of Friedländer (see note 9) 305. Even Wilamowitz (see note 2) 367, grants that Eryximachus has some ideas. The agreement between his "Wissenschaftslehre" and that of Plato has been most thoroughly discussed by Sybel (see note 20) 26 ff. His admiration for Eryximachus' doctrine is perhaps exaggerated, though P. Cesareo (*I due Simposi in rapporto all'arte moderna* [Palermo, 1901] 114; cf. also Gildersleeve [see note 1] 110) is mistaken in claiming that Sybel identified Eryximachus with Plato; he clearly saw the limitations of the physician's thought (cf. 27 with 30). The physician indeed rests his case at the point from which Plato takes his flight, as Friedländer says (*ibid.*), who has also pointed to the unfortunate tendency of the critics either to admire or to condemn the speakers altogether ([see note 9] 299, note 2).

[30] Taylor (see note 9) 218, characterizes Eryximachus as the speaker who treats the cosmic aspect of Eros, but cf. above note 20. For the relation of Socrates' speech to the preceding ones, cf. Bury (see note 3) lvii ff. That the speech of Aristophanes is a satire on the theories of Eryximachus and of physicians in general is a contention of Bury (*ibid.*, xxxi ff.) which I do not find convincing; Wilamowitz (see note 2) 367 seems to agree with Bury.

[31] Cf. Bury (see note 3) *ad loc.*

than those of the others, Socrates excepted; at least, Eryximachus reasons and is conversant with philosophy. There may be ambiguities and inconsistencies in his oration. Still Socrates reserves for him the compliment that he "fought well" (193E–194A). This praise, even if touched with irony, cannot be discounted, for Socrates notes whether the others speak "sufficiently and well" (177E).[32] The statement must mean that to Plato, Eryximachus was not the least noteworthy of the speakers.

Contrary to the contention, then, that the physician is represented as a pedant, that he makes a fool of himself whenever he starts discussing a medical topic or when he elaborates the main subject of the evening, he is portrayed realistically and with sympathy. This result, I think, squares well with the fact that Eryximachus, in addition to giving the speeches that have been considered so far, plays an important rôle throughout the symposium. If one analyzes the framework of the dialogue carefully, he realizes that the physician is by no means just one of the guests among the others, but is a prominent figure at the banquet.

First of all, Eryximachus is responsible for the decision that the symposium be not devoted to excessive drinking, which would make it impossible that speeches be given at all. On his advice the company resolves that everybody drink only according to his pleasure (176D–E).[33] Moreover, it is he who moves that the flute-girl be dismissed and that the entertainment be conversation rather than music (176E). And it is he again who suggests that each guest make a speech in honor of Eros (176E–177D).[34] To be sure, "the tale is not his," as he says himself (177A). Phaedrus has always wondered why none of the poets or sophists has ever given to Eros the praise due to him, and he has often expressed his astonishment to Eryximachus, his friend and lover (177A–C). But from Phaedrus' protestation no action would ensue here and now, were it not for Eryximachus. If Phaedrus is "the father of the subject"

[32] For the interpretation of the statement made in 177E, cf. Friedländer (see note 9) 299. Socrates' unqualified approval of Eryximachus can be fully appreciated only in comparison with his pretended praise of Agathon's speech which he immediately retracts (198A–B).

[33] Cf. above p. 154. Bury (see note 3) vii says that the potations are restricted on the proposal of Pausanias. But the latter asks only for deliberation (σκοπεῖσθε 176A) and is apparently not aware of a good way to reach the ease which he wishes to enjoy (*ibid.*). Taylor (see note 9) 211 is right in stating that "on the advice of the physician Eryximachus" it is resolved that there be no enforced deep "potting."

[34] This fact, of course, is generally recognized. The statement of Wilamowitz (see note 2) 362 that Phaedrus "das Thema stellt" is obviously only a slip.

(177D) that will be discussed, Eryximachus, one might say, is "the father of the debate" that is about to take place. Intent on prescribing the proper diet for his friends, on checking their bad desire and on encouraging their good one, and being the good doctor that he is, he knows when the right moment has come for action. He has diagnosed that these people who are disinclined to drink would be willing to listen to his condemnation of drunkenness (176C). He also diagnoses that the present occasion provides the opportunity for doing a favor to Phaedrus by celebrating Eros (177C).[35] For he feels sure that the guests will be delighted to praise this god: they are all lovers and in love (177D–E). The physician is not mistaken in his judgment. His motion that the banquet be celebrated by speeches on Eros is unanimously accepted (177E–178A).

But it is not only the introductory scene which is dominated by Eryximachus; even later he continues to play an outstanding part. Together with Phaedrus, he is the president of the banquet. Whenever the speeches are formally introduced or concluded, either Phaedrus or Eryximachus is addressed; whenever difficulties arise or a diverting chat sets in, one of the two intervenes or is drawn into the conversation. Pausanias addresses Phaedrus (180C; 185C), and so do Agathon (197C; E) and Socrates (212B; C). Phaedrus also puts an end to the quarrel between Socrates and Agathon (194D–E), and he authorizes Socrates to talk as he pleases (199B–C). Eryximachus, on the other hand, is the "guardian" (189A) over the speech of Aristophanes, who directs his oration to him (189C; 193D). Socrates turns to Eryximachus before and after Agathon's talk (194A; 198A–B).[36] Last but not least, when Alcibiades threatens to make himself president of the banquet (213E) and urges the company to drink, Eryximachus saves the situation: he induces him to follow the procedure agreed upon at the beginning and to give a

---

[35] In 176C, note the words: ἐπειδὴ οὖν μοι δοκεῖ οὐδεὶς τῶν παρόντων προθύμως ἔχειν πρὸς τὸ πολὺν πίνειν οἶνον, ἴσως . . . ἧττον ἂν εἴην ἀηδής, and again in 177C; ἐν τῷ παρόντι πρέπον μοι δοκεῖ εἶναι ἡμῖν τοῖς παροῦσι. To observe the καιρός is one of the main tasks of the physician, as is evident from the Hippocratic writings, cf. Edelstein (see note 22) 114 [109*].

[36] Robin (see note 6) xiv seems astonished that Eryximachus fails to assume leadership in the conversation, while he characterizes Phaedrus as president of the banquet who is addressed by all the speakers. This has been shown to be erroneous. Incidentally, Socrates, though he addresses Phaedrus, also turns to the whole company (212B–C), and Alcibiades simply addresses the guests (215A), either because he considers himself president of the banquet (Robin, *ibid.*), or because the subject introduced by Eryximachus has been given up in favor of a new topic.

speech like the others (214A–C). Spurred on by Eryximachus, Alcibiades decides to praise Socrates (214D).[37]

In all the various acts of the symposium, then, Eryximachus appears as a person of distinction, a fact strangely neglected, it seems, by all modern interpreters in their evaluation of his rank among the guests. This physician is not simply on sufferance in the company with which he feasts.[38] He is their peer, nay, in some respects, their superior. For he exercises a certain authority over them. Within the framework of the dialogue, he is indeed more important than anybody else. Pausanias and Aristophanes and Socrates and even Agathon, the host, are but speakers; occasionally they participate in the interludes. Phaedrus assumes his place as president only through Eryximachus; it is mere politeness that he, to whom Eryximachus has given credit for his suggestion of the subject, is honored as the originator of the speeches. Eryximachus, however, lays the foundation for the whole contest. He holds the conversation together at the point where it is in danger of breaking up. As there would be no encomia of Eros without him, there would be no praise of Socrates without his insistence.

Now that the exceptional rôle of Eryximachus has become evident, one can hardly help asking whether it may be of some significance that it is a physician who is given such a prominent position. Of course, it could be merely by chance that Eryximachus stands in the foreground of the scene. It may be that Phaedrus really talked to him in the way described; it may be that Eryximachus did suggest a eulogy of Eros at a banquet of which Plato had heard, and that he acted as president of the gathering because he had introduced the motion that led to the contest of speeches. On the other hand, even supposing that there was some historical evidence on which Plato based his report, he has surely taken great pains in describing Eryximachus and in portraying the

[37] That Socrates, too, is asked whether he agrees to Alcibiades' speaking (214E) seems natural and merely polite; it does not detract from the weight of Eryximachus' words. Bury (see note 3) xxiv has pointed out that in the "third act" account is taken only of Agathon, the host, Eryximachus and Socrates. Robin (see note 6) LII thinks that Eryximachus' rôle in the scene in question only serves to emphasize the contrast between Alcibiades' originality and adventurous fantasy, and the mediocrity of the physician of the "juste milieu." Such an interpretation, however, hardly does justice to the significance of Eryximachus' intervention.

[38] Contrary to Gildersleeve, cf. above p. 153. If among those who leave the symposium, Phaedrus and Eryximachus alone are mentioned by name (223B), this is again an indication of their importance within the framework of the dialogue as well as a feature that stresses their moderation (Bury [see note 3] xxviii).

physician. Twice he shows Eryximachus acting in this capacity, at the very beginning when he advises against μέθη (176c–d), and in the middle of the piece when he cures Aristophanes' hiccoughs (185d–e). In the final part, again, Alcibiades solemnly refers to Eryximachus as a physician (214b). One is never allowed to forget that he is a doctor. Could this be without meaning, just a fortuitous circumstance?

Yet, as Jowett says: "If it be true that there are more things in the *Symposium* of Plato than any commentator has dreamed of, it is also true that many things have been imagined which are not really to be found there."[39] I should hesitate to suggest an answer to the question raised, were it not certain that for Plato, the physician was an exemplar, that in his ethical inquiries he used the medical art as a simile. That Plato's thought is tinged by medical concepts has often been maintained during the past few decades.[40] As a matter of fact, it has been contended that medicine influenced him as deeply as did mathematics: while the latter shaped his natural philosophy, the former is said to have molded his ethical doctrine. From medicine, it has been assumed, Plato took the distinction between art and chance, between conscious and purposeful actions and haphazard decisions; the dignity of a practical science to which he wished to raise ethics already had been realized in the science of medicine. Even the definition of the aim of moral endeavor, which is based on the concept of an innate good of the soul, seems indebted to definitions of medical treatment that are based on the concept of an innate good of the body. Whether such assumptions are correct or not, it is a fact that for Plato the relationship between the physician and his patient served as a model of human relationship, and it is with his use of this parallel alone that I am here concerned.[41]

[39] Jowett (see note 10) 524.

[40] One of the first to deal with the subject was H. Nohl, *Sokrates und die Ethik* (Tübingen, 1904) 34 ff. The discussion of the problem has been placed on a broader basis by E. Hoffmann, "Der gegenwärtige Stand der Platonforschung," Anhang zu E. Zeller, *Die Philosophie der Griechen* (2.1, fifth edition) 1070 ff. Cf. also W. Jaeger, *Paideia* 2 (Oxford, 1944) 131; 145; 321 f., and Taylor (see note 9) 217.

[41] In another paper I propose to deal in detail with the general bearing of medicine on Platonic ethics and at the same time to investigate the use of the simile of the physician in early and late Greek philosophy. Generally speaking, it seems to me that the distinction between τέχνη and τύχη is to be found not only in medicine but also in other arts, just as the innate good of the object is a concern not only of the physician but also of other artisans; e.g., *Gorgias* 503e, and P. Shorey, *The Idea of Good in Plato's Republic*, University of Chicago Studies in Classical Philology 1 (Chicago, 1895) 227. It is most of all the general analogy between body and soul that has influenced Plato's thought. [See below, p. 349 ff.—Ed.].

Plato finds occasion to mention the physician in his discussion of rulership (*Politicus* 293A–C); for the physician, to him, is the ruler of his patients. Whichever method of healing he may employ, whether he follow books or not, whether he be poor or rich, he is called a doctor, if he has knowledge of medicine and acts for the benefit of the sick. All prescriptions which such a man gives, even those which mean temporary harm or pain, are considered justified because he is an expert in his art, and people submit to his ordinances. This common attitude toward the doctor indicates the criterion of right rulership. It is not the social standing of the ruler, nor the attestation of his prescripts, nor their specific content that matters; it is his knowledge alone that decides about his fitness. The example of the physician, to be sure, is not the only one through which Plato clarifies this view. He refers also to the trainer (294D), to the captain (297A), and finally to the weaver (308D). But the physician is the most representative type of the ruler and remains in the foreground of the discussion. He is mentioned together with the trainer (295C) and the captain (298A ff.), he alone is selected when the general definition of rulership is given (293C), and Plato says expressly that his art provides an especially good example of right rule (293B; cf. 296B–C).[42]

Moreover, there is apparently one characteristic of rulership that can be brought out solely by looking at the "image" of the physician. He does not only command, he sees to it that his patients understand the rules given and follow them voluntarily. Certainly, the slave doctor behaves differently. Without asking the sick for an account of their diseases, he prescribes like an autocrat what he thinks necessary (*Laws* 720C). Not so, however, the freeborn doctor. He talks to his patients, he learns from them and in turn instructs them. He gives no prescription until he has persuaded the sick, and he leads them on by persuasion (*ibid.* 720D–E). For his leadership rests on persuasion, not on force (*ibid.* 722B). It is true that if the slave doctor were ever to meet the freeborn doctor and to witness his procedure, he would burst into laughter and say with contempt that the patient wishes to regain his health, that he does not wish to become a doctor himself (*ibid.* 857C–E). Yet it is exactly

---

[42] Note the words: τοὺς ἰατροὺς οὐχ ἥκιστα νενομίκαμεν. L. Campbell, *The Sophistes and Politicus of Plato* (Oxford, 1867) *ad loc.*, translates "and physicians more especially." H. N. Fowler's translation (Plato 3 [Loeb] 1925), "And physicians offer a particularly good example," seems more adequate.

the aim of the good doctor to educate his patient as well as to heal him, and in this respect he is the model of the true ruler.[43]

The simile of the physician, then, has indeed great significance for Plato, though at the same time its limitations must not be overlooked. It is the statesman or the lawgiver rather than the philosopher whom he compares with the physician. Quite a different human relationship prevails between the philosopher and his pupil and the statesman or lawgiver and the citizen. For while the statesman is, or ought to be, an expert who rules over men through a knowledge which he has but they lack, or governs and educates them by means of laws, the philosopher does not exercise any rule, nor is he supposed to teach others the truth which he has in his possession. The philosopher, as Socrates says himself, practices the art of the midwife. He has no wisdom within himself, he can only help his fellows to bring forth their own knowledge (*Theaetetus* 149A ff.). Later philosophers glorify the philosopher as the physician of the soul. To Plato, however, philosophy is not a kind of medicine tending the patient on his sickbed and putting him under the spell of sound and salutary tales through which he will be able to void his vast overload of sins and fill instead "his fearful emptiness of righteousness" (Philo, *Quis rer. div. heres*, 297). To Plato, the philosopher is not a physician, sitting in his clinic where people come with their sickness that he may lecture them and heal them through his words, imparting wisdom to them (Epictetus, 3.23.30). The Platonic philosopher is but a humble helper in the search for truth; unlike the statesman or lawgiver, he has no authority over men, nor does he strive for it.[44]

[34] For *Laws* 720c ff. and 857c, cf. also W. Jaeger, *Paideia* 3 (New York, 1944) 215. I am not sure that Plato's account is historically correct in all respects. The distinction between slave doctors who treat slaves and freeborn doctors who treat freeborn patients is not warranted by the evidence available. On the other hand, the good doctor did hold converse with the sick, even though he did not educate them to be physicians, and medical men even wrote books on diseases for the use of laymen. Nor can there be any doubt that the physicians considered their relationship to their patients as that of a ruler to his subjects. Cf. in general Edelstein (see note 22) 102; 105, note 1 [98*; 100,* note 20].

[44] As far as I know, it is only in *Phaedo* 89A that Socrates is said to act like a physician. But here, diagnosing his listeners' diseases—they are perturbed by the objections raised—he heals them through an exhortatory speech, not through philosophical teaching. In an analogous way, the simile is applied by Protagoras, who states that in education the sophist changes the soul by the use of words, just as the physician changes the body by the use of drugs (*Theaetetus* 167A). The difference of the simile of the physician from that of the midwife has not sufficiently been stressed

The comparisons of the philosopher with a midwife, of the statesman with a physician, occur only in the later works of Plato, the *Theaetetus*, the *Politicus*, the *Laws*. Yet they express in a pregnant form a
belief that is inherent, I think, in all Platonic writings. The earlier dialogues, always ending with a negative result, are full of Socrates' protestation that "he does not know." The theory of recollection of the truth
rests on the assumption that the knowledge resides in man's own
thought. The method of the philosopher, as it is finally evolved, is that
of dialectics, and it is his art of dialectics which Socrates likens to the
art of midwifery (*Theaetetus* 161E). Even in the *Gorgias* where two arts
are distinguished, the one dealing with the body, the other with the
soul, it is legislation and justice, not philosophy, that are compared with
gymnastics and medicine (464B). Nor is the fundamental distinction
between philosopher and statesman impaired by Plato's assertion that
one day the king must become a philosopher, or the philosopher a king,
if the state of affairs in this world is ever to change for the better. In
the exercise of their functions as philosopher and statesman there would
still be the difference between authoritative rule and dialectical investigation. If the statesman rises above the sophist, the philosopher rises
above the statesman in more than a geometrical proportion (*Politicus*
257B).

The bearing of the simile of the physician having been outlined, it
should now be possible to conjecture with some assurance whether the
rôle of Eryximachus in the *Symposium* has any meaning in regard to its
content. That Plato, in depicting Eryximachus, was guided by his view
of the physician's art as a model seems obvious. Eryximachus rules over
his patients by virtue of his knowledge; he persuades them so that they
obey him voluntarily. When he has learned from the guests what their
complaints are, he gives his advice and they in turn are persuaded and
obey him (176D). When Aristophanes turns to Eryximachus and informs
him of his sickness, the physician enumerates in detail three possible
means of treatment, and thus instructs Aristophanes how to take care
of his ailment; he does not prescribe any one treatment in an autocratic
manner.[45] Nor are Eryximachus' friends less aware of the fact than is

---

by Hoffmann (see note 40) 1075. Incidentally, Zeller ([see note 40] 637, note 2)
claims that *Republic* 489B–C identifies the philosopher with the physician. Yet apart
from the fact that only one detail is selected for comparison, in the passage in question the philosopher is viewed as the ruler of the many.

[45] Much has been written on the meaning of this episode which causes Eryxi-

Plato that the physician is a ruler, that he must be esteemed as such. When Alcibiades is asked by Eryximachus: "What are we going to do?" he answers: "Whatever you command, for it is necessary to obey you; the leech is of the worth of many other men" (214B).[46] Of course, I do not mean to claim that all the features of Plato's interpretation of the doctor's relationship to his patients are woven into this dialogue. The representation of Eryximachus is not a paradigm of the medical art. But the essential characteristics of the good doctor are sharply accentuated in his portrait. He prescribes, the others follow his instructions. His wisdom is superior; the others, in their failings, acquire insight from him that they themselves do not possess. They are led to grasp the truth by persuasion.

And is this not exactly the experience of him who listens to the various speeches given at the banquet? Each of the speakers talks with authority, in a dogmatic fashion. Their teaching is non-dialectical and therefore unphilosophical. Even Socrates is not in his usual mood. Although he chides Agathon for believing that wisdom could flow from one person into another as water flows through wool from a fuller cup into one that is emptier (175D), later on he himself imparts the knowledge that he has obtained from Diotima with the assurance of the initiated. And could not all of the speakers say what Socrates says at the end of his oration (212B): of this I am persuaded and of this I try to persuade others? For they no less than Socrates have indulged in the recounting of mythical tales of the truth of which one cannot be sure, but can only be persuaded, and can only hope to persuade others.[47] Besides, their speeches are encomia (e.g., 177E), eulogies of a god or

---

machus to speak in place of Aristophanes. Within the context of the whole, the scene may have been introduced so as to make the intended order of the speeches appear incidental, cf. K. Reinhardt, *Platons Mythen* (Bonn, 1927) 63; Friedländer, *Platon* 1 (Berlin and Leipzig, 1928) 187 f., but it also serves to underline the position of the physician at the banquet.

[46] The verse from Homer (*Iliad* 11.517) is also quoted in the *Politicus* (297E), cf. above p. 166.

[47] That the content of the *Symposium* is mythical has been acknowledged by Friedländer (see note 45) 207 and by Wilamowitz, who has especially stressed the non-dialectical character of its teaching ([see note 2] 360) and the fact that Socrates speaks only of persuasion ([see note 22] 170 f.). P. Frutiger, *Les Mythes de Platon* (Paris, 1930) 112 ff., judges differently, but he fails to account for the features just referred to. To be sure, the myth told by Socrates is a "true myth," based on the *logos*, while the others are not (cf. Friedländer, *ibid.* 207 f.). Fundamentally, however, all orations are unphilosophical, at least from the standpoint of the Platonic system.

demon, just as Alcibiades' oration is an encomium (214D) of Socrates, who embodies the ideal of the good man. Such encomia the *Republic* leaves to poetry as its sole and justifiable province after Homer and the tragedians have been expelled from the city (607A). In the *Symposium* they are recited in competition with the works of poets and sophists who have neglected their duty of praising Eros (177A–B).[48] They are composed with that true rhetorical art which is allied with kingly statesmanship and uses myths for the persuasion of the many (*Politicus* 304C–D). Although they are so wondrous that one forgets oneself in hearing them and wishes them to be retold again and again, they do not convey the truth in philosophical terms; nor are they capable of doing so on account of their subject matter. For Eros leads man to the vision of the beautiful which he beholds but with "the eye of faith and desire,"[49] while it is thought that enables him to ascertain the good through dialectics, and thus to know.

That the physician, the exemplar of authority that persuades, is given such a significant rôle in the *Symposium*, is, I suggest, an intentional device of Plato. It is meant to emphasize the singularity of the content of this dialogue, the specific character of its method and instruction. Many other features of the framework of the *Symposium* seem to serve the same purpose.[50] With the exception of Socrates, no philosopher is present at this banquet at which speeches are prescribed as a kind of diet for those who feel unable to drink as much as would fit the occasion. Even if these people are highly educated and cultured, they are not investigators of the truth in their own right. Nor do they belong to the inner circle of Socrates' friends; they are outsiders, living far apart from the man who is the wisest of his generation, or, like Alcibiades, unable to submit to his guidance. Even those who retell the conversation are among the least noble of Socrates' pupils; Aristodemus, who apes him in externals (173B), and Apollodorus, a crazy fellow (173D), not a sober thinker but rather a passionate enthusiast who cannot control his emotions (*Phaedo* 117D). Finally, the people to whom the story is told are businessmen, men of the practical life (173C). It is as if Plato, by giving such a setting to his work, had attempted to treat with irony the teach-

[48] The relation of the passage in the *Republic* to the *Symposium* has been pointed out by Friedländer (see note 45) 142; the rhetorical character of the speeches has been stressed by Jaeger (see note 40) 180.

[49] Cf. Jowett (see note 10) 533.

[50] For the interpretation of the framework of the dialogue, cf. also Friedländer (see note 9) 295 ff.; Wilamowitz (see note 2) 359 f.

ing of that dialogue which to so many generations has seemed his greatest on account of the seducing splendor of its beauty. Perhaps he was aware of the fact that if it were taken as his final word, as his deepest insight, reason might find it difficult to assert the supremacy which he attributed to thinking, even above the claim of beauty.

THE METHODISTS*

Beside the Dogmatists and the Empiricists, the Methodists were the most important school of physicians in Imperial times. The school's literary legacy is lost, with the exception of isolated books by Soranus, of which there survive: in Greek, *Soranus*, ed. J. Ilberg, Leipzig, 1927, CMG IV, and in Latin translation, Caelius Aurelianus, *De morbis acutis et chronicis* (for editions, see Ilberg, "Vorläufiges zu Caelius Aurelianus," S.-Ber. Sächs. Ges. phil.-hist. Kl. LXXVII 1925, H. 1,7). The numerous fragments have not yet been collected. Moreover, there is no study of Methodist doctrine based on an attempt to relate it to general developments; the only work to date has been concerned with chronology and with individual physicians belonging to the school. The most complete material is to be found in the histories of medicine (J. F. K. Hecker, *Geschichte der Heilkunde*, Berlin, 1822, I, 394 ff.; K. Sprengel, *Versuch einer pragmatischen Geschichte der Arzneikunde*, Halle, 1823, II³, 28 ff.; H. Haeser, *Lehrbuch der Geschichte der Medizin*, Berlin, 1863, I³, 268 ff., 304 ff.; R. Fuchs, "Geschichte der Heilkunde bei den Griechen," in Neuburger-Pagel, *Handbuch der Geschichte der Medizin*, Jena, 1902, p. 328 ff.).

I. ADHERENTS TO THE SCHOOL; QUESTIONS OF CHRONOLOGY

The following are mentioned as adherents of the school: Thessalos, Themison, Proklos, Reginos, Antipatros, Eudemos, Mnaseas, Philon, Dionysios, Menemachos, Olympikos, Apollonides, Soranus, Julianus (Galen X 52–53 K.). Most of these physicians are also enumerated in the pseudo-Galenic εἰσαγωγή (XIV, 684 K.; Ὀλυμπιακός should read

* "Methodiker," Pauly-Wissowa, *Realenzyklopädie der klassischen Altertumswissenschaft*, Supplementband VI, Stuttgart: Metzler, 1935, cols. 358–73.

In this translation, words like Dogmatic, Empiricist, Methodist, Skeptic have been capitalized when they seem to refer to definite schools rather than general concepts.—Ed.

'Ολυμπικός, cf. M. Wellmann, *Hermes*, LVII, 406, 4). Mention is also made of M. Modius Asiaticus (Kaibel, *Epigrammata Graeca*, 306. 116). For the times, lives, and teachings of the individual physicians, cf. corresponding articles in the *Realencyclopädie* and M. Wellmann, 396 ff. Concerning Meges, whom he also mentions, cf. p. 176 below. More extensive lists include doubtful or untrue data.

The founder of the Methodist school is generally taken to be Themison of Laodicea, a pupil of Asclepiades of Bithynia, whose opinions he merely transformed in his new doctrine. Thessalos is believed to have then completed the systematization of Methodist teaching at the time of Nero. This theory has most recently been voiced by Wellmann, 396. 401. 405. This point of view is based on the pseudo-Galenic εἰσαγωγή, the author of which says: μεθοδικῆς δὲ ἦρξε μὲν Θεμίσων ὁ Λαοδικεὺς τῆς Συρίας παρ' Ἀσκληπιάδου τοῦ λογικοῦ ἐφοδιασθεὶς εἰς τὴν εὕρεσιν τῆς μεθοδικῆς αἱρέσεως, ἐτελείωσε δὲ αὐτὴν Θεσσαλὸς ὁ Τραλλιανός (XIV 684 K.).

This, however, cannot be so, for Galen himself, who once designated Asclepiades, Themison, and Thessalos as the ones to whom the elements of Methodist thinking should be traced back (οἷς sc. λόγοις . . . ὧν ὁ Ἀσκληπιάδης καὶ Θεμίσων καὶ Θεσσαλλὸς ἔθεντο τὰ στοιχεῖα XVIII a 256 K.), calls Thessalos the founder of the school (τὸν τῆς αἱρέσεως αὐτῶν [sc. τῶν μεθοδικῶν] ἄρξαντα Θεσσαλόν I 176 K.), and the Methodists the pupils of Thessalos, or Thessaleans (τοὺς τὴν Θεσσαλοῦ πρεσβεύοντας αἵρεσιν, οἱ ἀπὸ τοῦ Θεσσαλοῦ X 305 K. οἱ Θεσσάλειοι X 269 K.). Themison is the man who, before Thessalos, planted the first seed (πρὸ τούτου ὁ τὴν ῥίζαν αὐτοῖς τῆς ἐμπληξίας ταύτης ὑποθέμενος X 52 K.), but was not the school's founder. This is corroborated by the statement of Celsus: "On the authority of the teaching of Themison, as they would like people to believe, certain physicians these days claim the following . . . a medicine . . ., which they define as a certain way, which they call 'method' " (quidam medici saeculi nostri, sub auctore ut ipsi videri volunt Themisone, contendunt . . . medicinam . . . quam ita finiunt ut quasi viam quandam quam μέθοδον nominant . . . esse contendant, 26, 12 Marx). Thus, according to Celsus, too, Themison is not the founder of the Methodist school; the Methodists merely cite him and represent their doctrine as the outcome of his, as an interpretation of his views. What Galen considers a fact, Celsus cites as the contention of the Methodists, namely, that Themison's teaching is the root of their method. Since Themison is not the founder of the school, but only the predecessor whose teaching constituted its point of departure, Celsus can even call the Methodists rivals of Themison (Themisonis aemuli 27, 17); had they been his pupils, they could not have been so designated. Celsus does not say who founded Methodism. According to him, Themison merely altered certain aspects of Asclepidean doctrine and thereby created his own doctrine (ex cuius [sc. Asclepiadis] successoribus Themison nuper ipse quoque quaedam in senectute deflexit, 18, 31–19, 1). As one of the followers of Asclepiades, however, Themison is a Dogmatist (as were all the other "aemuli Asclepiadis" 20, 24).

Soranus, too, denies that Themison founded the Methodist school. Caelius Aurelianus describes the treatment of phrenitis according to the tenets of the school (haec est secundum methodum curatio phreniticae passionis) and then gives the opinions of other schools and their leaders (dehinc aliarum sectarum principes quid ordinaverint persequamur, *m. a.* I 11, 99). He speaks about Diocles, Erasistratos, Asclepiades, and finally about Themison, counting him, therefore, among the leaders of other sects, and not as belonging to the Methodist school. Yet Themison does have a special relationship to Methodism: quomodo Themison scribens celerum passionum curationes antiquorum peccatis assentiens quaedam incondita dereliquit, nam necdum purgaverat suam sectam et ob hoc phreniticorum ordinans curationem quibusdam erroribus implicatur, ipsius quoque inspicienda sunt singula (16, 155). When he wrote the work which Caelius cites, Themison already had a school of his own; but, in Caelius' opinion and in the opinion of the Methodists, he was still making mistakes, which he later, after purging his sect, was able to avoid. For, haec nunc Themison phreniticis curandis ordinavit, sed post ex methodica secta multa bona contulit medicinae (165). Later on, he adopted some of the tenets of the Methodists, thereby freeing his own system of errors. Thus Soranus, too, is of the opinion that the Methodist school arose independently of Themison and was not founded by him; indeed, in Soranus' view, it was rather Themison himself who was influenced by the Methodists. It remains uncertain whether Soranus, too, saw Themison's teaching as the point of departure of the Methodists. He claims, on the contrary—as Celsus and Galen do not—that Themison learnt from the Methodists; that he was, in fact, a follower of Thessalos; and that he calls Thessalos to witness (Themison . . . in quibusdam errare cognoscitur nondum sectam methodum respiciens, *m. ch.* II 1, 57; veterum methodicorum . . . alii solutionem ut Thessalus manifestat atque eius decessores ut Themison, II 7, 96: Themison vero iudicavit attestante Thessalo, II 13, 188). According to Soranus, Themison's development was a complicated one. In his youth, he was a pupil and follower of Asclepiades (cf. also *m. ch.* I 4, 140. 5, 179). Then he founded his own school, which he later remodeled in accordance with Methodist doctrines, so that on many questions he wrote like a Methodist (*m. ch.* V 2, 51) and was unable to abide by his own law (*m. ch.* I 5, 179).

The consensus among Celsus, Soranus, and Galen in their statements about Themison renders untrustworthy the single contention in opposition to them, that of the pseudo-Galenic εἰσαγωγή. Themison cannot be the founder of the Methodist school. Since Themison's school was not the Methodist school, Themison's pupils were not Methodists; and for this reason Meges was not a Methodist, Wellmann 405 to the contrary. But is Thessalos the originator of Methodism, as Galen says and as Soranus indicates by speaking of Thessalos and his followers (Thessalus et eius sectatores, *m. a.* I 1, 22) when he means the Methodists? To what period is the founding of the school to be attributed?

Thessalos was the most esteemed physician of the time of Nero; eadem aetas Neronis principatu ad Thessalum transilivit (Pliny, *n. h.* XXIX 6), and he dedicated one of his books to Nero (Galen, X 7 K.). His exact dates are not known, but even if, at the height of his success in Nero's reign, he was over sixty years of age, he can scarcely have founded the Methodist school before the end of the second, or beginning of the third, decade A.D. How far do the other assertions about chronology coincide with this?

Celsus says that physicians of his own time, of his generation (medici saeculi nostri, 26, 12), gave the name "method" to the medicine they taught (26, 23 ff.). The term "method," then, was first used by physicians of Celsus' generation, and the school must have been founded by them. Celsus writes toward the end of the reign of Tiberius, around 30 A.D. Thus the school can have arisen at the beginning of the first century A.D., at the earliest. It is not possible in any case to place the founding of the school at the end of the Republic, still less in the year 40 B.C. (Wellmann 396; there is no longer any foundation for this dating. Wellmann is of the opinion that Antonius Musa, who treated the Emperor Augustus in 23 B.C., altered Themison's doctrine. But since Themison was not the founder of the "method," and since his is not the Methodist doctrine, this is of no relevance for the Methodist school. Moreover, Antonius Musa seems not to have altered the doctrine of Themison but that of Asclepiades, of whom both he and Themison were students. According to Celsus, Themison also [ipse quoque 19, 1] altered Asclepiades' teaching. Others, then, did so, too. Pliny, *n. h.* XXIX 6 related that Asclepiades' sect, like all the earlier ones, was abandoned. If he is referring to changes made by Themison and then to others made by Musa, then, contrary to the opinion of Wellmann, an emendation is called for: sed et illa [sc. placita Asclepiadis] mutavit). It is certain that the Methodist school was founded, at the earliest, at the beginning of the first century.

The prerequisite of the "method" is the doctrine of Themison, of whose dates no exact information has come down to us. It is certain only that he heard Asclepiades teach (auditor eius [sc. Asclepiadis] Themison fuit, Pliny, *n. h.* XXIX 6). Asclepiades came to Rome in 91 B.C. at the latest (cf. Wellmann, *Ilbergs Jahrb.* XXI 1908, 685). If he was then about thirty years of age (I assume a somewhat different age from Wellmann 396, who places Themison's prime in 90–80 B.C.), he may have lived to about 30 B.C., for he died in extreme old age (suprema in senecta, Pliny, *n. h.* VII 37). It is not recorded when Themison was his pupil. If, as would be natural, this occurred when he was young, perhaps at the age of twenty (Themison . . . seque inter initia adscripsit illi [sc. Asclepiadi], Pliny, *n. h.* XXIX 6; according to Soranus, Themison, as a young man, was still entangled in the errors of Asclepiades [in iuventute, *m. a.* II 12, 84]), and if he heard Asclepiades teach shortly before the latter's death, the alterations he made in the doctrine would fall roughly into the second decade of the first century A.D., for he made them as a man of over sixty (in senectute, Celsus 19, 1; procedente vita, Pliny, *n. h.* XXIX 6). Themison's own school cannot have been founded much earlier, for Celsus says that it had happened recently (nuper, 19, 1); and he uses this dating when speaking of Themison in another passage (105, 27), as he does of Cassius (28, 23). Since Themison's new doctrine is the prerequisite of the "method," this latter arose, at the earliest, in the second decade of the first century A.D., and perhaps not until the third decade. Themison, at that time, would be a man of over seventy years of age, and he may thus still have learnt from Thessalos and the "method," as Soranus claims. From this point of departure also, therefore, one arrives at about the same foundation date as on the presupposition that Thessalos was the founder of the school. There is nothing to contradict the contention that Thessalos was the founder of the "method." Even if Asclepiades' death is placed in 40 B.C., as would follow from Wellmann's, in itself not entirely convincing, dating,

177

Themison's own doctrine would on the same premises have originated in the first decade of the first century A.D. Themison, then, would have been over eighty if the "method" was founded after 20 A.D.

But why does Celsus not mention Thessalos? Why is he silent concerning the founder of the "method"? In the context in which he wrote, he was not obliged to mention the originator of the school. There is almost an element of disdain in the way he speaks of certain physicians who represent the "method," just as Celsus in general rejects the Methodist system completely.

It is highly probable that Thessalos originated the "method." The single contradictory evidence (Galen XIV 684 K.) is, in any case, of doubtful credibility since it is based on the presupposition, which is certainly false, that Themison was the founder of the "method." It seems to go back to an interpretation of the Galen passage from which the pseudo-Galenic writing itself derived the list of followers which it was to hand down (Galen X 52 f. K.), incomplete though it was. As Galen says, Themison laid the foundation of the "method" before Thessalos was active, and this gave rise to μεθοδικῆς δὲ ἦρξε μὲν Θεμίσων . . . ἐτελείωσε δὲ αὐτὴν Θεσσαλός . . .; moreover, the importance of Thessalos in the founding of the school was established by Galen's other statements.[1] But it is also possible that Thessalos was only later singled out as chief representative of the "method" and elevated to the position of originator of the school for objective reasons. Perhaps at the beginning the Methodist school attached its doctrine just as little to the name of a single individual as did the Empiricists, taking their name rather from their principles (cf. Deichgräber, *Die griechische Empirikerschule*, Berlin, 1930, 43, 11). Perhaps Celsus, writing as a contemporary, was following this tendency when he named no names. Then Soranus and Galen, surveying the historical development from a considerable distance in time, adduced names, just as later it was thought possible to name founders of the Empiricist school.

The school, probably founded by Thessalos at the beginning of the first century A.D., had numerous adherents down to the end of the sec-

[1] Galen's historical statements, therefore, are manipulated along doxographic-isagogic lines, in conformity with the tendency of the pseudo-Galenic writing (cf. Diller, *Hermes* LXVIII 176–77). If one is unwilling to presume a direct dependence because of the probable chronological closeness of the two writings, one would have to think, here and in the following discussion, of a common antecedent and of versions varying in accordance with the authors' individuality.

ond century. Although the Methodists quarreled among themselves over almost every important question and interpreted the basic doctrines in different ways (οἱ . . . ἄπαντες ἀλλήλοις τε καὶ τῷ Θεσσαλῷ διηνέχθησαν Galen X 35 K.), the external unity of the school was preserved. The pseudo-Galenic writing, εἰσαγωγή, places three men, Olympikos, Menemachos, and Soranus in opposition to the other Methodists and says that they had quarreled with the aforementioned over certain points (διεστασίασαν δὲ περί τινων ἐν αὐτῇ Galen XIV 684 K.). Apparently, then, the others were more agreed among themselves, and the difference between these three and the rest of the Methodists was particularly great. It is for this reason that there was talk of a transformation or reformation of the "method" by Olympikos, and on the strength of this passage he and his followers were called young Methodists in contrast to the old Methodists (Wellmann 406 ff.). For this the words offer no basis, especially since disputes over questions of doctrine were so frequent among the Methodists. The opposition between the parties seems to have been taken from the same pseudo-Galenic writing from which the list of adherents of the school and the chronology of its founding were derived. For Galen first enumerates Thessalos, Themison, and a number of Methodists and says that their various doctrinal views should perhaps be spoken of later, and, together with those just cited, Menemachos, Olympikos, Soranus, and Julian should also be discussed (ἀλλὰ τῆς μὲν ἐκείνων διαφωνίας ἴσως ἄν ποτε καὶ ὕστερον εἴη μνημονεῦσαι, καὶ σὺν αὐτοῖς γε τοῖς νῦν εἰρημένοις τοῦ . . . Μενεμάχου καὶ . . . Ὀλυμπικοῦ—καὶ Ἀπολλωνίδου καὶ Σωρανοῦ καὶ . . . Ἰουλιανοῦ Galen X 53 K.). As in the lists of members of the other schools, not all the names mentioned by Galen are repeated, and the order is somewhat altered. But the contrast drawn between just these two groups goes back, patently, to the Galenic text. Galen himself gives no hint that the divergence from the "method" of the physicians cited later in the passage was greater than that of the others, and there is no other evidence for this contention. We must, therefore, assume that the school, in spite of all practical differences, preserved its unity toward the outside.

II. Doctrine

Statements about Methodist doctrine are to be found, above all, in Celsus and Galen (πρὸς Τρασυβοῦλον περὶ ἀρίστης αἱρέσεως I 106 ff. K.; περὶ αἱρέσεων τοῖς εἰσαγομένοις scr. min. III ed. G. Helmreich, Leipzig,

1893, 1 ff.) and in the pseudo-Galenic εἰσαγωγή (Galen XIV 674 K.; on the material as a whole, cf. Wellmann 400. 406). None of the surviving accounts gives the complete doctrine, but by drawing upon them all it is possible to reconstruct the system.

The dietetics of the healthy, which the Methodists taught as did almost all ancient physicians, resembles that of the other schools. From the single short account which has been preserved, it becomes clear that the Methodists paid as much attention as did the Dogmatists and Empiricists to human individuality and to differences of climate and location: estque etiam proprium aliquid et loci et temporis istis quoque auctoribus (the Methodists; for these words are contained in a polemic against their point of view): qui, cum disputant, quemadmodum sanis hominibus agendum sit, praecipiunt, ut gravibus aut locis aut temporibus magis vitetur frigus, aestus, satietas, labor, libido; magisque ut conquiescat isdem locis aut temporibus, si quis gravitatem corporis sensit, ac neque vomitu stomachum neque purgatione alvum sollicitet (Celsus 28, 28–34; the wording [istis auctoribus] makes it impossible to designate this, as does Wellmann 399, as a fragment from a Dogmatic writing by Themison).

In contrast to this, the teaching concerning the treatment of the sick differs basically from Empiricist and Dogmatist theory. For the Methodists believe that it is unnecessary to know what part of the body is sick or, indeed, what may have caused the illness. The patient's age, constitution, and habits, as well as the climate and location, are matters of indifference for the treatment. The disease alone is the teacher of what one needs to know (Galen III 12, 14–20). The physician, therefore, needs no anatomical or physiological knowledge, no general or special etiology. He simply observes certain general conditions (communia, κοινότητες) of the body. There are three such common conditions: the body's dryness, its fluidity, and a mixed condition, as well as variations of this in the various stages of the disease: . . . medici . . . contendunt nullius causae notitiam quicquam ad curationes pertinere; satisque esse quaedam communia morborum intueri. si quidem horum tria genera esse, unum adstrictum, alterum fluens, tertium mixtum, nam modo parum excernere aegros, modo nimium, modo alia parte parum, alia nimium: haec autem genera morborum modo acuta esse, modo longa, et modo increscere, modo consistere, modo minui (Celsus 26, 12; cf. Galen III 12, 20–13, 12). There are, therefore, really only three diseases, and they are diseases of the whole body. As far as the names of these common conditions are concerned, all Methodists are in agreement, but they interpret them variously. While some determine the dry and fluid according to the natural excretions, many others declare dryness and fluidity to be states of the body: τινὲς μὲν γὰρ . . . ταῖς κατὰ φύσιν ἐκκρίσεσι παραμετροῦσι τὸ στεγνὸν καὶ τὸ ῥοῶδες, ἰσχομένων μὲν αὐτῶν στέγνωσιν ὀνομάζοντες τὸ πάθος, ἀμέτρως δ' ἐκκρινομένων ῥύσιν. ἄλλοι δέ τινες . . ., οὐκ ὀλίγος χορός, ἐν αὐταῖς τῶν σωμάτων ταῖς διαθέσεσι τὰ πάθη φασὶν εἶναι καὶ μέμφονταί γε δεινῶς τοῖς εἰς τὸ κενούμενον ἀποβλέπουσιν (Galen III 23, 6–12; cf. X 35 K.).

Treatment follows immediately from the common conditions observed and consists of the physician's attempt to induce the condition opposed to the disease. He must make a dry body moist and dry out a moist one. The treatment is directed toward the whole body, for it is the whole body that is sick. The goal may be reached in various ways, depending on the varying common conditions and the stages of the illness: cognito igitur eo, quod ex his est, si corpus adstrictum est, digerendum esse; si profluvio laborat, continendum; si mixtum vitium habet, occurendum subinde vehementiori malo. et aliter acutis morbis medendum, aliter vetustis, aliter increscentibus, aliter subsistentibus, aliter iam ad sanitatem inclinatis (Celsus 26, 18; cf. Galen III, 13, 12–19). According to this principle alone are the patient's regimen to be chosen and medicines to be given whose properties the physician knows from experience (Galen I 119 K.). Only the common conditions need be observed (horum observationem medicinam esse, Celsus 26, 23).

In surgery, too, some Methodists believe it possible to practice on the basis of nothing more than the three above-mentioned common conditions (καὶ πειρῶνταί γ' οἱ μὲν τῶν κατὰ δίαιταν νοσημάτων, ἔνιοι δὲ καὶ πάντων ἁπλῶς δύο κοινότητας ἐπιδεικνύναι καί τινα τρίτην μικτήν Galen III 12, 23–13, 2). Most of them, however, adopt special common conditions of surgical relevance and distinguish two kinds of intervention, according to whether a foreign body has penetrated the body from outside, or a tumor has formed within the body: αἱ δὲ ἐν χειρουργίαις κοινότητες κατὰ τὴν τοῦ ἀλλοτρίου ὑπεξαίρεσιν. διττὸν δὲ τὸ ἀλλότριον, ἤτοι γὰρ ἔξωθέν ἐστιν, ἢ τῶν ἐν τῷ σώματι, τὸ μὲν ἔξωθεν ἁπλοῦν, τρία δὲ εἴδη τῶν ἐν σώματι (Pseudo-Galen XIV 681 K.; cf. Galen I 193 K. for a short list of the common conditions relevant to surgery; scr. min. III 15, 8 ff. Sext. Emp. Hypotyposes, I 238). There are, therefore, four common conditions in surgery that warrant intervention. Wellman 400 maintains that the surgical common conditions originated only with Thessalos, or were at least differentiated late, since Celsus says nothing about them in his account of the Methodist school. But in the introduction to his work, in which he also speaks about the Methodists, Celsus only discusses the dietetic doctrines of the various schools—as he expressly emphasizes (19, 4)—and therefore deals with Methodist surgery just as little as with the Empiricist and Dogmatist varieties. Since Galen's statements regarding Methodist doctrine agree with those of Celsus, insofar as a comparison is possible, it is permissible to fix the surgical common conditions described by him and later writers as belonging to the original doctrine of the school. That the Methodists should at first have been unconcerned with surgery, as Wellmann contends, is, in itself, improbable. The prophylactic condition belongs, as a sort of appendix, to the surgical common conditions: ἔστι δὲ παρὰ τὰς ἐν χειρουργίαις τέσσαρας κοινότητας καὶ τὸ λεγούμενον προφυλακτικὸν εἶδος, ὃ καὶ αὐτὸ εἰς κοινότητα τάττεται ἐπὶ τῶν δηλητηρίων καὶ τοξικῶν καὶ ἰοβόλων πάντων καὶ δακετῶν . . . (Pseudo-Galen XIV 682 K.; this differentiation may be of late origin, cf. below p. 185). It thus included poisoning and similar cases.

The physician must not only know, however, that in the presence of certain phenomena a dry or moist regimen must be ordered and medicines prescribed which will evoke an opposite state, and that foreign bodies must be removed. The important thing for him is to know to what extent he should change the regimen, which medicines should be used and in what doses, and how extensive the surgical intervention should be. In surgery, there follows from each common condition an absolutely fixed procedure to be carried out on a predetermined scale: τὸ μὲν ἔξωθεν, ὡς σκόλοψ καὶ βέλος καὶ πᾶν ὅπερ ἀλλότριον, ἐνδείκνυται τὴν τελείαν ἐξαίρεσιν. τῶν δὲ ἐν τῷ σώματι τὸ μὲν τῷ τόπῳ ἀλλότριον ὡς ὑπόχυμα . . . ἐνδείκνυται τὴν μετάθεσιν ἢ ἀποκατάστασιν εἰς τὸν ἴδιον τόπον. τὸ δὲ τῷ μεγέθει ἀλλότριον ὡς τὰ ἀποστήματα . . . τὰ μὲν διαιρέσει μόνῃ χρῆσθαι, τὰ δὲ περιαιρέσει τελείᾳ τῶν περιττῶν τὸ δὲ τῇ ἐλλείψει ἀλλότριον οὐχ ὡς περιττεῦον, ἀλλ' ὡς ἐνδεές, οἷον τὰ κολοβώματα . . . τὸ ἀναπληροῦσθαι ἐπιξητεῖ καὶ ἐνδείκνυται (Pseudo-Galen XIV 681 K.). The various cases are thus arranged under the various common conditions, and, for these, exact instructions are given on the correct extent of the intervention at any given time, so that the surgeon, on observing the common conditions, immediately knows what he must do.

In dietetics, the prescription of medicaments is more complicated. Although the Methodists differ from the Dogmatists and Empiricists as far as theory is concerned, in practice their behavior is similar (e.g.,

Galen III 20, 2 ff.). It is axiomatic for them, it is true, that treatment must bring about the condition opposite to the existing one, but they do not give the same medicine to everyone. They take the patient's age into consideration. Although, primarily, they prescribe for the whole body, they do not use the same medication for different parts of the body, as one would expect from their theory that the diseased organ is of no importance. And yet, unlike the Dogmatists and Empiricists, they claim not to depend on etiological knowledge or on observation of the age and constitution of the patient or of the season, on the basis of which the latter differentiate between drugs (e.g., Galen III 6, 10 ff. 19, 20 ff.). In theory, they depend solely on the common conditions and the stages of the disease. But sicknesses are subordinated to the three main common conditions, the solid, the fluid, and the mixed condition, in correspondence to the different natures of the affected organs, as in surgery. Thus φλεγμονή is broken down into a dry and a mixed disease. The dry disease comprises inflammations of the hand, foot, arms and legs, of the thighs, and every other part of the body with no external excretion; to the mixed form belong diseases of the mouth, eyes, and nose (Galen III 29, 25 ff.). In this way, a variation in treatment is attained which corresponds to the variation in the underlying common condition, with the result that the Methodists have to treat on just as individual a basis as the others. And, in the same way, depending on the different organs affected, all diseases will have belonged to different common conditions, and, by virtue of this fact, a different treatment was called for in each instance.

Further, the intensity of the common conditions determines the dosage of medicaments (τὸ μέγεθος τῶν κοινοτήτων . . . ἐνδείκνυται μέγεθος βοηθημάτων Galen I 194 K.). If the Methodists, like all the others, did not employ the same drugs for young and old (Galen III 20, 3 ff.), nor in all seasons (*ibid.* 20, 16 ff.), they needed only to assume the common conditions of disease, which, after all, always vary in individual cases, vary in degree in youth and age and in the different seasons; then, from this variation of the common conditions, they could derive variation of treatment. Thus, in practice, there again followed from a single observation what the Dogmatists and Empiricists gathered from a multitude of observations.

In addition, dosage of medicaments and the regimen were arranged according to the stage reached by the disease (οἴονται τὸν καιρὸν τοῦ νοσήματος ποτὲ μὲν τὴν τροφήν, ποτὲ δὲ τὴν ποιὰν τροφὴν ἐνδείκνυσθαι Galen I

183

211 K.). Celsus had already noted that treatment must be varied not only according to the variation in basic common conditions, but also according to the various stages (26, 21 ff.). Thus, on the basis of a system which appears to take only what is common to all into consideration, an individualized treatment is nevertheless possible. (On Methodist drug theory, on the formulation of the patient's regimen, and on surgery, cf. also the Handbooks and especially Th. Meyer-Steineg, *Das medizinische System der Methodiker*, Jenaer medizinhistorische Beiträge, Jena, 1916, where these questions are discussed from the point of view of medical context.)

The Methodists believed that all the fundamentals of treatment could be represented as knowledge (ἔνδειξις), not merely as observation (τήρησις). They agreed with the Dogmatists that experience was not enough for the physician, and for this reason they opposed the Empiricists. On the other hand, they did not, like the Dogmatists, derive their knowledge from logical deliberations but from the very phenomena from which the Empiricists gained their experience; they claimed an ἔνδειξις τῶν φαινομένων. Thus, in justifying their tenets, they take up a peculiar middle position between Dogmatists and Empiricists (Celsus 26, 26 ff., Galen III 14, 8 ff.). Yet, since they rely on the absolute validity of their knowledge and since, in theory, they do not allow for individual conditions, the author of the pseudo-Galenic εἰσαγωγή rightly says: οἱ δὲ μεθοδικοὶ καὶ δι' ὅλου ἐπιστήμην αὐτὴν (sc. τὴν ἰατρικὴν) ἀποκαλοῦσιν (XIV 684 K.). At the same time, their system did not have many tenets. They could claim that they were able to teach everything a physician has to know in six months (Galen III 15, 13), and they considered it the greatest advantage (τὸ μέγιστον ἀγαθόν) of their doctrine that a Methodist had to learn so little (Galen 14, 17 ff.).

III. Objections to the Doctrine; Philosophical Presuppositions; Historical Dependence

Opponents of the Methodists raised serious objections to their doctrine. They attempted to show that Methodism was not an independent system, but, according to one's interpretation of the theory, either an exaggerated Dogmatism or a pedestrian kind of Empiricism. It was further objected that the neglect of any observation of season and locality and the failure to take human constitutions into consideration signified a narrowing of medicine which placed the treatment of

184

human beings on the same level as the treatment of animals (Celsus 27, 17 ff.). The controversy also pointed up the contradictions between Methodist theory and practice (e.g., from the Empiricist point of view, Galen III 188, 24 ff.; from the Dogmatic, 22, 19). Finally, the basic concepts of Methodism, the common conditions and the stages, as well as the manner of deduction from them, were subjected to detailed criticism and declared philosophically untenable (e.g., Galen I 162 K.). There is no record of the way in which the Methodists defended themselves against these attacks, though it is certain that they did defend themselves and did it well. For in the accounts of their opponents, which furnish our only knowledge of the Methodists, the Methodists' answer to the accusations leveled against them is deliberately withheld. Thus Galen at one point has the Empiricist raise objections, the refutation of which by the Methodist is presupposed in the attacks of the Dogmatist (cf. III 26, 10 ff. with 21, 4 ff.; on the other hand, it is not possible to decide with certainty whether the introduction of the prophylactic common condition [Galen XIV 682 K.], which seems to be tacked on to the surgical ones, is not provoked by the opponents' argumentation [Galen III 18, 24 ff.]; in that case the polemic would be justified, and a defense would have been impossible before the doctrine was modified.)

Difficulties certainly exist, and therewith the possibility of objections. The mixture of Dogmatist and Empiricist principles is unclear, and the rejection of everything that older medicine had tested is difficult to understand. Above all, the fundamental principle of Methodism, the ἔνδειξις τῶν φαινομένων, seems full of contradictions. All knowledge is supposed to be derived from the phenomena, yet it should be more than observation, ἔνδειξις not τήρησις. How can something more than observation come from the phenomena? Knowledge, after all, can only result from logical argumentation (concerning ἔνδειξις as a logical concept of the Dogmatists, cf. e.g., Galen III 5, 17 ff.; on τήρησις as an Empiricist concept and on its distinction from the Dogmatist ἔνδειξις, ibid. 7, 1 ff.). How can the Methodist defend himself?

Sextus Empiricus, who believes Skeptics can only belong to the Methodist school of physicians, since it is the only skeptical one (Hyp. I, 236), says: ὥσπερ οὖν κατὰ τὴν ἀνάγκην τῶν παθῶν ὁ σκεπτικὸς ὑπὸ μὲν δίψους ἐπὶ ποτὸν ὁδηγεῖται, ὑπὸ δὲ λιμοῦ ἐπὶ τροφήν, καὶ ἐπί τι τῶν ἄλλων ὁμοίως, οὕτως καὶ ὁ μεθοδικὸς ἰατρὸς ὑπὸ τῶν παθῶν ἐπὶ τὰ κατάλληλα ὁδηγεῖται, ὑπὸ μὲν στεγνώσεως ἐπὶ τὴν χαύνωσιν, ὡς καταφεύγει τις ἀπὸ τῆς διὰ ψύχος ἐπιτεταμένον πυκνώσεως ἐπὶ ἀλέαν, ὑπὸ δὲ ῥύσεως ἐπὶ τὴν ἐποχὴν αὐτῆς, ὡς καὶ οἱ ἐν βαλανείῳ ἱδρῶτι πολλῷ περιρρεόμενοι καὶ ἐκλυόμενοι ἐπὶ τὴν ἐποχὴν αὐτοῦ παραγίνονται καὶ διὰ τοῦτο ἐπὶ τὸν ψυχρὸν ἀέρα καταφεύγουσιν (238). Thus he parallels the rule according to which the Skeptic acts and the principle by which the Methodist heals the sick. And just as for him the language of the Skeptical and Methodist schools are in complete agreement (239), so he interprets the ἔνδειξις τῶν φαινομένων Skeptically too: καὶ τὸ τῆς ἐνδείξεως ὄνομα ἀδοξάστως παραλαμβάνει (sc. ὁ μεθοδικός) ἀντὶ τῆς ἀπὸ τῶν φαινομένων παθῶν τῶν τε κατὰ φύσιν καὶ τῶν παρὰ φύσιν ὁδηγήσεως ἐπὶ κατάλληλα εἶναι δοκοῦντα, ὡς καὶ ἐπὶ δίψους καὶ ἐπὶ λιμοῦ καὶ τῶν ἄλλων ὑπεμίμνησκον (240). As every emotion necessarily extorts its own gratification by bringing about the opposite condition, so does the sick man's dehydrated body demand fluid, and the moist body dryness. It is this law, inherent in the phenomena, that the Methodist physician follows when he cures his patient by giving fluids or by drying the bodily fluid up, always inducing a condition opposite to the existing one. He calls this law of the phenomena ἔνδειξις τῶν φαινομένων. The Methodist, then, is able to defend himself against the accusations leveled at him by a recourse to Skeptical philosophy; indeed, Skeptical philosophy clarifies what in Methodism seems obscure and open to criticism. But then all fundamental concepts of Methodism must be capable of Skeptic explanation. Methodist medicine must be interpreted as a transposition of Aenesidemean Skepticism (Wellmann was the first to note the influence of Skepticism on Methodism, which he remarked on in connection with the opinion of Sextus [403]. But he does not state whether he agrees with Sextus and draws no conclusion from that influence—insofar as he acknowledges it—for the interpretation of the Methodist system).

The Skeptic declares that the phenomena are the only true things; that they exist is not disputed (*Hyp.* I 21–22). Thus the Methodists pay homage to nothing but the phenomena (Galen III 16, 9 ff.). Concerning everything but phenomena the Skeptic withholds judgment: he does not claim that the hidden is unknowable, but he has as yet no knowledge of it and it does not concern him (*Hyp.* I 236). Thus the Methodist leaves unanswered the question whether the hidden can be apprehended or not; he does not deny the possibility, as does the Empiricist (Galen III 14, 14), for it is of no consequence to him. It is true, the Skeptic does not doubt the possible existence of a cause, but he believes knowledge of the cause to be impossible, just as there exists for him no sign of the hidden (*Hyp.* III 13 ff. II 97 ff.). The Methodists deny all etiological knowledge; they renounce all semiology, all physiology, and anatomy. The Skeptic is aware of the difficulty inherent in the concepts of common condition and proof, and he uses them only insofar as they correspond to the phenomena and the principles of action derived from the phenomena (*Hyp.* I 237. 240. II 228). If one presupposes that the concepts have the same connotation for the Methodists, the latter's statements become understandable and convincing (Galen I 190 K. gives a Methodist discussion of the common conditions which is completely Skeptic in its argumentation). The same is true of the concepts of the whole and the part (*Hyp.* II 215 ff.). Each of these points of view, indeed the whole system, is really Skeptic.

In the Dogmatist schools of medicine, Dogmatic philosophy came to fruition, and, in the Empiricist school, academic skepticism (cf. *Quellen und Studien zur Geschichte der Naturwissenschaften* III [1933] 253 ff. [195*]). Methodism exploited Aenesidemean Skepticism, thereby absorbing the last Hellenic philosophy into medicine. The very name μέθοδος indicates a Skeptic stance: treatment consists of following the path prescribed by the phenomena (cf. Wellmann 403). At the same time, the Skepticism of the Methodists determines their peculiar middle position between Dogmatist and Empiricist medicine. The Skeptic standing at the end of a long development of thought, brings nothing new to it; rather, he tests its formal reliability, everything that has gone before being contained in his thinking. His conduct is similar to that of others, even though it is determined by a different law. In like manner, only the rationale of Methodism differs from that of the preceding schools; behavior remained unchanged.

The philosophical basis of Methodism is, then, Skepticism. But in what way is Methodism dependent on the preceding and contemporary medical doctrines? What medical problems provoked it? Methodism is shaped by the Themisonian system and, thereby, by the doctrine of Asclepiades—all the testimony agrees in this. And Themison stands as the point of departure of Methodism because it was he who introduced the concept of common conditions into medicine. Galen says: φαινομένας γοῦν εἰπὼν εἶναι τὰς κοινότητας ὁ σοφώτατος Θεσσαλός, ὀλίγον ὕστερον οὐ μόνον οὐδένα τῶν ἔμπροσθεν ἰατρῶν ἰδεῖν αὐτάς φησιν, ἀλλ' οὐδὲ τὸν πρῶτον γεννήσαντα Θεμίσωνα. τούτῳ γὰρ οὖν δὴ μόνῳ παραχωρεῖ, καθάπερ πατρὶ τέκνα γνήσια τὰς τερατώδεις ἐκείνας κοινότητας (Galen X 35 K.). Themison modified the Asclepiadan system by turning the atoms and pores into common conditions (on Asclepiades and Methodism, cf. Wellmann 398, 3). Since

Themison was the first to formulate the concept of the common conditions, the Methodists were obliged to consider their own doctrine an interpretation of his system, as Celsus says, or to see in him the root of their own doctrine, as Galen puts it. They merely gave a Skeptical interpretation to Themison's common conditions (φαινομένας γοῦν εἰπὼν εἶναι τὰς κοινότητας).

But why did they interpret them Skeptically? This was the time when Empiricists and Dogmatists were arguing over the question how it was possible to gain knowledge. The latter claimed that logic is the constitutive element in knowledge and allotted only limited significance to experience, while the former derived all knowledge from experience. Asclepiades, Themison's teacher, by denying that anything at all can be observed repeatedly in exactly the same way (Galen III 9, 9 ff.), exaggerated the arguments against the possibility of basing knowledge on experience alone. This threatened the very foundations of Empiricist medicine, and indeed of all Empiricism, which is only feasible on the assumption that one can observe objects which are constant in themselves. At the same time, the uniqueness of the individual was strongly emphasized and thereby a new difficulty brought out for the physician and his work. For he is obliged to know and to treat individuals, since all human beings are different. If the same thing is never repeated, how is he to know what he should do in the single case? The Dogmatists and Empiricists had taken individual conditions increasingly into account, although they tried to comprehend them in general terms. They presuppose that individuals are uniform as individuals and that, after all, a general knowledge of them would therefore be possible. Age and constitution constantly necessitated a variation in treatment, but patients of the same age or the same constitution required the same treatment. The teaching of Asclepiades rendered this escape impossible.

The problems were rendered more acute by the confrontation with Hippocratic skepticism and empiricism. The Hippocratic physicians had taught a medicine which was completely oriented toward the individual human being and what was right for him. They had renounced all generalized knowledge. For them, each person was so incomparable that the physician could only be guided in his actions by what he observed in the individual case (*Quellen und Studien* 256 [199*]). Dogmatists and Empiricists interpreted the Hippocratic writings, and it was inevitable that the old teaching, which had been accepted as dogma, gradually found itself in opposition to the opinion of the schools. The authority of Hippocrates added still more weight to the demand that the individual be considered absolutely unique.

No solution of the difficulties could possibly come from Dogmatism or Empiricism. Skepticism offered a way out, for in Skepticism there was the same rejection of all general principles, the same limitation to the here and now, as in Hippocratic empiricism (Quellen und Studien, loc. cit. [199*]). If the physician acted on Skeptical principles and made the afflictions of the human body the law governing his treatment, he was not letting himself be directed by a principle derived from his experience, or from his intellect, and then applied to his patient; on the contrary, each case suggested to the physician a suitable individual treatment. The physician then went solely by the patient he was treating. This satisfied the demand that had been made, while, at the same time, medicine was transformed in the mode of Hippocratic empiricism.

There is only one essential difference between the Hippocratic and the Methodist solutions to the problem. The Hippocratic physician found treatment difficult because of the necessarily individualized character of knowledge and treatment, which allowed no criterion in medicine except the patient's subjective experience (αἴσθησις τοῦ σώματος); the Methodist, on the other hand, could claim with a good conscience, that there was nothing simpler than treatment. For in raising to a principle the Skeptics' law that necessity resides in the afflictions of the body, he freed the physician from that indefinite, subjective criterion. The Methodist was aware that his doctrine ran contrary to the Hippocratic, but that it was also nothing but a modification of it. Hence, he turned the first aphorism of Hippocrates round and said: ἡ μὲν τέχνη βραχεῖα, ὁ δὲ βίος μακρός instead of ὁ μὲν βίος βραχύς, ἡ δὲ τέχνη μακρή (Galen III 14, 24 ff.; accordingly, Hippocrates too is interpreted as a Skeptic in Diogenes Laertius IX 73).

IV. CONTEMPORARY AND LATER OPINIONS OF METHODISM

In the first century A.D., Methodism was more highly regarded in Rome than were Dogmatism and Empiricism. The Romans preferred Methodist medicine because, in the first place, it employed fewer drugs and because the regimen it prescribed gave greater consideration to customary activities or left them unchanged. This was decisive for the school's reputation, for the history of Methodism was determined by the judgment of the Romans, the master race, whose relationship to medicine was quite different from that of the Greeks. From the outset, they refused strenuous and harshly disruptive treatment; the first Greek surgeon to come to Rome was hated for the brutal treatment he prescribed (Pliny, *n. h.* XXIX 6). The medicine which the Romans themselves had recorded depended on few drugs, but ones which were supposed to act quickly and be as pleasant to take as possible. Asclepiades himself owed part of his success to the circumstance that he prescribed only pleasant remedies and that he was willing to equate the easy with the true (Pliny, *n. h.* XXVI 7. Celsus 104, 27 ff.). The Methodists, through Themison, took over much of Asclepiades' practical medicine. Besides, it was consonant with their basic principle that the patient always be given what was bound to be pleasant in his particular condition: the dehydrated body was given fluids, the body which was too full of fluid was relieved of the oppressive superfluity.

But the Methodist school was also something new. Thessalos, who called himself the conqueror of all previous physicians (ἰατρονίκης, Pliny, *n. h.* XXIX 6), wrote in the dedication of his book to Nero: παραδεδωκὼς νέαν αἵρεσιν καὶ ὡς μόνην ἀληθῆ διὰ τὸ τοὺς προγενεστέρους πάντας ἰατροὺς μηδὲν παραδοῦναι συμφέρον πρός τε ὑγείας συντήρησιν καὶ νόσων ἀπαλλαγήν (Galen X 8 K.). This pleased the people of the first century A.D., for they demanded new things. Just as the Greek model was forsaken in poetry, just as in all matters men sought out paths of their own, the medicine of the period, too, was required to accomplish the heretofore unattained if it was to find approval. The Methodists were only speaking the language of their time when they boasted of revolutionizing medicine.

This attitude met with condemnation as early as the second century A.D.; archaism requires that people be better educated. The Methodists conceded that they must adapt their doctrine to the new views, but they did not on that account relinquish any fundamental tenet of their system. Soranus, it is true, reinstated etiology and physiology in medicine, but he said: τὸν μὲν οὖν φυσικὸν ἄχρηστον ὄντα πρὸς τὸ τέλος, φερέκοσμον δὲ πρὸς χρηστομάθειαν (CMG IV 4, 6–7; cf. C. Aurelianus, quoted in Meyer-Steineg, *op. cit.*, 45 ff.). Thus, it was only for the sake of his education that the physician need be versed in these matters; and through this adjustment, Methodist doctrine was sufficiently transformed to be able to persist in the new era. Galen, who as a strict archaist considers it effrontery when someone like Thessalos contradicts an aphorism of Hippocrates (Galen X 8 K.), only attacks the Methodists of the first century; Soranus, on the other hand, and those who follow him are clearly, in his opinion, the Methodist physicians with whom it is possible to have discussions, because in many matters they have been converted to the truer view (Galen III 26, 19 ff.). Galen's accusations, however, are unjust; they are unhistorical. Methodism was as justified in the second century in adapting itself to the educational ideal of the time as it had been in insisting on its originality in the first century A.D.

In spite of these objections to the Methodist school, however, its objective significance was never disputed. Not even Galen doubts that the Methodist school is the most important school of physicians beside the Dogmatist and Empiricist schools, and he always puts these three schools in the very center of his discussion. Thus the pseudo-Galenic εἰσαγωγή admits three basic medical doctrines: the Dogmatist, the Empiricist, and the Methodist (Galen XIV 678 K.); and medicine is classified in this manner in the compendiums down to Isidore of Seville (*Etymologiae* IV 2). Soranus' version of Methodism was considered the standard version because it agreed with the spirit of the later centuries; he had restored Methodism to the norm, and his works, like those of Hippocrates and Galen, were translated into Latin because of their factual significance.

Even in the Middle Ages, Methodism still counted, and its ideas were the subject of discussion (cf. P. Diepgen, *Geschichte der Medizin*, 1923, I² 100 ff. II 7. 43. 53. 56). At the beginning of the Renaissance, on the other hand, little value was attached to the Methodist system, as we are told by Prosper Alpinus, who expounded the doctrine in detail at the beginning of the seventeenth century, once more taking up the earlier intense concern with it (*De medicina methodica libri XIII*, 1609). Even in the seventeenth and eighteenth centuries, Methodism still had some influence on medical development (cf. Diepgen III 48. 71).

Since the nineteenth century Methodism has been only of historical interest. Medical historians, down to K. Sprengel 28, see in it one of the most important and most magnificent systems of ancient medicine (Haeser I 268. Fuchs I 328. Pagel-Sudhoff, *Einführung in die Geschichte der Medizin*, Berlin, 1915, 92. M. Neuburger, *Geschichte der Medizin*, Stuttgart, 1906, I 303). Less favorable judgments have been passed by the philologists, who deem it less important than the doctrines of the Dogmatists and Empiricists (Wellmann 397. A. Rehm and K. Vogel, *Exakte Wissenschaften*, Gercke-Norden, II Heft 5⁴, 1933, 75).

PART TWO

EMPIRICISM AND SKEPTICISM IN THE TEACHING OF
THE GREEK EMPIRICIST SCHOOL*

Already in antiquity there were disputes as to whether the teaching of the Greek Empiricists, like the school itself, was Hellenistic, or whether it could be traced back to an earlier time. The school, which takes its name from its principle, not from its founder, contends that Akron of Agrigentum was the first Empiricist, and that Philinos and Serapion had indeed propounded the doctrine earlier than the others, but later than he (p. 43, 1 ff. DG.).[1] Hippocrates too counts as an Empiricist (fr. 310 DG.); in the opinion of the Empiricists he had already taught the truth in almost all matters (fr. 103 DG.). Pliny likewise calls Akron of Agrigentum the first Empiricist (fr. 5; cf. 7a, b, d DG.). According to these statements, then, Empiricist medicine existed already in the fifth century before Christ. Celsus, on the other hand, states that Serapion was the very first to declare that rational methods were of no concern to medicine, which he based on experience and experiment alone (fr. 4 DG.). Others think that Philinos was the first to separate the Empiricist school from the Logicians (fr. 6; 7c DG.). According to this view, then, the Empiricist school and its teaching are only Hellenistic, and their derivation from Akron is a deliberate archaization to make the school appear older than that of the Logicians (fr. 6 DG.).[2]

Empirical medicine was certainly not first taught in the Hellenistic Empiricist school. The Hippocratic writings already require that the

* "Empirie und Skepsis in der Lehre der griechischen Empirikerschule," *Quellen und Studien zur Geschichte der Naturwissenschaften und der Medizin*, Band 3, Heft 4, Berlin: Julius Springer, 1933, pp. 45–53 (pp. 253–61 of the volume).

In this translation, words like Dogmatic, Empiricist, Methodist, Skeptic have been capitalized when they seem to refer to definite schools rather than general concepts.

[1] DG. = Karl Deichgräber, *Die griechische Empirikerschule*, Sammlung der Fragmente und Darstellung der Lehre, Berlin, 1930.

[2] Θέλοντες δὲ ἀπαρχαίζειν ἑαυτῶν τὴν αἵρεσιν ἵνα ᾖ πρεσβυτέρα τῆς λογικῆς ῞Ακρωνα τὸν ᾿Ακραγαντῖνόν φασιν ἄρξασθαι αὐτῆς. Concerning the derivation from Timon (fr. 7d; p. 43,3 DG.), cf. ftn. 19, below. For Isidor of Seville, Aesculapius is the first Empiricist, just as Apollo is the first Methodist and Hippocrates the first Logician (fr. 8 DG.).

physician rely on experience alone, that only that which can be proved by experience be considered true. All rational methods are consciously rejected. Thus, even though the Empiricist school only originated in Hellenistic times, empirical medicine existed earlier.[3] Empedocles gave a philosophic justification of the requirement that one be guided by experience only, and his doctrine influenced the physicians. It is for this reason that the Empiricist school could be derived from Akron, that is, from the Sicilian physicians influenced by Empedocles. Empirical medicine is indeed not a phenomenon typical of the Hellenistic period.[4]

In the Greek Empiricist school, however, empiricism as a concept is given a Hellenistic interpretation. In Hippocratic empiricism, experience had been the observation of every effect of every single factor on every individual; one determined how the individual behaves in relation to what he eats and drinks and does. Since only the unique occurrence can be apprehended, it is not possible to decide what should be done in the future from one's experience of the past.[5] Hellenistic empiricism, on the other hand, is the observation and recording of what may be seen often and occurring in like manner; the unique occurrence lies outside scientific knowledge. From many similar experiences it is then possible to determine how one should act in the future in similar circumstances. Experience brings, if not certainty, at least a measure of assurance.[6] Again, in Hippocratic empiricism, it was admitted that

[3] Cf. DLZ [Deutsche Literaturzeitung] 1931, 1117–18. For this reason, the Empiricists were justified in making Hippocrates an Empiricist; it was merely a question of which Hippocratic writings one believed authentic.

[4] Cf. DLZ 1931, 1118–19. One should not think of Democritus. Cf. ftn. 17, below.

[5] CMG [Corpus Medicorum Graecorum] I, 1, 51,19 ff. ἀναγκαῖον εἶναι ἰητρῷ περὶ φύσιος εἰδέναι καὶ πάνυ σπουδάσαι, ὡς εἴσεται, εἴπερ τι μέλλει τῶν δεόντων ποιήσειν, ὅ τί τέ ἐστιν ἄνθρωπος πρὸς τὰ ἐσθιόμενά τε καὶ πινόμενα καὶ ὅτι πρὸς τὰ ἄλλα ἐπιτηδεύματα, καὶ ὅ τι ἀφ' ἑκάστου ἑκάστῳ συμβήσεται. DG. says (pp. 271–72): "Here (in ancient medicine, which in DG.'s opinion barely touches the problems which are later clearly recognized) the opinion prevailed that experience was concerned with the realm of the recurrent, not of the permanent, and that it lacked an objective, generally valid, standard." But medicine has a standard: the individual reaction of the patient (41,19 ff.). This reaction can be ascertained, though it is not something permanent or recurrent, but something unique (according to 51,18 ff.). Further, the individual reaction of each patient to each foodstuff and each activity must be ascertained (51,22 ff.). The physician is aware of the difficulty of treating isolated cases where there is no preceding experience (41,22 ff.).

[6] Cf. the exposition of Empiricist theory in DG., p. 291 ff., especially pp. 295, 297, and the Fragments, p. 103,17 ff. The concept of experience is clearly influenced by Aristotle (cf. e.g., Metaphysics A I; DG. p. 274).

what cannot be experienced can, at least in principle, be explained through hypotheses. But medicine needs no such hypotheses; everything the physician has to know can be seen, even the causes of diseases (CMG I 1, 36,15 ff.; 45,25 ff.).[7] Hellenistic Empiricism teaches that there is no knowledge of the invisible, since no experience of it is possible; and it is therefore not possible to know the causes of disease (e.g., fr. 14 DG.). Such a theory of experience corresponds to Hellenistic skepticism.

Sextus Empiricus, it is true, denied that the Empiricist school was skeptical; he designated the Methodist school of physicians as the only one the Skeptic might join (*Hypotyposes* I 236 ff.). He was motivated to this rejection of the Empiricists by the fact that they claimed that the invisible was unknowable, which the Methodists did not dare to say (236).[8] They alone refrained from judging hastily whether the hidden is unknowable or not; instead, they limited themselves to the phenomena, and in the manner of the Skeptics they learned from the phenomena whatever seemed useful. Just as the Skeptic let himself be directed in his conduct by his emotional responses, so the Methodist physician allowed the conditions he observed in the patient to point the way to be followed in treating him. All orders given by the Methodist physician were based on what the patient felt (239). Furthermore, the Methodists even used words in the same way as the Skeptics (239–40). There existed, therefore, complete agreement between these two schools; it was the Methodist school, not the Empiricist, which suited the Skeptic better than any other school of physicians.

Yet if Sextus does not consider the Empiricist school skeptical, his opinion is determined by his particular concept of skepticism. At the

---

[7] One observes the fluids which are in the body; one observes that food produces in man similar fluids and that health and sickness are determined by the resulting mixture.

[8] Zeller, *Philosophie der Griechen* III, 2 (5), 49,1, does not believe that the statement quoted is Empiricist, since it is formulated in a conditional clause. But its Empiricist character is attested to elsewhere (fr. 14 DG.). From Sextus' words it follows at most that perhaps not all Empiricists advocated such a doctrine (cf. ftn. 24, below). At one point Sextus says: if the younger Academicians consider all things to be unknowable, they perhaps distinguish themselves from the Skeptics in this too (*loc. cit.*, 226). To be sure, not all Academicians held this view (Zeller, *loc. cit.*, III, 1, [5], 531–32). Here, too, then, Sextus apparently wants to make a similar distinction by means of the conditional form, though the distinction is concerned only with the problem of knowledge. Just as all Academicians manifestly (προδήλως) differ from the Skeptics in their judgment of good and evil (*loc. cit.*, 226), so do all Empiricists differ from the Methodists in their actions (cf. below, p. 198).

197

beginning of his work he declares that among philosophic investigators, some claim to have found the truth, others believe it cannot be found, still others search for it (I 2). Those who are specially called Dogmatists, the Aristotelians, the Epicureans, the Stoics, and others, are the ones who believe they have found the truth. That things are not understandable is taught by the schools of Kleitomachos, Karneades, and the other Academicians. The Skeptics search for the truth (3). The true Skeptic, then, knows nothing; he merely seeks to know something. For this reason, Sextus is unwilling to assert any of his propositions positively; he is willing only to state his opinion on each matter as he understands it, and as it seems right to him at the moment (4).[9] The Academy is in error: if only because it *asserts* that things are not knowable, it is not skeptical. Its negative judgment is no less dogmatic than the positive doctrines of the Dogmatic schools, and the Skeptic must not bind himself to any opinion. The Academy is also in error in that it affirms in direct opposition to Skepticism that judgment can be certain at least in questions of ethics (I 266 ff.).

If Sextus rejects Academic philosophy as not skeptical, he must reject empiricist doctrine for the same reason. Just as the Academy maintained the unknowable nature of all things, the Empiricist school maintained the unknowable nature of at least all hidden things. Just as the Academy recognized a certain sureness of judgment in ethical questions, the Empiricist school by dint of comparing many experiences acquired a knowledge which transcended the isolated phenomena and suggested rules for medical conduct.[10] Empiricist medicine thus contradicted true skepticism as understood by Sextus. According to the doctrine of the Academy, however, Empiricist medicine was skeptical, and this Academic form of the theory of experience was Hellenistic.[11]

---

[9] (περὶ δὲ τῆς σκεπτικῆς ἀγωγῆς ὑποτυπωτικῶς ἐπὶ τοῦ παρόντος ἡμεῖς ἐροῦμεν) ἐκεῖνο προειπόντες, ὅτι περὶ οὐδενὸς τῶν λεχθησομένων διαβεβαιούμεθα ὡς οὕτως ἔχοντος πάντως καθάπερ λέγομεν, ἀλλὰ κατὰ τὸ νῦν φαινόμενον ἡμῖν ἱστορικῶς ἀπαγγέλλομεν περὶ ἑκάστου. The meaning of skepticism is thus interpreted quite literally (cf. also the definition, I,7). Skepticism is by no means resignation, but the determination to engage in constantly renewed investigation.

[10] It is "an active skepticism, always striving to overcome itself in order to arrive through regulated experiences at a kind of conditional certitude" (Goethe, *Werke*, Weimar 1887 ff., 42², 258). That is, the Empiricist school differs in both theoretical knowledge and practice from Skeptical philosophy, while the Methodist school is in agreement with it in both.

[11] DG. is thinking only of the influence of Pyrrhonist skepticism on the Empiricist school (p. 279 ff.); on this point, cf. ftn. 19, below. In any case, the shaping of Empiricist theories, as Sextus testifies, is affected by the Academy, which in the Hellenistic period is indeed the representative of skepticism. The Pyrrhonist skep-

Yet, if empirical medicine existed before the Hellenistic Empiricists, the skeptical attitude, too, can be detected in classical times. For the Hippocratic empiricists teach that it is impossible to learn medicine quickly, because in medicine there cannot possibly be any rigid tenets. "Everyone who has learnt to write in the one way in which it is taught understands everything connected with it. And those who write can all write in the same manner, because that which is the same and is done in the same way cannot now, or ever, become its opposite but is always perfectly uniform and completely independent of the circumstances of the moment. Medicine, however, does not do the same things now and in the next moment; it acts differently in regard to the same individual, and its actions are opposed to each other."[12] Thus Sextus rejects every firm statement, every doctrine, as Dogmatic and therefore untrue; he is only willing to say how things appear to him at the moment, while the Academic Skeptics wrongfully dare to make pronouncements of general validity.[13]

The physician arrives at such a skeptical attitude because in every case he can rely only on the experience he gains at this moment and from this individual, because the sole criterion is how the patient feels whom he happens to be treating. Theoretical considerations as to the nature of man are well suited to the art of writing, but not to medicine.[14] Action can only be directed by what the moment teaches. The Skeptic, as Sextus says, allows his actions to be determined only by reality as it is now, while the Academician admits statements of general validity.[15]

tics form no school even though some individuals may tend toward the doctrine more than others (Zeller, loc. cit., III, 1 [5], 499–550). They do not believe in the possibility of positive statements, nor in a convincing or reliable definition of good (Zeller, loc. cit., 506).

[12] ἰητρικὴν οὐ δυνατόν ἐστι ταχὺ μαθεῖν διὰ τόδε, ὅτι ἀδύνατόν ἐστι καθεστηκός τι ἐν αὐτῇ σόφισμα γενέσθαι, οἷον ὁ τὸ γράφειν ἕνα τρόπον μαθὼν ὃν διδάσκουσι πάντα ἐπίσταται. καὶ οἱ ἐπιστάμενοι πάντες ὁμοίως διὰ τόδε, ὅτι τὸ αὐτὸ καὶ ὁμοίως ποιεύμενον νῦν τε καὶ οὐ νῦν οὐκ ἂν τὸ ὑπεναντίον γένοιτο, ἀλλ' ἀεὶ ἐνδυκέως ὅμοιόν ἐστι, καὶ οὐ δεῖ καιροῦ. ἡ δὲ ἰητρικὴ νῦν τε καὶ αὐτίκα οὐ τὸ αὐτὸ ποιέει καὶ πρὸς τὸν αὐτὸν ὑπεναντία ποιέει, καὶ ταῦτα ὑπεναντία σφίσιν ἑωυτοῖσιν (π. τόπων τῶν κατ' ἄνθρωπον ch. 41 VI 330–32 L.).

[13] There is also agreement in details. Thus the equivalence of the various opinions is advanced, even if only incidentally, as an argument against Dogmatism, and the principle of the uniqueness of the individual is formulated concisely (cf. DLZ 1931, 1117–18).

[14] ἧσσον νομίζω τῇ ἰητρικῇ τέχνῃ προσήκειν ἢ τῇ γραφικῇ (π. ἀρχαίης ἰητρικῆς CMG I, 1, 51, 13). It follows from the preceding statements that these words are to be understood as I have interpreted them. Cf. also Problemata IV, 1931, 114 [108*].

[15] The Methodist doctrine of medicine (cf. p. 197), then, corresponds to classical skepticism, whose true successor it is in theory and practice. Knowledge of the hid-

The classical empiricist, then, has the same medical approach as Sextus. It differs from that of the Academician, and therefore from that of the Hellenistic Empiricist, but the problems are the same for both. The difference in the solutions is no more than a difference in the concept of experience in Hippocratic and Hellenistic medicine. In that it is empirical and skeptical the Hellenistic school recalls older systems; only the particular form of its doctrine is typically Hellenistic.

It is also indicative of its Hellenistic character that the Empiricist school justifies skeptical medicine philosophically and refutes its opponent philosophically. The edifice of medical science is constructed according to the categories of philosophy; the concept of experience is reduced to its component parts by philosophical analysis; the possibility of scientific experience is proved. Dogmatic doctrine is refuted by confronting opinion with opposing opinion and by exposing vicious circles, by demonstrating *regressus ad infinitum*, or by pointing out the absurdity of assertions. Even its pragmatism, which rejects as useless and therefore valueless much of what its opponents accept, is philosophical. Only occasionally does the mere fact that the phenomena contradict it, or fail to prove it, decide against an assertion.[16]

While the skepticism of the Hellenistic physician is a philosophical conviction, the Hippocratic physician is a skeptic by reason of his medical experience and knowledge. For him there are no rigid tenets in medicine because in the sphere of medical action anything can mean anything, because in health and disease nothing is steadfast. Remedies vary in effect; pains arise in both similar and dissimilar ways. Purgations do not always purge but work in various ways; indeed, possibly they do not even act in a manner contrary to constipating drugs. Pains are caused by cold and by warmth and are removed by cold and by warmth. This countering effect of all remedies, this conversion of all things into their opposites, is the consequence of the nature of the human body. Man is constantly changing. To cure him, therefore, a constantly different intervention, a constantly new kind of procedure is required. Everything has the effect peculiar to it as long as the body is able to assimilate the material taken into it; the extent of its ability to do so is determined by the body's own individual nature. If it is un-

---

den, which the Empiricists call impossible, is for the Methodists useless (fr. 27 DG.); similarly, the Hippocratic empiricists attribute no medical significance to the invisible, knowledge of which they concede to be hypothetically possible (cf. p. 196).

[16] DG. has described the rationale of Empiricist theory and the refutation of the Dogmatic doctrine clearly and comprehensively (pp. 281 ff., 288 ff.).

able to assimilate the material, effects of the opposite kind arise. The physician's art consists in knowing how much each body can tolerate. One must tell oneself that everything which alters the present condition is a remedy; but what in the present circumstances constitutes a remedy can only be recognized in each individual case (*De locis in homine*, ch. 43–45, VI 336–42 L.).

Thus the Hippocratic empiricist is a relativist. But he is not, like Protagoras, a relativist from the conviction that man's knowledge is limited, that things can only be apprehended as they appear to each individual observer. Moreover, the empiricist physician does not believe that generally valid knowledge is possible. But he does not doubt it, as does Gorgias, because the intellect judges the same things in various ways and therefore does not recognize the truth.[17] Finally, the empiricist physician only trusts experience; but for him experience does not give firm results nor general definitions of things, as it does for Empedocles. The skeptical empiricism of the classical physician is discovered in medical practice itself and is derived solely therefrom.[18]

The later Empiricist school did not adopt these medical doctrines. At first, Hellenistic medicine was dogmatic because the philosophy of the time was dogmatic. The physician's personal experience was unable to prevail over philosophical conviction, and empirical skepticism was forgotten. Only when dogmatism was overcome in philosophy by skeptical reaction did an undogmatic, skeptical medicine reappear. Philinos and Serapion founded the new school. Yet the connection between medicine and philosophy was still so strong that medicine did not reach back to classical medical skepticism; rather, leaning on the Academy, it created a new medical skepticism based on philosophical principles.[19]

---

[17] Gorgias and Protagoras are true skeptics. Other philosophers are only later interpreted as skeptics (cf. Zeller, *Philosophie der Griechen* III, 1 [5], 494 ff.). Beside Plato, Democritus belongs to this group (cf. R. Walzer, *Galens Schrift über die medizinische Erfahrung*, SB Berl. 1932, 17–18). Only in this sense, not because of his theory of experience, is he important for the Empiricist school (cf. ftn. 4 above).

[18] This classical empiricism is medicine's own creation and, it seems to me, its original contribution to the development of Greek thought. If the Greeks have a dislike for the individual and a preference for the typical (Burckhardt, *Griechische Kulturgeschichte* III, 428–33), the counter-balance is provided by medicine, not by geography, history, or another science. It has been contended that philosophy took over the antithesis between experience and knowledge, between art and accident, from medicine. But it is impossible to decide this question because one cannot tell from the extant material where the antithesis makes its first appearance (cf. Pohlenz, *Der Geist der griechischen Wissenschaft*, Berlin, 1923, 8, and DG. 272 ff.).

[19] Hellenistic Empiricism, though unoriginal, is nevertheless important because from it philosophical ideas which would otherwise be lost can be recovered: in study-

From this skepticism of the Greek Empiricist school there finally emerged a new philosophical skepticism. According to tradition, Empiricist physicians were the leaders of the new Pyrrhonism.[20] But the doctrine of this new skepticism contradicted that of the Empiricist school: the two were incompatible.[21] How is the tradition to be understood?

As Hellenistic scientists the Empiricists interpreted classical medicine, which was different from their own, but similar to the new skeptical teachings. They read Hippocrates, they wrote the first commentaries on the Hippocratic works, they cited the authority of Hippocrates against the authority of Herophilos and Erasistratos.[22] At first the Aca-

---

ing it, one becomes acquainted with Academic skepticism. To what extent Empiricism also reflects Pyrrhonist skepticism, it is scarcely possible to determine. The derivation of the Empiricist school from Timon must mean that much of his skepticism passed over into the Academy, which was presumably aware of Timon's significance for the establishment of skepticism, as well as of the significance of Pyrrhon (cf. Zeller, *loc. cit.*, III, 1 [5], 507).

[20] Zeller (*loc. cit.*, III, 2 [5], 19) says: Several of the spokesmen of the new Pyrrhonism were physicians, and as such are expressly counted amongst the leaders of the Empiricist school; and though it is probably not true of all, the same can be assumed of many others.

[21] Zeller contends (*loc. cit.*, III, 2 [5], 18–20): "As far as its historical origin is concerned, the skepticism of Aenesidemos and his school can be traced back to two sources: to the doctrines of the Empiricist physicians and to the precedent of Pyrrhon and the new Academy. . . . But the Empiricist school from the very beginning tends unmistakably toward skepticism. It preferred to have nothing to do with inquiries into the causes of disease and into the specific effects of each medicament, because such inquiries either fail to fulfil their purpose or are dispensable for the practical ends of medicine in view of the usefulness of drugs already established by experience. This is an expression of the same distrust of human cognitive powers and the same limiting to the practically useful in relation to this particular science, that, raised to a general principle, was the distinctive feature of skepticism." I have attempted to show why this contention is not tenable. Zeller minimizes the difference between the Skeptics and the Empiricist school in questions of cognition (cf. ftn. 8 above) and overlooks the difference in matters of practice. He likewise underestimates the agreement between the Methodist school and the Skeptics (cf. pp. 197–98 above) and the difference between the new Academy and Pyrrhonist skepticism, because he is concerned only with questions of epistemology. Even though individual Academicians fail to assert that things are unknowable, they nevertheless believe in the persuasive power of the good, which one must know in order to act and to live happily (Zeller, *loc. cit.*, III, 1 [5], 531–33), cf. also Gellius, *Noctes Atticae* XIV, 6, concerning the dogmatism of the Academy.

[22] The need for interpretation of ancient works is already implied in the Empiricist concept ἱστορίη (DG. 301). At the close of the Hellenistic period there is generally speaking an increasing preoccupation with fifth century authors. Lykos wrote a commentary on π. τόπων τῶν κατ' ἄνθρωπον (fr. 316 DG.), i.e., on a basic writing of classic empiricism.

demic skepticism of the school was untouched by the discussion of these so very different views; but clearly the ever increasing preoccupation with the old medical skepticism gradually eroded the transmitted teaching. The better the meaning of Hippocratic skepticism was understood, the greater became the tension between the doctrine of the day and the still exemplary ancient theory. The rise of the Methodist school marked the triumph of ancient medical skepticism over the Hellenistic skepticism, which the physician had merely taken over from the philosophers. The rise of the new philosophical skepticism, which leaned on the views of physicians, constituted an infiltration of ancient Hippocratic thinking into philosophy.[23] Any physician who, in spite of the confrontation with Hippocrates, in spite of Pyrrhonist skepticism, remained an Empiricist was obliged at least to change the old Empiricist doctrine in decisive points. If some of the Empiricist physicians no longer claimed that what cannot be experienced cannot be known, if they more and more attempted to limit the concept of experience to the individualism which even the school advocated, this change was an attempt to solve the inner contradiction between the old and new doctrines.[24]

The peculiarly Hellenistic character of the Greek Empiricist school, then, does not consist in the circumstance that its doctrines were first proclaimed in Hellenistic times. There were empiricist and skeptic physicians before Serapion and Philinos. It is only the form of the Skeptical and Empiricist doctrines—and finally their reshaping through the confrontation with the classical—that is Hellenistic.

[23] DG. says (p. 280): "The fact that skepticism turned toward medicine and that medicine, conversely, accepted skepticism is rooted in the structure of both. Medicine operates in a realm which admits unconditionally valid knowledge only to a limited degree (cf. 362; the point here is that it is never possible to prove which of the many relevant circumstances has caused recovery): it is therefore not an exact science." R. Hönigswald, *Die Philosophie des Altertums*, Berlin, 1924, 386, also points out the connection between medicine and skepticism. But both authors only speak of it in reference to Hellenistic medicine. I have tried to show that already in classical times medicine had produced a skepticism of its own, though it is true that in Hellenism, medicine and philosophy do interpenetrate.

[24] That not all late Empiricists can have conceded that what cannot be experienced is unknowable I conclude from the statements of Sextus (cf. ftn. 8 above). DG. (310 ff.) describes how, in the course of the controversy with the Methodists, the Empiricist concept of individual experience evolved. Yet here, though individuality is a consideration in treatment, it never becomes the starting point for it, as it does with the Methodists. The Empiricist treats according to his knowledge, the Methodist according to how the patient feels, even though both explain the diseases themselves along the same lines.

GREEK MEDICINE IN ITS RELATION TO
RELIGION AND MAGIC*

I n the historiography of Greek medicine religious and magical healing, in general, are dealt with only occasionally and very briefly. No one
will deny that, throughout antiquity, incubations played an important
rôle, nor will it be disputed that incantations, at least in later centuries,
were of great importance. But since these are factors abhorrent to modern science, they are not interesting to the modern historian either.

The neglect of religious and magical medicine seems the more
justifiable because, according to the prevailing opinion, Greek medical
art itself dispensed with religion and magic. Traces of these, if they are
to be found in any period at all, soon became "rather of the drapery
than of the body of medicine."[1] Religious cures, "the half-world"[2] of
scientific medicine, and magical rites, its superstitious caricature—so to
speak—are said to have been rejected by the Greek physicians themselves. The abrogation of religious and magical thought is therefore
considered even as characteristic of the Greek attitude and as significant
for the difference between it and the Roman mode of thinking.[3] There
is no need for more than a perfunctory consideration of those unscientific conceptions.

It is true, religion and magic are very seldom, almost never, mentioned in Greek medical treatises; if they occur, they are usually discussed in a negative sense. At first glance it seems, therefore, safe to
conclude that they were of no importance, at least up to the time of
Galen. Later, while Galen's rational medicine was still preserved in the

* *Bulletin of the Institute of the History of Medicine*, 1937, vol. 5, pp. 201–46.
I wish to express my gratitude to Mrs. H. Cherniss for revising my English.

[1] T. Clifford Allbutt, Greek Medicine in Rome, London, 1921, p. 31: "In Greece
the theurgic invocations of Apollo Paean, of Chiron, of Aesculapius, seem soon to
have become, as in the Oath, rather of the drapery than of the body of medicine."
[2] W. W. Tarn, Hellenistic Civilization, London, 1930, p. 272.
[3] T. Clifford Allbutt, l. c.: "In Rome, and not during the Republic only, theurgic,
or hierurgic, or magical craft 'and those who used curious arts' were of the body of it;
drugs and operations were but auxiliaries."

encyclopedias, the new and prevailing spirit of medicine was that of religion and magic. But those centuries are called the decadence of ancient medicine. There is hardly another term used to describe this period, so strong is the conviction that scientific medicine cannot have anything in common with religious and magical forces.[4] Some scholars recognize the fact that religion and magic became apparent only in the Byzantine epoch but began to influence medicine long before Galen.[5] They date the decline earlier. According to them the rational treatment of Coan and Cnidian physicians was already contaminated in the fourth century B.C. For Hippocratic medicine did not outlive Platonic methods; from the Hellenistic era on it became speculative and even superstitious. Thus medicine, like all the other sciences, collapsed long before the close of antiquity.[6]

Now it is easy to argue that from a purely historical aspect these limitations and valuations cannot be accepted. Medicine, imbued with religion and magic or freed from both of them, medicine after Galen or

---

[4] H. O. Taylor, Greek Biology and Medicine (Our Debt to Greece and Rome), 1922, especially p. 122. Identical in its principle is the representation of the history of Greek medicine in Gercke-Norden, Einleitung in die Altertumswissenschaft, II, 5[4], Exakte Wissenschaften v. A. Rehm und K. Vogel, Leipzig, 1933. Cf. also U. v. Wilamowitz-Moellendorf, Die Griechische Literatur des Altertums (Die Kultur der Gegenwart, I, 8[3], 1912, p. 250). Ivan Bloch, Byzantinische Medizin (Handbuch der Geschichte der Medizin, herausgegeben v. M. Neuburger und J. Pagel, Jena, 1902, I, p. 508). A certain superiority of Greek medicine over the Roman is thereby acknowledged even for the latest centuries, cf. Gercke-Norden, l. c., p. 77 and M. Neuburger, Geschichte der Medizin, II, 1, 1911, p. 3. Cf. also S. Runciman, Byzantine Civilization, London, 1933, pp. 132; 237.

[5] M. Neuburger, l. c., pp. 3–4.

[6] W. H. S. Jones, Hippocrates, with an English translation (Loeb Classical Library), I, 1923, p. 8: "[In Greek medicine] the two methods, that of Greek philosophy and that of modern science, stand face to face. The struggle between them was, for the time being, short. Medicine, almost the only branch of Greek science scientifically studied, was worsted in the fight, and medical science gradually degenerated from rational treatment to wild speculation and even quackery and superstition. The transcendant genius of Plato, strong in that very power of persuasion the use of which he so much deprecated, won the day. The philosophic fervor which longed with passionate desire for unchangeable reality, that felt a lofty contempt for the material world with its ever-shifting phenomena, that aspired to rise to a heavenly region where changeless Ideas might be apprehended by pure intelligence purged from every bodily taint, was more than a match for the humble researches of men who wished to relieve human suffering by a patient study of those very phenomena that Plato held of no account. So for centuries philosophy flourished and science languished, in spite of Aristotle, Euclid and Archimedes." Withington in his contribution to W. H. S. Jones, Malaria and Greek History, Manchester, 1909, pp. 154 sq., expresses the same opinion, although he gives a different explanation.

in the Hellenistic period is, after all, Greek medicine; Greek medical literature is, indeed, an accumulation of the most different writings.[7] One must depict the facts as they are without any prejudice and properly determine the share which each of the different forms of treatment had in reality.

But this is not enough. There are not only "three lines of possible approach which may be described as the secular, the magical and the religious,"[8] each one of them of equal historical value, and each strictly separated from the others. That religious medicine at least changed a good deal by taking over results of scientific medicine, by becoming more rational, is a fact generally believed.[9] Yet an influence of religious and magical ideas on science is also conceivable. It can be denied only if it is true that the conception of medical art necessarily devoid of any religious and magical content was adopted by the ancient physicians. Whether this was generally the case is not to be decided without further proof; the reticence concerning religion and magic, even their rejection in many cases, does not suffice as an argument. For these are ambiguous instances which have to be interpreted first. Such an inquiry is also important, since religious healing and magical rites used by patients throughout antiquity and relied on in ever-increasing measure presented if not a theoretical, at least a practical problem to the physicians. Did the physicians recognize the practice of priests and magicians as a means outside their own activity or did they renounce it as being worthless and even false? Their reaction must have depended largely on their theoretical attitude toward religious and magical ideas.

These are the problems involved in the relation of Greek medicine to religion and magic. It is with their discussion and with the description of the historical situation that I shall try to deal, testing the char-

---

[7] Charles Singer, Greek Biology and Greek Medicine, Oxford, 1922, p. 80–81, is quite right in stating: "That mass [of Greek medical learning] contained much dross, material that survived from early as from late Greek times which was hardly, if at all, superior to the debased compositions that circulated in the name of medicine in the middle centuries. The recovered Greek medical writings also contained some material of the purest and most scientific type."

[8] W. R. Halliday, The Treatment of Disease in Antiquity (in "Greek Poetry and Life," Essays presented to G. Murray, Oxford, 1936, p. 277). But he, too, calls Galen "the last Greek medical scientist of antiquity. Man's mind had moved from a scientific toward a religious and magical view of the universe." (p. 293).

[9] Cf. R. Herzog, Die Wunderheilungen von Epidaurus, Philologus, Supplement XXII, III, 1931, pp. 145–147; cf. also O. Weinreich, Antike Heilungswunder, Religionsgeschichtliche Versuche u. Vorarbeiten, VIII, 1, 1909, p. 110.

acter of Greek medicine in regard to the explanation and to the treatment of diseases. In doing this I cannot base my argument on any continuous ancient debate of the subject; no such book is preserved. It is necessary to rely on single phrases to be found in the different writings and to take them as a clue to the underlying general ideology. This is a laborious procedure. A vast material must be collected and the judgment must be always restricted and modified. But no other way is left for an approach to the problem which is so important for the adequate interpretation of Greek medicine.

I. The Explanation of Diseases

By the Hippocratic as well as by the later physicians, the causes of illnesses are held to be first of all the effect upon the human body of cold, warmth, sun, air, and climate. This, no doubt, is a natural explanation and to many physicians it means this and nothing more. A follower of Anaxagoras in the fifth century B.C., an Epicurean or Skeptic in the Hellenistic centuries and later, each considers the celestial phenomena as appearances of nature, devoid of God.[10]

But this, to be sure, is not the only, not even the most usual meaning expressed by those conceptions. The Hippocratic book on the Sacred Disease states: "This disease . . . comes from the same causes as others, from the things that come to and go from the body, from cold, sun, and from the changing restlessness of winds. These things are divine, . . ."[11] Later, for physicians who follow Plato and Aristotle, the divinity of sun and stars and climate is unquestionable; nor are the forces of the lower world, air and water, deprived of divinity.[12] The Stoic physicians firmly believe in the divine character of the forces of nature. On the other hand, the interpretation of the gods as natural powers is very common and very Greek. Some declare that "the Phoenicians had better notions about the gods than the Greeks, giving as an instance that to Asclepius they assign Apollo as father, but no mortal woman as his mother. Asclepius . . . is air, bringing health to mankind and to all animals like-

---

[10] Cf. the corresponding medical theories p. 210.

[11] Jones, l. c., II, p. 183: Αὕτη δὲ ἡ νοῦσος . . . γίνεται ἀφ' ὧν καὶ αἱ λοιπαί, ἀπὸ τῶν προσιόντων καὶ ἀπιόντων, καὶ ψύχεος καὶ ἡλίου καὶ πνευμάτων μεταβαλλομένων τε καὶ οὐδέποτε ἀτρεμιζόντων. ταῦτα δ' ἐστὶ θεῖα, . . .

[12] E.g., Plató, Laws, X, 899b; Aristotle, On the Heaven, 288a 4–5.

wise; Apollo is the sun, and most rightly is he named the father of Asclepius, because the sun, by adapting his course to the seasons, imparts to the air its healthfulness." But the answer is that: "The argument was as much Greek as Phoenician; for at Titane in Sicyonia the same image is called both, Health and . . . thus clearly showing that it is the course of the sun that brings health to mankind."[13] All these instances reveal how utterly different are the ancients' conceptions of natural phenomena from those of modern times.

If this is so, the adequate interpretation of the terminology used in Greek medicine becomes very difficult. In his book on the Sacred Disease the author employs nothing but the terms sun and cold and winds and no theological vocabulary whatsoever. It is only in the differentiation of his conception from that of the others that he refers to the elements as divine.[14] Were it not for reasons of polemics, then,—that he wants to make clear his position against those who declare special diseases to be divine—he would scarcely even mention his belief in the divinity of the elements. Thus, natural and religious expressions are used as equivalents.[15] Whether this is so or not depends in every case on the philosophical and scientific outlook of the man who is writing.

As for dogmatic physicians of the Hellenistic schools the religious connotation of their words can safely be assumed. For they are more or less related to the Platonic, Aristotelian or Stoic philosophy. Only Em-

[13] Pausanias, Achaia, XXIII, 7 (Pausanias, Description of Greece, with an English Translation by W. H. S. Jones, Loeb Class. Library, III, 1918, p. 309): . . .ὸ ἐγνωκέναι τὰ ἐς τὸ θεῖον ἔφασκε Φοίνικας τά τε ἄλλα Ἑλλήνων βέλτιον καὶ δὴ καὶ Ἀσκληπιῷ πατέρα μὲν σφᾶς Ἀπόλλωνα ἐπιφημίζειν, θνητὴν δὲ γυναῖκα οὐδεμίαν μητέρα. Ἀσκληπιὸν μὲν γὰρ ἀέρα γένει τε ἀνθρώπων εἶναι καὶ πᾶσιν ὁμοίως ζῴοις ἐπιτήδειον πρὸς ὑγίειαν, Ἀπόλλωνα δὲ ἥλιον καὶ αὐτὸν ὀρθότατα Ἀσκληπιῷ πατέρα ἐπονομάζεσθαι, ὅτι ἐς τὸ ἁρμόζον ταῖς ὥραις ποιούμενος ὁ ἥλιος τὸν δρόμον μεταδίδωσι καὶ τῷ ἀέρι ὑγιείας . . . οὐδὲν δέ τι Φοινίκων μᾶλλον ἢ καὶ Ἑλλήνων ἔφην τὸν λόγον, ἐπεὶ καὶ ἐν Τιτάνῃ τῆς Σικυωνίων τὸ αὐτὸ ἄγαλμα Ὑγείαν τε ὀνομάζεσθαι καὶ . . . δῆλα ὡς τὸν ἡλιακὸν δρόμον ἐπὶ γῆς ὑγίειαν ποιοῦντα ἀνθρώποις. This opinion is the more important since Peripatos and Stoa had a conciliatory attitude toward common religion, the latter even trying to combine the popular belief with its philosophical theory. I am, however, only concerned with the problem of what Greek gods mean to the different periods and groups of men, not with the question of whether they were originally nature-gods or not.

[14] Cp. 1; cp. 22.

[15] Cf. Herodotus, II, ch. 24, where the author says in one statement (Herodotus, with an English Translation by A. D. Godley, Loeb Class. Library, I, 1926, p. 301): "During the winter the *sun* is driven by the storms from his customary course and passes over the inland parts of Libya. Now to make the shortest conclusion, that is all that need be said; for to whatever country this *God* is nearest, or over it, it is to be thought that that land is the thirstiest and that the rivers in it are diminished."

piricists and Methodists of those centuries can be said to think in purely
natural terms. For they are followers of the new Academy or of the
Pyrrhonean Skepsis. But what about the Hippocratic physicians whose
philosophical standpoint is hardly known, what about the average
physician who is a practitioner and not a trained scientist with a philosophical background?

The Hippocratic author, expressing his opinion that sun and cold
and winds are divine, does not give any proof of his assumption. Apparently he is not concerned with objections which could be raised
against such a belief. At first glance it seems to follow that he is making
a statement generally accepted in his time. But no doubt, in the fifth
and fourth centuries B.C., when this book and all the other Hippocratic
writings were probably written, there were men who believed that the
sun and moon and all the natural appearances are only corporeal bodies.
To them the processes going on in the world are not influenced by God.
This disbelief, as it is called by Plato, is widespread even in the fourth
century B.C.[16] At the same time, however, the average Greek, asked
whether God exists or not, truthfully asserts the existence of the gods.
He points to the evidence of the earth, the sun, moon, and stars as instances of deity and divinity. Concerning all the celestial phenomena,
concerning the years and months and all the seasons, he does not deny
that "all things are full of gods," as Thales said. According to him nobody is foolish enough to disregard this belief.[17] In other words, the disbelief in the divinity of those powers of nature is restricted to a certain
group of people, to the enlightened, but it is not at all self-evident nor
is it the attitude of the average man. For this attitude is relatively new
and rather suspicious: "The first man to put in writing the clearest and
boldest of all doctrines (concerning the natural explanation of the
phenomena) was Anaxagoras. But he was no ancient authority, nor
was his doctrine in high repute. It was still under seal of secrecy, and
made its way slowly among the few only, who received it with a certain
caution rather than with implicit confidence. Men could not abide the

---

[16] Plato, Laws, X, 866e; Sophistes, 265c.

[17] Plato, Laws, X, 886a; d/e; 899b/c. It is remarkable that Plato says, whether
in earnest or in jest, that these theories are familiar in Athens but unknown in Crete
(886b). They are certainly in contrast to the old religious attitude. For "it seems
the first men in Greece thought those only to be gods whom many of the barbarians
honour to-day—sun, moon, earth, stars and heaven." φαίνονταί μοι οἱ πρῶτοι τῶν
περὶ τὴν Ἑλλάδα τούτους μόνους τοὺς θεοὺς ἡγεῖσθαι οὕσπερ νῦν πολλοὶ τῶν βαρβάρων, ἥλιον
καὶ σελήνην καὶ γῆν καὶ ἄστρα καὶ οὐρανόν. (Plato, Cratylus 397c).

natural philosophers and 'visionaries,' as they were then called, for that they reduced the divine agency down to irrational causes, blind forces, and necessary incidents."[18] The Hippocratic author is quite right, then; his conviction does not need any detailed proof. For it is still more usual to understand the natural powers as divine than as merely natural; the opposite theory is the one which, in general, has to be demonstrated. It is the philosopher who must ascertain the divine character of the world against those thinkers who disagree with such an opinion; the ordinary man may still speak of it as carrying its own evidence.

From this fact it follows, of course, that in the Hippocratic writings one cannot possibly interpret all the natural terms as devoid of any religious meaning. It is not necessary to dwell on the fact that it is from the book on the Sacred Disease that the statement about the divinity of the natural quality derives, from this very enlightend and critical treatise as it is usually called.[19] All the same, the assumption is justified. With the exception of a few books the Hippocratic writers in general do not renounce the divinity of nature, even if they do not mention it expressly. They are, apparently, not atheists, as they would have to be if they embraced the opposite theory.[20] Even less can it be assumed that

[18] Plutarch, Nicias, ch. 23 (Plutarch's Lives, with an English Translation by Bernadotte Perrin, Loeb Class. Library, III, 1915, p. 291): Ὁ γὰρ πρῶτος σαφέστατόν τε πάντων καὶ θαρραλεώτατον περὶ σελήνης . . . λόγον εἰς γραφὴν καταθέμενος Ἀναξαδόρας οὔτ᾽ αὐτὸς ἦν παλαιὸς οὔτε ὁ λόγος ἔνδοξος, ἀλλ᾽ ἀπόρρητος ἔτι καὶ δι᾽ ὀλίγων καὶ μετ᾽ εὐλαβείας τινὸς ἢ πίστεως βαδίζων. οὐ γὰρ ἠνείχοντο τοὺς φυσικοὺς καὶ μετεωρολέσχας τότε καλουμένους, ὡς εἰς αἰτίας ἀλόγους καὶ δυνάμεις ἀπρονοήτους καὶ κατηναγκασμένα πάθη διατρίβοντας τὸ θεῖον. The possible forerunners of this disbelief are discussed very briefly, its novelty being stressed also in Plato's Laws, X, 886c/d. I am well aware that Aristophanes (Peace, v. 410 sq.) says the Greeks are given into the hands of the barbarians because they do not sacrifice to sun and moon. But it is quite a different problem whether sacrifices were made to these powers or whether these phenomena were considered to be divine at that time. And certainly Socrates, a contemporary of Aristophanes, did not want to investigate the meteorological phenomena, because they are *divine*, but was interested in *human* things alone, namely in ethical problems (Xenophon, Memorabilia, I. l. 12).

[19] Cf. e.g., U. v. Wilamowitz-Moellendorf, Griech. Lesebuch, I, 2, Text, Berlin, 1926, pp. 269–70: "Der aufgeklärte Arzt bekämpft die übernatürliche Natur der Krankheit . . . Aber nicht minder liegt dem Verfasser an der Einheitlichkeit der Naturauffassung, an der Wissenschaft, die auch für seine Beurteilung der Heiligen Krankheit massgebend ist." Cf. also Jones, l. c., II, p. 129.

[20] The merely natural explanation of the heavenly bodies was reason enough for calling the philosophers atheists (Plato, Laws, XII, 967c). Yet, as far as I can see, there is no proof for Heidel's assumption that the physicians also are named in antiquity a godless crew, certainly not because of their attacks against magicians (cf. Proceedings of the American Academy of Arts and Sciences, Vol. XLV, 1910, Footnote 47).

the average physicians abandoned the old inherited belief in the divine character of sun and air and seasons. Their mental attitude was still nearer to that of the people who, unable to endure the atheistic philosophers, expelled them even from Athens,[21] and who were always suspicious of the natural explanation of phenomena if it excluded the recognition of divine power. It is true that "it was not until later times that the radiant repute of Plato, because of the life the man led, and because he subjected the compulsions of the physical world to divine and more sovereign principles, took away the obloquy of such doctrines as these, and gave their science free course among all men."[22] For even in later centuries Epicureans were banished from the cities because of their atheism; throughout antiquity, the natural explanation of the world remained a bold venture. The average man recognized God's ways in the movements of heavenly bodies and so, ordinarily, did the physician.[23] It is evident then that all the external influences which are held responsible for the origin of diseases are in general not understood as merely natural. Sun and moon and stars and seasons are material to the modern mind, but to the ancients they are gods.

Now the question arises as to how the explanation of illnesses by inner factors, by the nature of man or of diseases, an explanation very common in antiquity too, must be interpreted. In answering it a certain difficulty, noticeable, I think, in the whole discussion of the subject of my inquiry, will become even more striking. The Greeks speak of nature as do the moderns. But what they mean by it, as what they mean by all their notions of natural phenomena, is different from the modern conceptions which in their definite form always arise in the modern mind at the mention of the terms.[24] Nevertheless, only these words can be used; step by step the distinct features of the ancient thought must

[21] Anaxagoras (Plutarch, Pericles ch. 32, The Law of Diopeithes); Protagoras (Sextus Empiricus, adv. mathematicos IX, 56); Diagoras (Aristophanes, Birds, v. 1073).

[22] Plutarch, Nicias, ch. 23, l. c.: ὀψὲ δ' ἡ Πλάτωνος ἐκλάψασα δόξα διὰ τὸν βίον τοῦ ἀνδρός, καὶ ὅτι ταῖς θείαις καὶ κυριωτέραις ἀρχαῖς ὑπέταξε τὰς φυσικὰς ἀνάγκας, ἀφεῖλε τὴν τῶν λόγων τούτων διαβολήν, καὶ τοῖς μαθήμασιν εἰς ἅπαντας ὁδὸν ἐνέδωκεν.

[23] Cf. Jakob Burckhardt, Griech. Kulturgeschichte⁴, III, pp. 324 sq.; II, p. 216, and Plato (Laws, X, 888b–e) who contends that nobody is able to continue in his disbelief " 'till old age."

[24] Not to mention the various meanings which the conception of nature had for the Greeks themselves; this problem cannot be dealt with here, cf. Heidel, l. c., pp. 95 sq.

212

be described in these same terms. In order to avoid any misunderstanding of the statements, it is necessary therefore always to remain cognizant of this difference between ancient and modern terminology.

From the fifth century B.C. on nature was conceived as a mechanical or dynamic power of its own without any divine manifestation. It was defined in this way by the followers of the physiologists in the pre-Socratic centuries and in Plato's time. Strato thought that nature, without the help of the gods, creates everything. The Epicureans, although believing in the existence of God, did not let him take part in the worldly processes. In the Academic philosophy nature was considered to be the necessity of movement; it was just in regard to diseases that such a conception was worked out most clearly.[25] Physicians imbued with those doctrines, then, cannot but contemplate the nature of man as devoid of God. Among the Hippocratic writers a few undoubtedly share such an opinion, the same ones who do not believe in the divinity of the elements. And the later Empiricists and Methodists do not recognize the divine impress of God either.

But certain as this is, the opinion that nature cannot be thought otherwise than as created and permeated by God is also to be found throughout antiquity. So it is said in the book on Airs, Waters, and Places: "I too think that these diseases are divine, and so are all others, no one being more divine or more human than any other; all are alike, and all divine, but each of them has a nature of its own, and none arises without its nature."[26] To this man, the distinction between divine and human and the different estimation of these two powers become meaningless because everything is equally divine. This does not imply that God acts directly and is responsible, by reason of His personal interference, for the single event. Such a possibility is expressly excluded. The individual disease has a nature of its own, but by this term its divine character is only expressed in another form; it is not done away with by being explained through nature. Individual nature therefore, since it does not contradict God, but is rather His essence, must be apprehended as created by God and as divine in itself. This conviction

---

[25] Concerning the physiologists cf. Plato, Laws, X, 889b; Sophistes 265c and Plutarch, De defectu oraculorum, 436d. Concerning Strato, cf. Cicero, Academica, II, 38, 121; De natura deorum, I, 13, 35; concerning the Academy cf. De natura deorum, III, 25, 65; 11, 27; 10, 24.

[26] Jones, l. c., I, p. 127 (slightly altered): ἐμοὶ δὲ καὶ αὐτῷ δοκεῖ ταῦτα τὰ πάθεα θεῖα εἶναι καὶ τἆλλα πάντα καὶ οὐδὲν ἕτερον ἑτέρου θειότερον οὐδὲ ἀνθρωπινώτερον, ἀλλὰ πάντα ὁμοῖα καὶ πάντα θεῖα. ἕκαστον δὲ αὐτῶν ἔχει φύσιν τὴν ἑωυτοῦ καὶ οὐδὲν ἄνευ φύσιος γίνεται.

is expressed also in the Hippocratic book on Regimen: "The nature of all things was arranged by the gods," and "all the things take place . . . through a divine necessity."[27] In the same way nature is thought of later. It is divine to the Platonic physician; to the Aristotelian physician it is at least demonic, the divine not being realized in an absolute degree.[28] The Stoic physician must find God everywhere in nature; for nature is identical with God; these are only different terms.[29] While there is a tendency to understand nature without referring to divine power, a more theological tendency also exists, nay even prevails, in antiquity.

This theological conception, however, seems to a certain extent self-contradictory. In the theory of the Hippocratic physicians rationalism and belief are interwoven with each other, naturalism and theology are combined into a unity; the same is valid for the ideas of the later physicians. Everything is natural, but in being so it is divine too, or to use another phrase it is supernatural; and proof of this is found in reasoning. The modern logical objection to such a theory apparently did not occur to the ancient mind; indeed, there was no opposition between God and nature.[30] At any rate, it seems impossible to contend that every form of supernaturalism was rejected by the Hippocratic physicians. On the contrary, they as scientists embraced a supernatural dogma.[31] Equally unfounded, I believe, is the statement that the gods were not dethroned by these men, yet that nothing was left to them

[27] Jones, l. c., IV, pp. 249–51: φύσιν δὲ πάντων θεοὶ διεκόσμησαν. 237: πάντα γίνεται δι᾿ ἀνάγκην θείην.

[28] Concerning Plato, cf. e.g., Sophistes 265c; concerning Aristotle, cf. E. Zeller, Die Philosophie d. Griechen, II, 2³, 1879, pp. 330 sq.

[29] Cf. e.g., Diels, Doxographi Graeci, 322b9–12.

[30] One is reminded of the most significant metaphysical idea of the seventeenth century which is characterized by Dilthey as "Halbheit des rationalen Supranaturalismus; Kompromiss zwischen Dogmenglaube und Vernunftwissenschaft." (Die Autonomie des Denkens im 17. Jahrhundert, Gesammelte Schriften, II, 1929, p. 283). In spite of all the divergence caused by the Christian conception of divine revelation the attitude of that time, as far as I can judge, is best compared with that of the Greeks.

[31] Th. Gomperz, Griech. Denker⁴, I, 1922, p. 257, says, "Mit ausserordentlicher Schärfe wird aber allem Supranaturalismus in zwei Erzeugnissen der Hippokratischen Schule (sc. the book on Water, Air and Places and the book on the Sacred Disease) der Krieg erklärt," although he admits that, according to the writers, "strenges Festhalten an ausnahmsloser Gesetzmässigkeit alles Naturgeschehens mit dem religiösen Glauben an einen göttlichen Urquell, aus dem im letzten Grunde eben dieses Naturgeschehen fliesse, vollkommen vereinbar sei." (p. 258). Concerning the book on the Sacred Disease and its attitude cf. p. 215, below.

but "the sole rôle of first cause in the physical world."[32] God is indeed deprived of any direct and special interference; he is not supposed to act arbitrarily. But what he loses on one side he gains on the other: everything, being a natural event, is divine.

This theory of supernaturalism does not go uncontested even in the Hippocratic writings. The divine influence is still recognized, but it is understood to be only one factor just as is nature, which is a power of its own. So the author of the book on the Sacred Disease says: "This disease is not in my opinion any more divine or more sacred than other diseases, but has its nature and origin."[33] And the same is repeated with the addition that the "origin of this disease, like that of other diseases, lies in heredity," that "the cause of this affection, as of the more serious illnesses generally, is the brain."[34] The conclusion is that "there is no need to put the disease in a special class and to consider it more divine than the others; they are all divine and all human. Each has a nature and power of its own."[35] What does this mean? It means that all diseases are divine in so far as they are caused by sun and air and winds, which

---

[32] W. H. Heidel, The Heroic Age of Science, 1933, p. 21. He recognizes that Greek science is not irreligious (p. 17) but the men of science maintain a common-sense attitude toward life (p. 20); for the time being the gods seem to be virtually excluded from the world of nature; so far as they receive a place in it, they find it under the shadow of Law or Custom (p. 21). Heidel, who stresses so much the importance of Greek medicine for the study of Greek science, does not refer to the author of the book on Regimen as a physician, but only as an intellectual leader (p. 21); this invalidates his argument concerning medicine. Almost all the more important Hippocratic books recognize the gods as a real factor in nature. It is impossible here to deal with every one of them. I need only refer to the book on Flesh in which the power of thinking is ascribed to warmth. The author apparently agrees with Diogenes of Apollonia (cf. K. Deichgräber, Hippokrates über Entstehung u. Aufbau d. menschlichen Körpers, 1935, p. 2, 10–14). Diogenes did not only expound the theological aspect, he bitterly opposed, as he had to, the physiologists, those men who thought they could explain everything by nature devoid of the divine spirit. In attacking them he maintains that the power of God creates the world, as Plato says (cf. Sophistes 265c). This, by the way, proves that the expression τῆς φύσιος τὴν ἀνάγκην cannot be understood as purely mechanical (contrary to Heidel, Proceedings, l. c., p. 100, 81), but it is rather to be understood in the sense of the book on Regimen. It is interesting that from the sixteenth century on some interpreters of Hippocrates refer to the book on Flesh if they want to prove the religiosity of the great physician (cf. Deichgräber, l. c., pp. 56 sq.).

[33] Jones, l. c., II, p. 139 (slightly altered): οὐδέν τί μοι δοκεῖ τῶν ἄλλων θειοτέρη εἶναι νούσων οὐδὲ ἱερωτέρη, ἀλλὰ φύσιν μὲν ἔχει καὶ πρόφασιν.

[34] Jones, l. c., II, p. 151: ἄρχεται δὲ ὥσπερ καὶ τἆλλα νοσήματα κατὰ γένος. 153: Ἀλλὰ γὰρ αἴτιος ὁ ἐγκέφαλος τούτου τοῦ πάθεος, ὥσπερ καὶ τῶν ἄλλων νοσημάτων τῶν μεγίστων.

[35] Jones, l. c., II, 183: ὥστε μηδὲν δεῖ ἀποκρίνοντα τὸ νόσημα θειότερον τῶν λοιπῶν νομίσαι, ἀλλὰ πάντα θεῖα καὶ πάντα ἀνθρώπινα. φύσιν δὲ ἕκαστον ἔχει καὶ δύναμιν ἐφ' ἑωυτοῦ.

are divine, as had been said before. They are human, apparently because they have their origin in heredity, in the organs of the body. It is impossible to admit the divinity of a special disease, for they are all divine; at the same time all diseases are human because of the influence of the body. The two spheres of the divine and of the natural are then fundamentally separate, although their influence is combined in every action.[36]

A similar theory has to be presupposed for the book on Prognostics. At the outset the physician is advised "to learn the natures of such diseases, how much they exceed the strength of men's bodies, besides whether there is any divine influence in them and to learn how to forecast them."[37] Divine influence and human nature again are separated as distinct forces. The nature of man is not in itself divine but the divine is thought to become apparent in the body. In what way this must be understood was already discussed in antiquity; the interpretations varied widely.[38] It seems to me that it is the spontaneous reactions which are signified by the word "divine." In one of the Hippocratic books it is stated: "In fact it is especially knowledge of the gods that by medicine is woven into the stuff of the mind . . . Physicians have given place to the gods. For in medicine that which is powerful is not in excess. In fact,

---

[36] Jones, l. c., I, p. x, without reference but, I think, mindful of these passages, says: "The fifth century B.C. witnessed the supreme effort of the Greeks to cast aside this incubus in all spheres of thought. They came to realize that to attribute an event to the action of a god leaves us just where we were, and that to call normal phenomena natural and abnormal divine is to introduce an unscientific dualism, in that what is divine (because mysterious) in one generation may be natural (because understood) in the next, while, on the other hand, however fully we may understand a phenomenon, there must always be a mysterious and unexplained element in it. All phenomena are equally divine and equally natural." This statement, I think, is not in accordance with the meaning of the Hippocratic author, as I tried to explain it. Everything is understood, even though it be in the form of a divine causality. On the other hand, the main theme of the book is not the uniformity of Nature, every aspect of which is equally divine (Jones, l. c., II, p. 135). It also follows from my interpretation that there is a difference in the basic theory between the book on the Sacred Disease and the book on Water, Air, and Places (contrary to Jones, l. c., II, pp. 130/1). Furthermore the thesis of Gomperz that the Hippocratic physicians rejected the belief in supernatural forces can certainly not be proved by the statement of this treatise; cf. n. 31, above.

[37] Jones, l. c., II, pp. 6–8: γνῶναι οὖν χρὴ τῶν τοιούτων νοσημάτων τὰς φύσιας, ὁκόσον ὑπὲρ τὴν δύναμίν εἰσιν τῶν σωμάτων ἅμα δὲ καὶ εἴ τι θεῖον ἔνεστιν ἐν τῇσι νούσοισι. Following the edition of Kühlewein, Jones omits the words concerning the divine, but they are contained in all the manuscripts. Cf. also Hippocrates, ed. Littré, VII, 1851, p. 312.

[38] Galeni in Hippocratis Prognosticum, ed. I. Heeg, CMG, V, 9, 2, 1915, p. 205, 28 sq. Erotiani Vocum Hippocraticarum Collectio cum Fragmentis, rec. E. Nachmanson, 1918, p. 108, 10 sq.

though physicians take many things in hand, many diseases are also overcome for them spontaneously."³⁹ The physicians then make room for the gods in regard to the spontaneous reactions of the body, which are considered as an interference of divine character, since they cannot be mastered by the human being. This is a theory unfamiliar neither to the fifth and fourth centuries B.C. nor to the later periods. Aristotle says: "There are a few to whom it seems that chance is a cause, but that it is not evident to human intelligence, since it is something divine and marvelous."⁴⁰ It is in this sense that the statement in this Hippocratic book and in the others can best be interpreted. The spontaneous reactions, which are not the effects of human efforts and which can only be acknowledged as facts, are mentioned very often in the book on Prognostics as well as in the book on the Diseases of Women, the author of which states that the physician has first of all to consider the possible divine influence, then the nature of women, and many other things.⁴¹ At any rate, many of the Hippocratic books, a greater number than identify God with nature, acknowledge the divine as a factor apart from nature, which is a power of its own.

No doubt in some treatises God is even entirely excluded from the bodily processes. For in the fifth and fourth centuries B.C. there are many people who believe in the mechanism of the nature of plants, animals, and human beings: "Nature produces them out of a certain spontaneous cause and without any creative intelligence."⁴² This, I think,

---

³⁹ Jones, l. c., II, p. 289: Καὶ γὰρ μάλιστα ἡ περὶ θεῶν εἴδησις ἐν νόῳ αὐτῇ ἐμπλέκεται. οἱ δὲ ἰητροὶ θεοῖσι παρακεχωρήκασιν. οὐ γὰρ ἔνι περιττὸν ἐν αὐτῇ τὸ δυναστεῦον. καὶ γὰρ οὗτοι πολλὰ μὲν μεταχειρέονται, πολλὰ δὲ καὶ κεκράτηται αὐτοῖσι δι' ἑωυτῶν.

⁴⁰ Aristotle, Physics, 196b, 5–7: εἰσὶ δέ τινες οἷς δοκεῖ εἶναι αἰτία μὲν ἡ τύχη, ἄδηλος δὲ ἀνθρωπίνῃ διανοίᾳ ὡς θεῖόν τι οὖσα καὶ δαιμονιώτερον. Cf. Aristotle, The Physics, with an English Translation by P. H. Wicksteed and F. M. Cornford (Loeb Class. Library), Vol. I, 1929, pp. 146–7 where the parallels are quoted. Chance in the Aristotelian discussion is identical with spontaneity, cf. l. c., p. 120.

⁴¹ E. Littré, Oeuvres complètes d'Hippocrate, VII, 1851, p. 312: περὶ δὲ τῆς γυναικείης φύσιος καὶ νοσημάτων τάδε λέγω. μάλιστα μὲν τὸ θεῖον ἐν τοῖσι ἀνθρώποισι αἴτιον εἶναι. ἔπειτα αἱ φύσιες τῶν γυναικῶν καὶ χροιαί. Heidel, The Heroic Age of Science, p. 18, characterizes this statement as the sort of curt remark that "one might perhaps expect to find in an unbelieving modern who wished to avoid offending sensibilities he respected but did not share." He points to the fact that later the divine does not occur, and this would be indeed an objection, as is already remarked by Galen (l. c., p. 208, 4–8). If one adopts the explanation I propose this objection is no longer valid, and the statement, obviously important, can be given its full value. Cf. also Hippocrates, ed. Littré, IX, 1861, p. 26; 28.

⁴² Plato, Sophistes 265c: τὴν φύσιν αὐτὰ γεννᾶν ἀπό τινος αἰτίας αὐτομάτης καὶ ἄνευ διανοίας φυούσης.

is even the more common attitude at this time. For the deification of the individual organism is a modern and advanced idea in these centuries, one that is not yet generally accepted. Only a few individuals already visualize that "all things were arranged in the body, in a fashion conformable to itself, by fire, a copy of the whole, the small after the manner of the great and the great after the manner of the small."[43] And they are physicians. But others, just because they adore God, are aware of the contrast between Him and man, "the one being utterly corrupt, the other being perfectly holy,"[44] They are physicians, too.

That the nature of everything is divine, that every process can only be understood as regulated by divine agency, is a conception which becomes current among men only in later times through Platonic, Aristotelian, and Stoic philosophy. It is, however, of the greatest importance that from the Hellenistic period on the religious rationalism is accepted by more and more scientists. For the mechanical and irreligious philosophy and science degenerated into avowed skepticism. The Epicureans do not care for a single and uniform explanation of the phenomena; they rejoice in manifold causes of the same event. The Empiricists refuse to explain anything because the human intellect cannot judge the causes and can discover only the proximate conditions. The Methodists deal only with the phenomena without considering causation at all. Scientific inquiry is restricted to dogmatic philosophers and scientists, who alone feel able to determine the causes and are interested in the understanding of facts. Galen says in his book on the Use of the Parts that "this is a sacred book which I composed as a true hymn of the God who has created us, in the belief that I am really pious not if I sacrifice many hecatombs of oxen to Him and burn thousands of talents of cassia, but if I first recognize myself and then explain also to the others the wisdom of God, His power, His excellence."[45] This statement is significant. The fact that Platonic, dogmatic philosophy recognizes the power of God in nature does not mean the end of science; it is rather

---

[43] Jones, l. c., IV, p. 247: πάντα διεκοσμήσατο κατὰ τρόπον αὐτὸ ἑωυτῷ τὰ ἐν τῷ σώματι τὸ πῦρ, ἀπομίμησιν τοῦ ὅλου, μικρὰ πρὸς μεγάλα καὶ μεγάλα πρὸς μικρά.

[44] Jones, l. c., II, p. 149: οὐ μέντοι ἔγωγε ἀξιῶ ὑπὸ θεοῦ ἀνθρώπου σῶμα μιαίνεσθαι, τὸ ἐπικηρότατον ὑπὸ τοῦ ἀγνοτάτου.

[45] Galen, De usu partium, III, 10, ed. G. Helmreich, I, 1907, p. 174, 6–13: ἱερὸν λόγον ὃν ἐγὼ τοῦ δημιουργήσαντος ἡμᾶς ὕμνον ἀληθινὸν συντίθημι, καὶ νομίζω τοῦτ' εἶναι τὴν ὄντως εὐσέβειαν, οὐχὶ εἰ ταύρων ἑκατόμβας αὐτῷ παμπόλλας καταθύσαιμι καὶ τάλαντα μυρία θυμιάσαιμι κασίας, ἀλλ' εἰ γνοίην μὲν αὐτὸς πρῶτος, ἔπειτα δὲ καὶ τοῖς ἄλλοις ἐξηγησαίμην οἶος μέν ἐστι τὴν σοφίαν, οἶος δὲ τὴν δύναμιν, ὁποῖος δὲ τὴν χρηστότητα.

the stimulus to perfection of scientific knowledge and empirical understanding. If God did not exist, the world would be governed by chance alone but not by intelligible laws or recognizable causation. Moreover, nature separated from God would not be capable of inspiring in man enthusiasm for scientific investigation. Dogmatic philosophy alone leads the philosopher to an understanding of the phenomena and the physician to an explanation of diseases by sun and air or by the nature of the body.

These considerations in themselves suggest that a belief according to which diseases are caused by demons cannot have had great bearing on Greek medicine. As a matter of fact there is, throughout antiquity, hardly one physician who accepts such a theory. The author of the book on the Sacred Disease, bitterly attacking those who trace epilepsy to the direct influence of a God or demon, does not give any indication that this opinion was held by physicians. He says that "those [men] who first attributed a sacred character to this malady were the same men who do it to-day, magicians, purifiers, charlatans and quacks."[46] A real physician apparently explained not even this disease by demons. The same thing is true of the fourth century A.D. when the physician Posidonius, very famous for his medical skill, is said to have denied that mania could be caused by a demon. There is no reason to suppose that this is a very unusual attitude; for the same opinion is expressed in Stephanus' Commentary to the Prognostics of Hippocrates.[47] And even in the seventh century A.D. physicians, it seems to me, no less than laymen, are convinced of the natural character of mental illnesses although at that time the demonological explanation is more and more emphasized.[48] And yet, concerning those affections the problem is at

---

[46] Jones, l. c., II, p. 141 (slightly altered): δοκέουσιν οἱ πρῶτοι τοῦτο τὸ νόσημα ἱερώσαντες τοιοῦτοι εἶναι ἄνθρωποι οἷοι καὶ νῦν εἰσι μάγοι τε καὶ καθάρται καὶ ἀγύρται καὶ ἀλαζόνες. Cf. On the Diseases of Girls (Περὶ παρθενίων), Hippocrates ed. Littré, VIII, 1853, p. 468.

[47] On Posidonius cf. Philostorgius, Ecclesiastical History, VIII, 10 (GSS Philostorgius, p. 111, 12 sq. Bidez). Stephanus in Scholia in Hippocratem et Galenum, ed. F. R. Dietz, I, 1834, pp. 71 sq. Dölger (Antike u. Christentum IV, 1934, p. 106) assumes that the explanation of Posidonius is not a common one. He himself remarks that Origines attacks physicians who explain mental diseases in a natural way (l. c., p. 96).

[48] Sophronius, Cyri et Joannis miracula, c. 54, Migne PG, 87, 3, 3624, says: τοῦτον δοκίμοις ἰατροῖς ὑπεδείκνυον, ἀπὸ πλήθους μελαγχολικῶν χυμῶν τὰς συνεχεῖς ἐπιληψίας ἐκείνας καὶ μακρὰς καρηβαρείας συμβαίνειν οἰόμενοι· ἑκατέρας γὰρ ὡς ἔγνωμεν ἔπασχεν, τὰς μὲν συνεχέστερον, τὰς δὲ ἐντονώτερον καὶ μακρότερον· ἀλλ' ὡς μίαν πρὸς πάντων ἀπόφασιν

least thoroughly discussed in medical books, whereas in regard to the other diseases and their causation by the wrath of God or evil spirits, with the exception of a few places, the subject is not even mentioned in Greek medicine. Some commentators note that, in Hippocrates' Prognostic, the word divine might be understood as pestilence since "this affliction seems to be caused by God."[49] Galen, dealing with the same term, remarks that "a few believe illness could afflict men also through a certain wrath of the gods and that they try to prove this opinion quoting the authors of the so-called irrational stories."[50] Whether Galen is thinking of physicians or only of laymen, whether these people explain mental diseases alone in this way or other illnesses too, cannot be ascertained beyond a doubt. These are, however, the only instances to be found in the works of Hippocrates and Galen and of the other medical writers. One is justified, then, in saying not only that the Greek physicians rejected the explanation by demonology but also that they did not take it seriously, that they treated the subject as negligible.

This attitude of the physicians is not an isolated one. The ancient philosophers also unanimously disagreed with the belief that diseases could be caused by demons. Not in Platonic or Aristotelian or Stoic philosophy, still less, of course, in the Skepsis are the demons held responsible for illness. Again the problem is scarcely mentioned; it seems unnecessary to deal with it very thoroughly.[51] Also the Neo-Platonists

ἤκουον ἀνθρώποις ἀνίκητον εἶναι τὸ νόσημα, πνεῦμα πονηρὸν καὶ οὐ μελαγχολικὸν χυμὸν ἔχων τὸ νόσημα. Certainly the physicians do not know in this case how to cure the disease; this however they sometimes do not know in the fifth century B.C. either. Apparently the Christian book wants to use the authority of the physicians as proof for the healing-power of the Saints and does not describe the actual situation correctly. Otherwise it would be hard to reconcile that the laymen originally believed in the natural character of epilepsy, yet, that the physicians are said not to have been of the same opinion.

[49] Erotian, ed. Nachmanson, l. c., p. 108, 18–19: διὰ τὸ τοὺς λοιμοὺς ἐκ θεοῦ δοκεῖν εἶναι.

[50] Galen, In Hippocratis Prognostic., l. c., p. 206, 3–5: ἔνιοι μὲν γὰρ οἴονται καὶ διὰ θεῶν τινα ὀργὴν γίνεσθαι τοῖς ἀνθρώποις νοσήματα καὶ λέγουσί γε μαρτυρίαν τῆς δόξης ταύτης παρὰ τῶν γραψάντων τὰς καλουμένας ἱστορίας ἄνευ λόγου. Cf. also Celsus, CML, I, 1915, p. 17, 15–16: Eodem vero auctore [sc. Homero] disci potest morbos tum (!) ad iram deorum immortalium relatos esse.

[51] One usually refers to Plato's Phaedrus, 244d, in order to prove that Plato, at least, explained diseases by the interference of God. But he is only speaking of mania, one of the gravest diseases and burdens, which, in this myth, he traces back to a kind of divine possession like the gift of prophecy and poetry. For Plato's theory on diseases, even on mental diseases, cf. Timaeus, 81e–86b. For the Stoics' cf. Diogenes Laertius, VII, 158. The Neo-Pythagoreans are the only philosophical sect of late antiquity which recognizes at least purifications (cf. Diogenes Laertius, VIII, 33).

disregard such a theory. Plotinus says: "They tell us they can free themselves of diseases. If they meant, by temperate living and an appropriate regime, they would be right and in accordance with all sound knowledge. But they assert diseases to be Spirit-Beings and boast of being able to expell them by formulae: this pretention may enhance their importance with the crowd, gaping upon the powers of magicians; but they can never persuade the intelligent that disease arises otherwise than from such causes as overstrain, excess, deficiency, putrid decay, in a word some variation whether from within or from without. The nature of illness is indicated by its very cure. A motion, a medicine, the letting of blood, and the disease shifts down and away; sometimes scantiness of nourishment restores the system: presumably the Spiritual power gets hungry or is debilitated by the purge. Either this Spirit makes a hasty exit or it remains within. If it stays, how does the disease disappear, with the cause still present? If it quits the place, what has driven it out? Has anything happened to it? Are we to suppose it throve on the disease? In that case the disease existed as something distinct from the Spirit-Power. Then again, if it steps in where no cause of sickness exists, why should there be anything else but illness? If there must be such a cause, the Spirit is unnecessary: that cause is sufficient to produce that fever. As for the notion, that just when the cause presents itself, the watchful Spirit leaps to incorporate itself with it, this is simply amusing."[52] This statement proves that even the latest philosophical system of antiquity, the one which is generally held responsible for so much superstition of the ancients, rejected the demonological explanation of diseases categorically. At the same time the polemic of Plotinus shows

---

[52] Plotinus, Psychic and Physical Treatises; Comprising the Second and Third Enneades, Translated from the Greek by S. Mackenna, London 1921, Vol. II, p. 235. (Plotin., Enneades II, 9, 14): καθαίρεσθαι δὲ νόσων λέγοντες αὐτοὺς λέγοντες μὲν ἂν σωφροσίνη καὶ κοσμίᾳ διαίτῃ ἔλεγον ἂν ὀρθῶς, καθάπερ οἱ φιλόσοφοι λέγουσι. νῦν δὲ ὑποστησάμενοι τὰς νόσους δαιμόνια εἶναι καὶ ταῦτα ἐξαιρεῖν λόγῳ φάσκοντες δύνασθαι καὶ ἐπαγγελλόμενοι σεμνότεροι μὲν ἂν εἶναι δόξαιεν παρὰ τοῖς πολλοῖς, οἳ τὰς παρὰ τοῖς μάγοις δυνάμεις θαυμάζουσι τοὺς μέντοι εὖ φρονοῦντας οὐκ ἂν πείθοιεν, ὡς οὐχ αἱ νόσοι τὰς αἰτίας ἔχουσιν ἢ καμάτοις ἢ πλησμοναῖς ἢ ἐνδείαις ἢ σήψεσι καὶ ὅλως μεταβολαῖς ἢ ἔξωθεν τὴν ἀρχὴν ἢ ἔνδοθεν λαβούσαις. δηλοῦσι δὲ καὶ αἱ θεραπεῖαι αὐτῶν. γαστρὸς γὰρ ῥυείσης ἢ φαρμάκου δοθέντος διεχώρησε κάτω εἰς τὸ ἔξω τὸ νόσημα καὶ αἵματος ἀφηρημένου, καὶ ἔνδεια δὲ ἰάσατο, ἢ πεινήσαντος τήκεσθαι, ποτὲ δὲ ἀθρόως ἐξελθόντος, ἢ μένοντος ἔνδον. ἀλλ᾽ εἰ μὲν ἔτι μένοντος, πῶς ἔνδον ὄντος οὐ νοσεῖ ἔτι; εἰ δὲ ἐξελήλυθε, διὰ τί; τί γὰρ αὐτὸ πέπονθεν; ἢ ὅτι ἐτρέφετο ὑπὸ τῆς νόσου: ἣν ἄρα ἡ νόσος ἑτέρα οὖσα τοῦ δαίμονος. ἔπειτα, εἰ οὐδενὸς ὄντος αἰτίου εἴσεισι, διὰ τί οὐκ ἀεὶ νοσεῖ; εἰ δὲ γενομένου αἰτίου, τί δεῖ τοῦ δαίμονος πρὸς τὸ νοσεῖν; τὸ γὰρ αἴτιον τὸν πυρετὸν αὔταρκές ἐστιν ἐργάσασθαι. γελοῖον δὲ τὸ ἅμα τὸ αἴτιον γενέσθαι καὶ εὐθέως ὥσπερ παρυποστῆναι τῷ αἰτίῳ τὸ δαιμόνιον ἕτοιμον ὄν.

that the Gnostic philosophy did accept such a doctrine of causation, a philosophy which combined Greek ideas with Christian religion. It is the Christians and the Jews who propagated these ideas at the end of Greek and Roman history as the Persians and Chaldeans had done in the very beginning.[53]

It is certain that philosophers and physicians do not believe demons to be the cause of disease. Not only is the scientific theory hostile to such an opinion,—this would explain only the attitude of the trained physicians, of the followers of the various medical schools—even the average educated man did not believe in the demonic character of diseases; his behavior as a patient was conditioned by this attitude. Modern interpretation is inclined more and more to claim that Greeks and Romans, in general, traced back the origin of diseases to possession by demons.[54] If this were correct, a queer contradiction of the data would arise. For these men are supposed to be the patients of physicians who apparently do not believe in demons, who do not even try to prove that in a special case it is the body and not a demon which has brought about the illness. Or did people call in only those unknown practitioners who did themselves believe in demons? But no physician could afford to do this. If the illness was caused by a demon, nothing could be done by the doctor. He must retire and give way to the magician. In such a case "he is expelled from the house" and the patient will say: "Oh, sir, leave

[53] Concerning the early Christian attitude toward diseases, cf. A. Harnack, Medizinisches aus der ältesten Kirchengeschichte, 1892, pp. 71 sq. The Jewish belief is most clearly formulated by Josephus, Antiquitates, VIII, 2, 5. Already Pliny traces the origin of magic back to Persians and Chaldeans on the one hand, to the Jews on the other. (Natural History, introduction to book XXX). The modern attempt to find magic in all centuries of Greek history is not convincing. Hopfner, (Realenzyklopädie d. klass. Altertumswiss., XIV, 1, pp. 301 sq., s. v. Mageia) collects the whole material; his survey only serves to prove that before the third century B.C. magic is not an important factor in Greek life. I do not presume to decide whether the situation was always different from that which is to be found in other countries and in primitive men, as Ed. Meyer assumes (Gesch. d. Altertums, I, 1⁵, pp. 93 sq.). So much is certain, that in Greece magic is revived only under foreign influences in later times (cf. Ed. Meyer, l. c., p. 98). Cf. Lucian's Tragodopodagra, v. 265 sq. Σύροι μέν ἐσμεν, ἐκ Δαμασκοῦ τῷ γένει.

[54] The modern interpretation is to be found in the article on Demons, RE, Supplement III, p. 267 sq.; p. 272, 38; cf. also Halliday, l. c., p. 281; E. Stemplinger, Sympathieglaube u. Sympathiekuren in Altertum u. Neuzeit, 1919, p. 5: "So ist das ganze Griechisch-Römische Altertum trotz Hippokrates erfüllt von dem Glauben an den Krankheitsdämon." The argument in these books is usually based on passages taken from poetry which cannot be acknowledged as the only and adequate instance in this problem. Moreover, it is again the mental diseases to which those passages mostly refer, and here the problem is a peculiar one, cf. p. 219, above.

me to pay my penalty, impious but wretch that I am, accursed and hateful to the gods and all the heavenly host."[55] After all, the physicians had patients; people must have thought them able to do something. The natural explanation of diseases must have been generally accepted.

The reasons for this acceptance can be ascertained by inquiring into the causes for the rejection of a demonological interpretation of disease. It is the author of the book on the Sacred Disease who says of the assumptions of the magicians that they "show, not piety, as they think, but impiety rather, implying that the gods do not exist, and what they call piety and the divine is, as I shall prove, impious and unholy."[56] The physicians then not only believe that they can explain diseases in another and more scientific way. They rely also on religious argumentation. For they hold "that a man's body is not defiled by God, the one being utterly corrupt, the other perfectly holy."[57] In slightly different terms Posidonius says the same thing in the fourth century A.D.: "men do not become ill through the affliction of demons . . . for it is not at all in the power of the demons to afflict the nature of men."[58] A god cannot pollute or possess the human body. The physicians apparently subscribe to the Platonic saying: "It is good since it comes into being by divine destiny."[59] In this way they adopt the Olympian religion and reject the chthonic cults; they adopt the pious reverence of the gods and reject purifications.

From the aspect of such a belief in antiquity, too, all magical rites are superstitious, as is revealed by Plutarch's discussion of superstition: "In the estimation of the superstitious man, [all the indispositions] of his body . . . are classed as afflictions of God or attacks of an evil spirit. For this reason he has no heart to relieve the situation or undo its effects, or to find some remedy for it, or to take a strong stand against it lest he

---

[55] Plutarch, On Superstition (Plutarch's Moralia, with an English Translation by F. C. Babbitt, Loeb Class. Library, II, 1928, p. 475): ἔα με, ἄνθρωπε, διδόναι δίκην, τὸν ἀσεβῆ, τὸν ἐπάρατον, τὸν θεοῖς καὶ δαίμοσι μεμισημένον. Cf. also Lucian, Philopseudes, 36.

[56] Jones, l. c., II, p. 145: καίτοι ἔμοιγε οὐ περὶ εὐσεβείης τοὺς λόγους δοκέουσι ποιεῖσθαι, ὡς οἴονται, ἀλλὰ περὶ ἀσεβείης μᾶλλον, καὶ ὡς οἱ θεοὶ οὐκ εἰσί, τὸ δὲ εὐσεβὲς αὐτῶν καὶ τὸ θεῖον ἀσεβές ἐστι καὶ ἀνόσιον, ὡς ἐγὼ διδάξω.

[57] Jones, l. c., II, p. 149, cf. n. 44, above.

[58] Philostorgius, l. c.: θεάσασθαι δὲ τὸν Ποσειδώνιον ἐν ἰατρικῇ διαπρέποντα. λέγειν δ' αὐτὸν ὅμως οὐκ ὀρθῶς οὐχὶ δαιμόνων ἐπιθέσει τοὺς ἀνθρώπους ἐκβακχεύεσθαι, ὑγρῶν δὲ τινῶν κακοχυμίαν τὸ πάθος ἐργάζεσθαι· μηδὲ γὰρ εἶναι τὸ παράπαν ἰσχὺν δαιμόνων ἀνθρώπων φύσιν ἐτηρεάζουσαν.

[59] Plato, Phaedrus 244 c.: ὡς καλοῦ ὄντος, ὅταν θείᾳ μοίρᾳ γίγνηται.

223

seem to fight against God and to rebel at his punishment."[60] Superstitious as this man is, he will use only rites and purifications, in contrast to the atheist, who "when he is ill, takes into account and calls to mind the times when he has eaten too much or drunk too much wine, also irregularities in his daily life, or instances of over-fatigue or unaccustomed changes of air or locality."[61]

For the Romans, too, the use of purification—the explanation of diseases by demons or gods—is superstition. It is Pliny who says: "To believe that there are a number of gods derived from the virtues and vices of man . . . indicates still greater folly. Human nature, weak and frail as it is, mindful of its own infirmity, has made these divisions, so that every one might have recourse to that which he supposed himself to stand more particularly in need of. Hence we find different names employed by different nations; the inferior deities are arranged in classes, and diseases and plagues are deified, in consequence of our anxious wish to propitiate them. It was from this cause that a temple was dedicated to Fever, at the public expense, on the Palatine Hill."[62] The Roman poet knows that "the mysteries of cruel magicians are abominated by the heavenly gods."[63] It is admitted that "our forefathers believed that purifications could remove the cause of every evil,"[64] the implication being that later, in the Roman Empire, at least the educated classes and all men who worship the Olympians reject such a be-

---

[60] Plutarch, On superstitition, l. c., II, p. 475: τῷ δὲ δεισιδαίμονι καὶ σώματος ἀρρωστία πᾶσα καὶ . . . πληγαὶ θεοῦ καὶ προσβολαὶ δαίμονος λέγονται. ὅθεν οὐδὲ τολμᾷ βοηθεῖν οὐδὲ διαλύειν τὸ συμβεβηκὸς οὐδὲ θεραπεύειν οὐδ' ἀντιτάττεσθαι, μὴ δόξῃ θεομαχεῖν καὶ ἀντιτείνειν κολαζόμενος.

[61] Plutarch, On superstition, l. c., II, p. 473: Νοσῶν θ' ὁ ἄθεος ἐκλογίζεται καὶ ἀναμιμνήσκεται πλησμονὰς αὐτοῦ καὶ οἰνώσεις καὶ ἀταξίας περὶ δίαιταν ἢ κόπους ὑπερβάλλοντας ἢ μεταβολὰς ἀέρων ἀήθεις καὶ τόπων. Plutarch in this passage is speaking of the atheist because he intends to contrast his behavior with that of the superstitious. But he presupposes the same attitude for the pious man.

[62] The Natural History of Pliny, II, 15, Translated by J. Bostock and H. T. Riley, I, 1893, p. 21 (cf. Cicero, De natura deorum, III, 63 and De legibus, II, 28): In numeros quidem credere atque etiam ex vitiis hominum . . . majorem ad socordiam accedit. Fragilis et laboriosa mortalitas in partes ista digessit infirmitatis suae memor, ut portionibus coleret quisque quo maxime indigeret. Itaque nomina alia aliis gentibus et numina in iisdem innumerabilia invenimus, *inferis* quoque in genera discriptis, morbisque et multis etiam pestibus, dum esse placatas trepido metu cupimus. Ideoque etiam publice Febris fanum in Palatio dicatum est.

[63] Lucan, The Civil War VI, 430–31: superis detestanda deis saevorum arcana magorum.

[64] Ovid, Fasti II, 35–37: Omne nefas omne mali purgamina causam credebant nostri tollere posse senes.

lief. It is emphasized, however, that "it was in Greece that the custom originated." In the same way Plutarch claims an alien origin for magic, which, he says, the Greeks took over "from the barbarians, learning their evil knowledge."[65] Certainly, the demonic conceptions are influential in Rome as well as in Greece, but they are consciously suppressed. Both nations assert the foreign character of those beliefs, as usual making another people responsible for them; even if purifications are used, they do not belong to that ritual which is recognized as the old and genuine religion.[66] To be sure, one is not justified in holding as the most characteristic feature of their behavior feelings which are held in contempt by men themselves. What is thought to be superstitious by the ancients cannot be interpreted as their general attitude toward disease.[67]

It stands to reason then that the Greek physicians understood illness as caused by sun and air and winds or by the nature of man, and that the average people accepted this explanation. Physicians and laymen, however, usually considered these factors as the expression of divine agencies; the merely natural interpretation was as rare and restricted as the superstitious belief in demons; both are exceptional cases, departures from the rule. It is not by chance that Asclepius is the god of doctors and of patients. He represents the rational theology in the Greek sense, in sharp opposition to every demonic religion, to magical rites and purifications, as the inscription on his temple in

[65] Ovid, l. c., 38: Graecia principium moris fuit. Plutarch, On Superstition, 166 ὦ βάρβαρ' ἐξευρόντες ῞Ελληνες κακά.

[66] Cf. J. Bernays, Theophrastos' Schrift über Frömmigkeit, Berlin 1866, p. 106. He stresses the fact that sacrifices for the sake of purifications, the latest in the development of Greek religion, are not on the same plane as the other sacrifices, even in the time of Theophrastos, who classifies the Orphic mysteries also among superstitious rites (in his characterization of the superstitious). Concerning earlier centuries and their dislike of purifications, cf. e.g., Plato, Republic, 364b, in regard to a later period cf. the Neo-Platonic polemic in the book of Porphyry, described by Bernays, l. c.

[67] The contention of the pious man that it is God who sends the disease, expressed already in the Homeric Epic (Cf. Odyssee, V, 394–97; IX, 409–11, also the pestilence in the first book of the Iliad is sent from God) must have been common to every period. But even in the epic no purifications are used, those which are mentioned concern only the usual preparation for prayers and sacrifices. (Iliad, I, 313, contrary to E. Rohde, Psyche⁹⁻¹⁰, II, 1921, p. 76, 1, who himself is more cautious in his judgment p. 71.) At any rate, the pious belief must be carefully differentiated from the theory that disease is a kind of pollution which has to be purified. These are two different attitudes. Already Hesiod says (Erga 102–4): νοῦσοι δὲ ἀνθρώποισιν ἐφ' ἡμέρῃ αἳ δ' ἐπὶ νυκτὶ αὐτόματοι φοιτῶσι κακὰ θνητοῖσι φέρουσαι σιγῇ, ἐπεὶ φωνὴν ἐξείλετο μητίετα Ζεύς.

Epidaurus reveals: "Pure must be he who enters the fragrant temple; purity means to think nothing but holy thought."[68]

II. The Treatment of Diseases

The myth of the god Asclepius says that of "those whosoever came suffering from the sores of nature, or with their limbs wounded either by grey bronze or by far-hurled stone, or with bodies wasting away with summer's heat or winter's cold, he loosed and delivered divers of them from diverse pains, tending some of them with kindly songs, giving to others a soothing potion, or, haply, swathing their limbs with simples, or restoring others by the knife."[69] The god in his treatment of diseases resorts to music, to drugs applied either internally or externally and to the use of the knife. The human physician is a surgeon and a pharmacologist, he invents the regulation of diet, in rare cases he has recourse to music. The therapy of Greek as well as of Roman physicians, is, then, throughout the centuries a scientific and natural one. But again it is necessary to determine the principles underlying the scientific and natural method of healing.

It is the aim of surgery and dietetics to influence the disease by the action and understanding of the physician. So far no other than human power is involved, yet, there is the problem to what extent the body can be helped at all from the outside, how much the healing-process as such depends not on what is done by the physician but on what is achieved by the bodily forces themselves. In other words, what value can be attributed to the medical art? The various physicians answer this question in different ways, depending on their different metaphysical standpoints. Plato remarks that all those who understand nature as a power of its own devoid of god at the same time deprive the different arts of their efficacy. Like heaven and the stars and the seasons, they

[68] Porphyry, De abstinentia Animae, II, 19: ἀγνὸν χρὴ ναοῖο θυώδεος ἐντὸς ἰόντα / ἔμμεναι. ἁγνεία δ᾽ ἐστι φρονεῖν ὅσια. I shall not discuss whether Asclepius was originally a chthonic Hero or not. There is no doubt that he came to be generally accepted by the ancient world as an Olympian.

[69] Pindar, Pythian Odes, III, 47–53 (The Odes of Pindar with an English translation by Sir John Sandys, Loeb Class. Library, 1927, p. 189): τοὺς μὲν ὦν, ὅσσοι μόλον αὐτοφύτων ἑλκέων ξυνάονες, ἢ πολιῷ χαλκῷ μέλη τετρωμένοι ἢ χερμάδι τηλεβόλῳ, ἢ θερινῷ πυρὶ περθόμενοι δέμας ἢ χειμῶνι, λύσαις ἄλλον ἀλλοίων ἀχέων ἔξαγεν, τοὺς μὲν μαλακαῖς ἐπαοιδαῖς ἀμφέπων, τοὺς δὲ προσανέα πίνοντας, ἢ γυίοις περάπτων πάντοθεν φάρμακα τοὺς δὲ τομαῖς ἔστασεν ὀρθούς. The translation of μαλακαῖς ἐπαοιδαῖς differs from the usual one, for the explanation thereof cf. n. 103, below.

say, animals and plants have been produced by the elements. "Not through reason nor through any god or art, but . . . through nature and chance. Art, however, later arising therefrom, comes into being later and is itself mortal since it is born from mortal things. Later on it creates some playthings which do not much partake of truth. . . . Arts which create something serious also are those which join their power with nature—like medicine, agriculture, and gymnastics."[70] Medicine, according to such an atheistic theory, undoubtedly belongs to those arts which accomplish something real, but medical art considered in this light is no longer a factor of its own. The result of its action derives from a source outside the art; the artist becomes simply the helpmate of nature. This is the theory expressed also by one of the Epidemiae: "Nature is the physician of diseases."[71] Thus, the power of nature is raised to its highest level, but in that case the physician must abdicate. If nature heals diseases then the physician ceases to do so. Such a theory is destructive of medical art.

No one will deny that "if nature be in opposition, everything is vain."[72] For "if a man demand from an art a power over what does not belong to the art, or for nature a power over what does not belong to nature, his ignorance is more alike to madness than to lack of knowledge."[73] These exaggerations aside, however, the reality of the art as a force which need not be derived from another force cannot be doubted. Neither chance nor spontaneous healing can contradict the proper value of medicine. Moreover, "if the medical art and medical men brought about a cure only by means of medicines, purgative or astringent, my argument would be weak. As it is, the physicians of greatest repute obviously cure by regimen and by other substances, which nobody—not only a physician but also an unlearned layman, if he heard of them—

---

[70] Plato, Laws, X, 889c–d: οὐδὲ διά τινα θεὸν οὐδὲ διὰ τέχνην ἀλλὰ . . . φύσει καὶ τύχῃ. τέχνην δὲ ὕστερον ἐκ τούτων ὑστέραν γενομένην, αὐτὴν θνητὴν ἐκ θνητῶν ὕστερα γεγεννηκέναι παιδιάς τινας, ἀληθείας οὐ σφόδρα μετεχούσας . . . αἱ δέ τι καὶ σπουδαῖον ἄρα γεννῶσι τῶν τεχνῶν, εἶναι ταύτας ὁπόσαι τῇ φύσει ἐκοίνωσαν τὴν αὐτῶν δύναμιν, οἷον αὖ ἰατρικὴ καὶ γεωργικὴ καὶ γυμναστική.

[71] Hippocrates, ed. Littré, V, p. 314, νούσων φύσιες ἰητροί. The author expressly says that to him nature is devoid of thinking and accomplishes everything without having learned it. This corresponds to the Platonic characterization of natural and irreligious philosophy and shows that the statement of the Hippocratic book can be linked with this theory. (Contrary to Deichgräber's reading S B Berl. 1933, 3, 52.)

[72] Jones, l. c., II, p. 263: φύσιος γὰρ ἀντιπρησσούσης κενεὰ πάντα. Although these words are used in regard to education, they are certainly valid in a wider sense too.

[73] Jones, l. c., II, p. 203: εἰ γάρ τις ἢ τέχνης ἢ ἃ μὴ τέχνη, ἢ φύσιν ἐς ἃ μὴ φύσις πέφυκεν, ἀξιώσειε δύνασθαι, ἀγνοεῖ ἄγνοιαν ἁρμόζουσαν μανίῃ μᾶλλον ἢ ἀμαθίῃ.

227

would say do not belong to the art. Seeing then that there is nothing that cannot be put to use by good physicians and by the art of medicine itself, but in most things that grow or are made are present the essential substances of cures and of drugs, no patient who recovers without a physician can logically attribute the recovery to spontaneity. Indeed, under a close examination spontaneity disappears; for everything that occurs will be found to do so through something, and this 'through something' shows that spontaneity is a mere name, and has no reality. Medicine, however, because it acts 'through something,' and because its results may be forecasted, has reality, as is manifest now and will be manifest for ever."[74] In this way the self-sufficiency of medical art is demonstrated on a rational basis contrary to the naturalists and disbelievers.

It is the usual attitude for the physician which is formulated in the first book of the Epidemiae: "The art has three factors, the disease, the patient, the physician. The physician is the servant of the art. The patient must cooperate with the physician in combating the disease."[75] Art and nature are thus properly evaluated. In the fight against illness, the knowledge of the physician is one factor, nature the other. Yet such a conception obviously presupposes a belief which gives God his share in the processes of the world. It is again the religious rationalist who, contrary to the atheistic thinker, has real confidence in his art. He notes equally and fairly the success and failure of nature. For nature, to him, has two different aspects: it not only heals, it also destroys. The physician, in some cases, can rely on it, in others he must fight against it.[76]

---

[74] Jones, l. c., II, pp. 199–201: Ἔτι τοίνυν εἰ μὲν ὑπὸ φαρμάκων τῶν τε καθαιρόντων καὶ τῶν ἱστάντων ἡ ἴησις τῇ τε ἰητρικῇ καὶ τοῖσιν ἰητροῖσι μοῦνον ἐγίνετο, ἀσθενὴς ἦν ἂν ὁ ἐμὸς λόγος. νῦν δὲ φαίνονται τῶν ἰητρῶν οἱ μάλιστα ἐπαινεόμενοι καὶ διαιτήμασιν ἰώμενοι καὶ ἄλλοισί γε εἴδεσιν, ἃ οὐκ ἄν τις φαίη, μὴ ὅτι ἰητρός. ἀλλ᾽ οὐδὲ ἰδιώτης ἀνεπιστήμων ἀκούσας, μὴ οὐ τῆς τέχνης εἶναι. ὅπου οὖν οὐδὲν οὔτ᾽ ἐν τοῖς ἀγαθοῖσι τῶν ἰητρῶν οὔτ᾽ ἐν τῇ ἰητρικῇ αὐτῇ ἀχρεῖόν ἐστιν, ἀλλ᾽ ἐν τοῖσι πλείστοισι τῶν τε φυομένων καὶ τῶν ποιευμένων ἔνεστι τὰ εἴδεα τῶν θεραπειῶν καὶ τῶν φαρμάκων, οὐκ ἔστιν ἔτι οὐδενὶ τῶν ἄνευ ἰητροῦ ὑγιαζομένων τὸ αὐτόματον οὐδὲν φαίνεται ἐὸν ἐλεγχόμενον. πᾶν γὰρ τὸ γινόμενον διά τι εὑρίσκοιτ᾽ ἂν γινόμενον, καὶ ἐν τῷ διά τι τὸ αὐτόματον οὐ φαίνεται οὐσίην ἔχον οὐδεμίην ἀλλ᾽ ἢ ὄνομα. ἡ δὲ ἰητρικὴ καὶ ἐν τοῖσι διά τι καὶ ἐν τοῖσι προνοουμένοισι φαίνεταί τε καὶ φανεῖται αἰεὶ οὐσίην ἔχουσα.

[75] Jones, l. c., I, p. 165: ἡ τέχνη διὰ τριῶν, τὸ νόσημα καὶ ὁ νοσέων καὶ ὁ ἰητρός. ὁ ἰητρὸς ὑπηρέτης τῆς τέχνης· ὑπεναντιοῦσθαι τῷ νοσήματι τὸν νοσέοντα μετὰ τοῦ ἰητροῦ.

[76] M. Neuburger, Die Heilkraft d. Natur, 1926, pp. 9–10, stresses the fact that in the Hippocratic books the healing power of nature is not exaggerated in a phantastic measure. He is also of the opinion that thereby the negativism and quietism is avoided which very easily results from too strong a belief in nature.

All these ideas, I think, are summed up in the statement "that there could surely be nothing more useful or more necessary to know than these things (sc. which the physician knows) and how the first discoverers, pursuing their inquiries excellently and with suitable application of reason to the nature of man, made their discoveries, and thought their art worthy to be ascribed to a god, as in fact is the usual belief."[77] For medicine is so great a power and is so mighty in itself that a god must have given it to mankind. The rational element contained in medical art is divine. Yet very seldom does this conviction lead to an exaggeration of the power of the art. In contrast to the conception that nature alone, not the physician, heals the disease, it is stated in one book: "By stitching and cutting, that which is rotten in men is healed by physicians. This too is part of the physician's art: to do away with that which causes pain, and by taking away the cause of his suffering to make him sound. Nature of herself knows how to do these things. When a man is sitting it is a labour to rise; when he is moving it is a labour to come to rest. In other respects too nature has the same qualities as has medical art."[78] The religious physician is usually aware of the limits of his art as his definition of medicine reveals: "In general terms, it is to do away with the sufferings of the sick, to lessen the violence of their diseases, and to refuse to treat those who are overmastered by their diseases, realizing that in such cases medicine is powerless."[79]

In later centuries the recognition of nature as a teleological power must have confirmed the advisability of the withdrawal of the physicians. Themison, who does not believe in teleology, is the first to pro-

---

[77] Jones, l. c., I, 37: οὐκ ἂν οὖν ἕτερα τούτων χρησιμώτερα οὐδὲ ἀναγκαιότερα εἴη εἰδέναι δήπου, ὡς δὲ καλῶς καὶ λογισμῷ προσήκοντι ζητήσαντες πρὸς τὴν τοῦ ἀνθρώπου φύσιν εὗρον αὐτὰ οἱ πρῶτοι εὑρόντες καὶ ᾠήθησαν ἀξίην τὴν τέχνην θεῷ προσθεῖναι, ὥσπερ καὶ νομίζεται.

[78] Jones, l. c., IV, pp. 253–55 (slightly altered): κεντεόμενοί τε καὶ τεμνόμενοι τὰ σαθρὰ ὑπὸ τῶν ἰητρῶν ὑγιάζονται. καὶ τόδε ἰητρικῆς. τὸ λυπέον ἀπαλλάσσειν, καὶ ὑφ' οὗ πονεῖ ἀφαιρέοντα ὑγιέα ποιεῖν. ἡ φύσις αὐτομάτη ταῦτα ἐπίσταται. καθήμενος πονεῖ ἀναστῆναι, κινεόμενος πονεῖ ἀναπαύσασθαι, καὶ ἄλλα τὰ αὐτὰ ἔχει ἡ φύσις ἰητρική. It is in accordance with the interpretation given in regard to the attitude of the physician that the book on Ancient Medicine states that the nature of man consisting of the mixture of the humors can and should be voluntarily altered by the physician. The same is valid for the book on the Nature of Man (Jones, l. c., IV, p. 10) and, I think, for more of the Hippocratic writings. But it is impossible again to deal with all of them in this connection.

[79] Jones, l. c., II, p. 193: τὸ δὴ πάμπαν ἀπαλλάσσειν τῶν νοσεόντων τοὺς καμάτους καὶ τῶν νοσημάτων τὰς σφοδρότητας ἀμβλύνειν, καὶ τὸ μὴ ἐγχειρεῖν τοῖσι κεκρατημένοις ὑπὸ τῶν νοσημάτων, εἰδότας ὅτι ταῦτα οὐ δύναται ἰητρική. As regards the restraint of Hippocratic physicians and the modern discussion of this problem cf. Jones, l. c., I, p. XVI sq.

ceed farther than the physicians before him and to write methodically about the treatment of chronic diseases. Erasistratos, admitting that nature does many things in vain, and Asclepiades, stating that nature cannot heal at all, are the only physicians whose treatment of some of the chronic diseases is especially mentioned.[80] This development is reflected by the change in the attitude of the doctor. For in the Hippocratic book it is said: "I should most commend a physician who in acute diseases, which kill the great majority of patients, shows some superiority."[81] In the books of the Methodists it is the chronic diseases "which bring those who have experience in medicine great and eternal fame."[82] In this case the merely natural and mechanistic understanding of nature brought about a progress in medicine; but this is an exception; in general, like in the explanation of phenomena, the Dogmatists are more progressive than the Methodists.

These considerations are of course important not only for surgery and dietetics, but also for pharmacology. In the treatment by drugs, too, the question arises how far the physician is able to help or must rely on the nature of the patient. On the other hand, there is a specific problem of pharmacology in connection with the efficacy of plants. Certainly herbs are prescribed as a means of natural therapy. If one remembers the ambiguity of the term "nature" in ancient medicine, one immediately realizes that in the administration of remedies also various attitudes must be differentiated from one another. All those men to whom nature is devoid of God also see in plants nothing but natural powers. But it is not only the superstitious layman, Pliny, who recognizes the grandeur and power of God, especially in the vegetable kingdom.[83] The great anatomist and physiologist Herophilus is said to

[80] Caelius Aurelianus, De morbis acutis et chronicis, ed. I. C. Amman, 1709, pp. 267–68: scribentium igitur medicinam nullus ante Themisonem tardarum passionum curationes principaliter ordinavit . . . Alii disperse atque de aliis passionibus scribentes . . . ut Erasistratus et Asclepiades. Themison autem tardarum passionum tres libros scripsit. As regards the attitude of Erasistratus and Asclepiades toward nature cf. Neuburger, l. c., p. 11 sq., who is not aware of the connection between these divergent theories and the discovery of the treatment of chronic diseases.

[81] Jones, l. c., II, p. 67: μάλιστα δ' ἂν ἐπαινέσαιμι ἰητρόν, ὅστις ἐν τοῖσιν ὀξέσι νοσήμασι, ἃ τοὺς πλείστους τῶν ἀνθρώπων κτείνει ἐν τούτοισι διαφέρων τι τῶν ἄλλων εἴη ἐπὶ τὸ βέλτιον. Cf. also the beginning of the Prognostic of Hippocrates.

[82] Caelius Aurelianus, l. c., peritis medicinae claram eternamque gloriam quaerunt. Cf. Aretaeus, ed. C. Hude, CMG, II, 1923, pp. 36, 4 sq.; p. 144, 3 sq.

[83] Pliny, Naturalis Historia, XIX, finis.

have called the plants "the hands of the gods."[84] This statement is not mere rhetoric. If nature is divine, the plants are divine too. Almost all physicians seem to agree with this. Some compose special remedies which are called sacred.[85] But Galen states in a more comprehensive sense: "One is right in saying that the plants act like the hands of the gods, since it is efficacious for the man who uses them to be trained in logical method and to have by nature a good understanding besides."[86] This interpretation, which accepts the divinity of the plants because of the divinity of the intellect in the human being who applies them, is just as characteristic for the Greek attitude as the more verbal explanation of Herophilus' statement.

Undoubtedly rationalistic supernaturalism revives the old conception according to which the power of plants contains something miraculous. But this does not mean the introduction of any magical belief. On the contrary, it hinders the acceptance of those ideas.[87] Galen expressly states that the Herophilean Andreas recorded magical rites to be used in connection with plants and that he was the first to discuss sorcery and such nonsense in medical books. Hippocrates, Euryphon, Dieuches, Diocles, Pleistonicus, Praxagoras, Herophilus, did not care for magical remedies. All the great pharmacologists, Crateuas, Heraclides of Tarent, Dioscurides, rejected those things. Andreas and Pamphylus and the men who followed them constituted a small minority; they were scholars

---

[84] Scribonius Largus, Compositiones, ed. G. Helmreich, 1887, p. 1, 1–3: Herophilus fertur dixisse medicamenta divinas manus esse. Cf. Galen, Opera ed. Kühn, XII, p. 966; Plutarch, Quaest. Symp. IV, 1, 3, 663c., the same is told about Erasistratos. Cf. also Nicander, Theriaca, v. 7.

[85] In Galen's works those named as inventors of divine remedies are: Antipatros, XIII, p. 136; Andromachos, XIII, p. 126; Archigenes in Aetius, III, 114 (CMG, VIII, 1, 1935, p. 305, 11 sq.); in regard to Rufus cf. J. Ilberg, Rufus v. Ephesus, Abh. d. Sächs. Akademie, XLI, 1930, p. 20.

[86] Galen, Opera, ed. Kühn, XII, p. 966: ἐάν τε πάλιν οἷόν περ θεῶν χεῖρας εἶναι τὰ φάρμακα καὶ τοῦτο ὀρθῶς ἐρεῖς. ἀνύει γὰρ μεγάλα τὸν χρώμενον αὐτοῖς ἔχοντα γεγυμνασμένον ἐν λογικῇ μεθόδῳ μετὰ τοῦ καὶ συνετὸν εἶναι φύσει.

[87] The mysterious effect of plants, still intimated at least in the Homeric Epic, was soon forgotten. The term φάρμακον, since the seventh century B.C., had no longer any magical meaning (cf. W. Artelt, Studien z. Gesch. d. Begriffe Heilmittel u. Gift, Stud. z. Gesch. d. Medizin, herg. v. Karl Sudhoff, 23, 1937, pp. 46 sq.). When in the beginning of the Hellenistic era more plants, especially those of the Orient, became known to the Greek physician, a new and strong influx of magic took place. For in the Orient magical rites were combined with the plucking of plants as well as with their preparation and use; and Egypt is, already in the Homeric poem, famous for its remedies (Artelt, l. c., p. 44).

rather than physicians; they were antiquaries.[88] These men, then, were an exception; they were isolated as were those who believed in the demonic character of diseases. And it is not venturous to assume that the same reasons by which the explanation of illness through demons was refused were responsible also for the attitude of the physicians in pharmacology.

But all the pharmacologists, nay almost all the physicians, believed in sympathetic remedies. They are to be found in Dioscurides as well as in Galen, in the books of Stoic physicians and even of Methodists. Is this not the reception of magic into medicine, and the first sign of decay? For, the Hippocratic books are free of those remedies, and it is only from the Hellenistic time on that they begin to be used. However, the sympathetic effect to the ancients is a natural phenomenon and proved by experiments, not by any magical theory. Even the Stoics understand it in this way and collect facts as proof of its reality; they do not rely on mere reasoning alone.[89] Unconvincing as the material seems to the modern it did convince even the Skeptics in antiquity. The only thing in the Stoic discussion that the Academic philosopher finds to agree with is the demonstration of sympathetic relations in the universe. For these are certain, although they must be explained, as the Skeptic believes, not by a divine spirit but by the spontaneity of nature.[90] Thus, from a teleological aspect as well as from a mechanical one sympathy is a reality.

That really experience is the basis of the judgment concerning the sympathetic or antipathetic effect is shown by the opinion about amu-

[88] Galen, Opera, ed. Kühn, XI, p. 795. Concerning Andreas cf. F. Susemihl, Gesch. d. Griech. Literatur in der Alexandrinerzeit, I, 1891, p. 817, 231; II, 1892, p. 421, 32. It is because of the rejection of those things by the medical profession that they are to be found only in the magical papyri which contain not the knowledge of physicians but prescriptions of folklore. What Galen relates about Andreas corresponds with Papyri Graecae Magicae, ed. K. Preisendanz, I, 1928, p. 168–69; cf. also Rohde, Psyche, l. c., II, p. 87, 3.

[89] Cf. E. Zeller, Die Philosophie d. Griech., III, 1³, 1880, p. 169, 2: "Unter der Sympathie verstehen die Stoiker nicht den magischen Zusammenhang, welchen der neuere Sprachgebrauch mit diesem Wort bezeichnet, sondern das naturgemässe Zusammentreffen gewisser Vorgänge in den verschiedenen Teilen der Welt." Cf. also n. 114, below.

[90] Cicero, De natura deorum, III, 11, 28: "Itaque illa mihi placebat oratio de convenientia consensuque naturae, quam quasi cognatione continuata conspirare dicebas, illud non probabam quod negabas id accidere potuisse nisi ea uno divino spiritu contineretur. Illa vero cohaeret et permanet naturae viribus non deorum, estque in ea iste quasi consensus, quem συμπάθειαν Graeci vocant; sed ea quo sua sponte maior est eo minus divina ratione fieri existimanda est."

lets. Soranus, for instance, rejects the wearing of amulets because his experience does not confirm the good results which others claim to have observed. He once admits amulets because of their psychological influence.[91] In the same way Galen accepts that alone which according to his experience has proved to be helpful and leaves all the other things to those who are able to prove them by their experience.[92] Thus, physicians try very carefully to exclude every allusion to magic; they go no farther than their own experience leads. Nay, they are aware that the use of amulets is a very ambiguous means and almost beyond the realm of medicine. It is characteristic that even a physician of the sixth century A.D. prescribes amulets only in those cases in which "no remedy of the art still has power."[93] But since the aim of medicine is to make healthy and to overcome diseases, "it is wonderful to win this struggle, and for that purpose to use everything which can possibly help,"[94] everything which is within human experience.

Yet, certain as it is that experience proves the sympathetic effect, this experience can be had only on the presupposition of a specific theory. One must at least believe that it is possible to connect two phenomena which happen at the same time. Otherwise the coincidence of facts will be understood as fortuitous and not as purposeful. It is for this reason that the Empiric physicians do not recognize sympathy, that only the experience of the Dogmatists and of a few Skeptics who do not cling too strictly to their views recognizes the reality of these effects. The belief in a teleological power of nature is presupposed by the belief in sympathy.

It is in accordance therewith that sympathetic influences are first mentioned in the writings of Theophrastus on natural philosophy.[95]

[91] Soranus, CMG, IV, 1927, p. 47, 17; 121, 26.

[92] Galen, Opera, ed. Kühn, XII, p. 573.

[93] Alexander v. Tralles, ed. Puschmann, II, p. 319: εἰ δὲ . . . μηδενὸς τῶν ἀπὸ τῆς τέχνης ἰσχύοντος . . . καὶ τοῖς φυσικοῖς περιάπτοις οὐδὲν ἄτοπον κεχρῆσθαι χάριν τοῦ σῶσαι τὸν κάμνοντα.

[94] Ibid., II, p. 474–75: καλὸν γὰρ νικᾶν καὶ πάσῃ μηχανῇ βοηθεῖν. Concerning the material preserved cf. L. Deubner, Greek charms and amulets, in Encyclopaedia of Religion and Ethics, ed. by J. Hastings, III, 1910, pp. 433–439.

[95] Theophrastus, Opera, ed. F. Wimmer, III, 1862, p. 92 (On Odor 63), p. 218 (Fr. 172, 3); p. 133, sympathetic effects in the human body are described, comparable to those already known by the Hippocratic writers (cf. Jones, l. c., I, p. 351, On Nutriment, XXIII). In the ps-Aristotelian Problemata (Aristotle 886a 24 sq.) probably written in the time of Theophrastus, examples of sympathy are described too. E. Stemplinger, l. c., p. 7, names the Pythagoreans, Empedocles, and Plato as forerunners of Theophrastus. The conception of sympathy goes back certainly to the

Theophrastus, although a Dogmatist and an Aristotelian, emphasizes the value of experience. He states that especially natural science, the objects of which are the bodies of the physical world, must start from experience; according to him it is perception which provides the material for human thought.[96] Thus, Theophrastus becomes interested also in things which are called fairy-tales by earlier thinkers. But he is the first who is unbiased enough not to think impossible from the outset what other people declared to be nonsense without any further inquiry. The discovery and utilization of sympathetic effects is a scientific advance not made until the fourth century B.C.[97] This fact explains why sympathetic remedies are still unknown to the Hippocratic physicians. Moreover, it shows that from the point of view of ancient medicine the use of such things cannot be determined as deviation from the true method. It is on a scientific principle quite different from that of magic that the use of sympathetic remedies is based in antiquity.

Later, with the rise of the Neo-Platonic philosophy and of the Christian religion, a change took place. The Neo-Platonists explained

---

period before the fourth century B.C. But it is Theophrastus who gives sympathy its place in natural science. Since he acknowledges its effect apparently on account of philosophical argumentations it is not the Stoics who have the first system of sympathy (contrary to Stemplinger, l. c.).

[96] Cf. Zeller, l. c., II, 2, 1879, pp. 813–14 and Überweg-Prächter, Die Philosophie d. Alterums[12], 1926, p. 403, where the relation between Theophrastus and Strato is stressed.

[97] Cf. Theophrastus, Inquiry into Plants, IX, 18, 4, 10; and in contrast to his statement Aristotle, History of Animals, 605a, 4–6, τὰ δ' ἐπιμυθευόμενα πέπλασται μᾶλλον ὑπὸ γυναικῶν καὶ τῶν περὶ τὰς ἐπῳδάς. I cannot deal with the problem whether the ninth book of the Inquiry into Plants is genuine or not. H. Bretzl, Botanische Forschungen des Alexanderzuges, 1903, p. 366, denies the authenticity of the last part "dessen nicht theophrasteischen Geist jeder (Botaniker) beim ersten Durchlesen fühlt." Rehm und Vogel, Exakte Wissenschaften, l. c., 5, 57, agree with him. But G. Senn, Das pharmazeutisch-botanische Buch in Theophrast's Pflanzenkunde (Verhandlungen d. Schweizer Naturforschenden Gesellschaft, Zermatt, 1923, II. Teil, pp. 201–02), opposes this opinion just as a botanist. The material at least is, according to him, genuine and the assumption of a "Pseudotheophrast" unnecessary. Manifold wordings of the book are now also proved by O. Regenbogen, Hermes 69, 1934, pp. 75 sq.; 190 sq., as far as the first books are concerned. Nothing indicates that the material, even if it is not collected by Theophrastus himself, does not go back at least to his school. So much is certain, that the interest in sympathetic remedies is rather an indication in favor of Theophrastus than against him. The rejection of incantations and of superstition (IX, 19, 3) in general is also in accordance with the attitude of Theophrastus. At any rate, it is not justifiable to omit the passages concerning sympathetic remedies, as is done in the edition of A. Horst in the Loeb Classical Library, 1916, p. 310.

sympathy not by physical but by psychic causes.[98] What had been physical thereby became spiritual. The Christian belief, on the other hand, separated God from nature; nature was no longer an animate being. Thus, effects which were in earlier times natural and empirical later became mysterious. And since they were supposed to be mysterious they were looked upon with suspicion or were forgotten by the physicians. Theodorus Priscianus says in the beginning of his book on physical remedies: "Nature is everywhere performing a great mystery," but "you will forgive me my work, oh my forefathers. The crude generation of our times is ignorant of the procedure of your investigations."[99] And it is Alexander of Tralles, a late physician of the decadent age, who states: "I should like to use all kinds of remedies, but because of the stupidity of the many of to-day who blame those who do it, I shrink from applying them."[100] The physician employing sympathetic remedies is now considered to be a sorcerer. In earlier centuries he was a scientist.[101]

In surgery, dietetics and pharmacology then Greek medicine is rational and hostile to magic. The same is true in regard to the use of music as a remedy for pains. The Sicilian physicians, like others, resorted to music as Caelius Aurelianus relates: "Others have approved of the use of songs, as the brother of Philistion also remarks in the XXII book on remedies, writing that a certain piper had played his melodies over parts of the body which, quivering and throbbing, were relaxed

---

[98] E. Zeller, l. c., III, 2³, 1881, p. 558.

[99] Theodorus Priscianus, Euporiston, ed. Valentin Rose, 1894, p. 250, 14: est enim in omni mundo natura quae operetur grande secretum; 250, 17–20: dabitis mihi veniam operis, patres priores. disputationum enim vestrarum rationes . . . aetas mundi rudis ignoravit. Cf. Pliny, N. H. XIX, 186: opus occultum, the hidden work.

[100] Alexander v. Tralles, ed. Puschmann, I, 1878, p. 573: ἐγὼ δὲ φιλῶ πᾶσι κεχρῆσθαι. διὰ δὲ τοὺς πολλοὺς τοὺς ἐν τῷ νῦν χρόνῳ ἀμαθεῖς ὄντας καταμέμφεσθαι τοῖς χρωμένοις τοῖς φυσικοῖς, ἔφυγον συνεχῶς χρῆσθαι τοῖς φύσει δρᾶν δυναμένοις. . . .

[101] It is significant for the derivation of the sympathetic remedies from experience concerning natural facts that they are usually called φυσικὰ or ἐμπειρικά. My attention was first drawn to this fact by a lecture of O. Temkin on Magic and Experience in which he emphasized the significance of these expressions (cf. also M. Neuburger, Gesch. d. Medizin II, p. 26). It is again in the magical papyri that the mysterious character of those things occurs first, the derivation of the healing power from nature being stressed. Here too, for the first time nature is revered as a deity who is not identical with the god governing the world but a demon who performs miraculous effects. Cf. K. Preisendanz, Philologus, 67, 1908, p. 474.

after the pain had been destroyed."[102] How this is to be understood becomes evident from the discussions of philosophers who were interested in the effect of music and from the judgment of Soranus about it. Gellius relates: "I ran across the statement very recently in the book of Theophrastus On Inspiration that many men have believed and put their belief on record, that when gouty pains in the hips are most severe they are relieved if a flute-player plays soothing measures. That snake-bites are cured by the music of the flute, when played skillfully and melodiously, is also stated in a book of Democritus, entitled On Deadly Infections, in which he shows that the music of the flute is medicine for many ills that flesh is heir to. So very close is the connection between the bodies and the minds of men, and therefore between physical and mental ailments and their remedies."[103] And Soranus asserts that those men were very stupid who believed that the strength of the illness can be expelled by melodies and songs.[104] There is no magical belief responsible for the use of music any more than magical powers are presupposed in the use of words. Diocles holds that one has to understand friendly consolation as incantation. For it stops the flowing of the blood when the wounded man is attentive and, as it were, connected with the man who speaks to him."[105]

At any rate in the administration of songs and in the use of words

[102] Caelius Aurelianus, De morbis acutis et chronicis, l. c., p. 555: "Alii cantilenas adhibendas probaverunt, ut etiam Philistionis frater idem memorat libro XXII, de adiutoriis scribens quendam fistulatorem loca dolentia decantasse, quaecum saltum sumerent palpitando, discusso dolore mitescerent."

[103] The Attic Nights of Aulus Gellius with an English Translation by J. C. Rolfe, Loeb Class. Library, 1927, I, p. 352–54: "Creditum hoc a plerisque esse et memoriae mandatum, ischia cum maxime doleant, tum, si modulis lenibus tibicen incinat, minui dolores, ego nuperrime in libro Theophrasti περὶ ἐνθουσιασμοῦ scriptum inveni. Viperarum morsibus tibicinium scite modulateque adhibitum mederi, refert etiam Democriti liber, qui inscribitur περὶ λοιμῶν in quo docet plurimis hominum morbidis medicinae fuisse incentiones tibiarum. Tanta prorsus adfinitas est corporibus hominum mentibusque et propterea vitiis quoque aut medellis animorum et corporum." It is by the expression modulis lenibus that the words μαλακαῖς ἐπαοιδαῖς in Pindar's Ode must be interpreted, cf. also Theophrastus, fr. LXXXVII, Wimmer: Ὅτι δὲ καὶ νόσους ἰᾶται μουσικὴ Θ. ἱστόρησεν ἐν τῷ περὶ ἐνθουσιασμοῦ, ἰσχιακοὺς φάσκων ἀνόσους διατελεῖν εἰ καταυλήσοι τις τοῦ τόπου τῇ φρυγιστὶ ἁρμονίᾳ. Sometimes the invention of this procedure was ascribed to Pythagoras, cf. Caelius Aurelianus, l. c.: "Alii denique hoc adjutorii genus Pythagoram memorant invenisse."

[104] Caelius Aurelianus, l. c.: "Sed Sorani iudicio videntur hi mentis vanitate iactari, qui modulis et cantilena passionis robur excludi posse crediderunt."

[105] Diocles, Fr. 92, Wellmann: Διοκλῆς ἐπαοιδὴν παρέδωκε τὴν παρηγορίαν. ἴσχαιμον γὰρ εἶναι ταύτην, ὅταν τὸ πνεῦμα τοῦ τετρωμένου προσεχὲς ᾖ καὶ ὥσπερ προσηρτημένον τῷ παρηγοροῦντι.

no magical belief is to be found. Every kind of incantation, too, is throughout antiquity rejected by physicians. In the Hippocratic book on the Sacred Disease it is said: "But perhaps what they profess (sc. in regard to incantations) is not true, the fact being that men, in need of a livelihood, contrive and devise many fictions of all sorts."[106] Galen declares all the incantations to be wrong.[107] Nay: "Animals like human beings can be cured not by vain words but by the reliable art of healing."[108] And in this respect the attitude of the Romans does not vary from that of the Greeks. For Celsus does not advise incantations, either; Varro warns against their use. The Roman law does not recognize as true physicians men who perform incantations.[109]

To be sure, incantations were never a means of the physician. The decadent age is in this respect not different from the fifth century B.C.[110]

[106] Jones, l. c., II, p. 147: ἴσως δὲ οὐχ οὕτως ἔχει ταῦτα, ἀλλ' ἄνθρωποι βίου δεόμενοι πολλὰ καὶ παντοῖα τεχνῶνται.

[107] Galen, Opera, ed. Kühn, XI, p. 792.

[108] Vegetius, ed. E. Lommatzsch, 1903, p. 199, 1–4: Aliquanti praecantatione tentant afferre remedia; quae vanitas ab aniculis solis diligenda est, cum animalia sicut homines non inanibus verbis sed certa medendi arte curentur (this general statement proves that the two incantations which are found in the text must be later additions, p. 306, 5–8; 10–11. The hostile attitude toward those remedies is confirmed p. 65, 3–5; 10–12.) Also in Gargilius Martialis only one incantation is mentioned (l. c., p. 309, 12 sq.). In the Mulomedicina Chironis, ed. E. Oder, 1901, p. 62, 7–10, incantations are rejected too. (Two exceptions p. 260, 4; p. 285, 4.) In Paelagonius, ed. M. Ihm, 1892, p. 90, 1, the incantation which is rejected by Vegetius (l. c., p. 199, 1–4) is given in detail. But the situation even in veterinary medicine is characterized by the remark of the editor of Paelagonius (§ 121, p. 154): "Utinam is qui Graeca hippiatrica congessit superstitiosior fuisset. Removit enim fere omnia harum superstitionum exempla, quibus Apsyrti liber refertus fuisse videtur. Unus codex Parisinus Milleri nonnulla servavit obscure scripta . . . Paelagoniana huius generis alia mox sequentur, quae ne Vegetio quidem digna visa sunt quae reciperentur. Immo is tamquam detrectatorem et contemptorem se iactat . . . etsi apud veteres magno in honore fuerint, ut vel Catonis . . . cantatio barbara testatur." One can only conclude that it is really impossible to ascribe to ancient physicians, not even to veterinaries, the use of incantations.

[109] Cf. Varro, Catus (Mommsen, Röm. Gesch. III⁶, 1875, p. 610). Digesta L, 13, 1. § 3 (The physician has the right to sue for his salary) non tamen si incantavit, si inprecatus est, si ut vulgari verbo impostorum utar, exorcizavit. non sunt ista medicinae genera, tametsi sint, qui hos sibi profuisse praedicatione adfirment. Cato, usually quoted for the Roman use of incantations, is not the only witness and his testimony has no value for the time in which Greek medicine was influential in Rome.

[110] The passages quoted above concerning the use of music are usually referred to as proof for the use of incantations in Greek medicine, cf. Wellmann, Die Fragmente d. Sizilischen Ärzte, 1901, p. 30a: "Ihr Heilverfahren . . . bestand, in Besprechungen . . . Beachtenswert ist ferner, dass Diokles gleichfalls ein Anhänger

Incantations are not only useless, and wrong, says Galen, they are out-side of the activity of the physician.[111] No one can perform incantations if he wants to be acknowledged as a good doctor: "It is not a learned physician who sings incantations over pains which should be cured by cutting."[112] This attitude does not signify a progress reached only in the time of the Hippocratic physicians. Homeric medicine is already opposed to such means, and the polemic of the book on the Sacred Disease only proves that in the fifth century B.C. problems must be discussed which before were not worth discussing.[113]

The rejection of incantations was the more difficult since not even those who trusted their validity claimed to have a reason by which their effect could be explained.[114] The men who performed incantations were priests, and even Plato admits that for the many it is not easy to come to a definite conclusion concerning the value of incantations.[115] But the Olympian religion remains strong enough to resist. Only the superstitious resort to incantations. A believer in magic may dare to state that disbe-lief in incantations proves disbelief in God; but even in the second cen-tury A.D. the answer is that this conclusion is rash, that, on the contrary, men who believe they can force God by their prayers are impious, as

jener Schule die ἐπαοιδαί zur Stillung des Blutes bei Wunden empfohlen . . . Es ist wahrscheinlich, dass die sikelische Schule diese populären Mittel der Volksmedizin aus pythagoreischer Lehre herübergenommen hat." Or it is said (RE, Suppl. IV, s. v. Epode, pp. 340–41): "Der Gebrauch der Epode ist in der antiken Welt nie geschwunden trotz der Gegner, die dagegen bei den Griechen selbst und bei den Christen auftraten. Schon im 5. Jahrhundert finden wir solche bei den Ärzten . . . Von späteren Ärzten welche ihren Gebrauch verwarfen, seien etwa Soranus . . . und Galen . . . genannt . . . aber diese Stimmen drangen nicht durch, da die volkstümliche Verwendung der Epoden von Anfang an auch von Ärzten oder solchen die dafür galten, übernommen wurde." Cf. also F. G. Welcker, Kl. Schriften, III, 1850, pp. 68 sq. I think it is sufficient to give the passages in full in order to prove that they have no magical implications whatsoever.

[111] Galen, Opera, ed. Kühn, XI, 792: μαγγανεῖαι οὐ περίεργοι μόνον, οὐδ' ἔξω τῆς ἰατρικῆς τέχνης, ἀλλὰ καὶ ψευδεῖς ἁπάσαι.

[112] Sophocles, Aias, 581–82: οὐ πρὸς ἰατροῦ σοφοῦ θρηνεῖν ἐπῳδὰς πρὸς τομῶντι πήματι.

[113] Contrary to Wilamowitz, Der Glaube der Hellenen, I, 1931, p. 29 (Schon im 5ten Jahrhundert) and Jones, l. c., I, p. 10.

[114] Alexander v. Aphrodisias, De Fato, cp. 8, Supplementum Aristotelicum, II, 2, 1881, p. 174, 20–25: ἄδηλα δὲ τὰ αἴτια ἀνθρωπίνῳ λογισμῷ ἐκείνων μᾶλλον ἃ κατά τινας ἀντιπαθείας γίνεσθαι πεπίστευται ἀγνοουμένης τῆς αἰτίας δι' ἣν γίνεται, ὁποῖα περίαπτά τέ τινα προσείληπται οὐδεμίαν εὔλογον καὶ πιθανὴν αἰτίαν τοῦ ταῦτα ποιεῖν ἔχοντα, ἔτι δὲ ἐπαοιδαὶ καί τινες τοιαῦται μαγγανεῖαι. τούτων γὰρ ὁμολογεῖται μὲν ὑπὸ πάντων ἄδηλος εἶναι ἡ αἰτία, διὸ καὶ ἀναιτιολόγητα λέγουσιν αὐτά. Not only incantations but all the other magical procedures are then justified by their empirical efficacy.

[115] Laws, XI, 933a.

they were called also in the book on the Sacred Disease.[116] It is not until the old religious feeling was weakened that foreign rites and superstition could get the upper hand. And it is important to note that Asclepius, the patron of physicians and patients, was for all pious men of these late centuries the symbol of Olympian religion.[117] If in antiquity nobody doubted that magic had its origin in medicine as Pliny relates,[118] the medical art of the Greeks and Romans has really freed itself from any magical ingredient. And this in spite of the necessary temptation to use everything which may help to cure the patient and in spite of the supposed empirical confirmation of the power of incantations. For even in the latest centuries it is on the efficacy of incantations in those cases in which the other remedies fail, that their use is based and excused. For the superstitious physicians themselves never forget that in performing incantations they transgress the limits of medicine.[119]

But what about the relation of physicians to the religious healing of diseases? What do they think about prayers and incubations, which were supposed by many people to help against illness in the same way as surgery and dietetics, remedies and music?

Prayers are not dealt with very often in medical books. In one of the Hippocratic writings it is said: "Prayer indeed is good, but while calling on the gods a man should himself lend a hand."[120] This is not an

[116] Lucian, Philopseudes, 29.
[117] Harnack, Medizinisches aus d. ältesten Kirchengeschichte, l. c., p. 72: "Das eigentümliche des Dämonenglaubens im 2. Jahrhundert besteht erstlich darin, dass er aus den dunklen unteren Schichten in die oberen, selbst in die Literatur, empordringt und eine ungleich wichtigere Sache wird wie ehedem, zweitens, dass er keine kräftige naive öffentliche Religion mehr neben sich hat, die ihn niederhält . . . Die ausserordentliche Verbreitung des Dämonenglaubens . . . (ist darauf) zurückzuführen, dass in der Kaiserzeit das Zutrauen zu den alten Religionen dahinschwand . . ." Concerning the foreign origin of incantations cf. e.g., Diodor, II, 39 (the Chaldeans), III, 58 (Cybele), Lucian, Demonax, cp. 23.
[118] Pliny, Naturalis Historia, XXX, 1: magicam natam primum e medicina nemo dubitat. But Pliny himself admits that incantations were rejected by the wisest (l. c., XVIII, 3–4).
[119] Cf. Alexander v. Tralles, l. c., II, 1879, p. 475 (the explanation of the supposed change of Galen's opinion concerning incantations); p. 579; p. 585. In this sense it must be understood that Ammianus Marcellinus (Res Gestae, XVI, 8, 2) speaks of an "anile incantamentium . . . quod medicinae quoque auctoritas admittit." Concerning the material preserved cf. again L. Deubner, Greek charms and amulets, l. c.
[120] Jones, l. c., IV, p. 423: καὶ τὸ μὲν εὔχεσθαι ἀγαθόν. δεῖ δὲ καὶ αὐτὸν συλλαμβάνοντα τοὺς θεοὺς ἐπικαλεῖσθαι. Cf. p. 447: "I have discovered regimen, with the gods' help,

ironical statement, for the same author declares: "So with this knowledge . . . precautions must be taken, with change of regimen, and prayers to the gods . . . that all dangers may be averted."[121] He firmly believes then in the power of prayers, although he thinks it necessary not
to rely on them alone where other means are available too. In the same
way the efficacy of prayers is presupposed in another Hippocratic treatise which refutes the theory that a certain disease can be understood
as holy. For "if we suppose this disease to be more divine than any
other, it ought to have attacked, not the highest and richest classes
only of the Scythians, but all classes equally—or rather the poor especially, if indeed the gods are pleased to receive from men respect and
worship, and repay these with favours. For naturally the rich, having
great wealth, make many sacrifices to the gods, and offer many votive
offerings, and honor them, all of which things the poor, owing to their
poverty, are less able to do; besides, they blame the gods for not giving
them wealth, so that the penalties for such sins are likely to be paid by
the poor rather than by the rich."[122] The belief that God would benefit
rich people more than poor ones because he receives greater offerings
from them is at least the basis of this argument. There is no reason to
assume that the Hippocratic physicians are opposed to the validity of
prayers.

At a later time no discussion of prayers is found in medical books,
Galen holding that it is better to recognize the power of God by understanding the world than by sacrifice.[123] This reticence concerning prayers
or even their renunciation does not involve, however, any hostility to
religion; it is in accordance with the attitude of the philosophers and
with that of pious men in general. From Socrates on it is held to be
offensive rather than reverent to ask favors of the gods. The pious man

---

as far as it is possible for mere man to discover it." Withington's opinion that the
book shows an irreligious attitude is certainly incorrect, l. c., p. 142.

[121] Jones, l. c., IV, p. 437: οὕτω γινώσκοντα χρὴ προμηθεῖσθαι καὶ ἐκδιαιτῆσθαι καὶ
τοῖσι θεοῖσιν εὔχεσθαι . . . ἀποτρόπαια τὰ χαλεπὰ εἶναι πάντα.

[122] Jones, l. c., I, p. 129: καίτοι ἐχρῆν, ἐπεὶ θειότερον τοῦτο τὸ νόσευμα τῶν λοιπῶν
ἐστιν, οὐ τοῖς γενναιοτάτοις τῶν Σκυθέων καὶ τοῖς πλουσιωτάτοις προσπίπτειν μούνοις, ἀλλὰ
τοῖς ἅπασιν ὁμοίως, καὶ μᾶλλον τοῖσιν ὀλίγα κεκτημένοισιν, εἰ δὴ τιμώμενοι χαίρουσιν οἱ θεοὶ
καὶ θαυμαζόμενοι ὑπ' ἀνθρώπων καὶ ἀντὶ τούτων χάριτας ἀποδιδόασιν. εἰκὸς γὰρ τοὺς μὲν
πλουσίους θύειν πολλὰ τοῖς θεοῖς καὶ ἀνατιθέναι ἀναθήματα ἐόντων χρημάτων πολλῶν καὶ τιμᾶν,
τοὺς δὲ πένητας ἧσσον διὰ τὸ μὴ ἔχειν, ἔπειτα καὶ ἐπιμεμφομένους ὅτι οὐ διδόασι χρήματα
αὐτοῖσιν, ὥστε τῶν τοιούτων ἁμαρτιῶν τὰς ζημίας τοὺς ὀλίγα κεκτημένους φέρειν μᾶλλον ἢ τοὺς
πλουσίους.

[123] Galen, De usu partium, l. c., cf. p. 216, 44.

is allowed only to express his gratitude; he may thank but can do no more.[124] The physicians, in adopting this attitude, follow the development of the religious feeling among the Greeks.

At the same period incubations have become the more recognized form of religious healing; they have replaced prayer, which is no more an adequate procedure. These incubations are dream-healings: either the way of curing is revealed to the patient or he is cured immediately by the god. Now, as regards mantic dreams, most of the physicians of all centuries admit their reality; they acknowledge even their divine character. In the Hippocratic Corpus "those dreams being divine and foretelling to cities or to private persons things evil or things good" are expressly named.[125] Herophilus distinguishes dreams sent by God from those which are natural. The Empiricists too reckon with the divinity of dreams; Rufus recounts such dreams as does Galen.[126] The Methodists are the only physicians who apparently do not believe in divine dreams; they never mention them. However, it seems justifiable to state that the great majority of Greek physicians recognize the divinity of dreams. And this is not at all astonishing, for almost all Greek philosophers did the same. Epicurus alone objects to such a theory, and it must be on account of Epicurean influence that the Methodists are the only physicians to disapprove of the value of mantic.[127]

Divine dreams are at first held to be unintelligible to physicians although dreams caused by physical factors can be interpreted by them. The Hippocratic author says: "such dreams as are divine have interpreters in those who possess the art of dealing with such things," namely in the priests.[128] Only the physical dreams are to be interpreted by physicians: "All the physical symptoms foretold by the soul, excess, of surfeit or of depletion, of things natural, or change to unaccustomed

---

[124] Cf. J. Bernays, l. c., pp. 104–105. Diogenes Laertius VII, 124 is heretical.

[125] Jones, l. c., IV, p. 423: Ὁκόσα μὲν οὖν τῶν ἐνυπνίων θεῖά ἐστι καὶ προσημαίνει ἢ πόλεσι ἢ ἰδιώτῃσι ἢ κακὰ ἢ ἀγαθά.

[126] Herophilus: Doxographi Graeci, 416, 14–22; Empiricists: Deichgräber, Die Griech. Empirikerschule, 1930, p. 78, 28; 95, 8; 149, 24; 150, 12; Rufus: Oribasius, III (CMG VI, 6, 1, 1931, p. 192, 3 sq.); Galen, Opera, ed. Kühn, XI, p. 341; XVI, p. 221; Asclepiades: Galen, Opera, ed. Kühn, II, p. 29.

[127] Cf. Cicero, De Divinatione, I, 5–6, where it is said that even Democritus adopted the belief in dreams. Concerning Pythagoras cf. Diogenes Laertius, VIII, 32; concerning the Stoa also Doxographi Graeci, p. 416, 10. Xenophanes and Epicurus resist the dogma. The old Academy acknowledged it, the new Academy was undecided in its judgment as was Panaetius (cf. Herzog, Die Wunderheilungen v. Epidaurus, l. c., p. 61).

[128] Jones, l. c., IV, p. 423.

things, these also the diviners interpret, sometimes with, sometimes without success. But in neither case do they know the cause, either of their success or of their failure. They recommend precautions to be taken to prevent harm, yet they give no instruction how to take precautions, but only recommend prayers to the gods."[129] Thus part of the realm of the diviners is in the fifth and fourth centuries B.C. usurped by the physicians and declared to be their own. But the priests are still the only interpreters of divine dreams.

Yet later on also physicians do interpret the divine dreams as well as the physical ones. The Empiricists and Galen do not ask the diviners about the contents of dreams, they understand them by themselves. This type of divination becomes a science of its own, and now "the divine prescriptions are simple and have nothing mysterious . . . ," they fall within medical reasoning.[130] At the same time a change in the theoretical understanding of dreams takes place. In the Hippocratic book, although it is the soul which tells beforehand what will happen, it is the body which causes the dreams.[131] But Herophilus declares dreams to be merely psychological phenomena; it is not the bodily changes but only the psychic changes that are manifested in dreams; these are the natural dreams which have to be separated from the divine.[132] His theory comes to be generally recognized even by the diviners. The book of Artemidoros, which is the most famous treatise on the interpretation of dreams, takes over its theory almost verbally from Herophilus.[133]

What are the reasons for the belief in the validity of dreams? They are partly philosophical but differ according to the various systems.[134] Yet the fact that the Empiricists also acknowledge the reality of divine

---

[129] Jones, l. c., IV, p. 423: ὁκόσα δὲ ἡ ψυχὴ τοῦ σώματος παθήματα προσημαίνει, πλησμονῆς ἢ κενώσιος ὑπερβολὴν τῶν συμφυτῶν ἢ μεταβολὴν τῶν ἀηθέων, κρίνουσι μὲν καὶ ταῦτα, καὶ τὰ μὲν τυγχάνουσι, τὰ δὲ ἁμαρτάνουσι, καὶ οὐδέτερα τούτων γινώσκουσι δι' ὅ τι γίνεται, οὔθ' ὅ τι ἂν ἐπιτύχωσιν οὔθ' ὅ τι ἂν ἁμάρτωσι, φυλάσσεσθαι δὲ παραινέοντες μή τι κακὸν λάβῃ. οἱ δ' οὖν οὐ διδάσκουσιν ὡς χρὴ φυλάσσεσθαι, ἀλλὰ θεοῖσιν εὔχεσθαι κελεύουσι.

[130] Artemidoros, Oneirocritos, ed. R. Hercher, 1864, p. 215, 1 sq.: τὰς δὲ συνταγὰς τῶν θεῶν ἤτοι ἁπλᾶς καὶ οὐδὲν ἐχούσας αἴνιγμα εὑρήσεις. Cf. in general A. Bouché-Leclerq, Histoire de la divination dans l'antiquité, I, 1879, pp. 295 sq.

[131] Jones, l. c., IV, p. 420.

[132] Herophilus, l. c., 416, 14: Ἡρόφιλος τῶν ὀνείρων τοὺς μὲν θεοπέμπτους κατ' ἀνάγκην γίνεσθαι, τοὺς δὲ φυσικοὺς ἀνειδωλοποιουμένης ψυχῆς τὸ συμφέρον αὐτῇ καὶ τὸ πάντως ἐσόμενον . . .

[133] Cf. Bouché-Leclerq, l. c., I. p. 297, who gives a thorough analysis of the book of Artemidorus and also names all the physicians and philosophers interested in the theory of dreams.

[134] Cf. e.g., Aristotle, On Dreams and n. 127, above.

dreams already indicates empirical proof too, for this school has no other valid principle. Accordingly it is sometimes expressly stated that "some dreams are prophetic for this is shown by experiment."[135] Nay, even the dream-interpreters rely on experience rather than on argument. They say that the validity of dreams can hardly be proved by reason but that it can be shown by experience.[136] Dreams, to the ancients, are a natural phenomenon even when they are considered to be divine, and as such they belong to natural science. There is then no reason for the scientific physician to object to healing by priests according to advice given in temple dreams.

But the physicians could not object to the miracles performed by the god either. For ancient dogmatic philosophy acknowledges the possibility of miracles. This depends on the fact that the natural laws are not held valid by the Dogmatists in every case but only in most cases. Exceptions are then always possible; things may happen for reasons still unknown, but they are not at all contrary to nature. Aristotle says: "It is the miracle, a thing contrary to nature but not contrary to nature as a whole, rather contrary to it as it appears in most cases. For in regard to the eternal nature which acts with necessity nothing comes into being contrary to it."[137] This sentence is valid for later generations too. Also the Stoic philosophers and the Neo-Platonists are able to understand miracles as nothing more than events whose causes are unknown. Dogmatic medicine, then, based on rational philosophy, cannot oppose religious cures; miracles are not excluded by its conception of science. The Empiricists, on the other hand, cannot disapprove of miracles since they acknowledge no general rules beyond experience. There is no sufficient reason to allow them to contradict those facts. Only the Epicureans, who try to explain everything and do not acknowledge the assumption that something can happen without an intelligible

s

[135] Galen, Opera, ed. Kühn, VI, p. 833: καὶ δή τινα μαντικῶς ὑπ' αὐτῆς (sc. τῇ ψυχῆς) προδηλοῦνται, καὶ γὰρ τοῦτο τῇ πείρᾳ μαρτυρεῖται.

[136] Artemidorus, l. c., p. 1, 11; 15–16 . . . περὶ ὧν ἂν ἔχω κατάληψιν, ἣν διὰ πείρας ἐπορισάμην, συγγράψαι . . . φέρων εἰς τὸ μέσον τὴν πείραν καὶ τὴν τῶν ἀποτελεσμάτων μαρτυρίαν, ἢ πᾶσιν ἱκανὴ γένοιτ' ἂν ἀντισχεῖν ἀνθρώποις, καὶ μέντοι καὶ πρὸς τοὺς χρωμένους μὲν μαντικῇ διὰ δὲ τὸ μὴ ἐντετυχηκέναι λόγοις περὶ τούτων ἀκριβέσι πεπλανημένους. Cf. p. 197, 12; 198, 14; 199, 1. Just because of their experimental basis dream-interpretations must not be identified with magic. Artemidoros therefore rejects every kind of magical belief and opposes magicians no less than do the doctors. Cf. p. 205, 25–206, 11.

[137] Aristotle, On the Generation of Animals, IV, 4, 770b9. ἔστι γὰρ τὸ τέρας τῶν παρὰ φύσιν τι, παρὰ φύσιν δ' οὐ πᾶσαν ἀλλὰ τὴν ὡς ἐπὶ τὸ πολύ. περὶ γὰρ τὴν ἀεὶ καὶ τὴν ἐξ ἀνάγκης οὐθὲν γίνεται παρὰ φύσιν. Cf. Zeller, l. c., II, 2³, p. 429, 3.

reason, are opposed to miracles.[138] Therefore, the Methodists, the physicians of late antiquity who were especially influential in Roman centuries, are the only ones who must reject religious medicine as well as magical medicine. But in general, physicians, as scientists, believe in miracles.

But doctors never expressly advise the use of prayers or of incubations.[139] It is possible only to infer from their theory that they must have acknowledged the validity of prayers and of dreams. This conclusion leads to a very strange problem. If religious medicine cannot be rejected by physicians, is it considered to be valuable in certain cases? And in which cases? Or is it that physicians only believe it possible to be cured by divine help but that they do not resort to it themselves? This would be strange too. But there is no indication to be found in the medical writings as to when patients should use religious medicine and when they should use human medicine. At least, there is no direct indication. Indirectly, I think, it can be deduced from the facts upon what occasions the physicians themselves allow their patients to go to the temple: It is the case of chronic diseases or of every disease which cannot be cured by human knowledge.

The negative attitude of the Greek physicians in many diseases has always been felt to be puzzling. They seemed to be satisfied with the statement that such and such a man can be helped no more. They

---

[138] Cf. Zeller, l. c., V, p. 697, 6; 704; 720. Dilthey (Das natürliche System der Geisteswissenschaften im 17. Jahrhundert, Gesammelte Schriften, II, 1923, p. 132) stresses the point that miracles could not be entirely discarded until the system of Descartes. The "Begriff von der ausnahmslosen Macht und Geltung der Naturgesetze . . . entstand erst, als durch Descartes alle psychischen Kräfte aus der Natur vertrieben worden waren." Concerning Epicurus cf. Lucretius, De Rerum Natura, I, v. 150–54.

[139] R. Herzog, Die Wunderheilungen v. Epidaurus, Philologus, l. c., p. 149; p. 61, believes, along with others, that the passage to be found in the book on Sacred Disease: θύειν τε καὶ εὔχεσθαι καὶ ἐς τὰ ἱερὰ φέροντας ἱκετεύειν τοὺς θεούς (Jones, l. c., II, p. 148) "auf die Incubation hinweise." Such an interpretation, however, spoils the argument used by the Hippocratic author. He has claimed that the patients if really possessed by god should not be purified; he adds "one should rather if such patients are to be found pray to the gods and bring them to the temples." For it is his belief that the possession by god, since it is divine, should not be driven away but revered. The Scythians behaved similarly for they revered those men who were possessed by a god (cf. Jones, l. c., I, p. 127). If incubations were advised by the author this would mean a kind of healing which is necessary only if such men are ill, a contention which the author starting from the presuppositions of his enemies tries to refute. The healing of diseases by prayer alone was not recommended before Christian times, cf. Epistle of James, ch. V, 14, 15, 16; The Acts, ch. XL, 20; ch. V, 15.

advised against treating patients who cannot be cured and believed it to be part of their art both to know in what cases the physician cannot accomplish anything and, in those cases, to refrain from doing anything. This, no doubt, is a very peculiar, even inhuman behavior. For it excludes the help of the physician in diseases which are gravest and in which his help is most needed. But such an attitude becomes immediately intelligible if the physician presupposes that the patient, if not treated by him, will go to the temple.

When the art of the physician fails, everybody resorts to incantations and prayers;[140] this phrase was frequently quoted in antiquity. It is especially true in chronic diseases, as it is said: "Those who are ill with chronic diseases and do not succeed by the usual remedies and the customary diet turn to purifications and amulets and dreams."[141] For, of course, one will not go to the god if the case is not serious. Therefore it is a topic of the temple-cures that the god could help when the physicians could not.[142] In a world in which the temples of Asclepius are open to everybody who is ill it need not be mentioned that the patient can and should go to the god if the human physician cannot do anything for him. It is sufficient to state in which cases the physician can do no

[140] Diodorus, Fr., XXX, 43. Dindorf: ἐκεῖνοί τε γὰρ [οἱ ἐν ταῖς μακραῖς νόσοις δυσποτμοῦντες] ὅταν ταῖς παρὰ τῶν ἰατρῶν θεραπείαις ὑπακούσαντες μηδὲν βέλτιον ἀπαλλάττωσι καταφεύγουσιν ἐπὶ τοὺς θύτας καὶ μάντεις, ἔνιοι δὲ προσδέχονται τὰς ἐπῳδὰς καὶ παντοδαπὰ γένη περιάπτων. Cf. Pliny, N. H., XXX, 98.

[141] Plutarch, De Facie in orbe Lunae, 920b: οἱ ἐν νοσήμασι χρονίοις πρὸς τὰ κοινὰ βοηθήματα καὶ τὰς συνήθεις διαίτας ἀπειπόντες ἐπὶ καθαρμοὺς καὶ περίαπτα καὶ ὀνείρους τρέπονται. Cf. the stories related about Pericles (Plutarch, Pericles, ch. 38), Bion (Diogenes Laertius, IV, 54), Cleomenes (Plutarch, Sayings of Spartans, 223 E), which prove that this attitude is not restricted to the lower classes or to any century. It is the general reaction of men (contrary to Rohde, l. c., p. 89 and Welcker, l. c., p. 69). Since the physicians did not acknowledge magical help to be possible, they were the more interested in that their patients resorted to religious medicine.

[142] Cf. Weinreich, Antike Heilungswunder, l. c., p. 195 sq. "Zur Topik der Wundererzählung, die Kunst der Ärzte versagt." A survey on incantations and the diseases in which they are used also shows that they are especially relied on in chronic diseases. Herzog, in his commentary to the tablets of Epidaurus (Die Wunderheilungen v. Epidaurus, l. c.) expressly mentions that the diseases cured by the god are those which are not or cannot be cured by human physicians. Later, when the chronic diseases are also treated by physicians, the religious incubations are more restricted to the revelation of remedies, and the type of illnesses dealt with in the temples changes (Weinreich, l. c., pp. 113 sq.). Still, the god performs miracles as in the case described by Rufus, cf. n. 126, above, and in this sense religious medicine of course could never be replaced by human medicine. For, as Rufus says: "If somebody were so good a physician that he could provoke fever (as the god can), there would be no need for any other procedure of healing."

more. The consequence that the patient then should try to find help with the god is self-evident and removes the responsibility of the physician, as it relieves his conscience. This, at least, is true in so far as the physician has no ground for objecting to the healing by the god, since he acknowledges divine cures as real and helpful. It is not by chance, then, that the Methodists were the first to treat chronic diseases regularly; they were the only physicians who objected to the possibility of divine interference. But in general, religious medicine is, throughout antiquity, a subsidiary of human healing by surgery, diet, drugs, and music.

To sum up the results of my inquiry: Greek medicine in its aetiology as well as in its treatment of diseases is rational and empirical. About this fact there can be no doubt. But this is Greek rationalism and empiricism: it is influenced by religious ideas. God and His action are powers reckoned with by the physicians in their theory and in their practice. Every form of magic, however, is rejected as useless and wrong. If it is explained at all, it is on account of a religious belief that the physicians renounce magical superstition. Certainly, in many cases the Skeptic in his resignation also refrains from magical ideas. But this resignation, then, is not restricted to the renunciation of magic alone. It means also the disapproval of every aetiology and is therefore destructive of medical science. Moreover, the majority of physicians belong to the Dogmatic school. The Dogmatists and the unknown practitioners are religious and hostile to magic, which is held to be superstition. From the beginning until the end of antiquity there is no change in the attitude of the physicians in this respect. The relation of medicine to religion and magic therefore cannot be used for distinguishing different epochs of medical history. Greek medical art is a science; it is the beginning of modern science and yet different from it in its foundation.

246

THE HISTORY OF ANATOMY IN ANTIQUITY*

Various testimonies report that Alexandrian physicians dissected and vivisected humans. For earlier times, such dissection or vivisection is not attested. Later, in the first century of Roman supremacy, dissections are still taken for granted by ancient writers; already in the Empire one hears that they are impossible to perform, and vivisection probably is no longer performed at all. Thus tradition has it that the dissection of human bodies began in Alexandria at the same time as vivisection, and that it ended in the first century A.D.

Modern scholars hardly accepted the accounts that have been preserved as they stand. Those who did accept without question the tradition contained in the few testimonies did so because in themselves these testimonies appeared to be reliable and above suspicion, and because they did not contradict one another. But it can easily be objected that the survival of these statements is merely accidental, that reports of dissections performed in pre-Alexandrian times may have been lost. Above all, many physicians considered it impossible that the Hippocratic physicians had not yet practiced anatomy. The knowledge of the body to be found in the Hippocratic writings, they contended, was only obtainable through dissection. It is true, this conclusion did not remain uncontested. Other physicians declared that all the Hippocratics knew about the human body could also be known without dissection.[1] No universally acceptable conclusion was reached. Nevertheless, the performance of dissections was attributed even to much earlier times: already the Homeric physicians were said to have dissected, and the basis for this hypothesis was once more the conviction that the knowledge of the body that the Homeric poems evince was not attainable

* "Die Geschichte der Sektion in der Antike," *Quellen und Studien zur Geschichte der Naturwissenschaften und der Medizin*, Band 3, Heft 2, Berlin: Julius Springer, 1932, pp. 50–106 (pp.100–56 of the volume).
[1] The various opinions are most thoroughly represented in "Die Geschichte der Anatomie," by R. von Töply, in *Handbuch der Geschichte der Medizin*, edited by Neuburger and Pagel, II, Jena, 1903, p. 175.

without dissections.[2] This claim too did not go uncontested; the knowledge of the Homeric physicians was attributed not to the practice of anatomy but to observation of human sacrifices, in so far as chance observations of injuries or of skeletons did not furnish sufficient explanation.[3] Thus the assertions contained in the tradition were expanded by means of indirect conclusions based on the knowledge displayed by the various centuries: the Alexandrian physicians were not the first to practice anatomy, dissections having already been performed by the Homeric and Hippocratic physicians. Such daring conclusions were drawn in an unhesitating identification of ancient and modern medicine: one could not imagine ancient medicine at any period without anatomy any more than one can think of modern medicine without anatomy. Without dissection all treatment seemed out of the question.

When, however, the historical approach elucidated the complete dissimilarity between ancient and modern medicine, there arose another, an opposite, objection to the tradition. It was said that the physician naturally needs a certain amount of knowledge of the body for his surgical practice, but this knowledge need not be comprehensive at a time when surgery is rudimentary. Ancient surgery confined itself in the main to operations on external organs; internal organs were seldom operated upon. The treatment of internal diseases did not depend on knowledge of the internal organs. Thus for Greek medicine, human anatomy was not the necessary presupposition for the treatment of diseases. Supposing that occasional autopsies really took place, they were of no importance for medicine. Greek physicians did not dissect systematically, and not as physicians, though perhaps as scientists and philosophers. The surviving accounts cannot be correct; not even in Alexandria did physicians practice anatomy, as little as they did before Alexandria or afterward.[4]

The weightiest objection raised against tradition was, however, the claim that in Greece dissection was utterly unthinkable. Religious

[2] This claim was first made by O. Körner (*Münch. med. Wschr.*, LXIX, 1922, p. 1484 ff.). While he here considers anatomy the only way to acquire knowledge, later he calls it one possible method beside others (*Arch. f. Gesch. d. Med.*, XXIV, 1931, p. 186).

[3] E. Fuld, *Münch. med. Wschr.*, LXIX, 1922, p. 1731.

[4] It is above all H. E. Sigerist who has based the interpretation referred to in the text on such arguments as the general dependence of medicine on historical conditions ("Geburt der abendländischen Medizin," *Essays on the History of Medicine*. Presented to Karl Sudhoff, Oxford, 1924, pp. 201, 195).

and magical concepts, veneration of the dead, and dread of the corpse were believed to have made dissection impossible.[5] Likewise, vivisection seemed unthinkable for humane reasons. One was unwilling to attribute so much cruelty to physicians, the helpers. The accounts of dissection and vivisection were declared to be wicked inventions by which one school sought to discredit the other.

Scholars then have objected to the tradition for the most varied reasons; and it is this fact that sets the task of a history of ancient anatomy. One must try to understand the meaning of the tradition and to justify it in the face of the objections which have been raised. Should the misgivings, which do not appear to be without substance, prove really valid, the tradition must be discarded. Should what tradition claims prove true, however, then one must try to understand why dissections came to be performed in Alexandria; one must investigate the conditions for performing dissections, their frequency, and the possibility of obtaining material. The method of such an investigation can only be a historical one. That considerations of a medical nature yield no results is already demonstrated by the various contradictory explanations which physicians have given in their attempts to understand the knowledge of the Homeric and Hippocratic physicians. The value of a tradition can only be judged through a historical understanding of the time from which it derives and for which it is valid.

I

In an account of the Dogmatic physicians of Alexandria, Celsus hands down as their viewpoint: "Necessarium esse incidere corpora mortuorum, eorumque viscera atque intestina scrutari; longeque optime fecisse Herophilum et Erasistratum, qui nocentes homines a regibus ex carcere acceptos vivos inciderint" (Celsus, ed. F. Marx, *Corpus Medicorum Latinorum* I, 21, 14–17; Prooemium, 23). According to Celsus, therefore, the Dogmatists considered the dissection of cadavers necessary; vivisection of humans seemed to them to be right and particularly useful. Herophilus and Erasistratus were by far the most meritorious, for they cut open criminals turned over to them by the king. Such vivisections are expressly attested only for the founders of the Dog-

[5] This thesis, as far as I know, was first stated by Welcker (*Kleine Schriften* III, Bonn, 1850, p. 218 ff.).

matic schools, almost in the style of a historical narrative; they are not pictured as necessary, as are dissections of cadavers. Thus vivisections seem no longer to have been performed after Herophilus and Erasistratus, or they were no longer possible. The school supported the demand for vivisections only theoretically, by declaring them to be right and by representing what the founders did as by far the best thing to do.[6] The Empiricists, the opponents of the Dogmatists, whose school originated in the Dogmatic schools of Alexandria, rejected dissection and vivisection (Prooemium, 40 ff.).

Celsus speaks of dissections and vivisections only in the account of the Alexandrian schools. In his statements concerning the earlier physicians they are not mentioned. From this one may conclude, it seems to me, that they did not occur earlier, that dissections and vivisections first took place in the Alexandrian schools. One can tell no more from Celsus' account. Celsus himself says: "Incidere autem vivorum corpora et crudele et supervacuum est, mortuorum discentibus necessarium" (*CML*, p. 29, 17–20; Prooemium, 74). Thus, like the Dogmatists, he demands dissections, and like the Empiricists, he is against vivisections; he says nothing about difficulties that might be encountered in dissecting.

A short time afterward, however, dissections are no longer possible. Rufus says: "We shall try to teach you how to name the internal parts by dissecting an animal that most closely resembles man. Of old this was more correctly taught on man" (*Oeuvres de Rufus d'Éphèse*, ed. Daremberg, Paris, 1879, p. 134, 10 ff.). He can no longer practice anatomy, much as he wants to. And the same is true for Galen. He advises studying the human body not only through isolated observations or out of a book. As he says: "It should be your task and your endeavor not only to learn the exact form of every bone from books, but eagerly to look on the human skeleton with your own eyes. This is very easy in Alexandria, so that the physicians of that area instruct their pupils with the aid of autopsy. One must try, if for no other reason, to go to Alexandria just for this" (*Galeni Opera*, ed. Kühn, Leipzig, 1821, II 220).

---

[6] Other attacks on vivisection were also directed against the founders of the Dogmatic school. Tertullian (*De anima*, ch. 10) says of Herophilos: "That physician or butcher who cut up six hundred corpses in order to investigate nature, who allowed himself to hate mankind for the purpose of acquiring knowledge, I cannot tell whether he really was able to explore what is inside the body, since what was formerly alive changes in death, a death not of the natural kind but one changed itself through the violence of dissection."

In order to study the human body on the human skeleton, one must therefore, as Galen says, go to Alexandria; only there is one taught by means of demonstrations. Galen himself can only perform animal dissection and has to refer his pupils to chance skeletal finds for their observations on men, as he adds.[7] In the Roman Empire, dissections are no longer performed at this time, except in Alexandria.

These are the essential testimonies concerning dissection and vivisection. The Alexandrians dissected and vivisected, and during the early Empire dissections at least were taken absolutely for granted. At the end of the first century and in the middle of the second, however, teaching from the human skeleton was still possible only in Egypt. Dissection began in the third century B.C. in Alexandria, and only in Alexandria was it still possible in the second century A.D.

Yet, one claims, the Homeric physicians already performed dissections. What the Homeric physicians knew about the body can only be inferred indirectly from the Homeric poems; certainly they will not have known less than the poet. Homer's statements about the body, about the internal and external organs, have again and again been admired. The poet seems to know the human body intimately and he describes it in the most graphic way. Whether he learnt what he knows from the physician, or recorded the people's common knowledge,[8] the physicians of that time knew the human body well. But how did they obtain this knowledge? Really through dissections? It is said that certain observations could not have been made except in dissecting cadavers.[9] The injuries resulting from wounds received in battle are never large enough to allow one to see and become acquainted with these organs as exactly as the description given presupposes. It is difficult to argue about how great injuries from weapons can be; to many physicians at any rate all the knowledge of the Homeric physicians seemed explainable by their observation of wounds. It will never be possible to say with certitude that certain observations could not have been made on wounded men. Yet that would be the necessary presupposition for the claim that in Homer's time wounds were not the only occasions for observing the human body.

Yet even if it were possible to presuppose as much, there would

---

[7] On this, cf. M. Simon, *Sieben Bücher Anatomie des Galen*, Leipzig, 1906, II, p. XIII.

[8] For the extent of the general knowledge of the body, cf. p. 261 below.

[9] O. Körner, *Münch. med. Wschr.*, LXIX, 1922, p. 1484 f.

251

still be no proof that the Homeric physicians dissected. Other ways could be imagined by which they arrived at their knowledge. Whether, in truth, human sacrifices furnished the first possibility of investigating the human body, as animal sacrifices did of investigating the bodies of animals, I do not venture to decide. Perhaps the priest looked upon a human whom he sacrificed just as dispassionately as on the animal which was offered up. The insensitivity of the people of those times to the cruelty of human sacrifice, their naive ability to see what interested them even when the sight was dreadful to them, or seems dreadful to modern man, does not permit the simple rejection of such an assumption. Before one's enemy, before the person condemned by God to death, all human feelings cease. How far callousness can go when one human being no longer looks upon another as his equal is shown in the frightful story told by Plato. Leontios, the son of Aglaion, on his way to town, sees some corpses on the place of execution. He wants to go up to them, but at first he feels this to be impossible. Finally, however, his eagerness gains the upper hand, he covers his head, runs up to the hanged men and shouts: "And so, unholy ones, feast your eyes on the beautiful sight!" (*Republic*, 439e–440a). Yet nothing certain can be said on the question whether the human sacrifices, which did indeed occur in Greece until a late period, really furnished the first insight into the structure of the human body.[10] In order to make a decision one would have to know what is not known, namely, whether the bodies of human sacrifices were cut to pieces, as were the bodies of animal sacrifices, whether the differences in character of the human organs were of religious significance, as were, though only after Homeric times, the differences between animal organs.[11]

But it seems certain to me that the Homeric physicians did not dissect, even if what they knew could not be observed from injuries. The reason is that one cannot conceive that anyone would have interfered at that time with the human body with the intent to gain scientific knowledge. One could not make such studies because conscious investigation merely for the sake of knowledge was still far from the naive mind of man, and above all because respect for the dead and dread of

[10] This kind of explanation has been stressed in particular by Fuld, *Münch. med. Wschr.*, LXIX, 1922, p. 1730.

[11] Cf. F. Schwenn, *Die Menschenopfer bei den Griechen und Römern*, Religionsgeschichtliche Versuche und Vorarbeiten, XV, 3, Giessen, 1915; and L. Hopf, *Die Anfänge der Anatomie bei den alten Kulturvölkern*, Abhdlg. z. Gesch. d. Med., IX, Breslau, 1904, pp. 23, 36.

cadavers were then too great for men to dare to interfere with them. One might offer up a human sacrifice to the god if he demanded it, one might leave a dead enemy or a criminal unburied, but one could not force oneself as yet to the extent of cutting open the dead body. A long development was required before the religious and magical opposition was overcome, and before dissections were thus, at a certain moment, rendered feasible.[12]

The knowledge of the Homeric physicians, it is contended, requires that they dissected; this conclusion does not seem possible. Similarly, it was claimed that the Hippocratic physicians dissected, for their great knowledge could not be explained in any other way. Yet other experts contradicted this claim, saying that the none too great knowledge of the Hippocratic physicians was easily explained by chance observations made during treatment.[13] The Hippocratics themselves never mention dissection of human cadavers. In their attempts to define the body, they make use only of external observation and of conclusions by analogy between human and animal organs. In the writing, *On ancient medicine*, the internal organs are described as they can be seen or palpated externally. The function of the internal organs is then determined by analogy to visible things: "But one must become acquainted with it from outside by way of what can be seen" (*Hippocratis opera, Corpus Medicorum Graecorum*, I, 1, p. 53, 12–13). It is already implicit in this analogy to visible things that the internal organs are counted among the invisible things and therefore are not rendered visible by dissection. In the writing, *On art*, diseases are classified according to visibility or invisibility. Against the visible the art is well armed. "But the art should not be helpless even where the less visible is concerned" (*CMG* I, 1, pp. 15, 17). And after a short description of the internal organs, it is said: "At least, when a person sees only with his eyes, it is not possible to know anything about the matter under discussion; for this reason I designated it not apparent, and the art too does not deem it apparent" (p. 16, 11–13). Since the "matter under discussion" refers to the internal organs, the writer cannot have seen them, not even at dissections. Against the invisible the physician is helpless. The consolation that the art need not be despondent when the curing of invisible diseases is at stake does not hide the fact that it is so in general. Those who make

[12] This claim can be substantiated fully only later in dealing with the religious opposition and its gradual decline, (cf. p. 274 ff., below).
[13] Cf. p. 247, above.

253

such imperfect attempts to define the invisible internal organs from the outside cannot have performed dissections, which reveal what is most hidden. But if the parts of the body are not determined by this method, the only means left is to draw analogies from animal findings to the human body. Thus, in *On the sacred disease*, a human organ is compared to that of the goat (*Oeuvres complètes d'Hippocrate* par E. Littré, Paris, 1839–61, VI, p. 366). The same thing occurs in *Epidemics* VI 6 (V, p. 309 L.). Similarly, in *On the heart*, the following proof is given for a particular statement about the process of drinking: "If a person mixes water with blue or red coloring and then gives the water to a very thirsty animal to drink, preferably to a pig, for this animal has no sense of the clean and beautiful, and if he then cuts open the animal's throat while it is still drinking, he will find the throat stained by the drink" (IX, p. 80 L.). Thus animal and human organs are again unhesitatingly compared. However, although the other statements perhaps refer to chance observations, in this writing the statement is verified by an experiment consciously set up. How unusual this was is shown by the words which follow the description of this vivisection: "But such an operation is not to everyone's taste"; still at this period, then, not every physician can perform such operations on animals without feeling revulsion. From the fact that here animal dissections are demanded it follows also, I think, that in another passage in the same writing, which speaks of the dissection of a "dead body," an animal, not a human being, is meant. The passage runs: "And if someone who understands the old method of excision takes the heart out of a cadaver, and if he opens one of the valves and closes the other, neither water nor air can be forced into the heart, at least not on the left side. For here the locking is rightly tightest. For in the left ventricle the intellect of man has its seat and governs the rest of the soul" (IX, p. 88 L.). Just as, earlier, the assertion made with respect to human drinking was immediately verified in the drinking of an animal, here too an animal heart may be meant, even though afterward a conclusion is reached as to the location, in the heart, of human understanding. Here, therefore, as in all other instances, it is a question of animal anatomy and animal analogy.[14]

[14] H. Haeser, *Lehrbuch der Geschichte der Medizin*, third ed., I, Jena, 1875, p. 129 f., discusses all the passages cited and declares it to be entirely possible that the knowledge on which they are based was gathered without dissections from observation made during treatment. If any passage, then the passage *On the heart*, in his opinion, points to dissections; it does not prove them. Why I interpret the passage differently I have attempted to show (cf. also Littré's notes on the passage in his

In two places in a Hippocratic writing there is, it seems to me, a presentiment of human dissections, a first inkling of their possibility, but not more. At the beginning of the writing *On the reduction of the joints*, the author presents his theory about a certain reduction. He once argued with other physicians about the handling of a case, and only with difficulty could he persuade them that the matter really stood as he claimed: "If one stripped the flesh from the arm at the shoulder, laying bare the place where the muscle contracts and then the tendon at the armpit and from the collarbone to the chest, it would be seen that the head of the humerus protrudes forward, although it has not fallen out" (*Hippocratis opera*, ed. Kühlewein, II, Leipzig, 1902, p. 112, 4–9). In other words, it is here stated that one would have purposely to lay bare a human organ, a part of the human body in itself not visible, in order to comprehend the correctness of the opinion advanced. But these words are no more than a thought, a possibility; the factual knowledge can have been gained while treating patients. Just as reference was made to an animal dissection to verify the theory of drinking, here the author says that one would have to cut open the patient to verify the formulated theory. There is no wound at hand in which what has been claimed may be seen; no one can at the moment be found on whom one could see the muscles; thus, it would be necessary to cut open a human being. In the same way, it is only a question of playing with a possibility when one is told at another point that the dislocation in question cannot be cured, "unless one proposed to cut into a human being, thrust one's hand into the cavity, and push outward from inside. One could do this on a corpse, but not in a living man" (pp. 174, 19–175, 3). The sole method of treatment that could effect a cure could only be carried out on a corpse; it is thought that one could cut the corpse open. Such a thought is an anticipation of the future, but the Hippocratic physicians themselves did not dissect humans.[15] They gained their knowledge from chance observation and from animal dissection.

The correctness of this statement is also proved, I believe, by the fact that contemporaneously with the Hippocratic physicians, and for some time subsequently, the philosophers and scientists were still de-

---

edition). If my interpretation is not correct, it would still be necessary to keep in mind the date of the writing which can scarcely have been composed before the middle or the end of the fourth century. For the state of the study of human anatomy at that time, cf. p. 281, below.

[15] As will be shown (cf. p. 275 ff. below), they too were prevented from dissecting by prejudices of a religious and magical nature.

scribing the human body in accordance with analogies based on animal dissection. The pre-Socratic philosophers occupied themselves intensively with the human body and its structure. Alcmaeon of Croton's discoveries, according to a reliable tradition, were supported by dissection and vivisection of animals.[16] Perhaps the other pre-Socratics too investigated the human body in the same way, if they did not merely engage in speculation about it. No statements by the investigators themselves concerning their methods have survived, but there is no indication of anatomies on humans. And the decisive fact is that Aristotle, to whom the internal organs of man are the "most unknown thing" in existence, still defines their nature not by means of human dissection but solely through analogy to the findings in animals. The external parts are known: "Best known are man's external parts, but it is just the opposite as far as the internal parts are concerned. For least known of all things is the structure of men's bodies, so that it is necessary to consider the individual parts, comparing them to the parts of other animals which they by nature resemble" (*Historia animalium*, ch. 16, 494 b 22–24).[17] If the pre-Socratic philosophers, if Aristotle, only apprehends the human body by drawing analogies, the Hippocratic physicians will scarcely have performed dissections. At least one would expect a reference to these dissections in Aristotle; he would have to evaluate the results and come to grips with this method as with all others. But, after all, the assertion that the Hippocratic physicians practiced anatomy is merely an unprovable contention. And if the Hippocratic physicians did not dissect, the Homeric physicians will certainly not have done so. Even later, the knowledge that dissection was possible and justified never disappeared once dissections had been performed, even when they were no longer feasible; Galen and Rufus speak of dissections although they could no longer perform any. It is only the findings of human dissection that were not bound to be retained; later too results were forgotten.[18]

[16] Cf. M. Wellmann: "Alkmaion von Kroton," *Archeion*, XI, 1929, p. 159.

[17] This passage, in which Aristotle speaks about his method, proves that he cannot have been familiar with dissections on human cadavers, and it is in accordance with this that one must interpret all other statements the meaning of which is not unequivocal. Incidentally, in the *History of animals* a human dissection is mentioned as a possibility that could not be realized.

[18] Thus the shape of the uterus, for instance, correctly described in accordance with anatomical studies, was later incorrectly described on the basis of abstract speculation. It is a mistake of Fuld's (*loc. cit.*) to assume that knowledge once gained could not have been forgotten and therefore to believe, because of the incorrect

What tradition relates seems then to be confirmed. Before Alexandria there were no human dissections. Only in Alexandria, as all testimonies prove, does human anatomy begin. Yet one literary and one factual objection remain. Galen, at the beginning of Book II of his *Anatomy* (II 280 ff. K.), reviews the writers who preceded him. Since the oldest book he knows is the work of Diocles (282), he attempts to explain to himself why there are no older works, how it came that the Asclepiads wrote no books about anatomy or about dissections. In earliest times, he says, medicine was a craft that was handed down from father to son. It was therefore not necessary at that time to write about things which everyone knew from childhood through practical training. Only when the art was imparted to people outside the family did it become necessary to write textbooks of anatomy. And the first of these textbooks, the first at least that Galen knows, is the *Anatomy* of Diocles. One must conclude that Galen at any rate was of the opinion that the Hippocratics had already dissected humans.[19] But it seems certain to me that, in forming such an opinion, he was only trying to explain the facts that he found incomprehensible. There were no anatomical textbooks among the Hippocratic writings. Hippocrates had worked anatomical instruction into the therapeutic books, which is of course much more correct than writing anatomical textbooks (282), for how could Hippocrates have done anything wrong? Yet the absence of all anatomical books before the time of Diocles still remained strange. To Galen, who considered dissection the best way to teach about the human body, it seemed inconceivable that the Asclepiads, that Hippocrates, who was wisest in all things, did not perform dissections. Consequently, he explained the absence of books by saying that in those ancient times when conditions were so different, textbooks were not yet necessary; and he does not forget to praise the olden times and to inveigh against the times in which he himself lives. The story itself betrays the purpose of the invention.[20]

views of the Hippocratics, that dissections could not have been performed in Homeric times.

[19] For, it seems to me, in relating the later dissections to the Hippocratic ones in this manner, Galen equates them. At any rate, as far as I know, he does not expressly attribute the first human dissections to the Alexandrians.

[20] If this explanation of the Galenic story were not accepted, one would have evidence that already the Hippocratic physicians dissected. But the testimony would not refute the results of the preceding investigation and would on their account have to be rejected. The final refutation will again be provided by the discussion of the magic and religious beliefs (cf. p. 275 ff., below).

More weighty is the factual objection that arises. One asks oneself whether the Hippocratic physicians could perform their task without dissections and the knowledge gained therefrom. Although it can never be demonstrated beyond any doubt that a particular theory could only be arrived at through anatomy, the feeling persists that all the chance observations would not provide sufficient material for knowing as much as the Hippocratics knew, and as much as one has to know to treat patients correctly. But there are in fact other methods besides dissections by which physicians in antiquity became, in their opinion, sufficiently acquainted with the human body. The Empiricists and Galen, who, not ignorant of dissections, yet did not perform any—the Empiricists because they did not believe dissection necessary, Galen because dissecting was not a practical possibility for him—nevertheless were able to acquire the knowledge of the human body which they needed. Galen describes in detail how one could investigate the structure of the body if one could not dissect. He said that even so it was not impossible to see the human skeleton: "I have very often seen human bones owing to the dilapidation of graves or memorials. Once even a river reached a grave which a few months earlier had been made without any particular care, destroyed it effortlessly, its surging carrying off the body of the deceased and bearing it a stadium length downstream, the flesh already decomposed but the bones still completely joined. At a point where the bank formed an inlet and a sort of backwater, the corpse was washed ashore. And it looked as if a physician had purposely laid it out for the instruction of a youth. But once also I saw the skeleton of a robber lying in the mountains, a little off the road. The robber had been killed by a wayfarer who had travelled together with him and whom he had attacked. And no inhabitant of the region was willing to bury him; rather, full of hatred, they rejoiced that the birds devoured him, tearing the flesh from his bones and, as it were, letting him lie there after two days for the purpose of instructing anyone wanting to see a skeleton" (II 221–22 K.). Only if these possibilities are barred does he advise animal dissection: "But if even in this way you are unable to get a look at a human skeleton, dissect a monkey and examine every one of his bones closely, removing the flesh" (II 222 K.). Galen, then, has a very high opinion of the instruction to be gained from such chance observations. He feels that it can even be a substitute for animal dissection, which means for all dissection. But this opportunity to learn existed for the Hippocratic and Homeric physicians too. If one had any interest at all in the human skeleton, one could become acquainted with it in this way without dissecting. What is valid for a time when dissection was no longer possible must also be valid for a time when there was as yet no dissection.

It is true, such occasions are important only for viewing bones. The internal organs can scarcely be seen in this way, and Galen too expressly refers to such chance finds only for the study of osteology. But the internal organs could become familiar during treatment. Just as Galen considers chance skeletal finds a sufficient substitute for dissection—only for didactic reasons not quite sufficient, as will be shown (cf. pp. 298 f., below)—the Empiricists believed that the observation of wounds and the view of the internal organs possible during treatment could be a substitute for dissection, They differentiated between the intentional dissections of the Dogmatists, performed on the dead or the living, and the chance dissection made possible by the occurrence of a major injury (K. Deichgräber, *Die griechische Empirikerschule*, Berlin, 1930, fr. 67). They thought that what one could see in such chance observations sufficed to provide all the knowledge a physician must have (Dchgr. fr. 68).[21] Certainly, what is valid for a time which is familiar with human dissection must also be valid for a time in which dissection was not yet practiced. If even the Empiricists thought they could renounce dissection because what could be learnt in medical practice constituted sufficient knowledge of the internal organs, then the Homeric and Hippocratic physicians must have been equally able to manage without dissections.[22] It was possible, therefore, to know the human skeleton and equally possible to know the internal organs of man in other ways than through performing dissections. The feeling that medicine without dissection cannot possess sufficient knowledge of the body is unfounded. Even though the knowledge of the Homeric and Hippocratic physicians was great, it is unnecessary to assume that dissections already took place at that time.

If the surviving accounts then testify that dissection and vivisection occurred first in Alexandria, there is no reason to assume these accounts are false, that they are fortuitous, that others have been lost which would perhaps have proved that dissections took place in earlier

[21] The significance of this polemic of the Empiricists against the Dogmatists I shall consider in detail in another context (cf. p. 286, below).

[22] For the particular arguments of the Empiricists, see the discussion of the reasons advanced in favor of dissection and against it (cf. p. 286, below).

times. It is believable that before Alexandria medicine managed without dissections: there were other, adequate, means of instruction about the human body. In the Hippocratic writings and in the philosophical and scientific investigations of the fifth and fourth centuries there is no reference to human dissections; it must rather be assumed that such dissections only began in Alexandria. And as the tradition relates, human dissection and vivisection soon cease to be performed: vivisection indeed seems to have occurred only at the beginning of the Dogmatic school; by the beginning of the Empire, dissections are no longer feasible.

II

The accounts concerning dissection are confirmed by comparing them with one another and with the accounts of the methods used by the scientists. This confirmation, however, does not insure them against the objections arising from certain general considerations. Moreover, in the accounts themselves much remains unclear, much is uncertain. One must try, by examining the objective considerations opposing the tradition, to better understand the tradition itself and to corroborate its correctness.

The data of the tradition are contested for general historical reasons. Greek physicians, it is contended, did not dissect because anatomy is not at all the prerequisite of ancient, as it is of modern, medicine. Anatomy had no closer relationship to ancient medicine than had, for instance, botany or zoology, for there was no necessity to study the internal structure of the organism. Occasionally scientists and philosophers may have dissected human cadavers; the physicians did not do so systematically, and not as physicians. Only the surgeon needed a certain degree of topographical knowledge, though not even his had to be comprehensive. Further, it is not even sure that dissections were performed at all. One has to ask oneself whether this view is correct; it seems to be further corroborated by the fact that in the opinion of not a few physicians instruction during treatment and by means of occasional finds was adequate. Why then should physicians have dissected at all?

Certainly knowledge of the body in antiquity is to be found not only among physicians, but also among philosophers and natural scientists. Indeed the people's relation to the body was quite different from today, and they knew the body much better than it is usually known

260

today. One must, however, realize in what respect the physician's concern with the body differs from the concern of the philosophers and natural scientists and from the general knowledge of these things. Only then will one also be able to decide what this knowledge means for medicine, whether one can really say that dissection as a method of gaining anatomical knowledge is only loosely bound up with medicine. One will be able to decide whether medical dissection was not required—if it was at all possible to dissect —because the physician needed to have exact knowledge of the body. For it would naturally testify to the correctness of the accounts if an essential connection could be proved between knowledge of the body and practical medicine. Otherwise one would be obliged to assume that though physicians needed knowledge of the body and its internal organs, they never made use of the best means of acquiring that knowledge, and such an assumption is not very probable.[23]

In antiquity, knowledge of the body is never exclusively professional knowledge, as it is now. Everyone knows the structure of the body. Homer depicts injuries down to the smallest detail. The poet knows the body accurately, and his audience must know it too if they are to understand his words at all. Aristotle says at the beginning of the *History of animals*, when he first turns to the description of man: "First one must look at the parts of man. For just as everyone judges coins according to those with which he is most familiar, so it is in all things. But man is of all living things of necessity the most familiar to us" (491 a 19 ff.). At least the externally visible parts of man are perfectly well known to everyone from his daily experience (494 b 21). And Gregory of Nyssa can still say in his work on *The creation of man:* "Everyone learns from observing himself the exact structure of his body, through sight, through living, and feeling; in this one's own nature is one's teacher" (240 c Migne). Ancient man is always intimately acquainted with his own body; that one must have such a precise knowledge of oneself is self-evident to him.

Knowledge of the body is also always interesting to him; he needs no particular professional interest to be attracted by it. This remains true throughout antiquity and in this respect there is no difference be-

---

[23] In my representation of the objections to the tradition I have purposely followed Sigerist's statements almost word for word (cf. p. 248, above). I am anxious to examine every objection raised so that afterward the tradition itself can be examined without reference to arguments not directed against the testimony as such.

tween educated and uneducated people. All want to hear about the body. Homer could not have described the fighters' injuries in such detail if his listeners had found no pleasure in such portrayals, if they had not enjoyed hearing such stories just as much as the narration of every other event in real life, the making of a shield, the preparation of a meal, the convocation of an assembly. This is so in later times too, however much the detailed treatment of the motifs may change. Exact depiction of the physical events therefore never disappears from heroic poetry; in this sense all description of battle scenes resembles the Homeric. Correspondingly, to the historians, the portrayal of the deaths of the heroes is of importance. It is a completely naturalistic picture; every detail is described, however gruesome and dreadful.[24] The people who read the books demanded such portrayals, because what happens to the body fascinated them. It is in this sense too that one should understand historians' descriptions of unique formations in the structure of corpses. Thus Herodotus tells, after he has spoken about the battle of Plataea: "But this too was still to be seen later, when the flesh of the corpses decomposed. That is to say, the Plataeans gathered the bones in one place, and there a skull was found which consisted of a single bone, without any suture. It was seen too, however, that the cheek and the piece above the cheek had teeth all in one piece, all out of one bone, the teeth and the molars. Besides, the bones of a man five ells tall were found" (IX 83). Just as the people who gathered together the bones of the fallen took an interest in their form and were capable of noticing and of recording the unusual,[25] similarly the "marvelous" and the unusual in the human body is of importance to the historian, whose subject is the portrayal of the great and marvelous deeds of men. He records it—just as he tells of an astonishing custom, presuming that his readers want to know such things too—because strangeness of the human body concerns them as does the strangeness of human fate. And one continues to find detailed reports of how the Egyptians embalmed the

[24] K. Sauer, *Untersuchungen zur Darstellung des Todes in der Griechisch-römischen Geschichtsschreibung*, Diss. Frankfort, 1930, who has pointed out the importance of the portrayal of death in historical writers, has noted that the picture given by Greek and Roman authors differs: the latter tend to expand and exaggerate the description of details. In any case, it is necessary in evaluating these descriptions also to remember the difference just mentioned.

[25] A story of this kind shows that it is not out of the question that priests looked at the human body during human sacrifices. If the story were not recorded, would anyone believe that people examined a skull found on a battlefield to discover its structure?

dead, in Herodotus (II 86), as in Diodorus (I 91), that is, in the fifth as well as in the first century B.C. The simplest and clearest expression of interest in the body one finds in the many nature stories, animal stories, and "marvelous stories" which abound throughout antiquity ever since books were written. They tell of the bodily structure of men and of animals, which interest man as much as he himself, and of which even the historian speaks.[26] Pliny characterizes well the ancients' feelings in his *Natural history*, in which he says, at the beginning of his description of living creatures: "The foregoing is a description of the world, and of the lands, races, seas, important rivers, islands, and cities that it contains. The nature of the animals also contained in it is not less important than the study of almost any other department, albeit here too the human mind is not capable of exploring the whole field" (VII 1).

This ever-enduring general interest on the part of the people, and their general familiarity with the human and animal body, probably narrows for the first time in medicine into a special professional interest and knowledge. For the physician, at all events, cannot treat his patients without increased knowledge of the body, even though he may not always have to know the body as thoroughly, as completely, as anatomy teaches him to know it, especially the internal organs. The knowledge inseparable from the treatment of diseases, and certainly from surgical treatment, is after all more than man's simple experience of himself. The understanding of the physician concerns certain definite data regarding health and disease in which he must be interested in order to know the body and its reactions in these respects. What people in general possess is a knowledge of the whole without any reference to particulars. There cannot have been any books containing this primordial knowledge of physicians; the beginnings of medicine lie before the centuries in which written records were made. But not even from the period in which writing began, and in which people may therefore have written medical books too, have such works survived. The Hippocratic books, the oldest writings of physicians to be preserved, represent the medicine of the fifth and fourth centuries. The philoso-

[26] As an example, Herodotus' description of a hippopotamus may be quoted (II 71). Of course that such descriptions are to be found in the writings of an early historian is also to be explained by the fact that at that time specialization in the sciences had not yet taken place. But they occur also later on, as I have shown, and in my context the decisive point is not why such descriptions are included in history books and not in other books, but rather that they are included at all and appeal to the reader.

phers' and scientists' investigations, which after all constitute the second professional narrowing of the general interest in the body, do go back to an earlier period, and fragments at least of the work of the pre-Socratics have survived. From Anaximander to Democritus, all these philosophers are occupied with the structure of the human and of the animal body. From pre-Socratic philosophy the preoccupation with these questions carries over into Platonic and Aristotelian philosophy and into the Hellenistic philosophical systems. Ancient philosophy throughout concerned itself with the same problems which, according to the tradition, were also tackled out of medical interest by the physician.

In the thought of the pre-Socratics, philosophical motives and the striving for factual knowledge were still inseparably bound together and it would be difficult to determine which interest was decisive for each individual. But their motive is certainly not the medical one, which makes a man who wants to cure diseases study the body because he believes that he cannot otherwise be of any help. Yet, while the pre-Socratics desire knowledge for the sake of knowledge, as philosophers and scientists, in Platonic philosophy, in the physiology of the *Timaeus*, the philosophic view detaches itself from the scientific view. Even when Plato makes use of results to which the scientists' and physicians' investigations have led, the important thing for him is the interpretation and arrangement of the facts. Contemplating man, like contemplating the world, proves the purposefulness of God's creation. It is only to prove this principle and to make it understandable that he discusses the structure of the human body at all in his context. The same is true in Aristotelian philosophy. Even when Aristotle speaks of man in the writing *On the parts of animals*, what he offers is a philosophical penetration and elucidation of the known facts. Indeed, even the late Aristotelian *History of animals* attests the empiricism of a philosopher.[27] In Hellenistic philosophy too, in both the Stoic and Epicurean systems, the theory of the human body—which forms an intrinsic part of philosophy—is not a matter of scientific investigation but is philosophy based on the insights gained by science. Facts are cited in order to demonstrate the school's philosophy. In an examination of the various points of view which may be important for anatomy, Galen says: "The man of natural science, who loves science for its own sake, uses anatomical

[27] Cf. F. Solmsen: "Die Entstehung der Wissenschaften," *Das humanistische Gymnasium*, 1931, p. 73 ff.

observation in one way; and in a different way the man who does not love it for its own sake but in order to prove that nature does nothing without purpose" (here the philosophers are meant, as Galen himself says in the subsequent sentences [II 286 K.]). As a physician influenced by the Stoics and by Plato, he naturally speaks of the proof of the teleological working of nature. But starting from a different point of view, one may wish to prove something different; the result of the investigation is not fixed. The only certain thing is that the philosopher does not contemplate man's nature for its own sake, but in order to verify his principles in that area of human knowledge also. Finally, preoccupation with the problems of the body is transmitted from philosophy into the last form of metaphysics created in antiquity, Christian religion. As the heir of philosophy, the Church too has a teaching concerning the nature of man. Like philosophy, she takes over the findings of the scientists, of the laity, and recasts them in accordance with her own principles, just as did the Stoics and the Epicureans, the Aristotelians and the Platonists. Gregory of Nyssa says: "But one can also read the information concerning such problems which scholars have painstakingly worked out in books and can gain an exact knowledge of everything. Some learnt through anatomy where everything inside us is situated. Others observed also the purpose of every part of the body and explained it, believing the knowledge of human structure that could be acquired in this way to be sufficient. But if a man wishes in addition that in these matters too the Church should be his teacher so that he is never in need of counsel from outside—it is the law of the blessed flock, as the Lord says, not to listen to a foreign voice—I will give instruction in these matters also" (240 c d Migne). A Stoic or an Epicurean too would in such questions have consulted only a textbook of his school, as a Christian is supposed to, or he would have read only the work of one of the physicians or scientists of his school. Not until the new Christian attitude has completely displaced the old Greek pagan one, not until it has become medieval-European, is there any dogmatic repression of human investigation. The elucidation of facts is not more conditioned by Christian doctrine than by any other philosophical doctrine. What the Church does is not more than, nor different from, what every ancient philosophy did.[28] The theory of the human body is always a part of philosophy.

[28] Even the assertion that man is formed in God's image still is interpreted merely symbolically (Gregory, *Oratio* I 275 b ff. Migne). That in my opinion the

For the pre-Socratics, philosophy was identified with knowledge of nature, as it was with all knowledge. For Plato this was no longer the case. Then Aristotle, in his old age, made room for independent scientific investigation.[29] One has as yet no over-all view of the history of this pure science. It was pursued for hardly longer than a few generations. That the human body too was the object of scientific interest is certain.

If human dissection was possible, then philosophers and scientists will have performed such dissections. But does this mean that every dissection was the result of scientific or philosophic interest? Must one not concede that the philosophers only dissected in order to prove or confirm their theories, and perhaps in order to check the facts found by others? Could not the scientists themselves, who were perhaps the first to perform dissections, work up within a short period all the material that has survived in the medical works? Can the physicians have been without any share in this research? If one attributes human dissections, provided they did actually take place, solely to philosophical and scientific interests, it seems to me that one is explaining them on too narrow a basis.

Tradition has it that the physicians dissected as physicians. A greater knowledge of the human body was of necessity important to them. The Hippocratic writings, however, the oldest surviving works of physicians, by no means generally consider knowledge of the body to be the prerequisite for treating internal diseases. In general, they explain disease by the humors in the body and by the way these are combined. Such a theory màkes it unnecessary to take the internal organs or their form and character into account. For a man's nature is not identical with his bodily organism, but with his humoral mixture, in fact, with the individual reaction of his individual humoral mixture to what he consumes. Thus, one is told in the writing *On ancient medicine:* "But it seems to me that if the physician is anxious to do what is needed, he must of necessity know this much about nature and earnestly strive

---

relationship of Church and philosophy must be understood in this way explains why I do not agree with R. von Töply's claim (*Studien zur Geschichte der Anatomie im Mittelalter*, Leipzig, 1898, p. 35): "These words cited from Gregory sufficiently characterize the spirit of the Church and its intentions. The community of the faithful is to be completely seqarated from the rest of the world. . . . The Church provides the faithful with all knowledge, even anatomy and physiology."

[29] This has been shown by Werner Jaeger (*Aristoteles*, Berlin, 1923, pp. 351, 358 ff.).

to acquire knowledge of it, namely, how a person relates to what he eats and drinks and to whatever else he does, and what are in every case the consequences for him" (*CMG* I, 1, p. 51, 18–23). The physician cures his patient by bringing about, or restoring, the right admixture of humors, not by making a sick organ healthy again. Consequently, he does not have to be acquainted with the body and its internal organs: according to this view, the anatomical structure of the body is for the physician a matter of indifference. Yet even on the basis of this theory, knowledge of the body again becomes necessary in a certain sense. For the humors move within the body. The structure of the single parts of the body determines whether the humors stand still in one or another place in the body, or are driven to one or another place. Thus even the writing *On ancient medicine* acknowledges an objective element in what influences every disease; it recognizes that the individuality of the organs is a factor in determining humoral mixture and the movement of the humors in the body (53, 1 f.). The physician must also know which ailments are determined by the properties of the humors and which by the structure of the bodily organs. What is meant by properties of the humors is, of course, the way they are combined and the strength of the composition: "By forms, however, I mean what is inside a man. One thing is hollow and from being broad it becomes narrow; another thing is spread out, another firm and round, then flat and hung high up, then again stretched out, long, thick, porous, and strong, then again spongy and light" (53, 3–8). For the different forms of the organs cause the humors to be drawn in this direction or that, and to run off from one place to another (53, 8–12). In another writing, *Places in man*, it is actually said: "The nature of the body must constitute the beginning of medical instruction" (ch. 2, VI, 278 L.). In accordance with this demand it is then shown how the nature of the individual organs determines certain reactions of the flowing humors. Organs of the body may become of particular importance in another way, when the humors are no longer thought of merely as the content of the body, no longer as dependent merely on the space in which they are contained, but are related to a definite organ which is seen as their source. Thus in *On the sacred disease*, the writing which locates the phlegm in the brain and makes it flow thence into the body, there is a detailed description of the brain (ch. 3, VI, 366 L.). And the fact that a writing, *On the heart*, is devoted to a full description of the heart must also be attributed to the importance of that organ for the combination of the humors which de-

267

termines the disease.[30] Thus, already in Hippocratic medicine, there are the beginnings of a union of the physician's art and knowledge of the body for the explanation of internal diseases. Even though knowledge of the body is not yet generally obligatory, even though it is demanded only in some of the Hippocratic writings, which are a collection of the most diverse, contradictory systems, at all events the demand is made that acquaintance with the body is essential if one is to understand the etiology of diseases.

The work of the physicians of the end of the fourth century has been lost. Nor have the works of the Hellenistic physicians survived. But it is possible to determine from secondary sources whether or not knowledge of the body was of importance for the Alexandrian schools. And Celsus states that the Dogmatic schools, which considered knowledge of hidden causes to be necessary for any treatment, teach that knowledge of the internal organs of the body is the prerequisite for correct treatment of internal diseases. The statement runs: "Since pain and the various kinds of diseases arise in the interior parts no one in their opinion can provide remedies for them unless he knows the internal organs" (Prooemium, 23). And further on he says: "For when pain occurs internally, neither is it possible for one to learn what hurts the patient, unless he has acquainted himself with the position of each organ or intestine; nor can a diseased portion of the body be treated by one who does not know what that portion is" (*Ibid.*, 25; transl. Spencer, Loeb Classical Lib., I, 15). And again: "External remedies too can be applied more aptly by one acquainted with the position, shape and size of the internal organs, and like reasonings hold good in all the instances mentioned above" (*Ibid.*, 26; *loc. cit.*).[31] For the Dogmatic schools, knowledge of the internal organs is therefore absolutely essential to the curing of internal diseases. No one can apply remedies for diseases located in the internal organs without knowing those organs. The connection between the physician's art and the study of the organs is here, therefore, no longer limited to surgical intervention. Also what is here

[30] I refrain from discussing the fragment (VIII, 538–40 L.) entitled, *De anatomia*, preserved in the *Corpus Hippocraticum*, the date and subject matter of which I am unable to determine.

[31] These arguments are brought forward in a discussion of vivisection. Since vivisection, too, is one means of investigating the body, arguments adduced to prove its necessity can also be taken as arguments in general in favor of investigating the body. Vivisection itself will be discussed later in a different context (cf. p. 283, below).

demanded is not just the occasional investigation of certain organs; rather, the connection is a generally valid one, and knowledge of all internal organs is intended. Knowledge of the body, formerly closely connected with etiology, now becomes the prerequisite for therapy.

The Empiricists rejected the methods and doctrines of the Dogmatists completely. But they too believed that the physician must know the human body in order to treat it. For the repudiation of vivisection and dissection as methods was not in any way based on the claim that knowledge of the body was unnecessary for the physician, but only on the contention that these methods did not accomplish the desired end and that they were in addition cruel and frightful. After discussing the Empiricist objections to the etiological theories of the Dogmatists, Celsus says: "Now the matters just referred to they deem to be superfluous; but what remains, cruel as well, to cut into the belly and chest of men whilst still alive" (*Ibid.*, 40; *loc. cit.*, p. 23). Vivisection is therefore not only superfluous but also cruel, for the subject dies, and so the physician still sees only the organs of a dead man (*Ibid.*, 40–42). All he succeeds in doing, therefore, is cruelly slaughtering a human being, and not in becoming acquainted with the internal organs of the living, which was his object (*Ibid.*, 43). And then one reads: "If, however, there be anything to be observed whilst a man is still breathing, chance often presents it to the view of those treating him. For sometimes a gladiator in the arena, or a soldier in battle, or a traveller who has been set upon by robbers, is so wounded that some or other interior part is exposed in one man or another. Thus, they say, an observant practitioner learns to recognize site, position, arrangement, shape and such like, not when slaughtering, but whilst striving for health; and he learns in the course of a work of mercy, what others would come to know by means of dire cruelty" (*Ibid.*, 43; *loc. cit.*, p. 25). The physician can, therefore, become acquainted with the internal organs through such chance observations also; he does not need the methods of the Dogmatists. Yet one must not, because of the contrast in methods, overlook the fact that in principle both Empiricists and Dogmatists consider knowledge of the body essential for the physician. For otherwise the refutation of the Dogmatic arguments could not be accomplished by showing that the Dogmatic method did not achieve its purpose and that everything that could be learnt in this fashion could, after all, be adequately and more easily learnt in a different way. The Empiricist too is anxious to grasp the position of the organs and their nature, but he learns about them in the course of treating patients, and indeed for him internal and external organs are of equal importance.[32] It is in this comprehensive sense therefore that one must understand Galen's account, in which he says: "This knowledge is so essential to physicians that not even the Empiricists, who wrote whole books against anatomy, dared to despise it. On the contrary, they joined in characterizing it as the most useful of knowledge, but they thought the nature of the organs could be learnt adequately from wounds as they occur on particular occasions" (Galen, II 288 K.; Dchgr. fr. 68 131, 9–14). They cannot have found the importance of this knowledge of the body in etiological evaluation; rather, they must, like Dogmatists, have judged it impossible to treat and cure without knowledge of the internal organs. For the Empiricists, in contrast to the Dogmatists, rejected all etiologies. One can therefore say with certainty what they meant by knowledge of the body, in spite of the absence of express documentation.

All Alexandrian schools, the Dogmatist schools as well as the Empiricists, taught that knowledge of the body is essential for the physician. This was merely initiated in Hippocratic medicine and became fully developed in Hellenistic times. But the Alexandrian schools went beyond Hippocratic medicine, for in Alexandria knowledge of the body became an essential prerequisite for practice. This alliance between medicine and anatomy then persisted in Greek medicine as long as the Hellenistic influence lasted. Only the motivation of it was not always the same: the therapeutic motive allied itself later on with a didactic one.

As Celsus already declares: to dissect dead bodies is necessary for those who are engaged in learning medicine (Prooemium, 74). In the first century A.D., Rufus of Ephesus wrote a textbook on the nomenclature of the parts of the human body. He starts by asking the reader, a student, what he learnt first in zither playing, in writing, or in all the other arts, and he answers that one always begins with the terminology (Drbg., 133,1–134,3). The inference is: "Will you not now begin medicine too by learning the names, first what to call each part of the body, then everything else that accompanies the instruction? Or do you find it sufficient when the person who shows it to you instructs you like a mute about what you want to know? To me, at least, this does not seem

---

[32] For a more detailed discussion of the bearing of these arguments on the history of anatomy as such, cf. p. 286 ff., below.

preferable" (134, 3–7). What Rufus says is a far-reaching transformation of that statement in the Hippocratic writing, *Places in man*, that the nature of the body must constitute the starting point of medical thought. For Rufus, however, knowledge of the body, at least in this context, has become something quite formal. The problem for him is the training of the young physician, not the treatment of disease, and it appears ill-bred, uneducated, not to be completely at home with the instrument on which one is supposed to play. This differs from the criteria of the Alexandrian schools, although it by no means excludes the possibility that Rufus too looked upon knowledge of the body as an unconditionally essential prerequisite for treating internal diseases.

Galen's doctrine unites the Hippocratic, the Hellenistic, and contemporary theories; it joins philosophy and science. It is his doctrine which together with that of Hippocrates becomes the dogma of subsequent times. Galen considered knowledge of the human body to be of great value; anatomy was important to him because it investigated external and internal organs: "Anatomy is of value for the recognition of every kind of function, whether of the body or of the soul, for through anatomy one acquires precepts. And it has another value besides for him who is desirous of extracting splinters or missile points in right manner, or who wishes to open something correctly, be it tumors or fistulas or abscesses that he wishes to operate on. This, as I said, is the most essential knowledge, and he who would be a good physician must be particularly well versed in it. After that he must be versed in the functions of the internal organs and, moreover, he must know why they are essential" (II 286 K.). In this connection it is immaterial that it is through dissection that knowledge of the organs is obtained; the important point is that, like the Hellenistic schools, Galen, for therapeutic and etiological reasons, cannot conceive of the physician devoid of knowledge of the body.[33] Later schools, later physicians, repeat what has already been said, scarcely adding to it; their work consists merely of reading and compiling. From Galen and the other authors whose writings they digest thoroughly, they take over the requirement of knowledge of the body, together with the justification of this requirement.

Physicians surely needed a greater knowledge of the body than is generally possessed by laymen. To them it is, above all, the data that

---

[33] For Galen's attitude toward anatomy and consequently the value he ascribed to knowledge of the bodily structure, cf. M. Simon, *op. cit.*, p. XIII ff.

are important, not their interpretation. In Alexandria, knowledge of the body is in fact essential, because it is believed that one cannot treat patients without it. Why then, if it was possible to do so, should the Alexandrian physicians not have practiced anatomy, systematically, as physicians? Otherwise they would have neglected to use the best means to learn about the body. It seems therefore altogether credible that they performed dissections for medical reasons, as the tradition has it. And they and later physicians then labored long to perfect the knowledge of the body. The tradition that from Alexandria on physicians dissected as physicians must be true.

Of course, there was interest in such investigations among others; not only physicians, but philosophers too were concerned with them. And the fact that these latter devoted themselves to such study could not be without influence on the anatomical knowledge gained. In antiquity, philosophy was in general not so rigorously separated from science as it is today. Rather, the two were always interrelated; the method of the one was not without significance for the other; one was conscious of this association and it was consciously pursued. As for every other science, this in itself was important for the science concerned with man, and its history too can therefore only be understood in connection with the history of philosophy. It is even more significant that philosophy made the investigation of the human body its own concern and thereby mingled pure research with the demonstration of speculative principles. This being so, a high degree of vigilance, a great sense of responsibility were necessary if objective judgment was not to be thwarted. But the greatest danger lay in the fact that the preoccupation of philosophers and physicians with the same problem led to a division of the anatomical investigations made. The body was not studied as a unit; some things interested only the philosophers, some only the physicians. In differentiating between medical and philosophical dissections, Galen says that for physicians anatomy served as a means of orientation: ". . . in the function of the internal organs and, finally, in their necessity, as far as these things are of importance to the physician in diagnosing diseases. For much is useful not to physicians but to philosophers, and in two ways, as has been said—either for the sake of knowledge itself, or in order to make manifest the art of nature, which is contained in every one of her parts" (II 286 K.). It follows that the philosopher does not need to know what interests only the physician, just as the physician does not have to know what is the concern only of the philosopher. This implies a division which is bound to be dangerous, for any investigation of an object is of necessity indivisible. When the unity of the object is destroyed by the investigative methods, many an important fact will remain unobserved because from the beginning it is excluded and disregarded, as irrelevant, as belonging to a different field.

Even if not all investigation of the human body is important for the physician, although he shares the discussion of such questions with the philosopher, there are nevertheless certain problems important for him as physician. On the other hand, philosophy's interest in investigating the human body made it impossible for the physician, as physician, to confront the totality of the problems. When he wished to investigate man's genesis, the original composition of the material of the body, the final purpose of the organs, he did so as a philosopher, not a physician. But only such exploration of the body was the domain of the philosopher, whether he engaged in it for purely scientific or for speculative reasons, to adopt Galen's terminology. Though in antiquity the physician in his interest in the structure of the body competed with the interest of people in general, though because of the fact of philosophical investigation and scientific knowledge he was not the only one to study the human body, this did not exclude a merely medical interest in anatomy.

III

In the face of the reports on dissection which have been adduced and have seemed more and more acceptable, it has been claimed again and again that dissection could never have taken place in Greece. Even though there were testimonies to that effect, they were not believed to be true; they were held to be either inventions or calumnies, because for the ancients reverence for the dead was a duty of the most binding sort. It was everyone's duty to see to it that a corpse was buried, and there existed no greater obligation toward relatives.[34] How then can it be possible that the ancients ravaged dead bodies in order to find out the structure of human organs? Fundamentally, such an attitude toward the dead was derived from old, magic views of the world. Man's body

[34] The testimony on men's feelings toward the dead and their duties to the corpse is most easily available in L. Schmidt, *Die Ethik der alten Griechen*, Berlin, 1882, II, p. 97 ff.

is inseparable from him; even after death he still feels what is happening to his body, just as he knows everything that is still said about him.[35] Indeed, the soul finds no peace in the underworld, it fails to gain entrance there, until the body is safely interred. If, therefore, one wants the dead man to find rest, one must see to it that his body finds repose. This repose must never be disturbed: every care is to be taken to protect the sanctity of the grave. The common people clung steadfastly to these old animistic concepts; the simple Greeks never forsook these ideas of death and the realm of the dead.[36] Truly, it must seem impossible that among such people dissections could have been performed.

But it would seem to me already a mistake to check the credibility of the reports on dissection by referring to the ideas held by the masses. Dissections are performed by scientists, by scholars. If, therefore, one wishes to judge whether or not the Greeks could practice anatomy, one has to ask what scholars thought about death, about life after death, and about the duties of the living toward the corpse. Whether it was possible or impossible to dissect depends on their attitude to these questions. They could dissect if they had overcome the magic view, the awe of the corpse, the concept that it was unclean. The opposition of the populace, the misgivings of the crowd, might perhaps make it difficult for scholars to obtain cadavers for dissection, but these difficulties could have been surmounted.[37]

Now, at any rate, the physicians who performed dissections seem not to have been conscious of those magical or animistic prejudices which in the opinion of modern scholars would from the very beginning have made dissections impossible. Celsus speaks at length about the reasons for and against performing dissections. When he talks about the dissections performed by the Dogmatists, he talks about the procedure as if it were a matter of course, as if there could be no opposition to it on human grounds; he says not a word about the emotions which it arouses. Celsus, on these questions, only reports the Empiricists' objections to the Dogmatists' doctrine of the necessity for dissecting. As he says, dissection, "even if not cruel," as is vivisection, is "none the less

[35] Hippias expresses this thought in a very naive way in the Platonic *Hippias Major* 282 a.

[36] On the Greek ideas of death, cf. E. Rohde, *Psyche*, Tübingen, 1921 (seventh–eighth edition) II, p. 336 ff.

[37] This is proved by the development which, at the end of the Middle Ages and at the beginning of the Renaissance, had strength enough to break down the opposition and prejudices of the people and led to the dissection of cadavers.

274

nasty" (Prooemium, 44). It is then a feeling of disgust that the destruction of corpses provokes; at any rate he mentions nothing else.

That dissections actually take place, Celsus does not doubt: like the Dogmatists, he demands them. He at any rate must believe that his account of the Dogmatists is correct and to be taken seriously; he cannot consider what he reports to be malicious slander. How much in general one took dissections for granted is to be seen also in the fact that in a philosophical writing Cicero can say: "We do not know our bodies; we are ignorant of the position of the parts and what power they have. Therefore physicians themselves in whose interest it is to know these things have recourse to dissection" (*Academica* II, 122, p. 133, 12 ed. Plasberg). For Cicero too, then, dissections performed by physicians are a matter of course.

In short, the dissections, the occurrence of which appears quite certain, were felt to be merely disgusting. They seem to have been resisted only by human emotions. One must try to understand how these emotions could be overcome, once the feasibility of dissections has been established. One must first ask how it was possible to overcome—to such an extent that they were no longer of any significance in scientific discussion—the earlier magic and religious concepts which assuredly held sway among the people at all times. One must ask whether or not scientists were really free of these concepts, and when they became free of them. Then it will be proved against all objections that it was possible for the ancients to perform dissections. The answer to these questions can only be found by inquiring into the philosophers' ideas of death and of man's duties toward the dead. For the scholar's *Weltanschauung* is determined by them.

Now, philosophy slowly eroded and finally completely abandoned the concepts in which the people continued to be enmeshed. At the beginning, it is true, no opposition is as yet manifest between popular and philosophical views; but in the philosophy of the fourth century a change begins which gradually leads to a complete transformation of the idea of death. Plato is the first to give clear expression to the new concept. In the *Phaedo*, Crito asks Socrates what his friends should do about his burial. With a quiet smile, Socrates replies: "As you wish, if only you really get possession of me and I don't escape you" (115 c). And then, turning to his friends, he says: "Men, I cannot persuade this Crito that I am the Socrates who now speaks to you and lays out what has been said in detail before you; on the contrary, he believes me to be the man whom he will soon see dead and for this reason he asks me how he should bury me." Crito did not believe what Socrates had said about the immortality of the soul in the preceding conversation. But the others at least should believe him: "Now you must serve as my guarantors to Crito, but the guarantee should be quite different from the one he gave the judges. For he guaranteed that I would remain here, while you must guarantee that I shall most certainly not remain here when I am dead, but shall depart and be gone. I ask this so that Crito may find it easier to bear, and when he sees my body being burned or buried he may not be distressed on my account, as though something terrible were happening to me, and so that he may not say at the burial that he is laying Socrates out, or carrying Socrates out, or burying him." And he comforts Crito: "You must be brave and say that you are burying my body; and bury it as you see fit and in whatever manner seems most appropriate to you." Socrates believes in the immortality of the soul; he believes that man is not body, but soul. Hence, the fate of the body is not germane to man's true being. In this dialogue, in which orphic concepts and Pythagorean doctrines unite with Socratic and Platonic thoughts, the separation of the soul from the body appears as the real goal of the philosopher, for the philosopher seeks to become what man really is. The body only fetters the soul; the liberation of the soul from the body, which death brings, is a deliverance. Therefore it is unnecessary to trouble oneself about the corpse: nothing that happens to the dead body need cause friends pain. Whoever asks how the body should be buried believes that the man he loved and the dead body he sees before him are one and the same, that the dead man can still feel what is happening to him. If Socrates nevertheless gives his friend permission to bury his body as he wishes and as best conforms with custom although it is not Socrates, he does so out of respect for the law, out of reverence for ancient custom, out of humanity, but not because he believes in it.

To this thought Plato held fast, still teaching the same doctrine in the *Laws*, the work of his old age. Man is not identical with the body; revering the body is therefore unnecessary, indeed in a certain sense pernicious, as Socrates already told Crito after trying once more to instruct him: "For you should know, dear Crito, that ugly words not only falsify the matter itself but also contaminate souls with evil" (*Phaedo*, 115 e). He states the laws for burial of the dead (*Laws*, XII, 958 d–959 a) and then continues: "But in all other matters one should trust the lawgiver, even when he says that the soul is entirely different from the body and that, in life, what constitutes each of us is none other than the soul, while the body which we appear to be merely follows the soul's lead. And, further, when he declares that it is well said of the dead that their bodies are their images but that the true personality of each of us is immortal, that it is called 'soul,' and that it departs to other gods to give its account . . . and no great help can be given a man once he is dead. All his relatives should have helped him while he was alive" (959 a–b). One should therefore not mourn immoderately, and one should not squander one's means on the burial of the corpse. One should spend the right amount, as a gift "on the soulless altar of the gods of the underworld" (959 d). Through death, the departed has only freed himself of the body and has gone to other gods. No one should believe that the soulless body he sees is the friend or brother, the father or wife for whom he mourns. If the ancient reverent regulations are preserved, prescribing that the corpse must be tended and interred with certain honors, the reason is again strictly one of piety, humanity, and perhaps also the wish to meet the beliefs of the people halfway. But such thoughts and such behavior do not represent the truth. Rather, the human being to whom we were attached and the corpse we see before us have nothing in common.

This Socratic and Platonic doctrine is binding on all later philosophers, however they may differ in interpreting the details. Diogenes the Cynic does not wish his friends to spend more money than necessary on him after his death. So he forbids them to bury him (Diogenes Laertius, 79, 52), differing in this from Socrates: "Diogenes was rougher; his feeling it is true was the same, but like a Cynic he spoke more harshly and required that he should be flung out unburied. Upon which his friends said: 'To the birds and wild beasts?' 'Certainly not,' said he, 'but you must put a stick near me to drive them away with.' 'How can you, for you will be without consciousness?' they replied. 'What harm, then, can the mangling of wild beasts do me if I am without consciousness?' " (Cicero, *Tusculan disputations* I, 43, 104; transl. King, Loeb Classical Lib., pp. 123–25).[38] Diogenes can behave in this way only because for him the dead body is no longer a person, because the corpse is for him

---

[38] Cicero, in this context, speaks in general of the absence of feeling in the dead; he too begins his accounts of the views of the philosophers with Plato's *Phaedo*. To be sure, what he then tells about Anaxagoras permits the conclusion that he too considered the place of burial unimportant, though not burial itself, as did Diogenes,

devoid of all feeling. He immediately exaggerates the attitude taken by Socrates; the Cynic sage is no longer filled with reverence for the old opinions, as was Socrates. He makes no concessions to custom; the opinions of the crowd are false and must be contradicted.

For Aristotle too it is self-evident that the real essence of man is the soul, although he does not see it as opposed to the body in the manner of Plato. For the fact that the soul can only truly exist when tied to matter, that there is no personal immortality, no separation of the soul from the body after which it departs to other gods to exculpate itself, these things change not one whit the essential superiority of the soul over the body. In spite of them it is the soul that is the divine, the essential; it is not the body that is the human being. It is for this reason that he says: "At any rate, when its Soul is gone, it is no longer a living creature, and none of its parts remains the same, except only in shape, just like the animals in the story that were turned into stone" (*De partibus animalium* I, 1, 641 a 19–21; transl. Peck, Loeb Classical Lib., p. 69). Even before, in a polemic directed against Democritus, one reads: "Now a corpse has the same shape and fashion as a living body; and yet it is not a man" (640 b 35–36; *ibid.*, p. 67). For Aristotle, therefore, a man's corpse is no longer the man himself.

The Hellenistic philosophers too are of the same opinion; they too no longer acknowledge the original, religious and magical concepts of the people. The Cynic Diogenes had merely forbidden his friends to bury him so that they might do nothing unnecessary; but Epicurus says: "Nor will the wise man think of his burial" (Usener, fr. 578).[39] What happens to the human body after death is of no concern. With death the soul is destroyed, the human being is completely annihilated. There is no immortality, no life after death, no punishment, no judgment. It would therefore be meaningless to bother about what happens to the corpse. Death has nothing to do with man.

Likewise the Stoic was necessarily indifferent to the fate of dead bodies. For him death was nothing more than the freeing of divine reason from ungodly matter. How then could he attach any significance to

---

for instance. It is impossible with regard to these problems to go beyond the Platonic testimony. Democritus' views may have been similar to those of Plato, to judge by the opinions of Epicurus (cf. below), but too little is known of his dogma to be certain of his opinion (cf. 55 B 1 Diels).

[39] This doctrine, according to various testimonies, survived in the Epicurean school (cf. Rohde, *op. cit.*, p. 332, 6).

what happened to the body after death? He can have no fear of a man's dead body; he can no longer see the man himself in it. It is true, he is more inclined to give in to the views of the people; he does not disregard their opinion, as did the Cynics; his attitude corresponds more to that of Socrates. But this does not alter the fact that for him the human being can no longer be identical with the body, which after death remains behind without a soul. Some Stoics adopted the Cynic interpretation completely. Thus Chrysippus, in his book about *Duties*, writes among other things about the duty to bury one's parents and says: "When one's parents die, one should bury them as simply as possible, for the body, like hair and nails, is nothing that concerns us, and we are not in need of such care and attention. For this reason they should use the flesh for food, if it is still usable, just as one should use one's own limbs, for instance an amputated foot or the like. But if the flesh is unusable, they should bury it and erect a gravestone, or they should burn it and scatter the ashes or throw them far away, and not go to any trouble, just as with nails and hair" (Arnim III, fr. 752). This statement shows the extremes to which a Stoic could go.

Hellenistic philosophers then follow the Platonic line of thought and unanimously relinquish the popular ideas about death and the popular reverence for, and awe of, the corpse. Any idea that a magic power might yet inhabit the corpse is lacking. The body of the living man is not the man himself; no more is the body of the dead man the dead man himself. With this all the religious and magical inhibitions which might keep people from touching the corpse fall away. The person is after all completely destroyed, totally without feeling; what happens to the corpse is of no consequence. If Celsus mentions no magic or religious objections at all that were raised in the Hellenistic discussion of dissection, this is in agreement with the general philosophical point of view. Men of science, standing in the tradition of Hellenistic philosophy, could not dread touching a corpse for any magic or religious reasons. If scientific considerations seemed to dictate the practice of anatomy, it was, as Celsus tells us, at most a natural feeling of disgust that kept them from dissecting cadavers; it was not dread of the unclean. Hellenistic physicians, then, could indeed dissect.

The decisive point is, however, that the Hellenistic physicians were the first who could do so. For only with Platonic philosophy does the transformation of the old ideas set in, removing the inhibitions and objections that at first necessarily made it impossible even to think of touching corpses or of cutting them up. Philosophical doctrine does not immediately shape men's feelings the moment it is proclaimed. It takes time for it to become of practical consequence, for it to be translated into actions. The new views of death, therefore, could hardly influence scientific methods before the end of the fourth century. All reports of dissections by physicians say that Herophilus and Erasistratus were the first to dissect. This traditional account is credible because it fits in with what one would expect from the general intellectual development. It was not yet possible for the Homeric and Hippocratic physicians to dissect; it is not by chance that there are no accounts of dissections from earlier times.[40] It was only when knowledge of the internal organs of the body had for the first time come to be really important for the physician, that it was possible to perform dissections, because the old ideas had changed completely. It was only then that one could gain a comprehensive knowledge of the human body.

Only the natural feeling of aversion, of disgust, at dissecting remained. But as long as men have still been capable of humane sensitivity, it has never been possible to dissect without a feeling of inner revulsion. No one, aware that the body into which he is cutting is the body of a human being, can do so without emotional resistance, even though his reason may refute all arguments and show him that his feelings are unreasonable. The Hellenistic physicians experienced this just as much as other people, but what they felt furnishes no evidence of what they did. In spite of all resistance, in spite of the feeling—which the Dogmatists must have had as much as the Empiricists—that dissecting was dreadful, horrible, revolting, they nevertheless learned to do it in the pursuit of knowledge, for the feeling of disgust had to be suppressed if they believed that thereby they were serving mankind. In words that cannot fail to arouse admiration, Aristotle had tried to convince the young of the nobility and value of an investigation which must concern itself with what is revolting and frightful. He says: ". . . for though there are animals which have no attractiveness for the senses, yet for the eye of science, for the student who is naturally of a philosophic spirit and can discern the causes of things, Nature which fashioned them provides joys which cannot be measured" (645 a 8–11; *ibid.*, p. 99). And then he goes on: ". . . in all natural things there is somewhat of the marvelous"

[40] It is at least, generally speaking, true that they were not able to dissect. The possibility that individuals did so can never be excluded, especially when one thinks of Anaxagoras and Democritus.

(645 a 17–18; *ibid.*, pp. 99–101). Just as Heraclitus invited his friends to enter with the words, "Here too there are gods," so one must approach the examination of each living being without distaste, for in all of them nature reveals herself. Nor is it only the examination of animals that confronts man with the dreadful and revolting: "If, however, there is anyone who holds that the study of the animals is an unworthy pursuit, he ought to go further and hold the same opinion about the study of himself, for it is not possible without considerable disgust to look upon the blood, flesh, bones, bloodvessels, and suchlike parts of which the human body is constructed" (645 a 26–30; *ibid.*, p. 101).[41] In this way the Aristotelian ethos of research in natural sciences already tried to counter man's resistance to what frightens and disgusts him and to subordinate it to the search for truth. It is this ethos which the Alexandrian physicians adopted.

In Alexandria, then, the possibility of dissecting human cadavers existed; in that respect the tradition is correct. Is tradition also right in giving the impression that the possibility did indeed exist in Alexandria, but no longer existed in the Roman Empire? To be sure, Celsus, who, in spite of many changes in doctrine dictated by the Roman way of life, followed by and large the Alexandrian medical tradition, still demanded dissections and gives the impression that they are feasible. But already Rufus and Galen declared any human dissection to be impossible in the European parts of the Roman Empire (cf. p. 250, above); only in Alexandria, nowhere else, could one still learn from the skeleton, as Galen says. The question arises, therefore, why dissection was no longer possible in the rest of the Roman Empire.

The explanation, it seems to me, lies above all in the abrogation of Greek ideas, in their transformation by Roman concepts. Greek philosophy had trained the scholar to feel no dread in the presence of a corpse, not to identify the corpse with the human being. And what is at stake is only the attitude of the scholar, for whom anatomy is necessary for his scientific training. That the point of view of the educated never became the point of view of the people was without significance for science. As long as it was pursued in the Greek states, it was proof against the popular convictions. And the scientists who wanted to dissect were also able to do so. But the situation changed when Greece and the world be-

---

[41] The significance of these statements within the context of Aristotelian philosophy is brought out fully by Jaeger's interpretation (*Aristoteles*, Berlin, 1923, p. 362 ff.).

came Roman. Neither Greek philosophy nor Greek science remained immune to this change, and the ideas of the new rulers gradually gained supremacy. At first, it is true, Greek ideas won a complete victory; for the Romans could only learn. In the beginning of the Empire, however, thought became Romanized, however Greek its form might remain. Now the Romans were always under the sway of magic and animism, much more so than the Greeks had ever been. For a while Epicurean philosophy had banished these notions; it had forcefully combated magic, the Romans' superstition, the fear of death, and the fear of magic power exercised by the dead, under which they labored. The opposition of knowledge to traditionalism engenders the passion of Lucretius, whose work latinized Epicurean philosophy. But at the beginning of the Empire Epicurean philosophy, which had always been the philosophy of the few, was completely driven out by Stoicism, which did not pursue the fight against superstition as vigorously. On the contrary, it favored superstition: it forgot all those tenets that, as in Epicurean philosophy, should have enforced the suppression of magic; in Rome, it was transformed, Romanized. Moreover, the climate of opinion became altogether less philosophical. Religious sentiment began to grow stronger again, becoming permeated with mysticism and superstition and affecting philosophy; the way was being paved for Christianity, and in the process Roman magical notions were given free rein. In no other legal system are the dead and their graves protected as in the Roman, and this protection Christian law took over from Roman law.[42] But since now magical notions again gained ground and not even the educated were under the influence of a free and enlightened philosophy but one that had fallen prey to a superstition, even the scholars no longer felt free to undertake dissections. Individuals, it is true, will still have wished to dissect; Rufus and Galen, in the tradition of Hellenistic science and ancient Greek philosophy, demanded that dissections be performed. But this demand was far from being the demand of all scientists, as it had been in Alexandria: beginning with opposition of the Empiricists to the Dogmatists, science had renounced anatomy in the schools of the Methodists and others, for scientific reasons. This is why what now seemed imperative to only a few individuals could no longer be carried out, especially in a milieu that had changed so radically: for Galen and Rufus, dissecting is no longer possible. The general demand for dissec-

---

[42] Cf. Th. Mommsen, *Römisches Strafrecht*, Leipzig, 1899, p. 812 ff.

tions voiced by the predominant Alexandrian schools could, in the beginning, be realized, because all scientists shared in it, and because inwardly they all felt free to dissect. What some individuals now demanded, even in opposition to their science and in opposition to prevailing opinion, could no longer be realized, because now the people and the state were against it too. The Hellenistic physicians had at least had the help of the kings, who were themselves schooled in philosophy. The Roman Empire permitted no dissections. Only in Egypt, as Galen says, not in the European provinces, could anatomy still be practiced; why it was possible there will be discussed later (cf. p. 300 ff. below). The latinized world at any rate allowed no dissecting, and it is not by chance that a Latin writer tells that even dissection of animals was sufficient grounds for convicting him of the practice of magic (Apuleius, *Apologia*, ch. 25 ff.).

In sum, the reports that have survived concerning the history of anatomy and its course in the post-Alexandrian period seem true: the history of anatomy is as tradition portrays it. In Alexandria it was possible to dissect; then dissection soon became less frequent; it was in many instances abandoned for scientific reasons; finally, it was generally rejected by men who were again under the sway of religion and magic.

The reports of dissections are not inventions; and the reports of vivisections are, I think, no less true. If dissection has been considered impossible for religious reasons, vivisection has been considered impossible because modern scholars were unwilling to impute such cruelty to physicians and ridiculed the testimony on vivisections as an accusation which cannot be taken seriously.[43]

Now, that vivisection is cruel even the ancient Dogmatists admitted, as is clear from the apology which Celsus weaves into his account

[43] It is surely strange that scholars could go so far as to deny the possibility of vivisection on the ground of humanitarian considerations. After all, physicians of the Middle Ages and of the present, too, have at least considered vivisection. Carpus (*Commentaria*, 1521, p. IV b) says: "For in our time anatomy is not practiced on living bodies, and yet the data would be found out much better in the living than in the dead, were it not that we recoil from such an enterprise because of its monstrousness" (cited by M. Roth, *Andreas Vesalius*, Berlin, 1892, p. 474; cf. also the other passages there cited). And H. Braus (*Anatomie des Menschen*, Berlin, 1929, p. 1) says of the art of dissection: "Its greatest disadvantage is that it can only be performed on the dead; times are past when the ancient investigator demanded, and received, living slaves as objects of his study." Why then among the ancients should mention of vivisection always have been made in the spirit of reproach?

of the procedure. In their opinion, Herophilus and Erasistratus acted in by far the best way in vivisecting criminals. And after the scientific justification for vivisection has been given, one reads: "Neque esse crudele, sicut plerique proponunt, hominum nocentium et horum quoque paucorum suppliciis remedia populis innocentibus saeculorum omnium quaeri" (*CML*, p. 21, 29–32; Prooemium, 26). Vivisection, then, is excused because it is practiced only on criminals and essentially for scientific reasons; it appears justified in that the torture of a few, and of a wicked few at that, aids all innocent generations.[44] In making his standpoint more precise, Celsus says: "As for the remainder, which can only be learnt from the living, actual practice will demonstrate it in the course of treating the wounded in a somewhat slower yet much milder way" (Prooemium, 75, Loeb, p. 41). The discussion of vivisection is thus shaped by the accusation of cruelty.

Christian polemics also, at a time when Galen only defended the right to dissect without being able to do so, passionately attacked vivisections which hardly occurred anymore, in order to expose the inhumanity and cruelty of the pagans. Tertullian says: "That physician or butcher (Herophilus) who cut up six hundred corpses in order to investigate nature, who allowed himself to hate mankind. . . . A death not of the natural kind but one changed through the violence of dissection" (*De anima*, ch. 10). Later, Fulgentius (*Mythologia* I, praef.) says: "Galen's family . . . is so ingrafted into almost all of Alexandria's narrow streets that one can count more little surgical butcher stalls than dwelling places" (transl. Ed.). There was general agreement that vivisection was cruel; but why should individuals nevertheless not have done what is cruel if they considered it necessary? Men are often forced to resort to horrible means in the pursuit of the good. Nobody can tell how man, even the most humane, should decide, and will decide, in such situations. If tradition attests that the Dogmatists, that Herophilus and Erasistratus, had the courage to perform vivisections, considering it cruel, but hoping in this way to save an infinite number of others, is one not obliged to believe it?

The people of the Hellenistic age, to be sure, were distinguished by their humaneness. When Theophrastus disapproves of animal sacri-

---

[44] Here, it becomes clear that vivisection is by no means a continuing necessity and practice. For the death of a few means the salvation of the men of all times. On the question of the frequency of vivisection and dissection, which is one of the most important in the history of ancient anatomy, cf. p. 296 ff., below.

fices, indeed of all bloody sacrifices—for they are not pleasing to the gods—one of his arguments is the kinship of man and beast. It might therefore appear still less likely that vivisection of men was practiced in a period which even rejected the sacrificing of animals to the gods. But the concept of humaneness which Theophrastus upholds is limited by the concept of necessity. According to his view, any slaughtering of animals is fundamentally to be rejected, and yet men are forced to kill animals for food. As much as possible, to be sure, one should refrain from eating the meat of animals; however, it cannot always be avoided. Men are bound to kill animals in order to survive, and for this reason it is also permissible to do so. Similarly, as Theophrastus says, one is allowed to kill human beings and to punish the criminal with death. It is only the unnecessary sacrifice, the unnecessary cruelty, that should be shunned.[45] If then the killing of human beings, and in addition of criminals who have forfeited their lives and whose killing was regarded as permissible and proper, if the killing of such men was the necessary condition for saving other, innocent, people, why should even the most humane scientist not decide to practice vivisection?[46] One would have to enter into a detailed examination of Hellenistic juridical and ethical views, in order to prove the tradition altogether correct. But equally precise inquiries would be necessary to justify contesting the tradition. In this context, it is impossible to go into such details. However, I am satisfied that the reports of vivisections are proved plausible by the fact that all the other reports with which they are interrelated are historically correct and because the counterargument, that rejects vivisection as inhumane, certainly does not stand criticism.

IV

If in Greece all the conditions for dissection and vivisection existed, contrary to the modern assumption, the simplest explanation of the fact that this was done for the first time in Alexandria seems to lie in

[45] Cf. Th. Gomperz, *Griechische Denker* III, 1931, p. 414 ff.; Zeller, *Die Philosophie der Griechen* III, 2, [fourth edition], Leipzig, 1921, p. 854 ff.

[46] It is clear in view of the Hellenistic concept of humaneness, which acknowledges no difference between man and animal, that vivisections of animals should, in principle, also be forbidden. And yet, one did vivisect animals, as is well known, because it was necessary.

the great, even decisive significance which knowledge of the human body then acquired. Dissection affords the most comprehensive and surest insight into the body: if such insight is considered indispensable for treatment, one will resort to dissections. But one may well object that the surest and best method often is not used, especially when the objectively best and most correct meets the strong resistance of external circumstances. One must, therefore, understand the exact purpose for which ancients performed dissections and vivisections and why they became necessary for them after other methods had long seemed adequate. Such understanding should at the same time furnish additional proof that they were actually carried out.

Celsus, in his account of the Dogmatists' dissections, says that they believed that one could not possibly treat internal diseases without a knowledge of the body: "ergo[47] necessarium esse incidere corpora mortuorum eorumque viscera atque intestina scrutari" (*CML*, p. 21, 14–15; Prooemium, 23). The dissection of cadavers, then, affords a scrutiny of the internal organs. But Celsus continues: "longeque optime fecisse Herophilum et Erasistratum qui nocentes homines ex carcere acceptos vivos inciderint considerarintque etiam num spiritu remanente ea quae natura ante clausisset eorumque positum, colorem, figuram, magnitudinem, ordinem, duritiem, molitiem, livorem, contactum, processus deinde singulorum et recessus, et sive quid inseritur alteri sive quid partem alterius in se recipit" (*CML*, p. 21, 15–21; Prooemium, 23–24). In other words, vivisection provides knowledge of man and his organs as they are in life. Dissection is not sufficient; vivisection has an advantage over it. Herophilus and Erasistratus acted best by far, because they vivisected. Or, as Celsus goes on to say, the advantage of vivisection is that it studies living man, not merely the dead, as does dissection, and without knowledge of the living it is not possible to treat the sick (Prooemium, 25). After all, it is the living whom one treats, and therefore one must know man as he is in life, not as he is in death.

The Empiricists rejected dissection and vivisection because they did not believe that the knowledge sought could be acquired in that

---

[47] Celsus, it would seem, simply infers that dissections are necessary because it is necessary to acquire knowledge of the body. But this falsifies the facts of history: dissections appear to be the necessary consequence only after they have once been performed. Theoretically, one could still have relied on conclusions by analogy, even later.

way. Dissection must be rejected because a dead man is not the same as a live one: "ne mortuorum quidem lacerationem necessariam esse . . . cum aliter pleraque in mortuis se habeant" (*CML*, p. 24, 21–23; Prooemium, 44). Vivisection must be rejected, apart from its horrors, because one cannot succeed in dissecting a human being alive: he dies under the physician's knife (Prooemium, 42). But, however right its aim, it is also unnecessary, because what one must know about man can be learnt from the living subject during treatment. Celsus himself considered dissection necessary, but this, as has already been shown, was for didactic reasons only. He thought that man's organs and their position could be better recognized in the cadaver than through occasional observation of wounds in the living. The rest, which can only be learnt from the living, should be learnt during treatment, not through vivisection (*Ibid.*, 74–75).

In this discussion, the particular problem which is decisive for the understanding of the rôle of dissection and vivisection becomes evident. It is knowledge of the living human being that is of fundamental importance. To that end, dissection of cadavers does not suffice: it is of value only in combination with vivisection, say the Dogmatists, or must at least be supported by it. The importance of dissection is limited: it must be supported—says Celsus in an attempt to find a compromise—though not by vivisection, yet by suitable observation of the living. Neither dissection nor vivisection is of any significance, according to the Empiricists, for the dead are no longer identical with the living, and it is the living patient whom one seeks to know, and whom one must know, if one is to treat him correctly.

To put it differently, the discussion about the value of dissection and vivisection is determined by definite philosophical and scientific theories about the nature of man. Is this nature changed in death, or does it remain unchanged? To what extent must allowances be made for these changes, if one wishes to learn from dissection and vivisection to improve one's treatment, and which methods can lead to such knowledge and which cannot? Thus the decision to be made about dissection and vivisection also turns, from being a purely medical problem, into a philosophical and scientific one. And in order to understand the formulation of the problem and its solution, one must go back as far as the philosophy of Aristotle.

In the first book of his work, *On the parts of animals*, Aristotle gives a quite general and systematic account of his position with regard to questions of zoology. After introductory remarks on the method to be used in every investigation, and therefore also in the present one (639 a 1–12), he proceeds to discuss the methodological problems peculiar to an investigation of nature (ἡ περὶ φύσεως ἱστορία). The question is whether one should investigate each substance (οὐσία) by itself, that is, whether one should discuss individually man and his nature, the lion, the ox, or some other animal, or whether one should consider collectively what is common to them. Aristotle chooses to treat together what is common, in order not to say the same thing in different places with inevitable duplication and without coordination (639 a 13–639 b 6). There follows a discussion of the relationship between factual description and etiology. This question too, he says, had before him not been dealt with systematically. He settles it in accord with his whole philosophy on the principle that being, not becoming, is decisive: for becoming is for the sake of being, not being for the sake of becoming (640 a 18–19). But in describing nature, the important thing is to catch not lifeless "being," but the force which informs this "being," its "power." It is by no means sufficient to grasp merely the material cause of "being"; the decisive factor is the final cause. Even in speaking about a bed or anything else, one would have to grasp the form rather than the matter. A bed is made of this or that, but it is made in this particular form and shape. For nature as form ranks higher than nature as matter (640 b 28–29). And then he says: "Does, then, configuration and color constitute the essence of the various animals and of their several parts? For if so, what Democritus says will be strictly correct. For such appears to have been his notion. At any rate he says that it is evident to every one what form it is that makes the man, seeing that he is recognizable by his shape and color." (640 b 29–35 transl. Ogle, *The Works of Aristotle*, Oxford: Clarendon Press, Vol. V). According to Aristotle, then, the human configuration, which, for his investigation of nature, is more important than the purely material explanation, has been resolved by Democritus into mere color and shape. But that is impossible, the objection being that "a corpse has the same shape and fashion as a living body; and yet it is not a man" (640 b 35–36; Loeb, p. 67). What Aristotle understands by "form," then, is not exhausted by external, spatial, or visible phenomena. A hand made of iron or wood is not a hand, or at least only in name, just as the physician in a portrait is a physician in name only. For such a hand can perform none of the movements which really characterize the hand (640 b 36–641 a 3). And from this follows the conclusion that: "Precisely in the same way no part of a dead body, such I mean as its eye or its hand, is really an eye or a hand" (641 a 3–5; transl. Ogle, *loc. cit.*). One must discuss a living creature in such a way as to grasp not the matter, but the specific function of the matter, just as one must in treating every other thing (641 a 14–17). When, however, it is part and parcel of the definition of the living creature that it has a share in the soul—and this means that it is capable of acting—one must apprehend just these qualities of the soul, this ability to act (641 a 18–19). And then he sums up his whole argument and gives its most poignant formulation in this sentence: "At any rate, when its Soul is gone, it is no longer a living creature, and none of its parts remains the same, except only in shape, just like the animals in the story that were turned into stone" (641 a 19–21; Loeb, p. 69).

It is clear how the matter stands. Atomism, the philosophy of Democritus, urges the scientist to investigate the external shape of things. The real world is made up of atoms; the true nature of things is constituted by them. For the naturalist, however, who unlike the philosopher seeks to grasp the world not through thought alone, but through observation, the reality of the phenomena consists only of their shape and color. This Democritean philosophy of nature is overcome by that of Plato and Aristotle, whose ultimate metaphysical insight— the recognition of the existence of the soul and of organisms—makes it impossible to look upon nature in as external a fashion, or to understand it as materialistically, as does Atomism. According to their view, nature is divided into various realms, in each of which the soul, the most elevated form of existence in the world, is realized to a different degree. The soul itself is not, as it is for Democritus, the result, so to speak, of matter, but rather that for which matter exists and in which it finds its meaning. Man can only be understood as an organism. The researcher, then, if he aspires to knowledge of man, must consider the capacities of his soul, his actions. Only in this way can he grasp man's nature, which, so different from that of other beings, is the real object of investigation. And in defining how man differs from the other organisms with which he belongs *qua genus*, one also comprehends the dissimilarities which constitute the species, man. Any research that is concerned with externals alone remains inadequate.

Every investigation of the dead is inadequate also. What matters is the life, the capacity of the soul to act. Where such a philosophical conviction determines the method of the scientist, only living man can interest him. Aristotle refutes the opposing point of view, that of Democritus, by objecting that there would in fact be no difference between the dead and the living if one needed only to recognize man's shape and color. A dead man still retains the same bodily form, yet he is no longer a human being. The dead man's parts, his eyes and hands, still have the same shape, but not the same "power." Therefore, what is important in the living cannot be the shape, which remains in death although the true substance of life has disappeared; it must be something else.

Such considerations, in point of fact, seem to remove all justification for dissecting dead bodies. And yet Aristotle's own knowledge is based in great part on such dissections, though they are dissections of animals. To some extent, then, he must acknowledge the value, and it is clear that in certain areas of knowledge it is possible for him to do so. For although the shape is not the essential aspect of an animal, it still belongs to it. Moreover, it does remain identical in death, and anatomy can therefore yield morphological results and is in this sense important.

However, according to Aristotle, dissection cannot lead to any further insights, at least not dissection of cadavers, because man also changes in death. Therefore, if one seeks to inform oneself about him, and if one believes that such information can be had only by cutting open his body, then one has to vivisect. One has to cut man open alive, just as formerly one cut up animals alive.[48]

It goes without saying that these considerations form the basis of the discussion concerning dissection and vivisection which Celsus preserved. The consequence of Aristotle's philosophy, of his argument against Democritus, is the demand for two kinds of dissection: the dissection to be practiced on the dead, which teaches only morphological data, and another practiced on the living, which teaches the functions, that which is truly worth knowing. The Dogmatic schools of Hellenistic times, which were always under the influence of the Aristotelian school, must have drawn this conclusion from Aristotelian thought. Even the counterarguments of the Empiricists echo Aristotelian arguments: for they are intent on knowing the living man. What they object to in vivisection is the inadequacy of the method: they prefer the investigation

---

[48] It is not without interest to compare with these Aristotelian thoughts the manner in which Plato compares the almost totally unchanged condition of the body, at least shortly after death, with the changelessness of the soul of the dead (Gorgias 524 b ff.).

of the human body and its functions during treatment. Substantially they argue, just as the Dogmatists argue, in favor of vivisection: the cadaver is unimportant, "since most things are altered in the dead" (Prooemium, 44; Loeb, p. 25). This is the Aristotelian argument against Democritus, but with one change: it is expressly conceded that one can learn the position of the organs in the cadaver. If the Empiricists nevertheless reject dissection of the dead, it is only because it seems unnecessary to them; observations which one can make by chance on corpses teach the same lessons.

The account by Celsus, then, which has been declared an invention and a calumny, adduces arguments and assumptions that are in agreement with philosophical arguments and assumptions. Apart from the history of philosophy, the history of anatomy is incomprehensible; when related to the former it becomes intelligible, and once this relationship is seen, the authenticity of the tradition too is confirmed. This is above all true of the reports on human vivisection. Because it was demanded by certain philosophical considerations, because it was by no means the sport of cruel men or the like, nor yet the sequel of blind indiscriminate investigation, but the consequence of the most exact deliberation, because it was bound to appear as the only possible road to knowledge, vivisection could be risked. For these reasons it was discussed and could be objected to only on methodological grounds as the Empiricists' polemic shows: the objections based on human considerations, would, by themselves, have had no meaning.

In the account which Celsus gives of Dogmatic medicine there is, it is true, an indication of a change in attitude toward the procedures which philosophical dogma and the consequences drawn from it really demanded. The Dogmatists, too, no longer vivisected human beings, although they considered it the most correct method of investigation; for them, only anatomy was absolutely essential. But Galen expressly differentiated between two kinds of anatomy, one studying the functions of the body, the other studying the parts (II 286 K.). Gregory distinguished quite precisely between an anatomy of position and an anatomy of purpose (*De hominis opificio*, 240 c Migne), that is, between morphological and functional results. This double goal still reflects the old problem whether man is body or soul, whether therefore one must have knowledge of the body, of matter, or of the soul, the living organism. For this reason, the anatomy of the dead, which alone can still be performed, cannot give complete and needed instruction concerning man, except insofar as animal vivisections at least are under-taken to replace human vivisection.[49] About Hellenistic medicine—for which the problem of dissection and vivisection has a degree of signifi-cance such as it has for the medicine of no earlier or later time—one can speak with little certainty, because the works of the period have all been lost. Nevertheless, such indirect sources as have survived at least make it possible to outline the course of development in general.

As I have shown, philosophical considerations provide the me-thodical basis for dissection and vivisection. And this is necessarily so, for the significance and value of the methods of the individual sciences always depend on philosophical arguments. But dissections and vivi-sections can be performed on animals; and on animals they were per-formed before the Alexandrian period. Why are they suddenly carried out on human beings in Alexandria? This is the decisive question in the history of anatomy; it is the final question which must be solved in order to prove the reality of human dissection and vivisection. And it would seem that just as the philosophical doctrine determines the judgment of physicians as to the dead and the living, so it is philosophy, not medicine, that determines the transition from animal to human dissection.

At the very beginning, knowledge of the human body was based on observations made during the treatment of diseases or through chance discoveries of cadavers. This first knowledge predates all con-scious investigation and research; it is by no means the knowledge of experts but a knowledge common to all.

When one was no longer satisfied with the observations one chanced upon, there began the conscious study of the human body. Such in-quiry, by which one tries to explore the constitution of the human body with exactitude and in a comprehensive manner, was undertaken rela-tively early, at any rate in the time of the pre-Socratics. Their investi-gation of the invisible, and this term includes the internal organs of the human body, rests on analogies. And therefore, even physiology, like all exploration of nature, was tied to the method of analogy. Nor did the Hippocratics proceed differently: they too explained the unknown by comparison to the known. Their observations, though still unscien-

---

[49] Even in late medicine one can find reflections of Aristotelian arguments, just as one finds them in Dogmatic and Empiricist medicine. So strong did the influence of Aristotelian philosophy remain in the natural sciences even at a time when quite different systems had long come to prevail in metaphysics and ethics!

tific and unsystematic, were nevertheless more than a mere recording of what one happened to find remarkable.[50]

Moreover, if, at first, analogical thinking related everything to everything and thus gained certain knowledge in the naive belief in a pervading unity of nature, later analogies with animals became particularly important for knowledge of the human body. That the study of animal organs was assumed to provide a clue to the knowledge of human organs, presupposes, of course, that in the last analysis man and animals are identical. Man, being a part of the world, of the animal world, can be compared to its other parts. This was the position even of Aristotle in his *History of animals.* It is true, he substantially refines the concept of analogy: he no longer takes the study of any chance animal as a basis for conclusions about man; rather, he relates the organs of certain animals to the same organs in the human; he bases the conclusion on the equation of functions. However, such conclusions, even in Aristotle, still presuppose the belief in a partial uniformity of nature, though no longer the belief in its all-pervading unity.[51]

It was only in Alexandria that conclusions by analogy were replaced by the method of dissecting. If one asks what is the principal difference between such analogical study of the human body and its study through human dissection, the answer would seem to be that dissection, through the very renunciation of such analogies, centers the investigation on the object itself. Thus the study replaces conclusions drawn from other empirical knowledge. Or, to put it differently, the one method is linked to extraneous data, while the other is not. The replacement of the one method by the other is to be understood through the history of scientific methodology as it now came into being.

In the later *Peripatos,* scientific conclusions based on analogy

---

[50] No study on the Homeric animal system has led to compelling results (O. Körner, *Die Homerische Tierwelt,* München, 1930). Of course, the Homeric poems too know of groups of animals. But the classification is implicit rather than conscious, and it would have to be conscious to be called a system in the strict sense of the word. Aristotle, it is true, did not deny that animal systems of various kinds had been outlined before his, but his objections to these "systems" show clearly that they do not correspond to the modern concept of a system, which is itself a creation of Aristotelian and Platonic philosophy. Disregarding the testimony of tradition, a science of zoology could, as Jaeger has shown, only come into being with Aristotle and in his late scientific period at that (*Aristoteles,* Berlin, 1923, p. 353).

[51] The principle of pre-Socratic and Aristotelian science has been thus formulated by O. Regenbogen (*Quell. u. Stud. z. Gesch. d. Math., Astron. u. Phys.,* Abt. B 1, 149 ff.).

came to be suspect. Aristotle himself, despite his opposition to Empedocles' overbold and all too poetical metaphors, had nevertheless to a large extent indulged in analogical conclusions, though with all the methodological refinements he deemed necessary. But already Theophrastus, in his study on plants, admitted such conclusions as proofs only between members of the same genus.[52] He says: "To insist at all costs on comparing what cannot be compared is an exaggerated [and harmful] undertaking because it embraces the danger that in the end one misses the approach most suited to the study of the object" (*Historia plantarum* I, 1, 4).

If, toward the end of the fourth century, the study of the human body is suddenly based on human dissection after centuries which had known only dissection of animals and conclusions by analogy with animals, this must, I think, be attributed to the same refinement in method that is to be found generally in all natural sciences of the period. If it had long been known that the human body is not completely identical with that of animals but on the contrary has certain features peculiarly its own, these differences were emphasized more and more in course of time. Thus the species of man became separated from the species of other animals, becoming almost a genus in itself. Where comparisons were still believed possible, they were no longer considered strict analogies, but mere similarities; a wish to draw comparisons at all cost seemed exaggerated and dangerous. At a certain point, therefore, the analogical method no longer produced results; one searched, I suggest, for a new method. And whereas in botany the refinement of method led to the stagnation of investigation, in zoology it led to progress that was to have the most far-reaching significance. For the dissection of the human body itself opened the way to undreamed discoveries.

Galen, reflecting on the history of anatomy, says that no textbooks of anatomy existed at the time of the Hippocratic physicians, nor did the physicians need instruction in anatomy. As he puts it: "In former times not only was there no need of anatomical instruction, but not even of books containing such matters. Such books, as far as I know, were first written by Diocles and after him by a few of the ancient physicians and also by not a few of the more recent ones" (II 282 K.). The first book about anatomy, then, according to the tradition as Galen

---

[52] This has been pointed out by O. Regenbogen (*op. cit.*, p. 155 ff.).

knew it, was written by Diocles, a contemporary of Theophrastus.[53] The tradition concerning the history of anatomical textbooks, as passed on by Galen, thus leads to the same period as does the historical consideration of methodology. It was also a disciple of Aristotle who is said to have written the first book with the title, *On skeletons* (περὶ σκελετῶν),[54] a title which, in the opinion of Galen (II 220 K.), is equivalent to anatomy. All chronological data too, therefore, place the decisive change in the way of looking at the human body and the dogma concerning it at the beginning of the Peripatetic school. And, as I have shown, the magical or religious prejudices, of whatever nature, by which an incision into the human body could still have been prevented no longer existed for the Alexandrian physician. The philosophy of this period considered experience the sole principle of knowledge. In sum, at that time, everything came together to suggest that the investigation of the human body be based no longer on conclusions by analogy but on experience derived from the object itself.

Later, the study of man was again supported by indirect conclusions. Even Galen describes man according to the findings in animals whenever he does not go back to teachings inherited from investigators who had still been able to open human bodies. But, compared to earlier times, he applied the method in a significantly different manner. While Aristotle had compared human organs to the organs of animals, in the belief that where the function is the same in man and beast, the organ of the one can be understood through the organ of the other, Galen relied on the study of those animals which he considered most similar to man. As he says: "For this purpose choose the monkeys which resemble man most closely. And these are the ones in which the thigh is not very long, and not the large ones which are called those with dogs' teeth. Then you will find that the other parts too are similar to those of man" (II 222 K.); besides the monkey, he considered also a certain number of other animals to be very similar to man, and these were the only ones he used in his anatomical studies.[55] Galen's method, then, contrasted

[53] On this matter, cf. K. Deichgräber, *Die griechische Empirikerschule*, Berlin, 1930, p. 274, ftn. 3.
[54] Clearchus of Soloi, see Athenaeus, *Deipnosophistae* 399 b, cf. Töply, "Geschichte der Anatomie," in Puschmann's *Handbuch der Geschichte der Medizin*, II, 1903, p. 181.
[55] Cf. M. Simon, *op. cit.*, p. XXXIII ff.

with that of Aristotle, implies an entirely new concept of comparing and classifying animals.

The history of ancient zoology and, above all, the history of the animal systems that were developed have not yet been explored sufficiently. Almost nothing is known about the various classifications and, in particular, about reasons for their being changed. I venture to suggest that the Galenic system deviates from that of Aristotle in part at least because there had been a change in the methods of investigating the human body. The motive for dissecting human cadavers is the conviction that human and animal bodies are incomparable. Once such a distinction has been recognized, and once it has led to separating the human species from the animal species, it is no longer possible for future researchers to take it for granted that man is a part of the animal kingdom, as one had done before. Aristotle's analogies to findings in animals gave him what he considered to be absolutely correct insight into the human body. Galen knew that the analogies to which he was led through dissecting whatever kind of animal he may have been studying were not absolutely true,[56] because he had learned that one is not allowed simply to draw analogies between creatures not resembling each other. The conclusion is safe only in the case of real uniformity or similarity. It is for this reason that he, or the system with which he is aligned, tried to find "animals similar to man," and that he only compared species which, as it were, represented an intermediate stage between the species of man and the species of animals. The unlimited comparison permitted by the old pre-Socratic doctrine of the uniformity of all creatures was replaced by the Aristotelian comparison of organs according to the concept of function; it was in turn succeeded, I think, by a new kind of comparison resting on a classification in which living things were arranged according to similarities and transitional forms.

It is easily understandable, indeed it seems necessary, that the dissection of humans should originate in Alexandria, and so does its coming to an end seem conditioned and required by the historical development of the sciences and of philosophy. The traditional account, which at first appeared to contain chance data, has proved to be well founded and correct. It is not by accident that nothing is known about dissections before Alexandrian times. Homeric and Hippocratic physicians did not yet practice anatomy; they did not need to, because what

[56] The matter has been dealt with in detail by M. Simon.

they wished to know, and needed to know, about the human body could also be learnt in other ways. They attached no importance as yet to a systematic knowledge of the internal organs, such as seemed essential later in Alexandria. But it was also in Alexandria that dissection could first be risked: for it was only in the Hellenistic period, and in connection with intellectual movements starting with Plato, that the old magical and religious beliefs had disintegrated to such an extent as to make dissection possible. And it was also in Alexandria that it became necessary to abandon the old methods of inquiry, for they had proved inadequate with the advance of methodological consciousness. And since the new approach being sought at that time could only be based on the direct study of the phenomena, there resulted the necessity to examine the human body itself, not merely the bodies of animals. It is as the accounts have it; dissections were performed and vivisections were performed; and just as tradition correctly records the time when dissections originated, so it records correctly the time when they ceased.

V

Since dissection and vivisection were actually carried out in antiquity, certain technical questions must finally be dealt with which are raised by the very fact that such dissections and vivisections were undertaken. To put it differently, one must ask where the material for these investigations came from, how frequently such studies were undertaken, how far they spread in the ancient world, and just where anatomy was practiced.

It is not too difficult to answer these questions as far as vivisection is concerned. That bodies for vivisection could be obtained only by coercion is not open to doubt: no one is likely to lend himself to it of his own free will. When Celsus therefore states that the kings handed over criminals to Herophilus and Erasistratus for scientific experiments, the statement surely denotes the only possible way to obtain human material for vivisection. Moreover, as I have indicated, the Dogmatic schools from the very beginning demanded not that vivisections be endlessly repeated, but that they be performed once for the benefit of future generations. They could only be performed where an authoritarian state interested in science provided the means for them, and for this reason they were performed only in Alexandria and at the beginning of the Hellenistic period, as Celsus tells.

297

As far as dissection is concerned, the questions of obtaining material, of frequency, and regional distribution are more difficult to answer. In these respects tradition is even more scanty than it is in regard to the history of Greek anatomy in general. This, however, is hardly due to the fact that many accounts were destroyed but, in the main, to the fact that most of the relevant data were not recorded. They were so self-evident to men and formed, as it were, part and parcel of their attitude toward life, so that there was no occasion for reflecting upon them. The interpreter, therefore, can but deduce what people's views must have been from a consideration of how men in general feel about such matters and attempt to correct what may be historically conditioned in his own opinion by what seems to be fitting for man in the ancient world. A human being, to be sure, can never be entirely indifferent to the cutting up of another human for scientific purposes. One need not think only of those to whom one feels closest; inured as one may have become to the horrible, one can still not come to the point where one accepts the dissection of the body, even of a stranger, with indifference and as a matter of course. It is these feelings to which Goethe gave expression in *Wilhelm Meisters Wanderjahre:* "Study was unpleasantly hindered by the constantly repeated complaint that material was lacking, that there were too few of the pale corpses which, for such high purposes, were wanted for the knife. In order to supply not enough, but as many as possible, harsh laws had been passed: not only criminals, who had in every sense forfeited their individual rights, but others too, physical and spiritual derelicts, were made use of. Rigor of enforcement grew with the need, and with it the revulsion of the people, whose moral and religious views of the world did not make it possible for them to renounce the belief in their own personalities and the personalities of those they loved. Yet the evil continued to grow, and people became confused and worried that not even the peaceful graves of their beloved departed ones were safe. Neither old men nor dignitaries, neither the lofty nor the lowly, were now safe in their resting-places; the grave adorned with flowers, the inscriptions meant to preserve a memory, nothing gave protection against profitable rapacity. The most painful of leave-takings seemed most cruelly troubled, and on turning away from the grave, one was already bound to fear the news that the quieted, bedecked limbs of the beloved were severed, carried off, and desecrated" (Bk. 3, ch. 3).[57] The

[57] The thoughts expressed here led Goethe to propose a "plastische Anatomie" which he described in detail in *Wilhelm Meister* itself and again set forth in a letter

feelings of people in antiquity will have been the same, perhaps less individualistic but all the more religious, even more concerned about the peace of the dead; at least the masses must have felt so. The difficulty of obtaining cadavers to dissect must, therefore, have been great.

However, the testimonies tell that these difficulties were overcome. Despite all obstacles, even medieval physicians were able, through the intervention of the state or robbery, to obtain the cadavers necessary for dissection; in the same way they succeeded in dissecting in the Renaissance and in modern times. Thus it was not impossible in Greece either. It must be added that dissections were certainly not more frequently performed in Greece than at the beginning of the Renaissance and in the Middle Ages, perhaps even more seldom. This seems to follow from the fact that the necessity for dissections was by no means universally recognized. Only the Dogmatic school insisted on them, while both the Empiricist and Methodist schools rejected them; when, later on, they were once more demanded, the demand was always made by individuals. Moreover, the fact that schools and individuals considered it right to dissect hardly meant that every physician had to dissect, any more than it meant this in the Middle Ages, in the Renaissance, and still later. In those periods too, dissections took place one or twice a year for the instruction of students at a university and for the purposes of research. It will not have been very different in Alexandria, even if one or the other great investigator out of scientific interest dissected more often. Finally, the Empiricists declared that anatomy could also be learnt from books. Galen vehemently attacked them on this account; he was surprised, and rightly so, that it was just the Empiricists who made such an assertion: "Here again we are astonished by the Empiricists' love of dispute. In regard to everything else, they claim that he who often observes the facts fundamental to medicine can imitate them better than if he gets only an occasional chance look at them. Similarly, they claim that he who has a job to do can do it better if he has done it often before. But then again they say that in anatomy alone one acquires sure knowledge of the things one learns through reading the investigations of the anatomists. And yet, not even someone who is shown the parts of the body by his teacher can remember them exactly

of February 4, 1832 (to Geheimrath Beuth in Berlin) with express reference to the *Wanderjahre*. Plastic anatomy was to replace dissection of cadavers through a study of representations of parts of the body.

299

if he sees them once or twice, but must see them repeatedly" (Dchgr. fr. 69, 131, 30 ff.; Galen XIII 607, 17 K.). This polemical remark is of basic importance for answering the question of the frequency of dissections. Books about anatomy came into existence when scientists began putting down the results of their research. If, in anatomical investigations, it is the results that are of interest, and if these results can be learnt from the books in which they were recorded, then further dissections are unnecessary. Here, too, then, independent investigation gives way to authority: the pupil simply learns established knowledge from his teacher, a method which modern science accepts only within certain limits but which was all-important in every branch of ancient learning. Consequently, dissections need not be repeated, even though it was considered necessary that they be performed once if any knowledge of the internal organs was to be gained.[58] It is true, not all ancient physicians shared this view. Many believed that dissections should constantly be repeated for pedagogical reasons, if not for the sake of research. Yet, the fact that there was no unanimity concerning the necessity for repeated dissections must have limited their frequency still more, and there were certainly only a few places of instruction where dissections were considered necessary for didactic reasons.

The great educational center for physicians in Hellenistic times and in the Roman Empire—that is in those centuries in which anatomy was of real importance—was Alexandria. This city, of the greatest significance for all Greek science, is particularly important for the history of anatomy. Physicians first performed dissections in Alexandria. This follows from the tradition, which traces them back to Herophilus and Erasistratus. It was the Dogmatic schools of Alexandria which always considered dissections necessary; Celsus' demand for dissections was based on the doctrines of Alexandrian scholars. Galen says expressly that one should go to Alexandria for the sake of anatomical studies. It was with regard to Alexandria that Fulgentius still speaks of the slaughtering of human beings, practiced according to the teaching of Galen.

In Egypt conditions as they had been in the beginning of the Hellenistic period remained the same for very long; even under the Roman Empire, there was little change in the form of life that had prevailed

---

[58] I cite two instances of dissections performed in late centuries because they attest how unusual the procedure had become: the dissection performed on the body of Hermogenes (cf. O. Immisch u. L. Aschoff, *Philol. Wschr.*, 42, 1922, 736 ff.) and that of bodies of German soldiers killed in the war (Galen, XIII 604 K.).

from early times. While the Egyptians lived according to their own laws, the Greeks stayed apart, and Greek science continued to flourish.[59] "Together with the first library of the world, Alexandria also retained throughout Imperial times a kind of leadership in scientific work, until the Museum perished and Islam destroyed the ancient civilization. It was not only the opportunities afforded, but also the ancient tradition preserved by the Greeks and their mentality, which kept the city pre-eminent; native Alexandrians, indeed, predominated in number and importance among the scholars."[60] Perhaps it was for this reason that in Alexandria it remained possible to practice medicine in the ancient manner. The works of the Alexandrian physicians of both the early and late periods have been lost; only the writings of people who lived and worked in the Romanized provinces or in Italy itself have been preserved. It is quite possible that these books do not represent Greek science as it was actually practiced by Greeks. When Galen advises the physician to go to Alexandria, it sounds as if he were intent on sending him to the seat of true instruction. While Galen himself was not able to perform dissections, much as he would have liked to, it was still possible to do so in Alexandria. In Alexandria, where dissections had been begun, they were still performed when, outside Alexandria, there had long since been no opportunity for them. To what extent dissections were ever performed outside Alexandria, whether in other cities they were not infrequent at all times, these are questions for which the data would seem to provide no conclusive answer.

[59] For the unique condition prevailing in Egypt, cf. Mommsen, *Römische Geschichte*, V [bk. 8, ch. XII]; and, of later studies, M. Rostovtzeff, *Social and Economic History of the Roman Empire*, Oxford, 1926, p. 255.

[60] Mommsen, *Römische Geschichte*, V 8 XII [p. 590].

THE DIETETICS OF ANTIQUITY*

Ⅰt is in the fifth century B.C. that ancient medicine first poses the question: How should a healthy man live in order to remain healthy? At this time physicians begin to understand the importance of the patient's mode of life for the curing of disease. They even try to cure the patient by merely rearranging his way of life, whereas formerly they used drugs or resorted to surgical procedures. But if one acknowledges that a sick man can become healthy by following a right way of life, one must conclude that a healthy man can become sick if he follows a wrong way, because clearly the condition of the body is determined by a man's way of life. He who would stay healthy must therefore know how to live rightly. Once this concept of health is recognized, its validity remains unchallenged throughout antiquity. From the fifth century B.C. to the last ancient century, the question how a healthy man should live in order to remain healthy is just as important a problem for medicine as the healing of the sick.

The physician's reply to the question is that a man should live as his health demands, that consideration of his health should determine his manner of life. But after all, when they are healthy, men must work to earn a living; they engage in politics; they are eager to win in one of the great games; they are interested in rhetoric, in art, in science; they want to participate in communal life. The regulation of their lives which the physician proposes therefore stands in opposition to reality. And if it is to prevail, it must contend with the exigencies and interests of daily life.

The physician demands this regulation on the basis of his conception of the essence of health. Everything a man does, every exertion he makes, and every intake of nourishment, influences his body and the elements which compose it. Exertion stimulates a bodily process by which materials are used up or eliminated; nourishment provides the body with materials which are assimilated to those already present and

* "Antike Diätetik," *Die Antike*, 1931, vol. 7, pp. 255–70.

thus change them. Beside exertion and nourishment, however, external conditions, such as the climate in general, the varying nature of the seasons, and the weather from day to day, also continually change the body and the composition of its materials. The latter must be in balance, or at least in a suitable relation to one another, if a man is to be healthy; every disturbance of the balance, any serious disproportion, brings sickness. From this it follows that exertion and nourishment must of necessity be consciously regulated and balanced in such a way that every excess is avoided, and the effect of external influences must constantly be neutralized by preventative measures. In order to stay healthy, therefore, a man must live according to a definite law; he may not do just as he likes. He must set definite limits so as not to do himself harm, and he must defend himself against the harmful influences whose cause he cannot remove.

But men cannot all live by the same law and remain healthy, for they are not all alike. Each individual has a different constitution, and his way of life must differ accordingly. A man is distinguished from another not only by the strength or weakness of his body; there is a difference depending, as well, on whether he is of slight or heavy build, whether by nature the mixture of elements in him is in balance or predisposed in any particular direction, whether he has a dry or a moist nature. A man is not even the same at all times of life: his age is a factor which must be considered in selecting food and choosing physical activity. Finally, a man's constitution is not the same each day nor in all seasons; variations in the seasons—extremes of temperature, changing wind conditions—alter the human body according to its age and constitution. Consequently, the regulation of life must be varied and adjusted to each season and even within the seasons if there are great changes. A person must be fed differently in winter and summer; in the spring he must exercise differently than in fall in order to remain healthy and to counterbalance the bodily changes induced by those in the external world. In addition, the regulation is different according to sex: the rules which are valid for men do not apply to women. The physician, with his insight into the nature of health, must therefore demand that people regulate their nourishment and exertions in accordance with all these factors.

But the man who wishes to live in accordance with the physician's requirements must have time at his disposal and be rich, in order to do everything he should. For only one who is not completely absorbed in any activity and can afford to do as he wishes can avoid every excessive exertion, always eat what is good for him at the proper time, stay quietly at home when it is hot, or be more active in sport when it is cold. Only the rich and independent, therefore, can live in a completely healthy manner. The average person can do only as much for health as his manner of life allows. His health is therefore much more threatened and exposed to greater hazards than that of the rich man. Ancient dietetics, from the beginning, takes cognizance of this social difference among men, which of necessity is of the greatest significance for their way of life. The majority are given only approximate directions corresponding to the exigencies of their lives, since it is not possible for them in any case to live in a completely healthy manner. These people must eat and drink whatever happens to be available, must exert themselves as necessity arises, must journey on foot if conditions demand it, or go to sea if their business requires it, expose themselves to heat and cold whether or not it is good for them. These people, who in all respects lead irregular lives, are counseled to divide the year into four main periods corresponding to the seasons, and to try on the whole to lead a different kind of life during each of these periods. In summer they should, as far as possible, favor moister foods, in winter drier ones. In the spring they should, as far as possible, perform physical exercises different from those done in the fall, and they should bathe and anoint their bodies in a manner appropriate to each season. In this way they can avoid the worst impairment of health. But only the man who does not need to be concerned with anything except his health can live in a perfectly correct manner. This healthy, wealthy person of leisure will observe himself and his body carefully even when he feels well, looks well, enjoys his food, and sustains every exertion with ease; even when nothing seems amiss. In accordance with certain symptoms which he has learned to recognize, he will immediately identify even the slightest disturbance of his health, whether already present or only suspected, and counterbalance it by precise regulation of diet and exercise (Hippocrates, *On regimen* 6. 594–606 L.). But even if, generally speaking, other physicians do not expect from the healthy such nervous attention to their well-being, they must nevertheless try to direct the independent, rich man (in contrast to people in general who lead unhealthy, irregular lives) toward a constant and precisely regulated life; this man must be guided only by his health. As a result of this, life becomes rigid and fraught with a peculiar anxiety. Men avoid everything that is unaccustomed or excessive, in accordance with the medical theory that health is a balance of the various forces affecting the body.

This dietetic system, thus, is determined by the social contrast between rich and poor—between the active and the idle. It takes into consideration the man who follows his trade, who visits the palaestra only when he has the time and who otherwise is engaged in his own pursuits, and the man who is not tied down by an occupation and can thus spend his life of leisure in the house and the gymnasium. This system does not yet accord a place in life to political activity, civic interests, or intellectual pursuits. It also rejects the agonistic ideal of physical training; the body should be exercised only to the extent which health requires. But in demanding that man should live only for his body and his health, not deviating from this mode of life unless forced to do so in his struggle for existence, the physicians advocate an attitude toward life that in the fifth century was no longer fully acceptable.

At the turn of the fifth to the fourth century, however, the physicians' dietetic doctrine has already begun to alter; for the mode of life has undergone further changes and new conditions have thereby been created. As Diocles says, in the morning a healthy person should wake at a definite time before dawn, when the food which he has consumed on the previous day is more or less digested. The time of waking varies according to the age of the person and the season of the year. After waking, he should remain in bed briefly until the heaviness and inertia of sleep have completely left the body. He should then rise, rub his head and neck, anoint his body with oil, and wash his face and eyes with water; the teeth should be cleaned of the remnants of food, the nose and ears oiled. After thus grooming himself, a man should set about whatever he is obliged, or wishes, to do. The physician cannot regulate his day; it is determined by what he must do, or cares to do (Diocles Fragment 141). Thus, whereas formerly every activity that made it impossible for a man to live only for his body and his health seemed forced on him, it could now be thought of as a matter of choice. Such choice probably extends not only to gainful business but also to political activities and intellectual pursuits. Dietetics can no longer ignore the reality of these forms of existence which have almost completely displaced a life concerned only with the body. Yet, the person who is not obliged to work, or does not wish to work, can still live for the body alone, without other interests; and this he should do if he would remain healthy.

For the independent man it is most fitting, after rising and performing the prescribed grooming, that he first take a walk. Upon returning, it is good for him to give some attention to his household affairs and to make the necessary dispositions concerning them until it is time to undertake the more serious care of his body. For this, youths and men go to the gymnasium for training; older men go to a bathhouse, or likewise to the gymnasium, to anoint themselves. When this is done, a carefully selected meal is eaten at home, toward noon, after which a short nap in cool shade is beneficial, although there should be no draft. Upon waking, some attention can again be given to household matters. Next a walk is taken, then a rest, and one returns to the gymnasium. Immediately after the exercises, which take the entire afternoon, one takes a bath or anoints the body, and goes home to the evening meal shortly before sunset. At this meal, too, only dishes selected in accordance with definite rules are served. Following the evening meal, one either goes to bed immediately or takes another walk before lying down. One should then sleep until dawn in a particular position—the only healthy one—keeping feet and body warm (Diocles, Fragment 141). This régime, embracing not only the course of the day, as formerly, but waking and sleeping as well, is recommended for every free day; and the man whose time is always at his disposal is well-advised to continue to live by these precepts, with only slight changes in exercise and food to allow for seasonal differences.

Taking part in social gatherings appears to be impossible in this scheme of life; none but a man's private concerns seem to exist, and even for them there is only a brief time twice daily. But the man about whom the physician talks has, after all, nothing to do except live for his health. To the free and independent man, the physician is a guide who leads him as he would if he were sick, without paying attention to anything but his body. All other men, however, must do at least something for the sake of their health in whatever way is possible for busy people, if they are not to become ill through their own fault. In this sense, they too remain in the hands of the physician.

Medicine in Hellenistic times, like earlier medicine, is concerned with the dietetics of the healthy. Indeed, at this time the doctrine of health is considered to be not only as important as therapeutics; it seems to be even more important than healing the sick. It is, after all, better not to let people get sick than to cure their diseases; similarly, the helmsman of a ship will be more eager to reach port before encountering a storm than finally to arrive in port after being buffeted by the storm and enduring many perils (Erasistratus, in Galen, 14. 692 K.). But now, the way in which the physician seeks to regulate life can no longer be the same as in earlier times, even though one is still supposed to live completely for one's health. Although the palaestra remains important in Greek life, as it does also in the Hellenized states, one can no longer imagine the healthy man of leisure spending the entire day there. For most people have become educated and take part in the brisk literary and intellectual life of this period. Because of this development, there is less time for the care of the body. The physician thus has to allow the healthy man of leisure time to devote himself to things other than his body—to reading and studying. Besides, more and more the old, set forms of life are beginning to be forsaken. With the economic ruin of the Greek cities, men who can afford to pay attention to nothing but their health become rarer and rarer. The bustling activity of politics and officialdom in the great states occupies the individual more and more; he becomes more restless and his life is no longer restricted to the confines of his city. Like the merchant and the soldier, the scholar, the scientist, and the writer now have a recognized place in society. They too, the physician thinks, must do something for their health. The day's routines are still interwoven with health regulations; everyone still goes to the palaestra when he can, even if life is no longer governed by concern for the body alone.

The penetration of Roman views into the Greek cultural sphere also brings a change in dietetics. Roman life is a life of activity. In the country the Romans are occupied as farmers or with the management of their estates; in the city they are engaged in business and politics. Even though physical exercise and games for adults and youths are taken just as much for granted, there is no gymnasium to which young and old resort daily. For the Roman, therefore, both ancient Greek and Hellenistic dietetics would be useless. When, in the second century B.C., Greek medicine finally begins to find acceptance in Rome in spite of strong opposition, it is, at the outset, reshaped in accordance with the living conditions of the now leading nation, permitting gymnastic exercise to yield to natural exertion. It takes the position that the daily routine should be regulated only in so far as this is possible for active people. Yet at the same time the claim that the healthy man who is free to do so should live for his health alone remains valid in the theories of the medical schools, however remote this claim is from reality.

In only one doctrine—and this was perhaps in connection with a turning away of medicine from dogmatic concepts to pure observation—was the assimilation of Greek medicine to the new way of life accomplished in such a way that the healthy man was freed from all medical supervision: one cannot prescribe laws to a man who is healthy and master of his own time, nor is it necessary. He needs no physician; he needs only to vary his way of life. He should sometimes be in the country, sometimes in the city, often on his estate. He should travel by ship, hunt, rest sometimes, but more often exercise his body. Inactivity induces old age prematurely; exertion extends the period of youth. It is sometimes good for a man to take cold baths, sometimes hot ones; to anoint himself, and sometimes not to. He may eat whatever is offered and whatever others are eating. He may go to banquets when he wishes to, though occasionally he must avoid them. At times he may safely overeat, if at other times he eats no more than he can tolerate. Eating twice a day is better than once, and as long as he can digest the food, he should eat as much as he can. Such a life is right and healthy. On the other hand, all kinds of athletics and prescribed nutrition are superfluous, for such training would necessarily be interrupted by the citizen's daily obligations and this would be harmful, and the body, which is accustomed only to regular and selected nourishment, would grow old early and sicken easily. Only frail persons of precarious health must be more cautious and must try, at least by means of certain precautionary measures, to protect themselves—by sleeping long hours, by taking walks, by exercise, and a correct diet. To this group most townspeople and almost all intellectuals belong (Celsus, 1. 1–2). In this doctrine of early imperial times, the nervous care and rigid caution resulting from ancient dietetics give way to a free and easy assurance. The leisured class no longer participate in intellectual life, and they again indulge more in physical pastimes. But the authority which dietetics relinquishes on the one hand by releasing the healthy is gained on the other hand by narrowing the concept of health in that fewer people are considered to be truly healthy. And it should be remembered that this solution of the problem is only one of many: other physicians proceed differently, and, in fact, the healthy man still does not rid himself of the physician.

Dietetics in the first century after Christ even regulates the entire lifespan of the healthy, from childhood to old age. It lays down a system for educating the young in which physical exercises and exertions are established in the same way as are the intellectual requirements suitable to each age. The principle is defended that scolding and shouting are harmful in the instruction of the young, while friendliness and patience on the part of the teacher contribute to the health of the pupils (Athenaeus, in Oribasius 3. 162 Drbg.). There was no consideration of such problems at the beginning of dietetics although, to be sure, Hellenistic dietetics must have dealt with them. Since from youth onward the development of mental and physical powers goes together, and since the free, independent man should find pleasure in his mind as well as his body, health lies for every age in the full realization of the mental and physical capabilities peculiar to it; however, although a man at the height of his powers is able to cope with the equally strong demands of internal and external nature, the older man must abandon physical exertion more and more and must turn to intellectual and artistic interests. The most beautiful old age is enjoyed by those who distinguish themselves by their education and knowledge, intellectual interests, by abstention from material pleasures, and by the harmony of their soul; by those who always have time at their disposal, and who delight in what people before them and they themselves have accomplished. For, what better friends could the intelligent man find, or with whom would he rather live, than those with whose works he occupies himself? What a joy, what an elation, for the soul it is to reflect on the world in the company of the great men of the past—the great philosophers, physicians, and men of science—and constantly to engage in debate with them! (Athenaeus, in Oribasius 3. 165–8 Drbg.). In this dietetic system, which clearly harks back to tenets of Hellenistic dietetics, the old somatic determination of health has been completely discarded. Only personal and material independence retain their importance in this doctrine. And busy people can live only by approximately correct rules.

With the ever-increasing Hellenization of Roman life in the second century A.D., with the acceptance of the classical age as exemplary, the dietetics of the healthy is again determined by the ideal of the man who lives for his health alone. The best life is that of the completely independent man who possesses a faultless body. Next best is the life of the man whose body is not altogether healthy, but who is free. In third place is the life of the man who has a healthy body, but who has a position or engages in some kind of activity, whether of necessity or voluntarily, either for the sake of making money or of gratifying passions or ambition. The worst life is the one lived with a sick body, in servitude and dependency (Galen, *Hygiene* 2.1). As to content, this dietetics recognizes the cultivation of mind and body as proper. Living according to gymnastic rules is decidedly rejected, even though, at this time and indeed earlier, in the first century A.D., the gymnasium was finding greater acceptance in Rome, and even Romans attended. In late antiquity, however, the physician only repeats and practices what earlier centuries have discovered; nothing is changed in the fundamental belief that the healthy, as well as the sick, are under his direction and that they must continually be doing something for their health if they are to remain healthy.

Thus, physicians wish to direct the life of the healthy individual with only his health in mind—or at least as far as this is possible. They have him withdraw from all activity that is not absolutely essential; they seek to involve him in a completely regimented life. In this way, they render him not only dependent, but virtually sick; he is well only if he lives a perfectly regular life. They increase his hypochondria still more by determining the effect of particular kinds of exertion and foods and, correspondingly, demanding a different combination of diet and exercise for each individual at all times of the day. Thus, chiefly by experience, but also by analogy and through rational deliberation, they evolved an extremely refined doctrine of nutrition. A distinction is made not only between the different qualities and effects of grains and fruits, meat and fish, wine and water; each of these categories is further broken down into particular kinds of food. Each of the various grains has its particular effect: wheat influences the body differently from barley. The same is true of the various kinds of meat, fish, wine, and the different qualities of water. With regard to grain, the soil on which it grows is significant; with regard to vegetables, it matters whether wild herbs or garden vegetables are being considered. Not only do the meats of different kinds of animals vary in effect, but there is a difference between the meat of wild and domesticated animals; what the wild animals feed on is important; and in the case of domesticated animals, it matters whether they are reared in the woods, in pastures, or in stables. Different parts of the animal benefit the human organism in different ways. Fishes vary not only according to their kinds and parts, but also according to whether they live in water that is swampy or clear, running or stagnant. Red and white wines—wines that are sweet or dry, or new or old; spring water, swamp water, rain water, and melted snow, all have different effects. Finally, attention is also given to the

311

effect of preparation on the nutritional value of foodstuffs. The distinctions made are sometimes exaggerated, but they provide an exact determination of the right food for every individual, at a given moment, according to his nature, age, sex, and the season.

In the same way, exertions and their effects are differentiated and investigated in detail so that a decision may be made as to which are beneficial and which should be avoided if the individual is not to become sick. Seeing and hearing, speaking and thinking, are considered natural exertions. They, too, influence the body—can harm it—and their injurious effects must therefore be combated; but used correctly, these faculties can be salutary. Thinking is as much an exercise for the soul as is walking for the body. Insomnia produces a different bodily condition from sleep; work affects the body differently from rest. Thus one should live a varied life and strive to balance even the natural bodily reactions. All sexual functions are exactly defined as to their influence on the organism, and a special regimen protects against their harmful consequences. Walking and the various forms of running count as exertions which, though natural, are nevertheless somewhat forced. Walks have a different effect according to the time of day at which they are taken, whether in the early morning, before or after meals, or before or after the gymnastic exercises. One may also walk at night and such walks make one slender. For some people, level paths are best; for others, paths which climb to a greater or lesser degree are recommended. All kinds of gymnastics and the various sports count as strenuous exercise, which can have a curative effect, depending on the individual's age, state of health, sex, and the time of year. At any rate, those who wish to remain healthy should participate in such activities only in accordance with these considerations. At a later period, certain bodily activities which in themselves constitute labor for men, such as digging, are used as therapeutic aids; and for women, housework and the supervision of maids are means for keeping healthy and vigorous.

Food and exertion are thus defined in detail as to their effect on health. They form the basis of the dietetic regulations which the physician prescribes for the healthy. A few remedies are added and these, again, are to be used according to the constitution of the individual, his age and sex, and the seasons of the year, in order to create a balance among the materials constituting the body. These remedies include baths, purgatives, enemas, friction, and anointing the body. But considerations of health should also influence the construction of the house in which one lives. The house should be built with a particular exposure in relation to the sun, or, if possible, one room should face in each direction so that one may live in different rooms at different times of the year; and indeed, according to the daily weather. Exposure to winds is considered; and attempts are even made to influence the planning of cities by hygienic considerations. The position of a city is important for the health of the inhabitants and for the kind of life they must lead. These stipulations, however, are of minor importance. What is decisive for dietetics for the healthy is the regulation of food and exertion, which must be, in so far as possible, different for each person and must take into account the wide differences in the effect of foods and various kinds of exercise.

In seeking to regulate diet, exertion, and even living conditions in so complicated a manner, the physician rendered man's health still more precarious than it must already have become by reason of his strictly ordered life. For not only a breach of regularity as such, but even the slightest deviation from one of these innumerable rules, was considered injurious to health. Since, however, the health regulation which the physician sought to impose made man a stranger to all activity and almost sickly because he did not dare deviate from a strict regimen, opposition was bound to arise. Those who took a positive attitude toward state and politics, toward literature and science, were as much bound to object as were the philosophers who rejected a life governed only by the laws of the body. There had already been opposition to the old gymnastics on the ground that its rules weakened men and left them no time for other interests; the attack was made in the conviction that the mind is more important than the body. This criticism of the gymnastic and agonistic ideal was transferred to medicine and to the ideal of life it projected. Plato expressed this in classical and final form in his discussion of the kind of medicine that cures the patient by reorganizing his way of life: In a truly well-ordered state, a certain occupation falls to everyone's lot, and in this he must of necessity engage; no one can afford to spend his life as an invalid, which is what happens when a man devotes himself entirely to health. In the case of the workman, one would laugh if this truth were questioned; in the case of the rich—those who seem to be the most fortunate—we are unaware of it (*Republic* 3. 406 c). All ages iterated this criticism of medicine. The grounds on which it was made changed; they were at times the joy of life and its pleasures. But the basic opposition to the demands of the physician remained.

Nevertheless, medicine held fast to the same ideal in every century and continued to require of men that they live, as far as possible, for their health. No criticism, or resistance, was able to overcome this ideal. The physician would not have persisted in his attempt to subordinate daily life to his authority—would not have fought for the right to regulate men's lives—if his demands had not, in some way, corresponded to men's feelings and needs. Were this not so, he would not have succeeded in controlling the life of the healthy individual by means of health regulations to a much greater degree than in modern times, when the healthy are almost completely emancipated from medical supervision. And that the physician enjoyed such success one must conclude from the fact that physicians continued to write on dietetics; this literature and the medical effort it embodies would otherwise be meaningless. The essence and prestige of the dietetics of the healthy in the final analysis rest on the value which ancient man attached to health. He consciously regarded health as a good—indeed as the greatest of all goods, at least of all external goods. For this reason he was willing to make an effort to maintain his health; of his own volition he sought out someone who could help him in this effort and placed himself under his orders. Poems and sayings of the post-Homeric period already evidence—along with a melancholy judgment of life, with doubt as to its worth—an almost exaggerated esteem for health, even above beauty, wealth, and inner nobility. Whereas in the epics man had prayed to the gods for fame above all, and also, later, for long life and a painless death, now the dominant wish was to be healthy; for without health all is as nothing. The physicians made this their philosophy when, turning to dietetics, they wished to prove its necessity; and they held fast to this tenet throughout all centuries: Without health nothing avails, neither money, nor any other thing (Hippocrates, *On regimen* 6. 604 L.). In the absence of health, wisdom cannot manifest itself; art cannot be revealed; there is no vigor to take up the fight; wealth is useless, the intellect ineffective (Herophilus, in Sextus Empiricus, *Adversus mathematicos* 11. 50). He who for the sake of ambition or passion chooses an active life, leaving himself little time for the care of his body, chooses to serve bad masters. Only the man who is completely free, by reason of fate or choice, can be shown how to live in health, how he may seldom fall ill, and how best to grow old (Galen, *Hygiene* 2.1). No one should voluntarily relinquish the possibility of living entirely for his health, for it is the highest of external goods. Almost all men who live the practical life acknowledge the justice of this evaluation, and not a few poets and writers agree with it (Sextus, *Adversus mathematicos* 11.49). In addition, it may be that at that time the fear of pain was greater and the reaction to it more primitive, and that people were therefore more anxious to prevent sickness. Besides, the belief in the superiority of the physically strong and the contempt for the weak and the sick, which had not yet been entirely overcome by the belief in intellectual superiority, must have strengthened the wish to be healthy. Furthermore, there was as yet no idea of vocation; within the social structure the heaviest physical labor was the lot of the slave; therefore, every free man had the opportunity to care for his body in ways which far exceeded what the active professional man can do for his health today. Finally, life was simpler than it is today, not as far removed from nature and the body. The development and value of dietetics were based on all these circumstances, and the physician succeeded in regulating life from the point of view of health without having to go from case to case, prescribing a way of life for each. He wrote books on diet for the laity from which everyone could learn for himself what was good for him. Thus, even though the rich man might have a physician constantly in his entourage, he was not obliged to ask the physician how he should live. Indeed, a man should know, learn for himself, what he needs: there is in fact no moment of the day or night in which he should not know what to do for the sake of his health. In walking and sitting, in taking baths and anointing himself, in eating and drinking, in sleeping and waking,— in every action and in all circumstances—he needs the counsel of medicine in order to live rightly and without injury to himself; yet to ask the physician about every detail is tiring, if not impossible (Athenaeus, in Oribasius 3. 164 Drbg.).

Nor was this general evaluation of health fundamentally altered by the philosophical systems. It is true that from the fourth century B.C. onward, these systems considered intellectual qualities to be the highest value; yet the value of health is never overlooked but is expressly recognized, as could never be the case in any modern philosophy except, perhaps, in a purely materialistic one. To the Socratics, health of the body is an aid to, and condition for, the right life of the soul. Academic and Peripatetic ethics considers it a good, although not the highest good; for each good must be assigned its particular place and value (Sextus, *Adversus mathematicos* 11.51). The Stoic tries to rely on himself and strives to be independent of all external matters, but at least he considers health to be desirable for the man who knows how to live rightly, even though health has no value in itself. That the Epicurean desires to be healthy is obvious: with regard to diseases, he consoles himself with the thought that the worst pains will soon end with death, that moderate pains often abate for a time, worse ones can be endured or done away with voluntarily, by suicide (Epicurus, Fragment 397). Only late, in about the third century A.D., does ancient philosophy turn toward the concept of inner life through which man is so alienated from the corporeal—or at least rendered so indifferent to it—that he neglects health together with physical, material values. Philosophy itself symbolizes the difference between the ancient and modern concepts of the value of health—and thereby of dietetics—by comparing the task of philosophy with the task of medicine. Error is a disease of the soul; true knowledge cures it. The philosopher therefore does for the soul what the physician does for the body. And as the healthy man is in need of the physician to remain healthy—or must be his own physician—every man needs philosophy, or must himself be a philosopher, to live rightly.

The value of health for the ancients thus remained constant throughout all periods. That is why medicine was able to make the same demands again and again on the healthy man's way of life, and why, despite all criticism, these demands were to a great extent met. Its doctrine—so much at variance with modern views—corresponds to a feeling for the body which the ancients never lost.

PART THREE

THE PROFESSIONAL ETHICS OF THE
GREEK PHYSICIAN*, [1]

Illiam Osler, for whom this lecture in the history of medicine is named, has many claims to fame. None is greater, I venture to think, than that, in the midst of a busy life devoted to the bodily welfare of man, he never for one moment forgot about man's intellectual and moral aspirations. An unexamined life, to use a phrase of Plato, he found not worth living. The physician and scientist turned historian, even philosopher, because he wanted to understand the meaning of human existence. And once he had made his own decision, he also felt impelled to speak out in advocacy of the "Way of Life" he thought he had discovered.

To his truly humanistic teaching—namely that the task and the dignity of the human being consist in the individual's willingness to live up to an ideal and to be of help to others—Osler finally gave expression in categories of William James' pragmatism, the philosophy that gained ascendancy in his later years. On the other hand, he was quite aware of the fact that his creed was not of today or yesterday, but took its origin and was put into practice long ago. When formulating his basic tenets for the last time, he characterizes as the heritage of Plato and as "the Greek message to modern democracy" that "need for individual reconstruction" with which "is blended the note of individual service to the community." At the same time, he pointed out that such an idealism once existed in Greece even in the daily pursuits of men of action. For to the ancient physician "the love of humanity

* Bulletin of the History of Medicine, 1956, vol. 30, pp. 391–419.
[1] The William Osler Lecture in the History of Medicine, Faculty of Medicine, McGill University. This lecture was given in the Amphitheatre of the Montreal General Hospital on December 9, 1955. It is here printed in a somewhat extended form, though substantially unchanged. I have added some footnotes referring to the pertinent literature and giving fuller documentation concerning certain points than was possible in the lecture.

[was] associated with the love of his craft—*philanthropia* and *philotech-nia*—the joy of working joined in each one to a true love of his brother."[2]

It is this appreciation of the humanism of the Greek doctor on the part of the humanist Osler that determined me to choose as my topic the professional ethics of the Greek physician. No other subject within my reach seemed more appropriate for a lecture in his memory. I wish to outline the various ethical positions taken by ancient physicians. In particular, it will be my aim to find out when and where the idea origi-nated that medicine itself imposes certain obligations upon the physi-cian, obligations summed up in the magic phrase "love of humanity." For, in my opinion, this lofty ideal was not the only one in antiquity that motivated the help proffered by medical men to those who suffer and are in distress. Over a long period of time other concepts of medi-cine and therefore other obligations and duties were held in high es-teem. Rome was not built in one day.

Now at first glance it may seem as if such a contention were in fact quite unwarranted. For is it not in one of the Hippocratic writings, the essay called *Precepts*, that the statement occurs which Osler quoted: "Where there is love of man, there is also love of the art" (ch. 6)? Is it not said in another Hippocratic book, the treatise *On the Physician*, that the doctor must be a "lover of man" (ch. 1)? And does not Galen, no mean judge in these matters, expressly assert that Hippocrates, Empedocles, Diocles, and not a few of the other early physicians healed the sick because of their love of mankind (*De Placitis Hippocratis et Platonis*, ed. I. Müller, p. 765)? In the classical age of Greek civiliza-tion, then, the ethic of philanthropy seems already to have been se-curely established.

But if one scrutinizes carefully the context in which the word "philanthropy" appears in the so-called Hippocratic writings just men-tioned, he realizes that it means no more than a certain friendliness of disposition, a kindliness, as opposed to any misanthropic attitude. A "philanthropic" doctor in the sense in which the term is used in the treatise *On the Physician* (ch. 1) will comport himself in a dignified manner; for aggressiveness and obtrusiveness are despicable; sour looks, harshness, arrogance, vulgarity, are disagreeable.[3] Likewise, the Hippo-

---

[2] *The Old Humanities and the New Science*, 1920, p. 62 f. For Osler's humanism and his adherence to James' pragmatism, cf L. Edelstein, "William Osler's Philoso-phy," *Bull. Hist. Med. 20*, 1946, pp. 280 ff.

[3] U. Fleischer, *Untersuchungen zu den pseudohippokratischen Schriften*

cratic *Precepts* (ch. 6) understands by the doctor's "philanthropy" his kindheartedness and his willingness to accommodate his fees to the patient's circumstances. He should also treat strangers and paupers, even if they are unable to pay him. That is, he should be charitable, recalling some of the benefits which he may have received himself in the past, or thinking of the good name that his charitableness is likely to make for him in the future. If he acts thus, if such "philanthropy" is present on his part, then also "love of the (medical) art" will be kindled in his patients, a state of mind that greatly contributes to their speedy recovery, especially when they are dangerously sick. No more—and no less—is implied by the famous aphorism: "Where there is love of man, there is also love of the art."[4]

"Philanthropy," then, in the two Hippocratic treatises designates a proper behavior toward those with whom the physician comes in con-

---

Παραγγελίαι, Περὶ ἰητροῦ *und* Περὶ εὐσχημοσύνης (Neue Deutsche Forschungen, Abt. Klass. Philologie), 1939, pp. 1; 54, seems to take φιλάνθρωπος to refer to "love of mankind." Yet Jones is surely right in translating the word as "kind to all," and μισάνθρωπος, the term contrasted with it immediately afterward, as "unkind" (*Hippocrates*, II, pp. 311; 313 [Loeb Classical Library]; cf. also E. Littré, *Oeuvres complètes d'Hippocrate*, vol. 9, 1861, pp. 205–7: *humain—dur*).

[4] The usual interpretation, "where there is love of man (on the part of the physician), there is also love of the art (on his part)," is refuted by the immediately following words: "For some patients, though conscious that their condition is perilous, recover their health simply through their contentment with the goodness of the physician." The previous sentence then must contain an assertion as to the patients' attitude, and it can only be "love of the art" felt by them in consequence of the doctor's philanthropy, contentment with the goodness of the physician, of which the author is speaking. In his opinion the question of fees discussed in ch. 6 has psychologically important consequences for the recovery of the sick. If the doctor is reasonable in his charges, or even willing to undertake the treatment without compensation, he creates an atmosphere of confidence that is helpful for the restoration of health. In the same spirit the writer, in an earlier chapter (4), has warned against discussing fees at the beginning of the cure because worry regarding fees is "harmful to a troubled patient, particularly if the disease is acute." Fleischer, *op. cit.*, p. 38, has clearly seen that the sequence of the statements made in chapter 6 points to the meaning: "wenn der Arzt Menschenfreund ist, sind die Menschen Freunde seiner Kunst." Nevertheless he tries to save the common interpretation, believing that the term "love of the art" is more often predicated of the representative of the art and that the latter's "wish for knowledge" forms the starting point of the discussion. But the context is quite a different one, as I have tried to show in the text. Nor is it "love of mankind" that is here made "the motive of medical practice." In *Precepts* too the author speaks of "love of man," having warned at the beginning of the chapter against "disdain of man" (ἀπανθρωπίη, "not to be unkind," Jones, *op. cit.*, I, p. 319; *âpreté*, Littré, *op. cit.*, vol. 9, p. 259). "Philanthropy" then appears here in exactly the same contrast as in the treatise *On the Physician*.

tact during treatment; it is viewed as a minor social virtue, so to say. And it was indeed in this way that the word, which later came to have such an exalted connotation, was commonly understood in the classical age and far down into the Hellenistic era.[5] Moreover, according to recent investigations, the book *On the Physician* was composed at the earliest between 350 and 300 B.C. *Precepts* cannot have been written before the first century B.C. or A.D. Neither the one nor the other treatise provides evidence for the ethics of the early Greek physician.[6] I trust that Osler, the scholar, would forgive me for dissenting from him in a question of interpretation and of chronology in which he followed the opinion of his time. I am sure he would not have wished me to put acceptance of authority before acceptance of the results of continued research.

As for Galen and his verdict, far be it from me to deny that even in the classical period there may have been men who dedicated themselves to medicine out of an instinctive compassion for the sufferings of their fellow men. But to assume that such a feeling, made conscious and, under whatever name, elevated to an ideal, could have extended to all mankind, would be the unhistorical projection of later concepts into an age entirely ignorant of them. To be sure, some of the Sophists taught that by nature all human beings—free, slave, and barbarian—are equal. The adherents of the rising enlightenment questioned existing conditions and extolled a natural or divine law of morality over the changing demands of the day. However, the time had not yet come to think in terms of obligations toward humanity.[7]

[5] The word φιλάνθρωπος originally was used only of gods and kings to denote their benevolent attitude toward men, i.e., toward their inferiors (or of animals who are friendly toward men). From the second half of the fourth century B.C. it began to be applied more generally and to be interpreted as kindliness and friendliness of individuals in their social contacts (cf. S. Lorenz, *De progressu notionis φιλανθρωπίας*, Diss. Leipzig, 1914, pp. 8 ff.; 14 ff.; 19 ff.; also J. Heinemann, *s. v.* "Humanismus," *Realencyclopädie der classischen Altertumswissenschaft*, Supplementband 5, 1931, col. 298). The contrast φιλάνθρωπος—μισάνθρωπος is usual in the fourth century (Lorenz, p. 25 f.); for the Peripatetic and Stoic interpretations of the term φιλανθρωπία as kindness, which is reflected in the Hippocratic respective treatises, cf. below, notes 19 and 20.

[6] For the late date of *On the Physician* and *Precepts* in general, cf. now Fleischer, *passim*, and below, notes 19, 20.

[7] W. W. Tarn, "Alexander, Cynics and Stoics," *Amer. Journ. Philol.*, *60*, 1939, p. 44, rightly says that even the cosmopolitanism of the fourth-century Cynics has nothing to do "with any belief in the unity of mankind or a human brotherhood." It is a negative rather than a positive creed (cf. also Heinemann, *loc. cit.*, col. 291).

Most important, those treatises of the *Corpus Hippocraticum* which were written during the fifth and fourth centuries B.C. and reflect the situation then prevailing, show clearly, I suggest, that even the best among the physicians were not concerned at all with such considerations as Galen imputes to them. Their ethics was not one of the heart or of inner intention. It was shaped by rather different values.

For the early Hippocratic books are concerned exclusively with a body of rules prescribing a certain behavior during the physician's working hours, with medical etiquette, one might say. It is explained how the doctor's office—his *iatreion*—should be set up, how it should or should not be equipped. Bedside manners are discussed, the right way to enter a sick room, to converse with the patient; whether or not to give a prognosis of the outcome of the disease if there is danger of a fatal issue. The surgeon is admonished not to make a show of the application of bandages or of operations, since to do what is proper is preferable to indulging in the mere display of one's dexterity. It is urged that a treatment once started should be completed, and that the physician should not withdraw his help from the sick so as to avoid blame or other unwelcome consequences.[8]

Such injunctions, and many more that could be cited, are dictated by the wish to uphold a certain standard of performance and serve to distinguish the expert from the charlatan. From Homeric times the physician had been an itinerant craftsman; even in the classical age, few physicians stayed in the cities of their birth or took up permanent residence elsewhere. Living here today, there tomorrow, they were not subject to the ordinary social strictures and pressures which result from

---

And the same holds true of the advocacy of the equality and kinship of men by Hippias and others (cf. Heinemann, *ibid.*, col. 287), or the "cosmopolitanism" to be found in Democritus and Euripides (cf. W. Nestle, *Vom Mythos zum Logos*, 1942², p. 380 f.). Lorenz' attempt to show that at least in the philosophical language of the fourth century philanthropy had the wider sense which it had later on (*op. cit.*, pp. 35 ff.), is refuted by the testimonies themselves. Still in Aristotle φιλανθρωπία is but an emotion, an instinctive feeling of friendliness and kinship that exists between men as members of the same species, just as animals of the same race feel akin to one another (cf. J. Burnet, *The Ethics of Aristotle*, 199, *ad* 1155 a 16 ff.; also H. v. Arnim, *Arius Didymus' Abriss der peripatetischen Ethik*, Sitzungsber. Wien, philos. hist. Kl., 204, No. 3, 1926, p. 107).

[8] For a more detailed picture of the rules of behavior, cf. L. Edelstein, Περὶ ἀέρων *und die Sammlung der Hippokratischen Schriften* (Problemata, 4), 1931, pp. 93 ff. [90* ff.] (this will be quoted as *Problemata*). Cf. also W. H. S. Jones, *Hippocrates*, II, Introductory Essay V.

323

the integration of the crafts into a community, and which tend to insure the reliability of the workmen. Besides, no medical schools existed; training was not required, everybody was free to practice medicine, the state did not issue any license. Under these circumstances abuses abounded and went unpunished. They could be prevented only by the individual's decision to make himself responsible before the bar of his own conscience, the conscience of a good craftsman, and this responsibility he assumed by the adoption of a strict etiquette. A great achievement indeed! For not only did the physician thus voluntarily establish a set of values governing sound treatment, he also gave, so to say, a personal pledge of safety to his patients, badly needed in a world that knew of no other protection for them.[9]

Yet at no point does the Hippocratic physician aim farther. Medicine to him is but the proper application of his knowledge to the treatment of diseases. "The medical art," it is maintained in one of the rare expositions of the character of medicine to be found in the *Corpus Hippocraticum*, "has to consider three factors, the disease, the patient, the physician. The physician is the servant of his art, and the patient must cooperate with the doctor in combatting the disease" (*Epidemics*, I, 11). In other words, it is the sole purpose of the good physician to achieve the objective of his art, to save his patient from the threat of death, if possible; to help him, or at least not to harm him, as the famous saying has it (*ibid.*). His ethic consists in doing his task well, in perfecting his skill; it is an ethic of outward achievement rather than of inner intention.[10]

As for the physician's motives in practicing medicine, he was engaged in it in order to make a living. Nor was there any conflict between his pecuniary interests and the exigencies of craftsmanship, as long as he remembered that love of money, of easy success, should not induce him to act without regard for the benefit of the patient, or, to speak with

[9] The term used by the true physician in setting himself apart from the charlatan is that of "expertness," which is at the same time "goodness" (ἀνδραγαθικώτερον καὶ τεχνικώτερον); cf. e.g., *Hippocratis Opera*, ed. H. Kuehlewein, II, 1902, pp. 236, 18–237, 1; and in general, *Problemata*, pp. 95–98 [92*–95*]. For the lack of supervision of the medical art on the part of civil authorities, cf. *ibid.*, p. 89 f. [87*].

[10] Here I am concerned only with the ideal of medical practice, as it emerges from the Hippocratic writings. How far reality could fall behind this ideal, how far the ancient physician could deviate from strictly medical considerations in order to attract patients, I have tried to show in *Problemata*, chs. 2 and 3 [65* ff. and 87* ff.].

Ruskin, that the good workman rarely thinks first of his pay, and that the knack of getting well paid does not always go with the ability to do the work well. If he learned to forget personal advantage for the sake of doing the right thing, he had, in his opinion, done all that was necessary.[11]

And society fully approved of such an attitude, as follows with certainty from a memorable passage in the first book of Plato's *Republic* (340 C ff.). The question there debated is whether self-interest is at the root of all human endeavor and therefore also of political activity. Parallels from the various arts, and especially the comparison with medicine, are used in order to decide the issue. The physician in the precise sense of the term is not a money maker or an earner of fees, Socrates holds, but a healer of the sick (341 C), just as it may be said of all the other arts that they were invented not for the sake of personal advantage, but rather for the purpose of performing a service, and most effectively at that. Medicine itself therefore has no concern for the advantage of medicine or of the physician, but only for that of the patient and his bodily welfare (342 C). Like every art, *qua* art, it looks out for the good of that which is its object. And when Socrates is asked rather mockingly: "Is this true of the shepherd also? Does he too have the good of his flock in mind?" (343 A ff.), he answers emphatically: "*qua* shepherd, yes." The fact that he sells the wool and makes money by so doing is not an intrinsic property of the art of shepherding; it belongs to another art, that of money making. For "if we are to consider it 'precisely' medicine produces health but the fee-earning art the pay, and architecture a house but the fee-earning art accompanying it the fee, and so with all the others, each performs its own task and benefits that over which it is set" (346 D). Yet the subsidiary art of fee earning cannot be entirely separated from the art producing health. "Unless pay is added to it," there would be no benefit for the craftsman, and consequently he would be unwilling to go to the trouble of taking care of the troubles of others. This is why everybody expects to make money with his craft, and why pay must be provided by those who benefit

---

[11] That the competent Hippocratic physician was willing to forego momentary success and easy gain follows e.g., from the surgical writings (cf. *Hippocratis Opera*, ed. Kuehlewein, II, pp. 168, 3 ff.; 175, 8 ff.; *Problemata*, pp. 97–99 [94*ff.], where I should not have quoted however a passage from the later *Precepts*.) The Ruskin quotation I have borrowed from P. Shorey (*Plato, The Republic*, I, [Loeb], ad 346 A).

from the craft. Otherwise the self-interest of the craftsman would not be satisfied (346 E–347 A).

All the interlocutors in the dialogue agree on this conclusion—and I think none of their contemporaries would have gainsaid their admission: the artisan has fulfilled his duty if he is intent primarily upon the aim of his art—that is, in the case of medicine, upon restoring health to the body—and thinks of his income afterward. No other obligations are incumbent upon him, no other personal qualities are demanded of him.[12] It is also clear that in the society of the fifth and fourth centuries, medicine is a craft like all the others and in no way differentiated from them. Completely free of any idealization of work as such, and considering it a dire necessity rather than an ennobling activity, the classical age judged all manual labor only by the standard of expertness and performance. What can, properly speaking, be called morality, it found realized in man's private life, and preeminently in his life as a citizen. Even medicine, therefore, remained impervious to moral considerations.[13]

But at this point your patience with my argument should be exhausted, and I must face the objection which no doubt will have been on your minds for some time: how does all this square with the content of the Hippocratic *Oath*? Certainly, the *Oath* prescribes a most refined personal ethics for the physician. It enjoins upon him a life pleasing to gods and men, a life almost saintly and bound by the strictest rules of purity and holiness. It makes him renounce all intentional injustice or

[12] In the Platonic passage referred to Socrates argues according to the beliefs generally held; the passage therefore is especially illuminating for the common attitude toward the crafts. Aristotle too maintains that the function of medicine is that of causing health, not of producing wealth (*Politics*, 1258 a 10 ff.), though by some it is wrongly turned into mere money making, as if this were the aim of medicine (*ibid.*). From the point of view of economic theory, medicine belongs to that "art of acquisition" which deals with exchange, and is "labor for hire" (μισθαρνία 1258 b 25).

[13] That the classical age did not know of the concept of "professions" but ranged the artist, the physician, and others with the common workmen or craftsmen (τεχνῖται) has been emphasized especially by A. E. Zimmern, *The Greek Commonwealth*, 1915², pp. 257 ff. For the contrast between the classical attitude toward work and the modern concept of the "nobility of toil," cf. H. Michell, *The Economics of Ancient Greece*, 1940, p. 14. It is because of the facts referred to that I cannot agree with W. Müri's statement that the Hippocratic physician is the "Vertreter des Standes" and as such "in seinem Auftreten nicht mehr ganz frei" (*Arzt und Patient bei Hippokrates*, Beilage z. Jahresber. über d. städt. Gymnasium in Bern, 1936, p. 35). W. A. Heidel's chapter on the medical profession (*Hippocratic Medicine*, 1941, pp. 26–39) also is vitiated by his failure to consider the particular social and moral values prevailing in the world in which the Hippocratic "doctor" practiced.

mischief. Here a morality of the highest order is infused into medical practice. Have not centuries upon centuries seen in the Hippocratic *Oath* the prototype of all medical ethics?

I trust that I am second to none in my appreciation of this document. Yet its picture of the true physician is evidence not of the thought of the classical era which I have so far considered, but of a movement which started in the latter part of the fourth century B.C.—the time when the *Oath* was composed—and extended through the Hellenistic period down to the time of Galen. Through it, the ethics of the medical craftsman was reshaped in accordance with the various systems of philosophy. The new standards characteristic of the second stage in the development of ancient medical ethics originated in a revaluation of the arts and crafts and in the transformation of the medical craft into a scientific pursuit.

To speak first of the change in attitude toward the crafts, Aristotle already raised the problem "whether artisans too ought not to have goodness, seeing that they often fall short of their duties through intemperance." But he decided that unlike the slave who is subject to "unlimited servitude," the artisan is subject only to "limited servitude," namely the performance of his particular job, and therefore is obligated only to do his task; his moral goodness is his own affair (*Politics*, 1260 a 36–b2; cf. *Nic. Eth.*, 1105 a 26 ff.). The so-called Pythagoreans of Aristotle's time, however, insisted on the moral implications of workmanship and considered it, if not a "noble toil" in the modern sense of the term, at least a matter of moral concern. They even claimed that "the good" could be achieved especially well through the crafts.[14] In Hellenistic philosophy such a belief became more widespread. Aristotle's successors distinguished the "happy life" and the "good life"—the one presupposing independent means, the other to be led by him who has

[14] The attitude of the Pythagoreans of the late fourth century toward the crafts I have discussed in *The Hippocratic Oath*, 1943, p. 60 [59*]. Their views are the more significant since, generally speaking, the fifth and fourth centuries considered the workman not only déclassé, but evinced a definite prejudice against him, contrary to the pre-classical generations, a prejudice to be found in aristocratic and democratic societies alike (cf. Michell, *op. cit.*, pp. 11 ff.; also M. Pohlenz, "Die Lebensformen, Arbeit und Erwerb" in *Der Hellenische Mensch*, ch. XIII, pp. 357 ff. That an exception was made in regard to the physician [*ibid.*, p. 359] is not attested). Among the few who at least maintained that for the poor it is shameful to remain idle rather than to work was the "historical" Socrates (cf. Pohlenz, *ibid.*, p. 358), whose teaching seems to have been important also for the development of a concept of professional ethics. Cf. below, note 39.

327

to have an occupation. In both, man is asked to fulfill the moral law. Finally, the Stoa recognized the acquisition of money through any kind of work as compatible with the moral order and taught that in whatever station in life one may find oneself, one can and must live up to the rules of ethics.[15] Such an entirely new appraisal of the crafts surely was facilitated by the fact that virtue or morality was increasingly identified not with the objective content of human actions, but rather with the inner attitude of the human agent. The principal criterion of right or wrong came to be found almost exclusively in the proper use of things, good, bad, or indifferent, rather than in the things themselves.[16]

Now, once it was realized that the craftsman can partake in virtue, the narrow limitations of the old ethics of good craftsmanship were swept aside. The moral issues latent in the pursuit of medicine, which the classical age had either failed to see, or failed to emphasize, were brought out into the open. The so-called deontological writings of the *Corpus Hippocraticum*, the *Oath*, the treatises *On the Physician*, *Precepts*,

---

[15] The Stoic philosophy of work, as it was formulated by Chrysippus, has been most adequately interpreted by A. Bonhöffer, *Die Ethik des Stoikers Epictet*, 1894, "Exkurs" IV, pp. 233 ff. For the importance of Stoic theories of the second and first centuries A.D. with regard to medical ethics, cf. below, pp. 340 ff. The Peripatetic doctrine concerning the life of the ordinary citizen and the art of acquisition is attested by Stobaeus (*Eclogae*, II, pp. 143, 24 ff.; 149, 21–23, ed. Wachsmuth, and Arnim, *op. cit.*, p. 90). I need not enter here into a discussion of the question whether the system outlined in Stobaeus can be traced altogether to Theophrastus (cf. Arnim, *op. cit.*, pp. 83 ff.), or whether it is influenced at least in part by Stoicism (R. Walzer, *Magna Moralia und Aristotelische Ethik* [Neue Philol. Unters., VII], 1929, p. 191 f.; also O. Regenbogen, *s. v.* "Theophrastos," *Realencycl.*, Suppl. VII, cols. 1492–94). However, it is important to note that the verdict of Aristotle's *Politics*, according to which workmanship may be noble or ignoble depending on how much or how little virtue it requires as an accessory (1258 b 38 f.), must be considered an interpolation along the lines of later Peripatetic ethics. For it is in contradiction to Aristotle's general position. That the sentence in question is an addition has been suspected for other reasons by W. L. Newman, *The Politics of Aristotle*, II, 1887, p. 203; the whole chapter in which the statement occurs differs in many respects from the rest of the text, cf. E. Barker, *The Politics of Aristotle*, 1946, p. 29, note 3.

[16] I should mention at least that at the turn of the fourth to the third century economic theory also began to consider the crafts in a new light. The Ps. Platonic dialogue *Eryxias* discussing the relation between wealth and virtue (393 A) entertains the notion that the crafts are not barter or "limited service," as Aristotle held (cf. above, note 12), but rather are to be classified under possession of wealth, and are thus more noble. The "expert pilot" and the "skilled physician" are the examples adduced (394 E); cf. M. L. W. Laistner, *Greek Economics*, 1923, p. xxviii f. The right, that is, the moral use of such "wealth" of practical skill forms the subject of a considerable part of the conversation reported in this dialogue, the only extant Greek treatise which deals exclusively with economic problems.

and *On Decorum*—the three latter composed in Hellenistic times, if not at the beginning of the Christian era—take up the various questions concerning medical ethics and try to give an answer to them from different philosophical points of view.[17]

Does not the practice of medicine involve the physician in the most intimate contact with other human beings? Is he not sometimes called upon to make decisions that reach far beyond the mere application of technical knowledge and skill? In the Hippocratic *Oath* that responsibility which is peculiarly the doctor's is defined in agreement with the way of life instituted by Pythagoras.[18] And what about the patient who is putting himself and "his all" into the hands of the physician? How can he be sure that he may have trust in the doctor, not only in his knowledge, but also in the man himself? Such confidence, according to the book *On the Physician*, can be aroused only if the physician asks himself what he should be like "in regard to his soul." Consequently the author of this treatise—perhaps the oldest known "introduction to medicine" which is posterior to the *Oath* by approximately two or three generations—prescribes for "the soul" of the physician self-control, regularity of habits, justness and fairness, a proper and good behavior, in short, all the virtues of the "gentleman." It is the doctrine of the Aristotelian school, I think, which is here adapted to medicine.[19]

Again, in the *Precepts* and in the book *On Decorum* it is the Stoic outlook which predominates. In the former treatise, gentleness and kindheartedness are commended. The physician ought to be charitable, especially toward him who is a stranger and in financial straits (ch. 6).

---

[17] The following analysis of the deontological writings, which go into minute details of medical practice, is not intended to be exhaustive. I shall simply consider a number of salient features that within the context of my discussion seem to characterize the teaching of these essays.

[18] For the Pythagorean origin of the *Oath* and its date, cf. Edelstein, *The Hippocratic Oath*, especially p. 59 f. [58* f.].

[19] Fleischer's dating of the treatise *On the Physician* in the third century (*op. cit.*, p. 56 f.) seems convincing to me. (H. Diller, *Gnomon*, *17*, 1941, p. 30, thinks it unlikely that the book was written after 300 B.C.). The short summary of ethics given by the "Hippocratic" author is usually related to the protreptic-paraenetic literature of the time (cf. J. F. Bensel, "De medico libellus ad codicum fidem recensitus," *Philologus*, *78*, 1922, pp. 102–4; also Müri, *op. cit.*, p. 37), or is linked in addition with the content of introductory manuals on the crafts which became common in the Hellenistic era (Fleischer, *op. cit.*, p. 54 f.). Yet, the right behavior of the physician is defined at least once in the typically Aristotelian manner as "a mean between extremes." ("In appearance let him be of a serious, but not harsh countenance, for surliness is taken for arrogance and unkindness, while a man of uncontrolled laughter

In keeping with such a kindly and tolerant attitude the good physician—the "fellow workman," as he is called (ch. 7)—must also be ready at all times to call in another physician as a consultant, and he must not quarrel with his confrères either. Thus, aspects of medical practice neglected in the *Oath* and in the essay *On the Physician*, are elucidated in the light of general moral considerations.[20] The essay *On Decorum*, on the other hand, though abounding in detailed advice on moral situations as they may arise in the course of a treatment, mainly discussed the "wisdom" of the physician. For "between wisdom and medicine there is no gulf; in fact, medicine possesses all the qualities

---

and excessive gaiety is considered vulgar"). Details of the precept also fall in line with Peripatetic terminology and doctrine. The concept of surliness (αὐθάδεια) is used here in the restricted and derogatory sense which it came to have in the Peripatetic school (*Magna Moralia*, 1192 b 31; Stobaeus, p. 146, 8, and Walzer, *op. cit.*, p. 161, n. 1). As Bensel already noted (p. 105), the word "vulgar" (φορτικός) is applied to him who indulges in excessive laughter, just as it is in *Nic. Eth.*, 1128 a 3 ff. Self-control (ἐγκράτεια) commended in the Hippocratic essay is treated as one of the main virtues in *Magna Moralia*, in contrast to the genuine Aristotelian ethics (Walzer, *op. cit.*, pp. 98; 106). The use of the term friendliness (φιλάνθρωπος, cf. above, note 3) agrees with that to be found in the Ps. Aristotelian treatise *On Virtue and Vices* (1251 b 35; cf. 1251 b 16; 1250 b 33; also Theophrastus *apud* Stobaeus, *Florilegium*, 3, 50). Finally, the ideal of the "gentleman" (τὸ δὲ ἦθος εἶναι καλὸν καὶ ἀγαθόν) remains valid throughout the history of Peripatetic ethics (Stobaeus, p. 147, 23). It is true, the ethics propounded in the book *On the Physician* is that of common morality, but as one has rightly said, the later Peripatos restored "bourgeois morality" (Walzer, *op. cit.*, p. 188). For the Peripatetic concern with the life of the ordinary citizen, cf. above, note 15. I should add that the Peripatetic flavor of the "Hippocratic" essay speaks for its being dated after 300 B.C.

[20] *Precepts* is usually held to be Epicurean in origin, cf. now Fleischer, *op. cit.*, pp. 10 ff. However Bensel, *op. cit.*, pp. 96; 98, rightly doubted an influence of Epicurus on any of the deontological writings because Epicurus (Fr. 196 ed. Usener) considers all forms of life which are not directed toward the happy life merely vulgar activities. Epicurean philosophy seems the only Hellenistic system that does not share in the rehabilitation of the crafts (cf. Philodemus, *On Oeconomics*, XXIII, 18 ff.). And indeed, the moral teaching of *Precepts* is Stoic rather than Epicurean. The term φιλανθρωπία, as it is used here (cf. above, note 4), corresponds to the meaning which the word has for the Chrysippean Stoa (φιλικὴ χρῆσις ἀνθρώπων [*Stoicorum Veterum Fragmenta*, III, 292 ed. Arnim]), and in its emphatically moral connotation differs significantly from the more utilitarian recommendation of φιλανθρωπία by the Epicureans (Philodemus, *op. cit.*, XXIV, 29). The injunction on fees laid down in *Precepts* is paralleled by Chrysippus' statements on fees for teaching (*St. V. Fr.*, III, 701). The definition of medicine as "habit" (ἕξις, ch. 2) is that of the Stoa(cf. e.g., *St. V. Fr.*, II, 393; III, 111). That the epistemological theories, too, are Stoic rather than Epicurean I hope to show elsewhere. The date of *Precepts* has been fixed by Fleischer (*op. cit.*, p. 24) in the first or second century A.D. At any rate, the book must be late Hellenistic.

that make for wisdom" (ch. 5), that is, wisdom "applied to life," "directed toward seemliness and good repute" (ch. 1), which should be carefully distinguished from its opposite, from false or sham philosophy. A physician who has the right kind of philosophy is indeed "the equal of a god"; his are all the virtues one can think of (ch. 5). To put it in the technical language of the Stoic school, to which the author of the the treatise owes allegiance, the true physician is the peer of the sage.[21]

Perhaps you are astonished at the fact that all these treatises which I have characterized briefly are so strongly imbued with philosophy. And thinking again of the Hippocratic *Oath* you may wonder why the ancient physician could not rest satisfied with the stipulation of his oath, which seems to tell him all he has to know about his duties. But the Hippocratic *Oath* originally was a literary manifesto, a programme laid down by one who wished to set matters right in accordance with his own convictions. It was not an oath taken by all physicians, if indeed it was ever taken at all by any one before the end of antiquity.[22] Throughout Hellenistic times and in the first centuries of the Christian era no common agreement existed concerning an ethical code binding for the medical practitioner. As was the case with the medical etiquette of old, so moral stipulations were accepted voluntarily. The writers of whom I have spoken were individuals trying to find out for themselves how to conduct their business in the right way. Just like Osler, they believed they could see their own work in truer perspective by taking

[21] The Stoic influence on the treatise *On Decorum* is generally recognized (e.g., Jones, *Hippocrates*, II, p. 270 f.) and has been traced in detail by Fleischer (*op. cit.*, especially pp. 78; 90: 101 ff.). The latter also dates the essay in the first-second century A.D. A reexamination of the background of the Stoic theories here adopted may perhaps lead to the assumption of a slightly earlier date. But this too I must leave for another investigation.

[22] Scribonius Largus, perhaps the first to mention the *Oath*, maintains that Hippocrates began medical instruction by administering this vow (*Compositiones*, p. 2, 27 f., ed. Helmreich). This of course is mere conjecture. Such books as Ps. Soranus, *Introductio ad medicinam* (V. Rose, *Anecdota Graeca et Graeco-Latina*, II, 1870) speak of a medical oath and of the oath of Hippocrates (pp. 244, 27; 245, 16 f.). In the fourth century A.D. Libanius (Κατὰ ἰατροῦ φαρμακέως, 9) refers to "the oath taken by physicians when entering upon the practice of their profession" (cf. R. Pack, "Note on a 'Progymnasma' of Libanius," *Amer. Jour. Philol.*, 69, 1948, p. 300), and many such oaths were in fact current (Pack, *ibid.*). That any of them were obligatory, cannot be proved. According to Ps. Oribasius, *Comment. in Aphorismos Hippocratis*, ed. Basileae, 1535, p. 7, the *Oath* was the first book to be read by the beginner, cf. K. Deichgräber, "Die ärztliche Standesethik des hippokratischen Eides," *Quellen u. Stud. z. Gesch. d. Naturwiss. u. d. Medizin*, III, 2, 1932, p. 93, n. 1, and the material there given on other oaths, p. 95, n. 33; p. 97, n. 42.

"the larger view." And in this endeavor where could they turn for instruction except to philosophy? Ancient religion had no moral or metaphysical message. In the vacuum that resulted from the disappearance of the city state, from the breakdown of the old ideal of civic virtue, philosophy alone could still provide guidance. It was, and it intended to be, not merely the domain of academics, but rather the inspiration of everybody who refused to get lost in doing his daily chores and was in search of standards on which to orientate himself. To be sure, adherence to whatever dogma seemed to the individual nearest to the truth did not yet make him a "philosopher-in-precept," and this holds also for the authors of the deontological writings. Philosophy gave them a *Weltanschauung* which enabled them to solve the task they had set for themselves.[23]

Yet I must turn now to a consideration of the other factor which, as I suggested before, was responsible for the acceptance of a philosophical ethic on the part of the physician: I mean the change of the medical art into medical science. Ever since the fifth and fourth centuries some physicians had interested themselves in the physiological and biological theories of the philosophers and had made use of them in their own work. Thereby they created scientific medicine, if I may use this term to designate the type of medicine that went beyond the practical application of traditional knowledge and demanded research into the nature of the body and of all the factors that may have a bearing upon it.[24] While throughout antiquity merely technical skill and empirical proficiency constituted the equipment of the average physician who as a craftsman was trained through apprenticeship with another physician-craftsman, the medical "scientists" studied philosophy. In the Hellenistic era they belonged to the various medical sects for which the unity of philosophy and medicine was axiomatic. And the new spirit in which medicine was thus approached soon made itself felt also

---

[23] It is usual to designate the ethics of the *Oath* as *"Berufsethos"* (cf. e.g., Pohlenz, *op. cit.*, p. 334); Müri uses this term in his analysis of the picture of the ideal physician, as it is given in the deontological writings (*op. cit.*, p. 39). In a loose sense, such a characterization is surely not unjustified. But it is important to note that none of the "Hippocratic" treatises here discussed considers the obligations of the physician as inherent in his medical task. They rather adapt philosophical ethics to medicine, cf. below, p. 337.

[24] For a more detailed interpretation of "scientific" medicine, cf. L. Edelstein, "The Relation of Ancient Philosophy to Medicine," *Bull. Hist. Med.*, *26*, 1952, pp. 301 ff. [351* ff.].

in medical practice. The ethics of these physicians became identical with that of the philosophical school to which they professed allegiance as scientists.

The first testimony to this effect is perhaps the Hippocratic *Law* written at approximately the same time as the *Oath*. Many physicians, the author of the short and almost enigmatic treatise holds, are physicians "by repute"; very few are physicians "in reality." Rather have the majority, "like the supernumeraries in tragedies," merely "the appearance, dress, and mask of an actor without being actors" (ch. 1). He who wishes to win the reputation of being a physician "not only in name, but in deed," must go through a proper training, that is, a philosophical training. Its result will also be "cheerfulness" and "joyousness," instead of "cowardice" and "rashness," which betray "helplessness" and "want of knowledge" (ch. 4). This is the Democritean ideal of theoretical speculation, according to which the man of true insight is at the same time necessarily the man of truly good character.[25]

While here the ethics of the scientific physician still remains vague and shadowy, it manifests itself in its fully developed form in the doctrine of the Hellenistic Empiricists whose sect was of the skeptic persuasion. The empirical physician therefore, like all skeptic philosophers, accepts the established rules of life which, though by no means representing absolute truth, have the sanction of probability. In accordance with the common aim of men, he practices medicine for the sake of

[25] In the interpretation of the *Law* I follow Wilamowitz, *Hermes*, *54*, 1919, pp. 46 ff. F. Müller's attempt (*Hermes*, *75*, 1940, pp. 39 ff.) to date the *Law* in the fifth century B.C. to me is unconvincing. As Fleischer says (*op. cit.*, p. 46), it is perhaps impossible to date the essay exactly, because many of its concepts became common stock in the discussion of moral problems. Yet the book cannot be earlier than Democritus, some of whose central ethical concepts are here presupposed, as Wilamowitz has shown. Nor will it be much later than the end of the fourth century, since unalloyed Democritean teaching did not long survive. Jones (*Hippocrates*, II, p. 275) connects the *Law* with the doctrine of secret medical societies, which he thinks might have existed in Greece, since at the end of the *Law* it is proclaimed: "Holy things are shown to holy men; to the profane it is not lawful to show them until these have been initiated into the rites of knowledge." But the description of "knowledge" through the metaphor of the mysteries is not uncommon with Greek philosophers (cf. E. Frank, *Knowledge, Will and Belief*, 1955, pp. 63 f.; 67). Wilamowitz, *op. cit.*, p. 49, already compared ἱερὰ πρήγματα in the *Law* with the ἱερὸν πνεῦμα that, according to Democritus, inspires the poet. Jones' translation of ἠδελφισμένος (*Precepts*, ch. 5) as "one made a brother" (of a secret society) involves an unnecessary change of the best manuscript tradition ἠδελφισμένως, for the meaning of which cf. Fleischer, *op. cit.*, p. 36.

reputation or of money, of neither of which he desires to have too much or too little, but just as much as is adequate and guarantees peace of mind. In his character and behavior he evinces tranquillity and gentleness. In his work he is not given to unnecessary talk, but prefers action; talking much or talking big is the habit of those who, unlike the empiricist and skeptic, believe in speculative theories. In his writings and in his research he is truthful, not intent on winning an argument à tout prix, or on displaying his conceit. On the whole, then, he follows in the wake of the day, relying on indubitable data of sense perception and experience; living thus, he lives like Hippocrates himself who, in the opinion of the skeptics, had of course been a skeptic, and as a skeptic had equaled the fame of Asclepius.[26]

Evidence on the ethical teaching of the early dogmatic sects is almost entirely lacking. A happy chance has preserved at least one testimony which bears witness to the preoccupation of Erasistratus with medical ethics. "Most fortunate indeed," he says, "wherever it happens that the physician is both, perfect in his art and most excellent in his moral conduct. But if one of the two should have to be missing, then it is better to be a good man devoid of learning than to be a perfect practitioner of bad moral conduct, and an untrustworthy man—if indeed it is true that good morals compensate for what is missing in art, while bad morals can corrupt and confound even perfect art."[27] Further details of the deontology of the Herophilean and Erasistratean sects may be contained in the writings of Galen, the great systematizer of medicine. At any rate, his little essay *That the Best Physician also is a*

---

[26] Cf. K. Deichgräber, *Die griechische Empirikerschule*, 1930, p. 322 f. Especially important is the statement, p. 82, 29 ff.: οἷός δ' ἐστι καθ' ὅλον τὸν βίον ὁ σκεπτικός, τοιοῦτός ἐστι περὶ τὴν ἰατρικὴν ὁ ἐμπειρικός. Ch. 11 of Galen's *Subfiguratio Empirica* treats "De moribus et dictis que debent esse in empericis." For the skeptics' conformance with the established laws, cf. e.g., M. M. Patrick, *The Greek Sceptics*, 1929, p. 51.

[27] Cf. Ps. Soranus, *Introductio ad medicinam* (Rose, *Anecdota Graeca et Graeco-Latina*, II, p. 244, 16–23): "Disciplinarum autem ceterarum minime sit expers [sc. medicus], sed et circa mores habeat diligentiam. iuxta enim Erasistratum felicissimum quidem est ubi utraeque res fuerint, uti et in arte sit perfectus et moribus sit optimus. si autem unum de duobus defuerit, melius est virum esse bonum absque doctrina quam artificem perfectum mores habentem malos et improbum esse. modesti si quidem mores quod in arte deest honestate repensare videntur, culpa autem morum artem perfectam corrumpere atque improbare potest." The *Introductio* which forms part of a collection of *Quaestiones Medicinales* (cf. Rose, *op. cit.*, p. 169), though hardly by Soranus, is based on good ancient sources. There is no reason to doubt the authenticity of the quotation from Erasistratus.

Philosopher gives an exhaustive account of later dogmatic ethics. It can be summed up in the demand that the physician should be contemptuous of money, interested in his work, self-controlled and just. Once he is in possession of these basic virtues, he will have all the others at his command as well (ch. 3). And how is such moral eminence to be achieved? Like Galen, the true physician must become a philosopher himself, an adherent of Plato, or rather of the Platonism of Galen's time, which was fused with Aristotelianism and Stoicism.[28]

With this short description of Galen's views I have come to the end of my analysis of the various attitudes taken by the scientist-physicians and by the craftsmen-physicians during the second stage in the development of medical ethics. The important consequence of the movement which I have described hardly needs reemphasis. The morality of outward performance characteristic of the classical era was now supplemented by a morality of inner intention. The physician—whether as an amateur philosopher or as a philosopher in his own right—had learned to regard his patient not only as the object of his art, but also as a fellow man to whom he owed more than knowledge alone, however great, can provide. He had learned to face him not only as a master of techniques, but also as a virtuoso in moral conduct.

Can one then go one step further and claim that between the end of the fourth century B.C. and the second century A.D. medicine had been elevated to the rank of the most philanthropic art? Have I answered also the specific question raised at the very beginning of my discussion? Have I uncovered the origin of the humanism which Osler admired in Greek medicine? It may almost seem so. For surely, in Galen's opinion, the physician who accepts his philosophy will be led to practice medicine out of love of humanity, the motive which Galen is willing to attribute even to Hippocrates, as I mentioned before. And since nowhere else, neither in the deontological writings of the *Corpus Hippocraticum*, nor in the teaching of any of the other medical sects, philanthropy is mentioned as the inspiration of the doctor, one should

---

[28] E. Wenkebach, "Der hippokratische Arzt als das Ideal Galens," *Quell. u. Stud. z. Gesch. d. Nat. u. d. Med.*, III, 1932–33, p. 372 f., stresses the influence of Hippocratic medicine on Galen's ideal as outlined in the treatise referred to. But although Galen identifies his philosophy with that of Hippocrates, one must remember that for him, Hippocrates and Plato agree in almost all points. Besides, he says expressly (ch. 3) that philosophy is indispensable for medical practice, just as it is for medical theory; in addition to logic and physics, the physician must take up the third part of philosophy, namely ethics.

conclude that it was dogmatic medicine, as formulated by Galen or maybe by one of his predecessors, which gave rise to medical humanism.[29]

But Galen's own appraisal of the possible motivations of medical practice, I am afraid, makes it impossible to rest satisfied as yet. For as he says (*De Placitis*, p. 763 f., ed. Müller) on the authority of the same passage in Plato's *Republic* to which I referred in my analysis of classical medicine, the physician's particular job is to take care of the health of the body, although it may be for a variety of reasons that he practices medicine. Some physicians engage in it for the sake of money, some for the sake of exemption from public duties—physicians in Galen's time were sometimes granted such privileges[30]—some few for love of mankind, just as still others for glory or honor. In so far as they are able to bring health to their patients, all of them are named physicians; in so far as they do what they do for different reasons, the one is called a "philanthropist," the other a lover of honor, the third a lover of glory, the fourth a lover of money. Therefore, Galen continues (p. 764 f.), the aim of the physician as physician is not glory or money, as the Empiricist Menodotus claimed; this may have been true of himself, but others in the past surely had different aims in mind. The motive of glory or money or of philanthropy is a matter of personal choice; it has no intrinsic connection with the pursuit of medicine.[31] For in regard to

[29] On the evidence of Galen's claim that "Diocles practiced medicine out of love of mankind" (cf. above, p. 320), K. Deichgräber, *Professio medici, Zum Vorwort des Scribonius Largus*, Abh. Akad. Mainz, Geistes- u. Sozialwiss. Klasse, 1950, No. 9), tentatively suggests that the association between medicine and philanthropy may be due to the influence of the Peripatos (p. 866, n. 1). Yet, for Aristotle, and even for Theophrastus, φιλανθρωπία is not "love of humanity" (cf. above, notes 7 and 19). As late as in Stobaeus' report on Peripatetic ethics the κοινὴ φιλανθρωπία, as it is called in contradistinction to the φιλία among friends (II, 121, 22; 120, 20), is not represented as one of the main virtues (cf. Heinemann, *op. cit.*, col. 298); it rather is a natural sympathy that prompts men to help other men in dire need and not think of themselves only (p. 120, 20–121, 22). Much as the Peripatos contributed to the Hellenistic concept of the unity of men, it was the Stoa that stressed the rational duties inherent in the idea of humanity (M. Pohlenz, *Die Stoa*, I, 1948, pp. 136–39). And even in the Stoic school justice was at first the obligation stressed in connection with cosmopolitanism; love of mankind came to be fully recognized only in the first century A.D. (Pohlenz, *ibid.*, p. 315; Bonhöffer, *op. cit.*, p. 106). I should be inclined, therefore, to believe that philanthropy became integrated into the ethical teaching of the dogmatic physicians not long before Galen's time, if indeed it was not Galen himself who accepted the ideal of philanthropy in accordance with his Stoic leanings.

[30] Cf. below, p. 346.

[31] In *That the Best Physician also is a Philosopher* Galen once speaks of medicine as a τέχνη οὕτω φιλάνθρωπος (ch. 2). The detailed refutation of Menodotus shows that

every craft it is necessary to distinguish between its common characteristics and those which belong to the individual practicing it. Failure to make this distinction is bad logic, irreconcilable with the tenets of Plato and Hippocrates alike (p. 765 f.).

This argumentation of Galen, so utterly devoid of ethical overtones or of any feeling of moral indignation, shows clearly that in his opinion philanthropy is not indissolubly joined with the practice of medicine. It is, so to say, a superfluity of riches on the part of the physician. What is expected of him is only that he should be an expert in medicine. However, no rules of behavior can be stated absolutely. For Galen as well as for all the other moralizing physicians medical ethics remains relative to the respective philosophies to which they adhere at their own discretion. Whoever differs from their views is a bad philosopher, to be sure, but he is not necessarily a bad physician or a bad man. Various motivations of medical practice, therefore, are quite legitimate; no one single or definite virtue is enjoined upon the doctor by his task. From the point of view of medicine, his specific morality is incidental rather than essential.

Does this amount to the admission that the ancients never identified medicine with love of humanity? That they did not know of any strictly professional medical ethics dictated by the aim of medicine itself? By no means. Almost a hundred years before Galen there must have been a clear realization of a medical humanism inherent in the task of the physician. Scribonius Largus, a writer of the early first century A.D., speaks of it as something quite self-evident to himself and his readers. It still remains for me to 'elicit the full meaning of the doctrine in question from the few sentences in which Scribonius alludes to it, to determine its historical antecedents, and to sketch its later fate.[32]

Scribonius has embodied his views on the moral conduct of the physician in the preface to his book *On Remedies*, in which he wishes to demonstrate the importance of treatment by drugs. Why is it, he asks (p. 2, 8 ed. Helmreich), that his colleagues refrain from the application of drugs? Are they unfamiliar with them? This would be just reason for

---

by the term in question Galen can only mean that medicine is "philanthropic" because it removes the sufferings of men.

[32] The fact that Scribonius upholds a humanistic ethics has often been noticed, of course; cf. e.g., J. Hirschberg, *Vorlesungen über hippokratische Heilkunde*, 1922, p. 35. A detailed analysis of Scribonius' views has recently been given by K. Deichgräber, *op. cit.* (cf. above, note 29).

accusing them of negligence. Or are they aware of the usefulness of drugs, yet deny their use to others? If so, they are even more culpable, "because they burn with envy, an evil that must be despised by all men, and especially by the physician who is himself despised by gods and men if his heart is not full of sympathy (*misericordiae*) and humaneness (*humanitatis*) in accordance with the will (*voluntatem*) of medicine itself" (p. 2, 15–19).

But the sympathy and humaneness "willed" by medicine imply more than that the physician should not withhold his knowledge from his patients. The true physician, Scribonius continues, "is not allowed to harm anybody, not even the enemies of the state (*hostibus*). He may fight against them with every means as a soldier (*miles*) or as a good citizen (*vir bonus*), should this be demanded of him. [As a physician, he cannot and must not fight or harm them], since medicine does not judge men by their circumstances in life (*fortuna*), nor by their character (*personis*). Rather does medicine promise (*pollicetur*) her succor in equal measure to all who implore her help, and she professes (*profitetur*) never to be injurious to anyone" (p. 2, 19–26). For, as Scribonius reiterates in conclusion, "medicine is the knowledge of healing, not of hurting. If she does not try in every way to help the sick with all means at her disposal, she fails to offer to men the sympathy she promises" (*hominibus quam pollicetur misericordiam*, p. 3, 5–8).

Obviously, according to Scribonius, the sympathy and humaneness required of the physician are due to everybody in equal measure. Humaneness (*humanitas*) for him is not merely a friendliness of behavior, it is a "proficiency and benevolence toward all men without distinction," it truly is "love of mankind," as *humanitas* was defined at that time in correspondence with the then prevailing meaning of the Greek word φιλανθρωπία.[33] Besides, sympathy and love of humanity constitute positive rules, and obedience to them supersedes all other allegiances that the doctor may have as a good citizen or as a soldier. They are the special obligation of the physician, which he cannot violate under any circumstances. Most important, the one and only right standard of conduct is enforced upon him by medicine itself, just as is the standard

[33] I am quoting the definition of *humanitas* which Gellius gives (*Noctes Atticae*, XIII, 17) as the one commonly accepted. Heinemann, *Realencycl.*, col. 306, has shown that in the literature of the first century A.D. the words *humanitas* and *humanus* and their Greek equivalents are used in the sense attested by Gellius.

of adequate knowledge. Unless he knows all that he ought to know and makes use of it for the benefit of the sick, he fails in his duty. He is as remiss, or even more so, if he does not fulfill his specific moral responsibility. Here, the ethics of inner intention and that of outward performance have become an inseparable unity; both are derived from the task to be achieved, from the "will" and "promise" of medicine itself, both are equally essential for medicine and the physician.

It is hardly by chance therefore that Scribonius calls medicine not merely an "art" or a "science," but a "profession" (*professio*, p. 2, 18; 27). This word, in the language of his time, was applied to workmanship in preference to the older and morally indefinite terms, in order to emphasize the ethical connotations of work, the idea of an obligation or a duty on the part of those engaged in the arts and crafts. It approximates most closely the Christian concept of "vocation" or "calling," except of course that for him who has been "called" to do a job his obligations are ordained by God, while for the member of an ancient profession his duties result from his own understanding of the nature of his profession.[34] But this difference of the ancient ethos of work from that of later ages does not lessen the strict validity of the rules to be observed. The true physician, Scribonius says, like a soldier, is "bound in lawful obedience to medicine by his military oath" (p. 2, 20–21). On the other hand, he who acts in a way unbecoming to a physician is a deserter, as it were; he is "deservedly despised by gods and men" (*diis hominibusque invisus merito*, ch. 199; cf. p. 2, 19: *diis et hominibus invisi esse debent*); he has "against the law transgressed the proper boundaries of the profession" (ch. 199).[35] He is, one might say, disqualified as a physician, for it is no longer up to him how he should conduct himself.

That such an ideal of medical humanism is foreign to the spirit of

---

[34] M. Weber, "Die protestantische Ethik und der Geist des Kapitalismus," *Ges. Aufsätze z. Religionssoziologie*, I, 1920, analyzing the meaning of the term *Beruf* or "calling" has pointed up its difference from the classical concept of work (p. 63). He has also noted, however, that in Latin, such words as *officium* (cf. also below, n. 42), *munus*, and *professio* (originally denoting, it seems, the duty of making a tax declaration) came to assume "eine unserem Wort 'Beruf' in jeder Hinsicht ziemlich ähnliche Gesamtbedeutung . . . natürlich durchaus diesseitig, ohne jede religiöse Färbung" (p. 63, n. 1).

[35] The simile of fighting and military service used by Scribonius is quite common in Latin philosophy (cf. e.g., Pohlenz, *Die Stoa*, I, 1948, p. 314); it also occurs in the language of the mysteries so often applied to knowledge in general, cf. above, note 25, and *Amer. Journ. Philol.*, 72, 1951, p. 430, n. 6.

Hippocratic ethics, Scribonius admits himself. Even in the *Oath*, which in his opinion is the work of Hippocrates, the "founder of our profession" (p. 2, 27), he can find his views at best by implication. For, as he puts it, Hippocrates forbids the physician to give an abortive remedy to a woman, "and thereby has gone a long way toward preparing the mind of the learners for the love of humanity. For he who thinks it to be a crime to injure future life still in doubt, how much more criminal must he judge it to hurt a full grown human being" (p. 2, 30–3, 2)?[36] But if Scribonius' concept of medical ethics goes in fact beyond the demands of the classical period, if it is distinct from the teaching of all the deontological treatises and all the medical sects I have discussed, where and when did it originate?

That Scribonius himself formulated the code of behavior which he upholds, I cannot believe; for he does not argue about it, nor defend it, he simply presupposes it and takes it for granted, as I pointed out before. In addition, reading his account one cannot fail to be reminded of the doctrine concerning human life and human obligations which characterize the Stoic philosophy of humanism evolved in the second century B.C. by Panaetius and embedded in Cicero's book *On Duties*, the manual of all later humanism, ancient and Christian, secular and religious alike. Here if anywhere in antiquity, a programme of a professional ethics was firmly established.[37]

For first of all, Panaetius, as Cicero represents him, accepted and even enhanced the more positive evaluation of the arts and crafts which earlier philosophers had made of them, granting that virtue has its place even among craftsmen. Medicine, next to architecture and education, is expressly mentioned and singled out by Cicero as socially acceptable, because it demands a high degree of insight and contributes something useful to life; it is therefore, he says, a "proper" (*honestae*)

---

[36] Scribonius concludes that Hippocrates apparently "thought it of great value for everyone to preserve the name and honor of medicine in purity and holiness, conducting himself after her design" (p. 3, 2–5). Thereby he translates into the language of his professional ethics the Pythagorean concepts of purity and holiness used in the *Oath* with reference to the art which the physician practices and to the life which he leads (ἀγνῶς δὲ καὶ ὁσίως διατηρήσω βίον ἐμὸν καὶ τέχνην ἐμήν). It is unwarranted, I think, to infer from this adaptation of the famous sentence in the *Oath* that Scribonius has a "religiös getönte Humanität" (Deichgräber, *op. cit.* [cf. above, note 29], p. 861).

[37] R. Reitzenstein, *Werden und Wesen der Humanität im Altertum*, 1907, p. 15, already suggested that the philosophy of Panaetius gave rise to a "*Standesethik*"; cf. also Heinemann, *op. cit.*, col. 294.

occupation for those for whose station in life it is fitting (*On Duties*, I 42, 151).[38]

But Panaetius' positive appreciation of the various occupations implies much more than a general approval of the activities indispensable for man's welfare and for civilization. Although philosophically speaking virtue is one and the same, and it is impossible to have any one virtue without having all of them (II, 10, 35 [Panaetius]), different aspects of this one and indivisible virtue in which all men share come to the fore in the various pursuits of human life and have to be practiced without fail. To give an example, the judge must always adhere to the truth, while the lawyer may sometimes defend the probable, even if this may not quite coincide with the truth (II, 14, 51 [Panaetius]). Obviously, here man's particular task imposes upon him certain obligations; each one has its own morality, from which there is no exception. For the judge is not permitted to indulge in any bias or favoritism out of friendship; while sitting as a judge, he is not supposed to act as a friend (III, 10, 43).[39]

If one asks why this should be so, the answer is that the individual who practices any occupation is playing a certain rôle. It may be one derived from chance circumstances, the place in society to which he is born and by which his inclination toward a particular career and also his opportunities for it are conditioned; it may be one which he assumes through his own free decision, through a deliberate choice of an occupation (I, 32, 115 ff.). But whether the rôle be inherited or chosen, one must act one's part as the rôle demands it, just as in the two rôles which

[38] In accordance with their own aristocratic prejudice and with the prejudice of the society in which they live, Panaetius and Cicero consider political and public activities the only ones proper for a gentleman (cf. M. Pohlenz, "Antikes Führertum," *Neue Wege z. Antike*, 2. Reihe, H. 3, 1934, p. 83 f.). The views of the older Stoics in this respect had been more liberal; cf. above, note 15.

[39] Panaetius surely was not the first to discuss the particular virtues pertaining to an occupation. His teacher, Antipater (*St. V. Fr.*, III, 61 f.), had engaged in a famous dispute about "business ethics" with his predecessor, Diogenes (*St. V. Fr.*, III, 49). The casuistry of the old Stoa insists on the fact that for the physician it is permissible to lie (III, 513), that neither he, nor the judge is allowed to indulge in commiseration "with the suffering of his neighbors" (III, 451). The beginnings of such a "differenzierende Ethik" may be traced even to the Sophists, and especially to the Xenophontian Socrates (cf. E. Norden, in *Hermes*, *40*, 1905, pp. 521 ff.; F. Wehrli, "Ethik und Medizin," *Mus. Helveticum*, *8*, 1951, p. 45 f.). However, the recognition that virtuous action may differ with different people and different positions in life is still a far cry from the acknowledgement of professional virtues. At any rate, they seem not to have been appraised systematically before Panaetius.

nature, in addition, has assigned to everyone—as a human being who has the same duties as all other human beings, and as an individual endowed with specific intellectual and emotional gifts (I, 30, 107 ff.)—one must live up to "the lines one has to speak." It is therefore that the judge must always utter the truth, that he is not permitted to listen to the voice of friendship, "for he lays down the rôle (or mask) of the friend when putting on that of the judge" (III, 10, 43). What is fitting for the one, is not so for the other.[40]

Now is this not fundamentally the way in which Scribonius views medicine and the obligations imposed by it? The rôle which the physician plays in the tragedy, or comedy, of life demands of him the virtue of humaneness, sympathy, or commiseration. His lines are to be spoken in this spirit. Consequently as little as Cicero's judge in his professional activity can ever be in a situation justifying his failure to cling to the truth—though there are other professions in which this virtue may sometimes come second—so Scribonius' physician must never neglect love of humanity and all the duties it entails. Certainly, commiseration and humaneness are not demanded of him alone; but they are his professional virtues, just as truthfulness is the distinctive virtue of him who sits in court notwithstanding the fact that it is required of everybody. Only when he steps out of his rôle, so to say, is the member of a profession free to follow another code of morals. The physician may take on the rôle of a citizen or of a soldier, and in that case he may fight and kill the enemy. Yet as long as he acts his professional part, he has to stick to his cue. Otherwise, he would cease to be a physician, in the same manner in which the judge who indulges in favoritism ceases to be the representative of justice.

The similarity between Scribonius' concept of a profession and that of Cicero, in my opinion, is so striking that the former can hardly be thought to be independent of the latter.[41] Perhaps Scribonius con-

[40] The discussion summarized in the text makes it clear that, in Cicero's view, each "profession" or career has its own ethos. The example of the judge is obviously used as particularly appropriate to Roman conditions; cf. also above, note 38.

[41] Deichgräber (op. cit., pp. 865 ff.) assumes that the ethics outlined by Scribonius is original with him, though with reference to ch. 199 he admits that "die Frage der professio der Medizin hat [for Scribonius] allgemeineren Charakter" (p. 859). This in itself is an indication, it seems, that he is merely applying to medicine a general theory of professional behavior. The physician to the emperor Claudius must surely have been familiar with Stoicism. He was the freer to accept Panaetius' teaching which did not influence the established medical sects, because he himself apparently did not belong to any of the schools of his age (Deichgräber, p. 865 f.).

sulted the same sources of which Cicero made use and found his inspiration there. Perhaps he drew from a lost treatise on medicine and its professional obligations influenced by Panaetius' Stoicism; treatises on other professions and their duties are known to have been written at the turn of the first century B.C. to the first century A.D. In whichever way Scribonius learned of the views of his predecessors, the principal tenets of the creed which his book attests for the first time must have their roots in the Stoic humanism transmitted through Cicero.[42]

As for the later history of this strictly professional kind of ethics, few testimonies are extant. The novelist Apuleius refers to certain physicians who hold it unfitting for "the medical sect" to be guilty of anyone's death, because they have learned that "medicine is sought out not for the purpose of destroying men but rather for that of saving them" (*Metamorphoses*, X, 11). His contemporary, Soranus, the great rival of Galen, mentions some colleagues of his who regard it as their duty to banish abortives not only because Hippocrates said one should do so, but also "because it is the specific task of medicine to guard and preserve what has been engendered by nature" (*Gynaecology*, I, 60).[43]

[42] E. Norden has drawn attention to the specific literature "De officiis judicis" which starts to appear around the middle of the first century A.D. (*Hermes*, 40, 1905, p. 512 f.). It differs from the usual type of "Introductions" to any given art in that here only the moral obligations of the judge are considered. With Cicero and his contemporaries the word *officium* comes to mean not only the objective task of an art, but also, if not preeminently, the duties incumbent upon the artist (cf. E. Bernert, *De vi atque usu vocabuli officii*, Diss. Breslau, 1930, pp. 25 ff.; 29 ff.; and above, note 34). Gellius mentions books on the juridical "office" in both Latin and Greek (*Noctes Atticae*, XIV, 2, 1). Panaetius and his pupils, Posidonius and Hecaton, wrote Περὶ τοῦ καθήκοντος; other Stoic books "On Duties" are known from Seneca (cf. H. Gomoll, *Der stoische Philosoph Hekaton*, 1933, pp. 27 ff.); the work of the artisan is considered as an *officium*, as a moral obligation, by Cicero (*De officiis*, I, 7, 22) as well as by Seneca (*De beneficiis*, III, 18, 1; cf. Gomoll, p. 77 f.). In the Stoic treatises just referred to the obligations toward one's country and toward other groups to which the individual may belong were set forth, or they were defined according to certain virtues. For the importance of philanthropy in late Stoic ethics, cf. above, note 29; below, note 45. The details of the general theory of professions as it was developed in the Middle Stoa I hope to discuss in an investigation of Stoic ethics. That the works on duties began to pay attention also to medicine is the more likely since physicians by this time were granted citizenship, and medicine was practiced even by free-born Romans (cf. K. H. Below, *Der Arzt im römischen Recht*, Münch. Beitr. z. Papyrusforschung u. antiken Rechtsgeschichte, 37, 1953, p. 20 f.).

[43] I should mention that Galen's refutation of Menodotus (cf. above, p. 336 f.) may be an indirect reflection of the fight about the new professional ethics. Menodotus was a pupil of the Skeptic Antiochus (cf. Deichgräber, *Empirikerschule*, p. 212), who leaned toward Stoicism and deviated in many respects from his school. Possibly his assertion that the physician's aim is money or honor was intended as the antithesis

While these passing remarks do hardly more than rephrase Scribonius' formulations, a poem composed by an otherwise unknown Stoic philosopher, Sarapion—he too lived in the second century A.D.—shows, I think, a certain evolution of the original theory. For in this poem, entitled *On the Eternal Duties of the Physician*, and inscribed on stone in the Athenian temple of Asclepius, the god of medicine and of the physicians, the god who prided himself most of all on his virtue of philanthropy, the "eternal duties" of the doctor are said to be: "First to heal his mind and to give assistance to himself before giving it to anyone [else]" and to "cure with moral courage and with the proper moral attitude."[44] Then "he would be like god savior equally of slaves, of paupers, of rich men, of princes, and to all a brother, such help he would give. For we are all brothers. Therefore he would not hate anyone, nor would he harbor envy in his mind." Here, the thought of Scribonius, the philosophy advocated by Cicero, is restated in the language of late Stoicism, in its new terms of human brotherhood, which indeed foreshadow the categories of Christian medical ethics.[45]

---

of the ethos of philanthropy. Also, Seneca's contention that men owe more to the physician than financial remuneration (*De beneficiis*, VI, 16, 1) may be a reference to physicians of the type Scribonius depicts, although elsewhere he acknowledges the fact that medical knowledge and moral goodness do not always go together (*Ep.* 87, 17). Finally, could not Pliny's notorious diatribe against the physicians best be understood if his judgment was determined by the humanistic ideal? For Pliny is careful in mentioning that all the crimes committed by physicians should be attributed to the individuals and not to the medical art (XXIX, 21 f.).

[44] Cf. P. L. Maas and James H. Oliver, "An Ancient Poem on the Duties of a Physician," *Bull. Hist. Med.*, 7, 1939, pp. 315 ff. The translation is Oliver's, whose emendation [αἰ]ώνια I also accept against Maas' [Παι]ώνια (cf. p. 320, n. 6).

[45] Maas in his commentary (*loc. cit.*, p. 323) says, *ad vv.* 12 ff.: "colore Epicteteus, ne dicam Christianus." It seems to me that the poem can be adequately understood within the confines of late Stoicism, that so often approximates Christian ethics. For the brotherhood of men cf. e.g., Epictetus, I, 13, 3 f.; Seneca, *Ep.*, 95, 52: "natura nos cognatos edidit . . . haec nobis amorem indidit mutuum." Sarapion enumerating man's various stations in life spells out Scribonius' claim that medicine does not judge men by their circumstances in life or by their personality. Both proscribe envy (Sarapion: [ʒᾶλος]; Scribonius: *invidentia*). While Sarapion derives from the brotherhood of men the duty not to hate anyone, Scribonius expresses the same thought positively through his concept of *humanitas*. (In the lines of the poem which I have omitted there are certain parallels with the deontological writings of the *Corpus Hippocraticum* noted by Oliver, p. 318, notes 2, 3; p. 320, note 4). Later Christian passages closely resembling the main drift of Sarapion's poem are to be found e.g., in L. C. MacKinney, "Medical Ethics and Etiquette in the Early Middle Ages," *Bull. Hist. Med.*, *26*, 1952, pp. 6; 11 f.; 27. Only one feature sharply distinguishes pagan humanism from the Christian attitude and that of the nineteenth-century

Finally the quintessence of pagan medical humanism was expressed by Libanius in a moving speech which medicine addresses to the young physician starting out on his career: "You desired to be one of the healers (of sickness), you had the benefit of having (good) teachers. Now, practice your art faithfully. Be reliable; cultivate love of man; if you are called to your patient, hasten to go; when you enter the sickroom, apply all your mental ability to the case at hand; share in the pain of those who suffer; rejoice with those who have found relief; consider yourself a partner in the disease; muster all you know for the fight to be fought; consider yourself to be of your contemporaries the brother, of those who are your elders the son, of those who are younger the father. And if anyone of them neglects his own affairs, remember that this is not permissible for yourself, and that it is your duty to be to the sick what the Dioscuri are to the sailor (in distress)."[46]

Is it by chance that the evidence concerning the survival of the humanistic ideal does not seem to go beyond the second half of the fourth century A.D.? Since on the whole the material for the history of medical ethics is so fragmentary, one hesitates to hazard judgment. Yet one may say with assurance that from the third century, Stoic philosophy—of which the doctrine of professional ethos formed part and parcel—ceased to have influence. The Neo-Platonists established Galen as the unchallenged authority in medicine. Through him, the philosophical ethics of the scientist-physician, which had never quite lost its appeal, came to predominate among the learned. Among the general practitioners of late antiquity, the teaching of the deontological writings of the *Corpus Hippocraticum* seems to have prevailed.[47] As for

---

humanist reformers (for whom cf. I. Galdston, "Humanism and Public Health," *Bull. Hist. Med.*, *8*, 1940, pp. 1032 ff.): pagan ethics lacks any recognition of social responsibilities on the part of the physician. Although sickness was understood in rational terms, and some diseases were traced to social conditions, even the gospel of brotherly love took account only of the relationship between the individual doctor and the individual patient. Immediate help rather than long-range improvement remained the watchword. In general, cf. O. Temkin in *Social Medicine: Its Derivations and Objectives*, ed. I. Galdston, 1949, pp. 3 ff.

[46] Κατὰ ἰατροῦ φαρμακέως, 6–7. Libanius writes in the vein of Cynic and Stoic popular philosophy, probably echoing older traditions. Already to Seneca and his generation, the physician had become "the friend" of the patient (*De beneficiis*, VI, 16, 1) sympathizing with him and loved in return as a friend (*ibid.*, 4–6); cf. above, note 43.

[47] Cf. e.g., the *Introductio* of Ps. Soranus, *op. cit.*, p. 245, 17; 22; 33. Even the late deontological writings soon became integrated into some of the collections of the Hippocratic works compiled in the Christian era; cf. Fleischer, *op. cit.*, pp. 108 ff.

the rising caste of especially privileged physicians—those who as city officials were granted immunity from public duties, and those who became court physicians—it is hard to believe that they should have been keen on following the precepts of brotherly love. As I mentioned before, Galen already noted that the city physicians accepted their position in order to be relieved from the staggering burden of "indirect taxation." The "courtly" ethics discernible even in his writings, according to which the physician will treat the emperor and his family, and all wealthy people for that matter, differently from what he proposes to do in the case of the poor, implies principles hardly compatible with Scribonius' love of mankind, or Sarapion's belief in the brotherhood of men.[48]

In the short span of time during which ancient medical humanism was current, once it had finally been formulated in opposition to the ideals of earlier generations, it most likely remained restricted to a small minority of physicians. Scribonius himself divined the slim chances for general acceptance of his belief and put the responsibility for this failure upon the patients. "Rarely," he says (p. 4, 9 ff.), "does anyone make an evaluation of the doctor before putting himself and his family under his care. And yet, if people have their portrait painted,

---

[48] For Galen's rules concerning treatment of the imperial family and of the rich, cf. e.g., *Opera Omnia* (ed. Kühn), vol. 13, pp. 635–38; 14, p. 659; also 12, p. 435. Surely, the distinctions here made became even more marked when the hierarchic structure of the empire was consolidated. The importance of the class of city physicians has been pointed up through Herzog's interpretation of an edict of Vespasian in which their privileges are set forth (*Urkunden zur Hochschulpolitik der römischen Kaiser*, Sitzungsber. Berlin, 1935, pp. 967 ff.; cf. also Below, *op. cit.*, pp. 23 ff.). Following perhaps the example of Augustus, Vespasian granted to all physicians exemption from taxes and from the burden of having soldiers billeted in their houses. Antoninus Pius revoked this edict and introduced a *numerus clausus* for the privileged physicians in each city (cf. Below, *op. cit.*, pp. 34 ff.); Galen's rather damning statement on those who practice medicine in order to be tax-exempt—to my knowledge never quoted in the pertinent literature—may throw some light on Antoninus' reasons for curtailing the benefits of Vespasian's edict. The imperial policy, in my opinion, was motivated by the recognition of the usefulness of medicine to the state, a topic widely discussed at that time (Quintilian, *Inst. Orat.*, VII, 1, 38; 4, 39; also Ps. Quintilian, *Declamationes*, 268). Herzog ascribes Vespasian's action to the recognition of medical philanthropy (*op. cit.*, p. 985), and restores the text accordingly (v. 6). Yet he himself concludes from the passages in Quintilian and from other statements that Vespasian invested physicians with the right to form corporations on account of "the usefulness of medicine" (p. 982 f.). It was not until Byzantine times that the privileges granted were made dependent on sufficient technical knowledge and on the morally unobjectionable character of the recipient (Below, *op. cit.*, p. 41).

they will first try to make sure of the artist's qualities on the basis of that which experience can tell, and then select and hire him." It is no wonder, therefore, he continues (p. 4, 15), that so many physicians rest content with little effort. Where no intelligent selection is made, where the good and the bad are held in equal esteem, "everybody will practice medicine as he sees fit" (p. 4, 24). The true reason for the relative ineffectualness of Scribonius' programme probably lies in a shortcoming which it shared with all the other ancient attempts to shape medical practice in accordance with moral concepts. None of them had the backing of institutions or organizations that had the power to enforce rules of conduct.[49] Yet, this very fact makes the achievement of the individuals who aspired to a medical ethics all the more impressive. It is praiseworthy indeed that under the given circumstances so many— some whose names history has recorded, and others whose identity has been obliterated—heeded Sarapion's appeal "to heal their own minds first" before giving help to their patients; that they were willing to forego material advantage for the law of their own conscience; that they took the initiative in raising and clarifying the moral issue, thereby laying the foundation for all later medical ethics.

It seems safe to add that among the ideals conceived by the ancients none was loftier than that which envisages love of humanity as the professional virtue of the physician. Even the Hippocratic *Oath* assumes full significance and dignity only if interpreted in the way in which it was understood by Scribonius and those who came after him. That this ideal of professional ethics also is the one most difficult to live up to goes without saying. In fact, one cannot help wondering whether unending failure rather than even momentary success must not be the inevitable fate of those who commit themselves in earnest to such a seemingly utopian doctrine. For does it not essentially amount to the demand that the physician should be a citizen of two states, as it were, the one here and now, where he has obligations to his country, the other "laid up in heaven," where he is obligated to mankind alone? How can such a conflict of duties ever be fully resolved?

No one saw this dilemma more clearly than did Osler, when in his last address, from which I quoted at the very beginning of my lecture,

---

[49] Throughout antiquity, medicine remained free from supervision by civil authorities. Even Roman law dealt only with cases of death attributed to the physician's treatment, or with questions of fees and similar contractual problems (cf. Below, *op. cit.*, pp. 108 ff.; also pp. 12 ff.; 63 ff.).

he extolled the ideal of ancient medical humanism and held it up as the ideal to be followed in the future. He spoke after the First World War, after the lights of civilization had gone out over the world. With intrepid honesty he acknowledged the fact that "scientific men, in mufti or in uniform" under the pressure of hostilities, of civic duties rightly or wrongly understood, had compromised their conscience.[50] In the atmosphere of modern nationalism and modern technology it had proved even harder than it may have been in the world of old to distinguish between the rôle of the physician and that of the citizen. Nevertheless, Osler was not shaken in his belief in the ideal, nay he staked all his hopes on a new effort to realize it.

"Two things are clear," he said, "there must be a very different civilization or there will be no civilization at all; and the other is that neither the old religion combined with the old learning, nor both with the new science, suffice to save a nation bent on self-destruction." Reforms are needed. "The so-called Humanists have not enough Science, and Science sadly lacks the Humanities." But even if this defect were remedied, still more remains to be done. What matters is to keep in one's heart and mind "the magic word 'philanthropy,'" love of mankind. Then, one day "the longings of humanity may find their solution, and Wisdom-Philosophia at last be justified of her children."[51]

Perhaps for those who have lived through the nightmare of another World War, who have witnessed the horrors of Fascism and Communism, an effort still greater than Osler's is required in order to have trust in ideals and in the future. If they seek for encouragement, they will find it ever anew, I think, in the sober appeal to good will and reasonableness which Osler made at the close of his memorable last speech, *The Old Humanities and the New Science*.

[50] *The Old Humanities and the New Science*, p. 13.
[51] *Ibid*., pp. 19; 34; 64.

348

THE RELATION OF ANCIENT PHILOSOPHY
TO MEDICINE*

I realize that the subject which I propose to discuss is somewhat alien to the topics to which your studies are devoted. Yet I venture to believe, and I hope not gratuitously, that my subject will seem to you meaningful at least and worth discussing. In our day it has become a commonplace to say that philosophy, the science of man, is to be based on physical science, especially on biology, physiology, medicine, and anthropology, that "the facts of man [are] continuous with those of the rest of nature."[1] Thus, understanding and conduct are to attain a firm foundation, and we flatter ourselves with the belief that in giving so much credence to medicine in the widest sense of the term we are developing tendencies inherent in ancient, in pagan thought. Did not the Greeks who worshipped the body consider man part of nature, different to be sure from animals and the world around him, but still, like all products of nature, obedient to the eternal laws of the cosmos?

At first glance, Greek philosophy seems to bear out the correctness of such a thesis. Whether we study the fragments of the Presocratics, or the writings of Plato, Aristotle, the Stoics, or the Epicureans, all these philosophers, idealistic and materialistic alike, discuss the structure of the human frame. Everywhere is man's mind seen in close relationship to his body. Various temperaments are differentiated in accordance with the variety of bodily constitutions. Shakespeare's words about Brutus, "His life was gentle, and the elements/ So mix'd in him that Nature might stand up/ And say to all the world, 'This was a man!' ",[2] seem well to express the Greek view. Moreover, philosophical

---

* *Bulletin of the History of Medicine*, 1952, vol. 26, pp. 299–316.

This paper was read in 1945 before the General Seminar of the New School for Social Research in New York. Preparing it for publication I have added some references to ancient sources and modern literature and have made a number of changes; but the argument has remained substantially the same.

[1] J. Dewey, *Human Nature and Conduct* [The Modern Library], 1930, p. 12; cf. p. 324.

[2] *Julius Caesar*, V, 5, 73–75.

books are full of physiognomic observations. The physical appearance
of the human being is used to diagnose his character. The diversity of
races, their achievements in art and culture are traced to physical environment. By nature, says Plato, are the Greeks fond of learning, the
Thracians and Scythians high-spirited, the Phoenicians and Egyptians
lovers of money.[3] And later philosophers make similar statements. Do
such views not clearly indicate that Greek philosophy must have learned
from Greek medicine? For from what source other than medicine can
its noted naturalism stem?

Indeed, modern interpreters are inclined to speak of an influence
of Greek medicine on ancient philosophical thought. I doubt the historical adequacy of such an assumption. I think that in antiquity, philosophy
influenced medicine rather than being influenced by it. Philosophical
insight guided the physicians in their biological, physiological, and
anthropological studies. And while in this respect philosophers were
the teachers of physicians, they even were their antagonists in the
struggle for leadership in the conduct of life, sternly rebuking the physicians' ambition to prescribe to man what he ought to do. The true
contribution of medicine to philosophy, I venture to suggest, lies in the
fact that philosophers found in medical treatment and in the physician's
task a simile of their own endeavor. The healing of diseases, as well as
the preservation of health, provided an analogy which served to emphasize the validity of certain significant ethical concepts and thus
helped to establish the truth of philosophy; therein consisted the most
fruitful relationship between ancient medicine and ancient philosophy.

Now, as regards the alleged scientific influence of medical research
on philosophical studies, one must first of all beware of imagining ancient medicine in the likeness of modern medicine and must remember
that medicine in antiquity was primarily a craft. The Homeric poems
group the physician together with the singer and the builder among
those craftsmen whom everybody welcomes, although "a leech is of the
worth of many other men for the cutting out of arrows and the spread-
ing of soothing simples."[4] Fundamentally the same situation prevailed
throughout all periods of ancient history. The average physician had a
certain technical proficiency; he knew medicine, as the phrase goes.
He acquired his skill through apprenticeship with another physician,
and when he became a master in his own right, he practiced his craft, or

---

[3] *Republic*, IV, 435 e–436 a; cf. *Laws*, 747 d–e.
[4] *Iliad*, XI, 514 f.; cf. *Odyssey*, XVII, 382–86.

art, as crafts and arts are always practiced, namely, in accordance with traditional views and usages. He prescribed remedies which had proved helpful before; he took care of wounds and other surgical cases in the way in which previous generations had taken care of them. While learning his trade he was not a "student of medicine"; while carrying on his business he was not a "scientist" applying theoretical knowledge to the case at hand. On the level of common medical practice biological and physiological inquiries were neither presupposed, nor were they actually made. There was not even an obligation to get any kind of training or to study at all; anybody could set himself up as a doctor without acquiring a license or undergoing an examination. It is therefore not astonishing that even in the second century A.D. there were physicians, at least in the country, who were unfamiliar with the difference between arteries and veins,[5] a difference that had been recognized five hundred years before. Yet they could well be successful and respected practitioners, for they relied upon experience, adroitness, and manual perfection, rather than on study or research.

It is in contrast to these craftsmen—the majority of physicians throughout Graeco-Roman civilization—that a relatively small number of medical men aspired to overcome the narrow limits of their craft. If it is characteristic of all Greek scientific achievement that it was the feat of individuals following the bent of their own minds, these doctors certainly were among the finest examples of unsolicited curiosity and delight in learning. Living mainly in the big cities of the ancient world, in the centers of culture, it was they who established the science of medicine as a thin layer over the vast body of merely technical and empirical skill. They patiently observed the courses of diseases, differentiated their various types, gave aetiologies, elaborated a theory of prognostics, formulated methodical rules of treatment. Doing all this, and much more than I can mention here, some of them also realized that the study of the human body must form the basis of medicine.

I have advisedly said that only some physicians acknowledged the need for such studies, for it was not until the very end of antiquity that biology and physiology were generally considered indispensable for medicine. And whether one peruses early or late medical authors concerned with these subjects, he immediately becomes aware of the fact that they were inspired by philosophy.

[5] Gellius, *Attic Nights*, XVIII, 10.

Even among the so-called Hippocratic writings of the fifth and fourth centuries B.C., the oldest surviving medical books, there are some treatises which deal with the nature of the human body. The doctrines here propounded clearly are adaptations of Presocratic theories, of Heraclitus, of Diogenes of Apollonia, and of others. The "Sicilian" physicians were adherents of Empedocles and of his doctrine of the four elements. Diocles, the "second Hippocrates," was an Aristotelian. In Hellenistic times, the medical sect of the Dogmatists, emphasizing the value of anatomy and biology, defended its position by reference to the doctrines of the Dogmatic philosophers and proceeded to explain the phenomena under investigation in accordance with their systems, Platonic or Aristotelian, Stoic or even Epicurean. In the same way the Empiricists, who denied that one can detect the hidden causes of the functions of the body or that such an understanding is useful for medicine, relied on philosophical arguments. They were followers of the Academic Scepsis. When subsequent to Galen, and largely through his influence, Dogmatic medicine became the representative medical system, and knowledge of biology and physiology was at last required of all scientists, a Platonizing Aristotelianism, modified by Stoic natural philosophy, became predominant in medical theory.

Only in one instance, as far as I am aware, was the assertion made that a true understanding of the nature of man can be gained not from philosophy, but from medicine alone. Yet to the Hippocratic author of *On Ancient Medicine*, who proffered this suggestion and who was perhaps himself influenced by the skepticism of the Sophistic movement, man's nature consists in his individuality; it is the sum-total of his particular reactions to food and drink; it is that which is incomparable and varies from case to case. Like later physicians in whose discussions the principle *individuum est ineffabile* was clearly formulated,[6] the Hippocratic writer was troubled by the problem of how the uniqueness of existing phenomena can ever be comprehended by any general theory, and he therefore rejected generalizations altogether. The doctor's insistence that the object of medicine is the individual patient, that the individuality of the phenomena constitutes their only reality, led to the formation of the Methodist school of medicine, the third of the Hellenistic sects, which, affiliating itself with the newly revived philosophy of Pyrrho, renounced the possibility of all general knowledge and pro-

[6] Cf. K. Deichgräber, *Die griechische Empirikerschule*, Berlin, 1930, p. 311.

fessed to be guided only by the Now and Here. Physicians of a similar hue in the first century B.C. had been influential in the restoration of Pyrrho's philosophy. Thus medicine to a certain extent counteracted the Greek predilection for the typical, the negligence of the particular. From the modern point of view, this may well seem to be its most outstanding contribution to Greek thought. But medical skepticism, consistently opposing any attempt at generalizing, also made the establishment of biology or physiology as a science illusory.[7]

It is fair to say, then, that only where medicine became allied with Dogmatic philosophy did physicians actually engage in scientific research concerning the questions of life and death, of health and disease, and that they derived the principles of their biological and physiological investigations from a more comprehensive view of the universe. Of course, I do not wish to imply that all Greek medical scientists were entirely unoriginal. Men like Herophilus or Erasistratus or Galen did not hesitate to interpret the nature of the human body in accordance with their own observations. They felt free to contradict specific philosophical doctrines and in some instances to evolve new theories. But in doing so, they philosophized, they were themselves philosophers, as in Galen's opinion the true physician should be. Even the change from animal anatomy to human anatomy, which certainly was brought about by physicians, was based by them on philosophical rather than medical argumentations.[8] Moreover, once it was admitted that the doctor must be an expert in matters concerning the structure of the human body, medical research led to the discovery of many new data. Dissections and experiments performed by physicians enriched biological and physiological knowledge and made it more precise, as well as more detailed. Yet it is not amiss to recall the fact mentioned before that up until Galen's time not all physicians were interested in inquiries of this kind. And even Galen himself did not believe a study of the entire body to be necessary for medical purposes. Nor did his medical writings impart to physicians more than a description of facts. Their explanation, the scrutiny of the organism as a whole, he put into his philosophical books, which he wrote as a philosopher for philosophers.

Under these circumstances, what Aristotle says of his own time

[7] For the development here sketched, cf. L. Edelstein, "Empirie und Skepsis in der Lehre der griechischen Empirikerschule," *Quellen u. Studien z. Geschichte d. Naturwissenschaften u. d. Medizin*, III, 4, 1933, pp. 253 ff. [195* ff.].

[8] Cf. L. Edelstein, "The Development of Greek Anatomy," *Bulletin of the Inst. of the History of Medicine*, III, 1935, pp. 241 ff.

seems indeed true of the entire history of Greek philosophy and of Greek medicine: physicians concerned with biology and physiology—that is, the ingenious and subtle ones, or the more philosophical ones, as Aristotle calls them in distinction to the great mass of doctors—took their departure from philosophy, just as truly systematic natural philosophy ended in a consideration of the principles of life, of health and disease, and of the constituents of the body.[9] Consequently the assumption of an influence of Greek medicine on Greek philosophy must be regarded, I think, as historically incorrect; modern naturalism and ancient naturalism are not identical. To call the Presocratics physicians and scientists rather than philosophers, as has become fashionable, or to say that from Empedocles on "it is impossible . . . to understand the development of philosophy without keeping the development of medicine constantly in view,"[10] is, I am afraid, a misrepresentation of the actual situation. It was as philosophers that the Presocratics embarked on the quest for the nature of things, and trying to detect the causes of all physical phenomena they also dealt with the human body. Nor is it meaningful to assume that Socrates, granted that he was an empiricist, learned the empirical method from medicine. The empiricism of the Hippocratics, as far as it was a conscious method, was itself derived from philosophy, as were their hypotheses concerning the nature of man. If one points to Plato's relation to contemporary physicians, one must at the same time admit that the physicians whom he may have followed were themselves imbued with philosophy. If one holds that biological research culminated in Aristotle's philosophy, one must realize that the concept of the organism which acts according to purpose was the discovery of the philosopher Aristotle. The doctors of his generation had no inkling of this and understood the body in terms of those early philosophies which the Platonic *Phaedo* and the Platonic *Laws* tried to combat for the first time. Nor does Stoic philosophy, as outlined in Cicero's *De Natura Deorum*, or Epicurean physiology, as described by Lucretius, indicate a preoccupation with medicine. Like physics, such studies in antiquity were the legitimate concern of philosophers and remained, even when taken over by physicians, philosophical rather than scientific inquiries. While astronomy and mathematics no doubt largely determined the course of ancient philosophy, medicine on the whole stayed within the boundaries laid down by philosophy. In its biological

[9] Aristotle, *De Respiratione*, 480 b 26 ff.; *De Sensu*, 436 a 19 ff.
[10] J. Burnet, *Early Greek Philosophy*, fourth ed., London, 1945, p. 201, n. 4.

and physiological theories it reflects the history of philosophy, but it does not explain it.

The same dependence of medical investigations on philosophical presuppositions is evident in the rare cases in which a medical treatise touches upon anthropological and ethical problems.[11] The famous Hippocratic book *On Airs, Waters, and Places* derives the human character from climatic conditions. The Asiatics are feeble, not war-like, but gentle, it contends, because in Asia the seasons are uniform and do not change either toward extreme heat, or toward extreme cold. Yet unlike Montesquieu, of whom this claim is reminiscent, the Hippocratic author does not believe that the form of the state also corresponds to natural conditions, such as the size of the country or the climate. To him laws, civic institutions, are an independent creation of the human mind, they have a causality of their own, they themselves create in man a second nature, as it were, so that in a monarchy even naturally brave and spirited people degenerate into cowards. It is Democritus who speaks through the mouth of the Hippocratic writer. Or again, Galen holds that all philosophers and all physicians are unanimous in assuming that the faculties of the soul depend upon the mixture of the elements of the body. Yet he warns his reader not to forget "the creative power of nature which shapes parts according to the traits of the mind"; he reminds him that "Aristotle dealing with this very subject wondered whether there was not a beginning more divine, something greater than just heat and cold and moist and dry. Wherefore I think it wrong of man to draw such rash conclusions in matters so great and assign to the qualities alone the power of shaping the parts. It is possible that these are nothing more than the instruments and something else the masterhand."[12] Moreover, Galen states, by choosing the right food and drink, by regulating his life correctly, man is able to attain virtue. And he is free to choose what is right; it lies within him to welcome the good, to admit and love it, to shun, to hate, and to flee the evil. To be sure, in Galen's opinion, Chry-

---

[11] How seldom medical writers dealt with the subject becomes clear from a perusal of the survey given by A. Rivaud, "Recherches sur l'anthropologie grecque," *Revue Anthropologique*, XXI, 1911, pp. 157 ff.; 457 ff.; XXII, 1912, pp. 20 ff. I should mention that physiognomic observations are to be found in Greek medical writings, but they are related to the state of the body rather than to that of the mind.

[12] *De Temperamentis*, II, ch. VI [I, pp. 635 f. Kuehn]; I am quoting the translation of the passage given by M. Greenwood, *The Medical Dictator*, London, 1936, p. 33. For the following reference to Galen, cf. *De Sequela*, ch. XI [IV, pp. 814 ff. Kuehn]; cf. also ch. IV [IV, p. 784 Kuehn].

sippus, the great Stoic philosopher, owed his right understanding of the world to the right mixture of the elements in his body. Nevertheless, he would not detract from Chrysippus' merit; for it was Chrysippus who by building up his body in the right way made himself understand the truth. Unlike Shakespeare, whose lines immortalizing the fatalism of a naturalistic view I have quoted in the beginning, Galen would not allow Nature to lay claim on Brutus' greatness. For the Greek physician agrees with Plato, who, though he emphasizes the fact that man's character is shaped by climatic factors, does not on that account dream of absolving him from the responsibility for his actions; or with Aristotle and other philosophers, who, much as they stress the importance of natural gifts, of habits and education, do not hesitate to proclaim man's freedom. He expressly denies the validity of the conclusion that the dependence of the faculties of the soul on the faculties of the body makes praise or blame of human actions unjustifiable.

At this point I beg your leave to make a digression. We are prone to quote the maxim *mens sana in corpore sano*, taking it to epitomize the ancients' conviction that only in a sound body can and will there dwell a sound mind. Actually Juvenal, whom we are quoting, says: "Let us pray that there be a sound mind in a sound body."[13] No ancient physician or philosopher, I think, would have believed that a sound body would or could so to say automatically produce a sound intellect and sound emotions. Galen's pronouncement on man's character, to which I have just referred, is, as he himself implies, typical of medical and philosophical thinking. It presupposes the acceptance of the Dogmatic concept of the soul, which through some of its faculties is the organ of emotions and mind, while through others it regulates the physical functions. The soul, moreover, or at any rate the mind, is considered a substance different from the body, even if modifiable by it. Philosophers more materialistic than Galen, denying the existence of spiritual substances, assumed at least the autonomy of man. Epicurus more vehemently than Plato or any idealistic philosopher defended human freedom. Stoic fatalism questioned man's freedom of action, not his responsibility for his character. It remained for Descartes to claim that the body was a machine, a mechanism that took care of all bodily movements and also produced emotions. It remained for Spinoza, elaborating on Descartes, to claim that "he, who possesses a body capable of the

[13] Juvenal, *Sat.*, X, 356: *orandum est ut sit mens sana in corpore sano.*

356

greatest number of activities, possesses a mind whereof the greatest part is eternal."[14] Descartes saw quite clearly that his concept of the working of the body contradicted the ancient concept of the soul. His new theory was based on Harvey's discovery of the circulation of the blood, from which it seemed to follow that the bodily functions went far beyond anything man had imagined before.[15] Later physicians continuing research along the lines suggested by Harvey, Descartes, and Spinoza, began to uncover the marvels of the body-machine. Medical insight began more and more to change the direction of philosophical thought. Ethics became allied with biology; the mind could now be considered an epiphenomenon of the body.

I am not asking who is right and who is wrong. I have made this digression only in order to accentuate the difference between the ancient and the modern situation. Ancient medicine neither in scientific nor in ethical matters made startling discoveries that heralded a new era; it voluntarily submitted itself to philosophy. This is perhaps one of the reasons for its failure as a science, great as it was as an art. On the other hand, the submission of medicine to philosophy may also in part account for the fact that in all investigations concerning an understanding of the body, as well as of the mind, the leadership rested unchallenged with philosophers.

But it is time for me to dismiss the consideration of these problems and to explain why, in spite of the affinity between medicine and philosophy stressed so far, the two could, as I stated at the very outset, have been opposed to one another in the controversy about the goal of life. To make this understandable, I must first of all remind you of the truism that to the ancients health certainly was one of the highest goods. Indeed, the Skeptic philosopher Sextus does not hesitate to say that to the common people, the men of practical life, health was the *summum bonum* at all times.[16] From post-Homeric centuries onward even poets and writers in ever-increasing numbers contended that without health nothing in this world has any value. To take such an attitude was well in accord with the inborn pessimism of the Greeks, their skeptical doubts as to the chances for happiness, their clear awareness of the tragic aspect of human life. Physicians generally sided with the many,

[14] Spinoza, *Ethics*, V, 39 (transl. by R. H. M. Elwes, *Philosophy of Benedict Spinoza*, p. 274).

[15] *Traité des passions*, I, article 1; 7; cf. *Discours de la méthode*, part V, 7 ff.

[16] Sextus Empiricus, *Adv. Mathem.*, XI, 49.

with the pessimists and skeptics. Since the fifth century B.C. they consistently proclaimed that, as Herophilus phrased it, "when health is absent, wisdom cannot reveal itself, art cannot become manifest, strength cannot fight, wealth becomes useless, and intelligence cannot be made use of."[17] And they urged that not only those who were ill, but also those who were healthy should follow the dictates of medicine, in order to remain healthy.

Their demand at first glance may sound reasonable enough. Yet it seems less convincing as soon as one begins to realize its implications. Since health was considered a balance of the various constituents of the human body, at every moment upset by man's actions, by his taking any food or drink, it had at every moment to be restored consciously. Consequently, a healthy person had to watch himself continuously, he had to subject himself to minute rules, he had to guard against any deviation from the prescribed regimen. Only thus could he be healthy and live long, he was told. An odd way of achieving health and longevity! One might well characterize it in the words in which Macaulay describes how oligarchical government achieves its stability, words which in fact are inspired by Plato's description of ancient dietetics. Oligarchical government, Macaulay says, "has a sort of valetudinarian longevity; it lives in the balance of Sanctorius; it takes no exercise; it exposes itself to no accident; it is seized with a hypochondriac alarm at every new sensation; it trembles at every breath; it lets blood for every inflammation; and thus, without ever enjoying a day of health or pleasure, drags out its existence to a doting and debilitated old age."[18]

But obeisance to such an ideal does not merely stifle enjoyment and pleasure; it makes man unfit for life. It makes him the slave of his body. He loses all freedom of action and decision; he cannot fulfill his duties as a citizen. Plato was not slow in pointing out all these dangers, nor did the Romans overlook them; their initial resistance to Greek medicine was to a large measure due to their opposition to doctrines which threatened to destroy normal political and civic life. Besides, such a regimen of precaution and concern with the body, as again Plato

---

[17] Herophilus *apud* Sext. Empiricum, *Adv. Mathem.*, XI, 50. For details of the medical theories here referred to, cf. L. Edelstein, "Antike Diätetik," *Die Antike*, VII, 1931, pp. 255 ff. [303* ff.].

[18] I am quoting Macaulay's remark from P. Shorey's note on the *Republic*, 406 b [Loeb].

reproachfully remarked, can be followed by the wealthy alone, by those who are not forced to earn a living. Physicians did not deny the correctness of this charge, but they dismissed the case of the poor as beyond repair and turned all their attention to the rich, the only ones who in their opinion could live a worthwhile life. And there is little doubt that many among the great and the wealthy heeded the advice of the physicians, especially in those centuries in which the city state began to lose in importance, or in which the political activity of the individual was diminishing, that is, in the Hellenistic period and in the time of the Roman emperors. Desiring health as they did, unhampered by any professional obligation, uninterested in being busy for the sake of being busy, the upper classes were free to live for their health, to indulge in the idolatry of the body endorsed by the physicians.

It was inevitable therefore that philosophers passionately fought against medicine and its glorification of health, just as they had opposed the agonistic ideal and the glorification of the athlete. More consequential even than their criticism of the political and social dangers which the teaching of medical dietetics promoted was their vigorous denial that health was the *summum bonum*, that it was identical with happiness, the aim toward which all human endeavor should be directed. Naturally, it is not my intention to contend that Plato, Aristotle, the Cynics, the Stoics, the Epicureans were altogether contemptuous of health. Before the slow disintegration of ancient culture set in, no Greek would have gone to that extreme; health remained a good to be at least preferred, as the Stoics put it. But philosophers were unanimous in their judgment that values other than health are superior. To give more emphasis to their point of view they even laid down their own rules for a proper regimen. What Plato in the *Republic* and in the *Laws* says about gymnastics, the education of children, the daily routine of men and women, what Plutarch sets forth in his charming little book *Advice on How to Keep Well*, serves to teach all and sundry how to live healthily without putting oneself into a strait jacket and without neglecting one's social and moral obligations.

To repress the dangers threatening from the leadership of physicians in society, Samuel Butler in his *Erewhon* made it a crime to be sick and therefore to be in need of medical care. Otherwise, the judge in the Erewhonian trial says, "the doctors should be the only depositaries of power in the nation, and have all that we hold precious at their mercy. A time of universal dephysicalization would ensue."[19] Butler's solution of the difficulty as he saw it may be ingenious, but it is hardly practicable. The problem was solved more reasonably and adroitly by Greek philosophers. Even Plato did not go beyond restricting the physician's practice to cases of emergency. However, he and Aristotle and all subsequent philosophers raised the question of who would determine what is valuable and what is not. The physician decides whether his patient ought to take walking exercise or not; he does not and cannot tell him whether he ought to be healthy or not, whether his life should be saved at all cost. In other words, the positing of aims lies with philosophy, not with the art of medicine, or with any other art or science, for that matter.[20] The physician therefore must mind his own business and not interfere with things that are beyond his reach. He may excel in preserving the health of those who wish to be healthy, in healing the diseases of those who wish to get well; but he cannot tell men what they should wish. In modern times, the physician has become the confidant of the healthy and of the sick, the expert of social agencies, the counselor of the judge, the authority to whom even the planners of foreign and domestic policies look up. To the Greek philosophers, he was no advisor on morals, justice, or politics. To them, medicine was not another form of education or philosophy. They clung to their prerogatives and insisted on their absolute sovereignty.[21]

Nevertheless—and this brings up the last aspect of my subject which I wish to discuss—whenever philosophers tried to interpret for the benefit of others the significance and meaning of their own endeavors, they could not find any parallel more illuminating than that of philosophy and medicine. Writers of all philosophical creeds gave a prominent place to the analogy of body and soul, to the similarity between the training of the body and the discipline of the soul, to the consideration of medicine as a counterpart of ethics, and, as I suggested before, it was perhaps in the usefulness of this comparison for the philosophical argument that lay the greatest debt of philosophy to medicine. What were

[19] Ch. XI (Some Erewhonian Trials).
[20] Cf. *Ethica Eudemia*, II, 2, 1227 b 25 ff.; cf. also *Ethica Nicomachea*, III, 3, 1112 b 12–16; *Magna Moralia*, I, 1, 1182 b 28–30. Cf. also Plato, *Laches*, 195 c–d.
[21] The dissension between physicians and philosophers is not taken into account by W. Jaeger, *Paideia: The Ideals of Greek Culture*, New York, III, 1944, pp. 3 ff.; this is one of the main reasons why I cannot agree with his evaluation of the role of medicine, cf. especially pp. 44 f.

the reasons for this peculiar predilection which philosophers showed for the medical simile? The frequency of references to medicine in philosophical books has, of course, often been noticed, but so far it has not found a satisfactory explanation.

Now, the starting point of all the comparisons between body and soul is perhaps not too difficult to understand. The philosopher, insisting on the value of the soul and proclaiming its superiority over the body, was faced with man's natural partiality to his body. He was therefore driven to contrast the two; he had to try to turn man's thought from his body and its interests to his soul and its concerns. In this attempt the Greek philosopher, while on the one hand finding his task especially difficult due to the Greeks' love of the body, gained on the other hand a specific advantage. From the fifth century B.C., that is, from the time when the discussion of ethical problems became an integral part of philosophy, medicine propounded the doctrine that the body needs conscientious care if it is to perform its functions properly. Philosophy therefore found in medicine a basis for exhortation which appealed strongly to the Greeks. Was it not obvious to conclude that what is true of the body must also be true of the soul, since body and soul are both parts of our being? That in fact it must be true to an even higher degree in regard to the soul which is so infinitely more precious?

Yet the protreptic appeal to the body and its medical needs, intended to enforce the dogma that the soul likewise needs care, was not merely emotional, it implied at the same time another purpose. In the beginning of the *Nicomachean Ethics*, Aristotle parallels his teaching concerning moral qualities with the teaching concerning health, because, he says, it is necessary to explain what is invisible by means of visible illustration.[22] The soul is invisible; knowledge about it is elusive. By comparing the soul to the body, that which is seemingly unreal is translated into comprehensible language. And if one remembers that in antiquity everybody was familiar with medicine—it was the only art or science about which everybody knew something; physicians wrote books for the general public; laymen discussed medical problems with their physicians; in short, medical knowledge was perhaps diffused more widely in Greek and Roman times than in any other period of history— one immediately realizes the particular forcefulness of such medical

[22] II, 2, 1104 a 13–14.

illustrations. In referring to medical insight the philosopher speaks of something that people can be expected to possess and that will help them to grasp the new kind of insight that they are expected to acquire through philosophy.

At this point, however, you may ask: how can medical knowledge, knowledge of the body, be helpful toward an adequate understanding of the soul? Are not body and soul essentially different? Is it not just the difference between the two which the philosopher tries to point out? My answer is that it is characteristic of Greek ethics that it conceives of the soul in the likeness of the body, that it visualizes the soul in very much the same way in which the body was understood, not on a highly technical level, to be sure, but rather in terms of that medical doctrine which was basic and almost universally accepted. The body has its desires, it strives to be filled, to be satiated. These bodily appetites in themselves tend to be extreme; they have no self-restricting limits. In order to prevent disease, to attain health, it is necessary to check the natural tendencies, to introduce measure, a standard by which to curtail the unlimited appetites. The desires of the soul, in the view of the Pythagoreans, of Plato, and of Aristotle, likewise tend to extremes; they strive unceasingly to be satisfied. Pythagorean ethics, Platonic justice, the Aristotelian doctrine of the mean, teach the measure, the standard by which the extremes of our passions are to be reduced to their right proportion. Nor did the body fail to provide an example when Cynics, Stoics, and Epicureans considered all natural activities of the soul, all natural emotions as bad, or even diseased. Does not language itself indicate the similarity of body and soul? Are not the emotions called by the same name, *pathe*, that denotes the sickness of the body? Is it not true—to use Lucretius' words—that "our soul itself has a flaw and that by this flaw an inward corruption taints all that comes from without, even though it were a blessing"?[23] And is it not equally true that the body and its natural functions are diseased? If man is not constantly on the lookout, he continually falls into disease, he is continually sick. This was exactly the theory on the basis of which the dietetics for the healthy was developed, as I have pointed out before. Like the body then, which must be made healthy, so the soul, sick by nature, needs purging, as Lucretius says, or treatment, as the Stoics contend, in order to be healthy.[24] Only in this manner can virtue be achieved, that state

[23] *De Rerum Natura*, VI, 17–19 [Loeb translation, adapted].
[24] *De Rerum Natura*, VI, 24; Chrysippus, Fr. 471 Arnim.

of eudaemonia which philosophers never tired of celebrating as "the health of the soul."

Important as the medical simile proved to be in all these respects, its deepest significance becomes apparent only in the consequences drawn from the analogies I have mentioned so far. To understand their full bearing it is necessary to recall one feature of Greek medicine that was obvious to the ancients, yet is rarely appreciated by modern interpreters. Greek medicine reversed man's natural beliefs; it had something paradoxical about it. It seems natural to suppose that we are healthy as long as we are not sick, that if we follow the instincts of our body we will be well. The teaching of Greek dietetics, the doctrine according to which every one, even the healthy person, must care for his body, ran counter to man's natural feelings. Moreover, it always remained strange to the ancients that man should renounce his rights over himself and should obey the physician, who reigns over him as the king reigns over his subjects, to borrow a phrase of Galen.[25] To accept such a rule again seemed unnatural, for the body is our own; we are its masters, and no one else. The irritation felt was aggravated by the fact that the free citizen, the rich man, had to follow the commands of a craftsman who often was a slave. Finally, the Greeks and Romans never ceased wondering about the paradox that by cauterizing and cutting, by doing violence to his body, man should achieve health, that good should come of something that in itself is painful and causes suffering.

It was precisely this paradoxical truth that reason and experience had taught man to accept in medical matters, on which philosophers seized for their purposes. You find the philosophers' teaching paradoxical, Epictetus asks. And he answers his own question by saying: "But are there not paradoxes in the other arts? And what is more paradoxical than to lance a man in the eye in order that he may see? If anyone said this to a man who was inexperienced in the art of surgery, would he not laugh at the speaker? What is there to be surprised at, then, if in philosophy also many things which are true appear paradoxical to the inexperienced?"[26] Indeed the whole range of the transvaluation of values that was brought about by philosophical ethics, could best be illustrated by the medical example.

The paradoxical quality of Cynic and Stoic teaching concerning natural feelings and emotions needs no emphasis. Their notion of the

---

[25] *De Methodo Medendi*, I, 1 [X, p. 4 Kuehn].
[26] Epictetus, *Dissertationes*, I, 25, 32–33 [Loeb].

"health of the soul" was as shocking, the very antithesis of the natural, as was the medical teaching about the health of the body. Nor did Lucretius deny that Epicurus' doctrine of "the healthy soul" seemed "somewhat harsh to those who have not used it, and the people shrink back from it."[27] By pleasure they understood something quite different from that which Epicurus considered pleasure. But did Plato's philosophy contribute less toward changing common beliefs? To be sure, he still upheld the old values; but did he understand them in the same way? Is it natural to believe that it is better for man to suffer injustice than to do injustice, if he must choose between the two? Plato found it necessary to turn man's neck, so as to make him see the light of truth.[28] Or is Aristotle's ethical theory opposed to a lesser degree to man's instinctive feelings? Can one immediately understand his contention that matters of conduct and expediency have nothing fixed or invariable about them, that moral qualities are so constituted as to be destroyed by excess no less than by deficiency?[29] Aristotle at any rate did not think this to be self-evident and took great pains to prove it.

Moreover, if man must acquire the knowledge needed to regulate his physical life from the physician, the expert, who has found it, if he must submit himself to his judgment, to his guidance, the same demand was made by the philosopher, and again it was upheld regardless of the social position of the expert, of the ruler, and of the ruled. It is true, Plato still believed that the individual by himself should and could find the truth. Socrates, to him, was not a physician; his help in finding the right answer was comparable to the assistance given by the midwife; man's knowledge is his own child, as it were. But wherever Plato tries to solve ethical questions within the framework of political theory, he finds no more cogent parallel to the position which the true statesman ought to occupy than that of the physician. Statesmen must rule, he says, "whether they are rich or poor, over willing and unwilling subjects alike, with or without written laws, just as physicians must prescribe cures with or without the patient's consent, and whether they do so on the basis of written laws or without them, and whatever they do, whoever they are, we call them physicians."[30] Aristotle, on the other hand,

---

[27] *De Rerum Natura*, IV, 18–20 [Loeb].

[28] *Republic*, VII, 515 c.

[29] *Ethica Nicomachea*, II, 2, 1104 a 11 ff.

[30] *Politicus*, 293 a–b. For Plato and the simile of medicine, cf. also L. Edelstein, "The Role of Eryximachus in Plato's Symposium," *Transactions of the Amer. Philol. Assoc.*, LXXVI, 1945, pp. 98 ff. [166* ff.].

bids us to be our own doctors, hitting the right mark through our own insight. With the Cynics and Stoics the philosopher himself became a doctor, the expert who diagnosed the disease of man. For the diagnosis of our passions, says Galen, cannot be entrusted to ourselves; it must be entrusted to other people, and "it is not just any chance person to whom this oversight can be given."[31] Ethics thus became *medicina mentis*, medicine of the soul; the philosopher came to rule over his client with absolute power.

Nor was the final point of comparison overlooked: the treatment cannot be soft and in accordance with our wishes; it must be painful, it must hurt. Plato insisted that the true statesman must be allowed to kill or to banish people, just as the physician is allowed to heal by cutting us, or burning us, or by causing us pain in any other way.[32] And while Lucretius was intent on lessening the bitterness of the remedy by adding "the delicious honey of the Muses,"[33] the Stoics delighted in emphasizing the harshness of the treatment. It may suffice to quote Epictetus: "Men, the lecture room of the philosopher is a hospital; you ought not to walk out of it in pleasure, but in pain. For you are not well when you come; one man has a dislocated shoulder, another an abscess, another a fistula, another a headache. And then am I to sit down and recite to you dainty little notions and clever little mottoes, so that you will go out with words of praise on your lips, one man carrying away his shoulder just as it was when he came in, another his head in the same state, another his fistula, another his abscess? And so it's for this, is it, that young men are to travel from home, and leave their parents, their friends, their relatives, and their bit of property, merely to cry 'Bravo!' as you recite your clever little mottoes? Was this what Socrates used to do, or Zeno, or Cleanthes?"[34] It is indeed true that this paradox, like all others, could best be made clear by the paradox of medicine, as Epictetus says.

I have come to the end of my analysis of the relation between Greek philosophy and medicine. Many intricate questions I could only touch upon. Many difficult problems I could discuss only in a general way. Details have still to be worked out. The characteristic differences prevailing in the various centuries must be marked more clearly. But

---

[31] *De Animae Perturbationibus*, I, ch. vi [V, p. 30 Kuehn] transl. by A. J. Brock, *Greek Medicine* [The Library of Greek Thought], 1929, p. 170.

[32] *Politicus*, 293 b.

[33] *De Rerum Natura*, IV, 22.

[34] *Dissertationes*, III, 23, 30–32 [Loeb].

this much, I think, can be stated safely: medicine did not influence philosophy by giving to it scientific information, nor did it help philosophy to find a solution of ethical questions. But medicine did serve philosophy as a means of explaining and of making acceptable to men that conclusion which philosophy itself had reached, that man can live without philosophy as little as he can live without medicine.

THE DISTINCTIVE HELLENISM OF GREEK MEDICINE*

A̲t least for one year, it was my good fortune to be Garrison's colleague. It was the last year of his life and the shadow of death had already fallen upon him; but the strength and charm of his personality
were unimpaired. When, after his death, I read in one of his letters the
advice he gave a young friend: "You must be frank in your statements
and still remain a gentleman,"[1] I believed I knew why I had been so
greatly impressed by our brief contact. The Colonel, except perhaps in
bearing, most unmilitary, was a truly civilized man. And gentleman
that he was in his life, he was a gentleman also in his work. He was not
satisfied with being a specialist. Much as he loved medicine and its history, the subject for him was part of the history of general culture. He
knew that in order to understand the position of the physician, one
must take account of the spirit of the age, which pervades the sciences
as well as the humanities, the fine arts no less than music, and bestows
a peculiar and unique character on individuals and peoples.

I recall my memory of Garrison not only to pay tribute to the historian in whose honor grateful friends have named the lecture that it is
my privilege to give. I also draw encouragement from it for the discussion of the topic I have chosen. In analyzing the distinctive Hellenism of
Greek medicine, that is the specifically Greek traits of medicine, the
achievements which set Greek medicine apart from Babylonian or
Egyptian medicine or medicine as practiced in any other period, I shall
be concerned with theories rather than with practical results; I shall try
to place what was achieved within the broader framework of Greco-
Roman civilization. Moreover, I propose to raise questions regarding
values and ideals which determined the patient's, as well as the physician's, attitude toward medicine and which themselves are largely
shaped by the outlook on life characteristic of Greeks and Romans.

Such a procedure is of course open to objections. Even granting

* *Bulletin of the History of Medicine*, 1966, vol. 40, pp. 197–255: The Fielding H.
Garrison Lecture for 1960.

that medicine is influenced by the time and place in which it is practiced and does not proceed in isolation, one may claim that its concern is always and everywhere the same. Its purpose is practical, its aim, to heal disease, by drugs or diet or surgery. In this sense, the distinctive character of the healing art of a civilization lies in the success of the treatment it provides for the sick. Its theories count for little; far less matter its dreams and aspirations outside the realm of medicine.[2]

I have no wish to minimize the importance of the practical achievement of the medical art. But I trust it is more than inability to deal with this theme that has led me to choose the other and attach to it equal, if not greater, significance. Although health and disease are coeval with man, they are experienced differently by different societies. Medicine and its development can be favored or hampered by social factors. The general intellectual movement can help or hinder the acquisition of medical knowledge. And since the physician is concerned not with dead matter or lifeless machines but with human beings, he is called upon to satisfy wishes and desires. He is asked to respond to hopes and fears as well as to bodily needs in the agony of the days, perhaps months, in which life is ending. None of these issues—constituting, as it were, the formal rather than the material aspect of medicine—can be neglected by the doctor who wants to carry out his task well. Without knowing how they were solved, the historian cannot estimate the full measure of medicine's past success.[3]

Such an evaluation of ancient medicine as I have in mind is a hazardous undertaking, first of all because the evidence preserved for it is scanty. For the commonly accepted attitudes of behavior, the facts of situations universally known are rarely stated explicitly in medical books or in the general literature.[4] Incidental remarks must be used to draw a generalized picture. Moreover, the subject has so far received little attention. Whenever one has attempted to delineate the distinctive character of Greek medicine, it is medicine of the classical age alone that has been dealt with.[5] And yet, did ancient medicine not extend over almost a thousand years, a span of time in which great social and intellectual changes took place? That all that should be said on so vast a topic could be ferreted out at one stroke and in the compass of one lecture, it would be foolhardy to believe. I therefore embark upon my discussion, not hoping for an exhaustive solution, but wishing to make a beginning, and realizing that all beginnings, as the ancient proverb has it, are small (Cicero, *De finibus*, V, 21, 58).[6]

I

Now, when one reads ancient medical literature, that is, when one directs one's attention not to medicine as it may have been practiced by the average physician, but as it was understood by the refined and accomplished doctor,[7] one is, to be sure, first of all impressed by the attempt to describe his cases and to conceptualize these descriptions. The Orient too possessed empirical information—and a vast store of it. The Greeks, borrowing data no doubt from their predecessors, turned it into knowledge. Where their forerunners had noted details, moments of sickness, as it were, they encompassed the whole process of illness.[8] And on the basis of such a comprehensive view, the majority of authors named diseases and studied their etiology. They recognized the importance of anatomical and physiological insight, they maintained that treatment depends on, and varies with, the explanation of the nature of the body and its constituent organs. The beginnings of such an attitude are exhibited in the Hippocratic Corpus. Hellenistic and later research develops it into a formal medical system. In short, the Greeks invented the science of medicine.[9]

That this scientism was one of the great achievements of ancient medicine has been denied of late. Classical medicine, one has said, was an art, not a science. The truly Hippocratic doctor was concerned with the patient, not with the disease. In fact, throughout antiquity, the good physician rejected the myth of scientific nomenclature; for him, the symptoms were the disease; he treated the patient, not the organs of the body. When etiological and anatomical thought became predominant, they were signs of decadence rather than progress and accomplishment.[10]

There is no gainsaying the assertion that theorizing is a danger to medical practice, that he who is concerned only with parts of the bodily frame and not with the human being as a whole will not be a successful physician. Nor were the ancients unaware of these facts. Having set forth the scientific approach to medicine, Aristotle says that men of experience, who have knowledge of particulars, succeed to a greater degree than those who have theory without experience and know only of universals, "for it is not man that the physician cures, except incidentally, but Callias or Socrates or some other person similarly named, who is incidentally a man as well" (*Metaphysics*, I, 981 a 18 ff.; Loeb). Yet if it is true that in treatment experience is indispensable and even superior to mere theory, it is also true that the "theoretician" is wiser than the experienced—for he knows the causes and the wherefores of the facts (981 a 24–29)—and is able to teach others what to do (b 7–9). Or as Celsus, summarizing the Hellenistic point of view, puts it, "this contemplation of the nature of things [in contrast to the nature of the patient], although it does not make a practitioner, yet renders him more apt and perfected in the Art of Medicine." Through it, Hippocrates, Erasistratus, and the others "did not . . . become practioners," they became "better practitioners" (*Prooem.*, 47; Loeb).[11]

Moreover, not only was it agreed upon among ancient scientists that experience at the bedside, as it were, was essential; they also tried to bridge the gulf that exists between universal insight and particular instances. Thus Cnidian medicine multiplied the disease entities. Instead of one type of pneumonia or of other illnesses, it assumed the existence of several kinds and thereby diversified abstractions and brought them closer to reality (*On regimen in acute diseases*, ch. 1). Another method, and the preferred one in the *Corpus Hippocraticum*, was the injunction that in treating the sick, the physician must take account of the disease and its "fashion" (hōrē), and, in addition, of the constitution of the patient—age, sex, physique—as well as of the concomitant circumstances—the seasons of the year, the place where treatment is administered, the occupation of the patient (e.g., *On the nature of man*, ch. 9). In medicine, therefore, it is impossible to lay down an absolutely fixed and invariable rule (*On places in man*, ch. 41). And Celsus, assenting to the proposition that medicine "admits of scarcely any universal precepts" (*Prooem.*, 63; Loeb),—despite his advocacy of rationalism in medicine (74)—gives a list of particulars underlying the generalities (70 ff.) which is almost identical with that to be found in the Hippocratic writers.[12]

Nor does anatomical thought ever come to predominate in ancient medical science. The Hippocratic books, generally speaking, consider knowledge of the structure of the human body a help to the physician; the functioning of the organs as such does not explain diseases. The work of the founders of human anatomy may have tended to divert the attention of the researcher from the whole to the parts of the body, as Galen was not slow in pointing out. But even he must admit that Erasistratus was not exclusively determined by merely anatomical considerations (*On the natural faculties*, II, 8), that instead he acknowledged the importance of the "faculties" in which Galen himself sees the true and individualizing cause of disease and the one to be combined with organic functions (II, 9). And Herophilus, the other leading anatomist, did, after all, trace illnesses not so much to their seat in organs as to the dyscrasia (*kakochymia*) of the humors. Thus the ancients always tried to strike a balance between the data of the given case and anatomy as well as physiology, considering the latter helpmates rather than guides of the medical practitioner.[13]

I do not say that everyone in antiquity saw the situation in the way I have represented it. There were those who rejected the explanations of diseases and the study of anatomy and physiology. They did so, however, because it seemed to them impossible on epistemological grounds to derive any certain knowledge from such investigations. What the physician can find out and needs to find out, they claimed, is to be gained from observations of a different nature. Nor shall I maintain that the attempts of the scientists to adapt universal formulations to individual instances were entirely successful. Galen remarks that all physicians agree that in the last analysis the individuality of the patient cannot be expressed in any formula; it is ineffable (*Methodus medendi*, III, 3; vol. 10, p. 181 f., ed. Kühn, also p. 159 f.). The same conviction inspires Celsus' contention that it is better to have a friend than a stranger as one's doctor (*Prooem.*, 73). The friend's familiarity with the patient supplies the data which abstract doctrine cannot provide. But even for the stranger the distance between learning and action was narrowed down by Greek medicine's endeavor to concretize as it were the concept of disease, be it that the process of abstraction was due to the constitution of disease entities or to the acceptance of physiological and anatomical theories.[14]

One does not need the testimony of Aristotle or Galen to realize that the problems which medical scientism faced were not peculiar to medicine. In every realm of human activity the application of general rules to particular cases has its difficulties, and different ancient scientists tried to solve them in different ways.[15] In jurisprudence the rigidity of the law led to a stress on the principle of equity, to a distinction between the written and the unwritten, the natural, law. Other sciences went in other directions. Nowhere, perhaps, was the attempt greater, more consistent, and as long-lasting, as in medicine. For it is only at the very end of antiquity that medical treatises turned into textbooks arranged by paragraphs, that diseases of the individual became cases to be decided by precedents, like legal cases. As Paulus of Aegina puts it, the ancient writers were too prolix: he will put his remarks into the form of a commentary on their writings, and his own work should be consulted as if it were a book of law (*Praefatio*). This legalistic turn, not uninfluenced, one is inclined to think, by the attitude of the Romans,[16] marked the end of genuinely Greek medicine. Now it had become a rigorous and undeviating science; before, it had been a science and an art at the same time, and this, I venture to maintain, was its first and perhaps most distinctive achievement.[17]

Like the origin of so many of the great historical accomplishments, that of medical scientism is nameless. But whoever it was who took the first step, he was not following a merely individual whim. Rather is medical science a Greek invention and born out of the same spirit which, in the Presocratic period, made sciences out of the riches of Oriental observations and accumulated data in the fields of mathematics, astronomy, geography, and history.[18] And from the beginning of its appearance in literature, medical theorizing was heavily in the debt of philosophy. Most of the doctrines proposed in the Hippocratic essays and the methods followed are taken over from Presocratic thinkers. The originality of the physicians appears in the adjustment of theory to practice which I have mentioned before. Moreover, scientific medicine quite naturally continued to grow under the tutelage of philosophy, which, in classical and Hellenistic times, did not divorce itself from the study of the human body and the exploration of scientific procedures. The demand for human rather than animal anatomy sprang from the philosophical analysis of the value of comparative research; physiological investigations were based on the philosophical concepts of organic life; rationalism, as well as empiricism, in medicine was founded on the same arguments that were invoked for philosophical rationalism and empiricism.[19]

Of course, the more complicated and detailed the actual research in anatomy and physiology tended to become, the more the physician turned into an expert on these matters and assumed the rôle of an adviser to the philosopher. What life is is a philosophical problem; where it is located in the body, however, is a medical issue to be decided only by the trained anatomist and physiologist. With regard to such questions, then, the philosopher has to learn from the physician, just as he is in need of instruction from the astronomer concerning the actual movements of the heavenly bodies, despite the fact that the principle of movement is worked out by philosophical reason.[20] But, to repeat, the foundation of medicine was laid down by philosophy; neither empiricists nor rationalists doubted this. That philosophy and medicine were in such a sense closely allied, was another distinctive characteristic of the Greek medical science.

It is true, such an assertion did not remain unchallenged in antiquity; it is being challenged nowadays. Among the ancients, the author of the Hippocratic treatise *On ancient medicine* considered philosophy incompatible with the medical art; Celsus, that is, Hellenistic historiography, celebrated Hippocrates as the physician "who separated this branch of learning from the study of philosophy" (*Prooem.*, 8; Loeb). Modern interpreters claim even more for medicine than that it had its own method, its own way of gaining pertinent insight. It was, they say, until the fourth century, the only natural science in the strict sense of the word. In contrast to the *a priori* speculations of Presocratic philosophy it built up an empirical theory of knowledge and performed genuine experiments. Doctors were the first to interrogate "Nature with an open mind, prepared to accept the answers she gives and to modify their practice accordingly."[21]

Now the latter contention is surely unwarranted. No Hippocratic book provides an empirical theory of knowledge, if by this term one means a set of generalizations based on particular data of observation or experiments. Even *On ancient medicine*, opposed as it is to philosophical postulates, is far from accomplishing such a feat. For it, nicety of truth allows of "neither number nor weight, by reference to which knowledge can be made exact, . . . except bodily feeling" (ch. IX; Loeb). That is, the investigator must, and can, find out only how a specific kind of food or drink affects the individual patient, whether it harms or strengthens him, how much or how little is detrimental or beneficial (ch. XX). To put it differently, things have no objective qualities; they become what they are through the reactions of the subject. Thus Protagorean skepticism is infused into medicine or seen as most fitting to its individualizing tendencies; all attempts at scientism, except with regard to what one can learn from the anatomical structure of the body (ch. XXII f.), are declared to be futile.[22]

As far as Hippocratic writers adhered to empirical views or performed experiments in illustration or confirmation of their views, they did not go beyond what can be found in the fragmentary remains of the Presocratics. And the same holds true of the proponents of a rational or, as one used to say later, dogmatic medicine. Nor can one find in these early writings an attitude toward nature that was peculiar to the doctor. Even the healing power of nature, undoubtedly known to them, became decisive for medical thought only after the teleological principle had been formulated by Platonic and Aristotelian idealism. The dogmatists of the Hellenistic era were indebted to philosophers for their discussions of mechanism and teleology, of qualities and faculties no less than of atoms and of the *horror vacui*. Empirical physicians, though they were wont to call themselves after their god, "experience," rather than any man, were followers of the Academic *skepsis*, just as the Methodists, granted that they helped to revive skepticism in the first century B.C., were of the Aenesidemean persuasion. The philosophical coloring of the Galenic system, the codification of ancient medicine, needs no emphasis.[23]

It stands to reason then that the development of Greek medicine cannot be separated from that of Greek philosophy. This was perhaps not an unmixed blessing. Historical hindsight can easily detect the impediments put in the way of medical science by philosophical speculations, nowhere more easily than in the fate of empiricism, which, under the impact of rational analysis, tended to become prematurely skeptical. But one may also wonder whether it would have been possible to give a permanent form to the scientific impetus, had philosophical reflection not helped to clarify it and to elevate it to a well-rounded and firm insight. Certainly it was submission to philosophy which gave to ancient medicine its consciousness of principles and methods, this unique quality that makes the books written so long ago still worth reading.

II

Why did Greek medicine follow a course so different from that of Oriental medicine, by which it was preceded? One is immediately ready to invoke in explanation the Greek genius, the creative power of individuals who shaped events. Far be it from me to underestimate the power of these factors. Yet I think that beyond them one can point to certain more particular features of the Greek social and intellectual setting that must have helped greatly to make medicine what it was to be.

The first of these features to be taken into account seems to be that medicine remained free from all legislative interference. In Egypt, says

Aristotle (*Politics*, III, 15, 1286 a 12 ff.), any change in treatment before four days have passed is prescribed by the doctor at his own risk. According to the code of Hammurabi, he who is unsuccessful in surgery will have his hands cut off.[24] Such prohibitive regulations make men cling to tradition and stifle the courage to attempt ever new things. Left unhampered, Greek inventiveness, not to say love of intellectual adventure, could unfold fully in the field of medicine and always seek improvement.[25]

It is, to be sure, natural that society should wish to call the doctor to account for his actions and not leave all responsibility to him alone. The ancients were well aware of this fact and marveled at the freedom they had granted to physicians. Their feelings often were expressed with sarcasm and irony. The doctor, says the comic poet Philemon (*Fragmenta comicorum graecorum*, ed. Meineke, IV, 1841, p. 68), is the only one permitted to kill and not to die for it; he is the only one to enjoy impunity for causing death, Pliny reiterates, for the situation did not change in the Roman world. Even physicians sometimes maintained that a supervision of medicine by the state would be of great value (Ps. Hippocrates, *Law*, ch. 1).[26]

And indeed, had the Greeks or Romans known of licensing physicians, they might have had fewer charlatans to treat their diseases, fewer doctors that were like supernumeraries in tragedies, as the Hippocratic writer puts it (*Law, loc. cit.*). Medicine then might also through Galen's efforts have reached a stage of unification much earlier than it actually did, for all departments of learning were ripe for such a simplification and the one empire favored it and supported it by the foundation of universities. As it was, differences of opinion reigned supreme. The *Corpus Hippocraticum* presents the most divergent views on essential problems. Hellenistic authors defend sharply conflicting theories and methods. For two or three centuries after Galen had inaugurated the "best sect," blending the best of the past with the results of his own research, there still remained room for the dissension between a qualitatively oriented biologism, rational and empirical at the same time, and an atomic mechanism which had skeptical overtones.[27]

But it was in consequence of the very same freedom that the ancients were able to develop the patterns of thought for later generations. And in regard to the relationship between patient and doctor, where freedom could so easily have turned into complete licentiousness and irresponsibility, the danger implicit in the social set-up was averted by

the creation of a professional ethics, unequaled in the Orient. Not that
the Egyptian or Babylonian physicians were unethical or necessarily
devoid of sympathy or love for their patients. But as far as standards of
treatment were generally acknowledged, they were, as I said, imposed
by the state; the kindness shown to the sick was the instinctive kindness
of the heart. The Greeks and Romans devised ethical rules from a scrutiny of the task of the physician, from a philosophical view of life, and
observed them as the expression of the code which is appropriate and
fitting for the devotee of the task of healing. This voluntary acceptance
of the moral law was not the least contribution they made to the constitution of medicine as an art and science.[28]

One must not, however, forget that although society did not restrict
the physician by legislation, it obviously cherished certain convictions
concerning his task and the manner in which it was to be carried out.
This is undoubtedly true of every society. It was especially true of the
ancients, who witnessed the rise of the arts and sciences, who dealt with
the problems involved, not only in recondite books but often enough in
public and private discussions, and who, as far as medicine was concerned, certainly took a lively interest in the subject and were not un-
informed outsiders but rather well informed and capable of judging the
experts. The consequences of such an attitude become especially clear
in the evaluation of the relationship between medicine and magic, that
pseudoscience from which the healing art is so often said to have sprung.

Whatever the situation may have been in prehistoric Greece, in
Homer's time the physician was already the member of a lay craft; he
was "a worker for the common weal" like the maker of spears, the
singer, the seer (*Odyssey*, XVII, 383–85). He remained throughout
antiquity a craftsman, an artisan, a scientist. As such, he was the representative of a knowledge peculiarly his own, not to be confounded with
the knowledge others had or pretended to have. First of all, therefore,
it was not his business to meddle with magic. "It is not a learned physician," says Sophocles (*Ajax*, 581 f.), "who sings incantations over
pains which should be cured by cutting"; a physician who uses incantations or exorcisms, the Roman law holds (*Digesta*, L, 13, 1; § 3), cannot
sue for his salary, for such things do not belong to medicine.

The verdicts quoted imply that not every physician refrained from
the behavior felt to be improper. How could it be otherwise, above all in
a world in which everyone who wanted to do so could set himself up as
a doctor? It is the more remarkable that the medical writings preserved,

376

from the fifth century B.C. to the end of antiquity, reject magic with one voice. In the majority of instances magic is rejected as a pseudo-science—the reason usually given by the rationalist; when its efficacy, though it remains inexplicable, is not completely denied—the position of the empiricist—it is still acknowledged that the physician proceeds by applying remedies, by using the knife, not by uttering words.[29]

In Egypt, in Babylon, in India, the demarcation line between a natural or rational treatment of disease and magical performances or religious rites was never clearly drawn. Medical treatises abound with incantations; none of the writers shows any awareness that in relying on such means he violates the law of medicine, nor are there critical voices outside the medical literature condemning him for proceeding in a manner unbecoming the physician.[30]

Did the Greek doctors of the classic age disentangle their art from magic driven by "the same impulse toward rationalism which had already driven the Milesian philosophers to disengage cosmogony from its mythical trappings?" The Greeks, no less than the Romans, surely were superstitious; and I have no wish to deny that some physicians contributed to the victory of light over darkness. But it can hardly be said that the medical art had at any time to be liberated by them from the shackles of magic. It was by definition, as it were, a human art. The rationalism of ancient life as a whole had given its fixed place to man's endeavor to overcome obstacles by powers which are in his own hands. Those who craved the assistance of other forces turned to other men supposedly experts in the use of supernatural means. The Greek doctors were more fortunate than their Oriental colleagues.

They were so also by the very fact that the position of religion in their world was different indeed from the one it occupied in the Orient. To be sure, the Greeks and Romans were hardly less religious than the Egyptians or Babylonians. Their cities too were filled with temples; market-places and houses were adorned with divine statues and pictures. But they knew no castes of priests preaching a dogma and wielding, directly or indirectly, political power. Men worshipped the divinities of their cities, their families, their guilds by paying respect to the divine might, not by professing a doctrine. Thus the possibility of a conflict between religion and medicine or, for that matter, science was greatly reduced and bound to be different from that characteristic of other cultures and other ages.

That disease should be treated by human skill was from the beginning of the historical era a demand that required no justification. Like all other arts, medicine was a gift bestowed by gods upon men and to be practiced, so to say, by their order and under their protection. And not to resort in this work to magical devices was a rule favored by the official Olympian religion, for until Oriental cults made their inroads into ancient life, until after their reception the religious temper changed, exorcisms and incantations survived in sectarian movements that were disdained by the intellectuals no more than by men who clung to the inherited tradition. The issue was, and could only be, to what extent diseases were caused by divine interference and to what degree they might be removed by divine intervention, an intervention to be brought about by prayers or incubations.

It goes without saying that in Greece, as well as in Rome, there was a time when diseases were thought to be sent by the gods. While Homer knows of such a divine cause only in the case of an epidemic disease (*Iliad*, I, 8–10), Hesiod says unambiguously that the diseases "come of themselves . . . come upon men continually by day and by night, bringing mischief to mortals silently; for wise Zeus took away speech from them. So is there no way to escape the will of Zeus" (*Works and days*, 103–105; Loeb). Here the natural explanation of illness is rejected altogether. But in the fifth century B.C. at any rate, such a view can hardly have had currency any longer. The Hippocratic writings discuss the divine origin of but one disease, epilepsy (*On the sacred disease*, ch. 1), and polemic against the supernatural explanation of mental diseases is occasionally to be found also in later medical treatises. For the rest, it is taken for granted that the causes of illness are natural. There cannot, then, have been a serious debate about this problem even among the laity and even toward the close of the pagan period.

It is another question entirely whether divine power can heal diseases, especially those against which human help is of no avail. The prayers that men silently addressed to the deity escape historical scrutiny. The popularity of the ancient healing cults, the thank offerings still extant, attest to the fact that in all centuries the ancients believed themselves able to secure divine assistance. Early medical authors remain silent on the matter. Only when speaking of the fear aroused by bad dreams, does a Hippocratic author venture to assert: "Prayer indeed is good, but while calling on the gods man should himself lend a hand" (*Regimen*, IV, ch. 87; Loeb). Incubations are not mentioned at all. Galen, on the other hand, confesses with pride the help he received from

378

Asclepius (T 458); he reports healings performed by the god on others (T 459), as had Rufus before him, because he thought the story "worth telling" (T 425).[31]

I see no reason to assume that the silence of the Hippocratic doctors implies disapproval of religious medicine. Disbelief in the divine in their time was rare indeed. They were amazingly clear-headed and frank in acknowledging the limitations of their art. The concept of a natural law that suffers no exception had not yet been conceived; the principle of infinite causation had not yet been dreamed of. Miracles, one is tempted to say, did not yet present a difficulty to human reason, any more than they did in the sixteenth century, when historical criticism for the first time examined the Christian religion and, setting aside the testimony of tradition, accepted the miracles of Christ as self-evident. As time went on, men became more doubtful. Skeptics challenged the miracles of Asclepius (T 416),[32] but ancient skepticism did not set out to overthrow the customs and beliefs pervading society. The Epicureans denied interference or concern with human affairs on the part of the gods. There still remained for the empirically minded investigator the fact of divine healing attested by good witnesses. The ancient rationalists, for whom Nature herself was divine, believed at least in the divine or prophetic nature of the dreams through which Asclepius more and more learned how to give his help. In short, given the ancient situation, given the peculiar kind of religion that prevailed, physicians could hardly be antagonistic to religious medicine and, where their own help failed, will have considered it an ally rather than an enemy. At any rate, they never fought against it, and they scarcely had any reason to do so. Within their own province they were never threatened by it.

Modern science arose in a milieu dominated by a dogmatic religion. That there is a conflict between science and religion has therefore become common opinion. In this struggle against religion and superstition the physician so often played a leading rôle that he has turned into a symbolic figure of the protagonist of enlightenment, of progress, of liberation from the shackles of the dark forces of reaction. The ancient physicians, on the whole, were satisfied with the world as it was. And indeed, it was an enlightened world that gave free scope to their work. The nineteenth century may have overestimated the rationalism of the ancients; the twentieth begins to underestimate it. It is not the overcoming of hostile forces that constitutes the glory of the ancient doctors; their fame rests and, to be sure, rests securely on the medical insight they obtained, on their concept of medicine as an art and science, on their elaboration of the patterns of medical thought.

III

Having discussed the scientific aspirations of ancient medicine as well as the factors favoring it, one may appropriately ask what this medical scientism promised to accomplish. In the broadest terms the answer to such a question must surely be that ancient medicine claimed to be capable of preserving man's health and of liberating the sick from the ills which had befallen them. But is so general a statement not a mere truism? What else can or should medicine do except preserve health and remove disease? Yet it is not a mere truism that the physician is needed for the preservation of health.

For Egypt and Babylon were unfamiliar with medical dietetics. To be sure, even there rules of living, of avoiding this or that, are to be found. Yet they are religious rules or taboos, which modern scholars not infrequently interpret as sanitary measures, and this they may, in effect, have been, although they formed part of divine worship. Nevertheless, there can be no doubt that to the peoples themselves they were religious rather than medical prescriptions. A rational dietetics is known to have existed outside Greece only in Hindu civilization.

If one compares the two, one does, however, become immediately aware of a characteristic difference. Hindu dietetics, by its very name, Ayurveda, holds forth the promise of longevity, it is "knowledge of long life"; a sound body is sought by the Yogi especially as a sound instrument of spiritual experience.[33] When the Greek doctor recommends dietetic means he is not concerned with the fact that it may prolong life. The main standard by which he measures human existence is the adult life. How to live in old age is a problem first mentioned in dietetic writings of the first century A.D. The art of "geriatrics," as it is now called, was, according to Galen, developed by "recent physicians" (*On hygiene*, V, 4). And the reason given for the necessity of a dietetics is, to speak with the Hippocratic author on *Regimen*, that "neither wealth nor anything else is of any value without health" (III, ch. 69; Loeb), or as Herophilus, who puts it more definitely, says in his *Dietetics:* "Wisdom cannot display itself and art is non-evident and strength unexerted and wealth useless and speech powerless in the absence of health" (Sextus Empiricus, *Adv. math.*, XI, 50).[34]

It needs no explanation, I presume, that the Greek physician speaks of all the goods of the earth where the Hindu doctor or the Hindu layman thinks of the art of contemplation through which one becomes conscious of the indestructibility of one's true self, of that part within man which is behind his individuation. Greek this-worldliness and Hindu other-worldliness are far apart. But it may at first glance seem strange that Greek medicine should pay little attention to the prolongation of life, to the old and their way of living. And yet it is not so strange after all, as soon as one recalls the typical Greek attitude toward old age, toward an existence beyond manhood, the time of full and undiminished physical vigor.

Old age is hateful not merely, or primarily, because it is wont to bring disease or at least to debilitate the body, not even because it is a life without pleasure, for it is "without golden Aphrodite" (Mimnermus, *Nanno*). No, there are many more disadvantages. Old age brings disappointment, a disappointment no one can escape. One loses one's friends, one finds oneself alone. One gets quarrelsome and bitter, for there is, on the whole, not much good in life. Things repeat themselves. Why, then, should one wish to live long? One does not even gain wisdom through age. The young show more sense than the old, and intellectual qualities decay together with the faculties of the body.

I do not say that there were no exceptions to such a sentiment. Solon's "As I grow old I am ever learning many things that are new" (Plato, *Amatores*, 133 C) symbolizes an opposing trend. And surely most men did, in reality, prefer living and living long to dying young. But generally speaking, the Greeks judged old age unfavorably.[35] The Romans, however, cherished and respected it. To them it was the age of authority, of true maturity. It is, I think, mainly a reflection of their influence, of the acceptance of their standards by Greek writers, that the care for old age was infused into dietetic medicine, which the Romans had at first bitterly opposed and had come to adopt only after some struggle. One must, of course, not leave other developments out of consideration. When after the breakdown of the city state, which demanded political participation as well as military service, the ideals of a professional life began to supersede that of the life of the citizen, and when a class of intellectuals and civil servants arose, the estimate of old age was bound to change. Age itself became more tolerable through the pursuits of the mind, which acquired a fixed place in the scale of values. The most beautiful old age, says Athenaeus, is that lived by him who is educated and has leisure to employ what he himself and others before him have accomplished. "What joy it is, reading in the works of the great men of the past, philosophers, physicians and all the other champions of learning, to reflect on this world and to be always in contact with their thought" (Oribasius, III, p. 165, 8 Daremberg). At any rate, it is clearly value outside of medicine that determined the beginning as well as the end of the history of ancient dietetics.[36]

And social valuations, I suggest, qualified in a peculiar manner also that unvarying task of the physician, the task of healing the sick, in which his art shines forth most clearly. Surely, when he is able to restore the sick to complete health, the patient will gladly receive the gift and ask no further questions. But what happens when this is not the case, when only the harshness of the disease can be ameliorated, the dangers it threatens avoided? Should the doctor under such circumstances go on with his treatment? Should or must the patient accept a life which is merely a prolongation of suffering?

Medical texts never discuss these issues. In the general literature they are discussed not infrequently. One is at first skeptical and believes that one hears the voice of an idealistic dreamer when one finds Plato asserting that it is better to die than to live in impaired health (*Republic*, III; 406 A-407 D). One may also think that it is a Spartan prejudice which leads one of their kings to pronounce the verdict: "The best physician is he who does not allow his patients to linger but buries them as quickly as possible" (Plutarch, *Apophthegmata Laconica*, 231 A). But even the sober and very unspartan Aristotle, in one of his books concerned with popular rather than philosophical morals, says: "Bodily excellence is health and of such a kind that, when exercising the body, we are free from sickness, for many are healthy in the way Herodicus is said to have been, whom no one would consider happy in the matter of health, because they are obliged to abstain from all or nearly all human enjoyments" (*Rhetoric*, I, 5, 10; Loeb, adapted). And from here it is but one step to the verdict of Euripides—an excellent verdict in Plutarch's opinion—with regard to "those who patiently endure long illnesses: 'I hate the men who would prolong their lives / By foods and drinks and charms of magic art, / Perverting nature's course to keep off death; / They ought, when they no longer serve the land, / To quit this life, and clear the way for youth'" (*Consolatio ad Apollonium*, 15; Loeb).[37]

Should one then assume that suicide was a recognized and fairly common escape from a life made intolerable and less than human by chronic diseases? That this was the case among the philosophically trained admits no doubt; the evidence preserved is plentiful and irrefutable.[38] That the decision was often taken also by average people is most likely. In cases of blindness it seems to have been almost a general phenomenon that men took their lives. It was not an ancient virtue to become adjusted to everything. Suicide, not condemned on principle by religion except within sectarian circles, was an honorable and required deed in certain situations of failure, whether failure in the life of the citizen or the individual. It was, when fate overpowered man, the only way in which the virtuous could prove himself to be virtuous.

One can be certain that ideals and reality clashed in this instance as they always do. Men cling to hope even where there is none left. As the moral of Aesop's fable of *The old man and death* puts it, "every human being is fond of life even if life has become miserable." On the other hand, one must not forget how readily Hippocratic medicine acknowledges the limitations of the medical art, how often the doctor is admonished not to treat diseases. Asclepiades, who charged medicine preceding him with having been "concerned with death," was the first to study chronic diseases systematically; it was only in later centuries that their cure rather than the cure of acute diseases became the outstanding accomplishment of the doctor. From every point of view it is true that the afflictions of illness were infinitely harder to bear in antiquity than they are in modern times. The willingness to give up a wretched life of physical suffering must have been correspondingly greater.

It follows that for good reasons the ancients were eager to learn the state of their illness, that they were convinced that the doctor owed them the truth about it. At least among the educated the decision to commit suicide in grave cases of disease was taken only after due consultation with the physician. But truth, I think, was asked for also in the last act, with which all medical treatment inevitably ends, the treatment of the dying, when all human help is of no avail. One sometimes says that the humaneness of the ancient doctor, his ethical consciousness as a physician, prohibited him from burdening with dire predictions those who were to die. Such a verdict is not borne out by the few statements that deal directly with the matter, nor is it in accord with the attitude toward death characteristic of ancient society.

That at all events it was not considered a duty to withhold the truth from the patient or to tell it only to relatives and friends is attested by the fact that certain remedies were given only after the physician had asked the patient to make his will, since he was facing great danger (Ctesias in Oribasius, *Collect. medic. reliquiae*, VIII, 8). Thus Aesop's *Ignorant doctor* tells his patient: "You will not arise the coming day; better put your things in order." How common this was, one learns from the dénouement: the patient survives, meets the doctor again, and blames him not for having asked him to make his will but for having been mistaken. Of course, it was considered illbred to be that blunt or to answer the inquiry of the patient as to whether he was going to die with the words: "Even Patroclus died, and he was a better man than you are" (*Iliad*, XXI, 107).[39] But blame for lack of manners must not be mistaken for the recommendation to withhold the truth.

Moreover, ancient philosophy was not merely an art of living but also an art of dying. It is not by chance that Christian authors in their "Art of dying well" were fond of quoting Seneca, who admonished men to die willingly and gladly.[40] But while the Christian had to know his fate in order that the priest might be called in and prepare the patient for his fight with the devil—now more eager than ever to ensnare the soul and bring upon it eternal damnation—the pagan wanted to know that the end was approaching in order that he might die nobly, that is, as befits a human being. He wished to take care of his affairs, to say good-bye to his family and his friends; he wished not to steal away but rather to face death as he had faced life—squarely. It was in the same spirit that he talked freely about death, did not try to hide from it, but gave it a place in life—death which to him was not as terrifying as it seemed to many another generation, which was not, at least for the majority of the ancients, the bridge to future punishment or rewards, but the brother of sleep that brings peace and relief from all suffering.[41]

Again and again the attempt has been made to outline the attitude of the physician merely on the basis of what one calls the demands of medicine. It has been said that he cannot, as a good doctor, tell the fatal truth to his patient. It has been claimed that medicine prescribes the duty of preserving life to the last moment, of making people live even when life is not worth living any more. I am not arguing that these ideals are at fault. I am arguing that history shows that they can be proved to be ideals by moral and metaphysical reasoning alone, as were the contrary ideals that prevailed in antiquity.

384

IV

Thus far I have looked at ancient medicine mainly through the eyes of the physician; I have tried to outline his scientific achievement, his obligations as they were shaped for him in the world in which he lived. It remains to shift the point of view, as it were, and to describe the reaction of society and of the individual. What place did medicine occupy in the social cosmos? How much use was made of it in the affairs of the day? Finally, what was its meaning for human life as it is acted out, to use the famous ancient metaphor, on the stage on which men make their passing appearance?

About the basic social situation there can be no doubt. The medical practitioner, working for a livelihood and working with his hands, preparing drugs or performing operations, was to the ancients a craftsman and, as such, belonged to the lower strata of the social order. And this was true throughout antiquity. It did not help his standing that in the classical and in the Hellenistic era he was usually a migratory worker, an "out-of-towner," and in Roman times a foreigner; in the Rome of Cicero no citizen had yet gone into medicine, while he would not scruple to become a lawyer, nor should one forget that in the empire probably more physicians were slaves than had ever been the case in Greece. From this fundamental social classification the individual could and did, of course, free himself. He who was a good doctor made a name for himself; he became famous; and fame was cherished by the pagans; it overcame even social barriers. Moreover, a city practice must have been more reputable than one in the country. In antiquity, the city was the center of life; the gradual increase in urbanization will, therefore, have generally raised the esteem in which the physician was held. As time went on, more opportunities opened. Cities came to engage physicians; as salaried officials they were persons of note. In the Hellenistic kingdom, in the Roman empire, one could be a court physician. A member of the court, whatever he does, is not a mere menial. Last, though surely not least, the scientific physician, the writer on medical topics, that refined type which, as Aristotle says, saw the connection between medicine and philosophy and studied his subject from that vantage point, was an intellectual, admitted to the society of other intellectuals. When they received recognition as a class, the physicians' renommée became greater too. They were now teachers, not merely of other craftsmen but of students; as researchers, they could be members of philosophical

385

schools, schools of medicine, even of the Lyceum, and finally in Rome of universities.[42]

The social status of the physician, then, was extremely varying, and it goes without saying that this was not without importance with regard to many practical problems. Not only do the country doctor and city doctor, and the court physician, treat their patients differently— Galen was quite outspoken on the matter[43]—the patients react differently to them; and since all medical treatment involves the issue of the physician's authority—to quote Galen again, the physician must rule over his patients as the king does over his subjects—the physician's rôle was not an easy one. He had no unchallenged way of commanding respect, for he lacked the magic wand that modern society has given the doctor, the university degree and the state diploma.

He did not even have the assistance he might have derived from being the representative of one of those arts which alone were exempted in antiquity from the common prejudice against "arts," I mean the "liberal arts," those considered necessary for the education of the truly human, and therefore free, man. Certainly, literature abounds with praise of the medical art. Had it not been invented, a Hippocratic writer says, and many historians shared his view, mankind could not have survived in the struggle for survival (*On ancient medicine*, ch. III). Plutarch can assert that medicine is more important than geometry, dialectic, or music (*De sanitate tuenda*, 122 C), that it is no less refined than any of the liberal arts (122 E). Galen proposes to prove that it is "the best of all arts" (*Protrepticus*). Roman writers such as Varro and Celsus even include medicine in their encyclopedias of the arts, together with agriculture, to be sure, and for utilitarian reasons. All praise, be it praise of the insight of the physician or of his usefulness, was of no avail. The seven liberal arts, the trivium and quadrivium, as at last canonized in the work of Martianus Capella, were grammar, dialectic, rhetoric, geometry, arithmetic, astronomy, and music. Medicine was not abstract and theoretical enough for ancient standards of approval.

However, notwithstanding social prejudices and literary and philosophical appraisals, should medicine not, in fact, have been the greatest of the human arts, since the ancients worshipped health? Health, one often says, was part of the Greek ideal of *kalokagathia*, of its aristocratic ethics. Only the healthy were considered fully human beings; the sick were inferior, weak, as the etymology of the Greek word implies. Thus a healthy life and consequently a life dedicated to health were absolute values. The physician, who procures and preserves health, must then have been highly regarded by everyone, even by the Romans when they came under the influence of Greek culture.

I have no intention of denying that the ancients valued health highly, as do all men by nature. They were also innocent of the Christian or Romantic glorification of disease. And once, indeed, in the seventh and sixth centuries B.C., the voices heralding health as the only stable good among the changes and vicissitudes of life became numerous. They must have struck a note in harmony with the ancients' character. For when the physicians in the fifth century B.C. worked out their system of dietetics, based on the belief that man is constantly liable to sickness and can prevent it only by following certain rules, they became preachers of the dogma that health is the foremost good, and they continued to be its champions to the end. There is no telling how far they succeeded, as they valiantly tried, in persuading the rich to live for their health alone. They certainly managed to make an impact on everybody, for dietary rules were followed in antiquity in large measure. The many books written on the subject, outlining what everyone can and must do, no matter what his station and occupation, are evidence of an active concern with health, greater than in modern times. Still it is not likely that medicine gained a foremost rank because it dispensed the goods of health and because health to the ancients was a good par excellence.

For, first of all, the common Greek ideal—the ideal of those who did not belong to the upper classes, had no independent means, and were not living a life of leisure—was, to speak with Aristophanes, not Hygieia but Plouthygieia, not health but wealth and health. Few even of the common people would, I suppose, have disagreed with the Hippocratic verdict that wealth without health has no great advantage or with Herophilus' extension of this assessment to all other goods. But, to put it their way, health and wealth—not to forget justice—were to them of superlative worth; to bring these superlatives into comparative harmony was their aim. It had to be, for the poor or the moderately well to do cannot dedicate their lives to health alone. It was not only Plato who pointed this out; the physicians themselves regretfully harped on the subject.

If one insists that in antiquity the decision on values did not rest with the lower class, it is even more certain that one cannot speak of a supremacy of the value of health. Philosophers and moralists of all centuries were unanimous in denying that health comes first, though, being

Greeks, they were quite willing to put it second or third. The recognition that health is an essential condition of happiness did not lead to the assumption that it is happiness. In the same way, the admission that disease impairs the enjoyment of everything did not involve the conclusion that it destroys all possibility of doing what one wants to do or should do. One did not mistake means for ends. Civic duties, moral and intellectual virtues took precedence over the goods and excellences of the body.

In view of these facts, it is hardly justifiable to speak of ancient medicine as an educational force, of the doctor as an educator. It is, of course, true that he identified himself with the ideal of health. But, as Aristotle implies, the physician can tell men how to be healthy but cannot tell them whether they should want to be healthy; this decision is in their own hands.[44] For the art of the user, that is, the ideals and convictions of man whom the arts serve, is superior to the aims and ideals which the arts themselves embrace. In so far as the ancients did live for their health, they did so because they wanted to do so. It was not the merit of the physician, any more than the credit for their military victories belonged to their gymnasts, though these made them strong in body and thus helped them to win their battles. The concept of the expert who advises the public and thus shapes the mind of society was foreign to antiquity.

Nowhere, perhaps, does this appear more clearly than in the fact that the physician did not even play a rôle where one would naturally expect him to have exercised his influence, I mean in the administration of justice. He was not called in to advise the judge or the jury, and he did not appear in behalf of the defense. Cases of insanity, of violent death, are, as a rule, conducted without the benefit of his advice. Court procedures in antiquity were dominated by what nowadays one would call the plaidoyer, by what the ancients called rhetoric. And from the fifth century B.C. on the "artistic proofs" were more and more stressed in comparison with the "artless proofs." That is, one tried to win the case through demonstrating probabilities, through influencing passions, through swaying the jury, not through gaining one's point by means of sensory, factual evidence. As little as antiquity knew the professional judge or prosecutor, just as little did it know the legal medical expert.

There is one last question that one must ask: what did medicine mean to the individual Greek and Roman? It is a question very difficult to answer. Hardly ever are the feelings of patients recorded in literature or on stone; honorary decrees erected by cities are eloquent in their expression of gratitude, but formal and stylized. The same is true of the literary appraisals of medicine and the physician, be they written in praise or as caricatures. Such statements, of course, abound. There is, on the positive side, Homer's assertion that a physician is worth many another man (*Iliad*, XI, 514). Although in its context it means no more than that in war the healer of wounds has a special usefulness, it was often quoted as a glorification of the whole healing art. The Pythagoreans claimed that medicine was the wisest of all human arts. On the other side of the ledger, derogatory remarks are equally outspoken. Medicine is an art that helps by inflicting pain and, in addition, asks for pay and receives it, a paradox the ancients never tire of marveling at. The doctor is also continually blamed for charging too much money, for being a busybody, for magnifying his merits. As Menander puts it, "physicians, you know, by way of building a towering reputation, are wont to diagnose insignificant troubles as greater ones and to exaggerate real dangers."[45] One resents the physicians' talking too much. One accuses them of hating men to be healthy, for that reduces their practice. If they are sick themselves, they do not keep their own rules. They are charlatans or pedants. If there were no physicians, no one would be more stupid than the grammarians, that is, the philologists.

One does not learn very much from these sayings except that men at all times have been the same. The fairest evaluation of the testimony is, I think, to consider it as reflecting two stages in the relation of the patients to the physician. When they are sick and in need of his help, they praise him to the heavens. When they have reached the harbor of safety, they make fun of him, and the more so as the more in their distress they have exaggerated his skill and elevated his capacities. An imperial decree of the year 370 A.D. puts the gist of the matter neatly: "The public physician should be decent and help the poor rather than be servile to the rich. We allow them to accept as much money as the healthy offer for their service, but not as much as the sick promise at the moment of danger" (*Cod. Theodosianus*, lib. 13, tit. 3, c. 8).

If one, then, does not learn much from these verdicts, one can perhaps conclude more from the fact that the ancients came to regard medicine as the one art that helps everyone without making any distinction of rank or person, without distinguishing even between friend and enemy. This was the rôle the physician's profession, one thought, demands of him. No doubt, it was, in fact, the rôle many physicians did play. And no greater tribute could be paid to any doctor than the tribute paid to him in the first century, that he is the friend of the patient, sympathizing with him and loved in return as a friend, for one owes to him more than money could pay for. Here all social prejudices are overcome, all barriers laid low through the gratitude of the heart for what the doctor as an individual can give to the individual patient in the hours of suffering, a suffering of the body and of the mind.[46]

In the same period, however, in which the patient's relationship to his physician was defined in words never to be surpassed in warmth, admiration, and respect, one notices an almost ironical turn of events. "A man who is thirty and still needs a doctor is a fool" said the emperor Tiberius (Tacitus, *Ann.*, VI, 46), and the statement is repeated with approval by others (Plutarch, *De sanitate tuenda*, 26). The hand of friendship extended by the physician then is here rejected. The individual assumes full authority over himself; he becomes entirely self-sufficient. Many and varied factors, I think, combined to bring about this change of temper.

One, of course, is the concern of medicine with the individual. If it is the individuality of the patient itself that counts most in the treatment, who could know the patient better than the patient himself? And since the educated knew medicine, as the phrase goes, why should they not take charge of the treatment to be administered? More important still, in antiquity disease, though it was never considered the consequence of sin as it was in Oriental cultures, came more and more to be considered a self-inflicted evil. All the handbooks on dietetics, in fact, presuppose this belief. Disease is unnecessary; it can be prevented if one lives in the right way. That such a belief was widely current is clear from anecdotes. Gorgias, when asked how it had been possible for him to live to a ripe old age, replied that he had lived with attention to health rather than to the wish of indulging himself. Democritus is reported to have said that one can preserve health through self-discipline, and the same opinion is attributed to Diogenes the Cynic. It is in the same spirit, I think, that Aristotle maintains: "old age is a natural disease, while disease is an acquired old age" (*De gen. anim.* V, 49, 784 b 33). That not only laymen or philosophers thought so is clear from Galen's claim that it is quite possible for man to keep free from disease. I used to be sickly myself when I was young, he adds, but I got over this bad habit. Even serious fever and infections can be avoided. The only necessary, unavoidable decay is old age (*On hygiene* V, 1; vol. VI, p. 309, ed. Kühn).

If this is true, if disease is an individual phenomenon due to an error of judgment, to wrong living, then it follows naturally that a truly educated man does not need a doctor and is, if nothing worse, a fool if he has to call upon one. And it is in this sense that medicine and philosophy are sisters (Tertullian, *De anima*, 2), that medicine is a second philosophy (Isidorus, *Orig.*, IV, 13). For both philosophy and medicine, if studied by man, will enable him to do the same thing, to lead the right kind of life. They show him the narrow path that leads to happiness.

No one, perhaps, has expressed this conviction more vividly and dramatically than Plutarch. Scholars and men in public affairs, he says (*De sanitate tuenda*, 27), are likely not to care about their health. Consequently misfortune often befalls them. It is the story of the camel and the ox. When the ox begged the camel to lighten his burden, the camel did not listen; and so the ox dropped dead. Or to express the moral of the parable in less homely language, man forces his mortal part, the body, to be partner to his immortal part, his soul; he tries to join the earthborn and the celestial element. This cannot be done. He who attempts it must in the end renounce everything he likes, reading and discussion and study. The aim should be "the even balance of a well-matched team" (cf. Plato, *Timaeus*, 88 B). We should feel that of the good gifts which fair and lovely health bestows, the fairest is "the unhampered opportunity to get and use virtue in words and deeds." Philosophy and medicine, medicine and philosophy, that is the answer to the human problem in sickness and health, as it is the answer to the question of the theoretical understanding of both. It is the most distinctly Hellenic characteristic of the ancients' attitude toward medicine.

NOTES

Editor's Note: On Thursday, March 24, 1960, Dr. Ludwig Edelstein delivered the Garrison Lecture before the American Association for the History of Medicine at its thirty-third annual meeting in Charleston, S. C. A complete manuscript of the text of the lecture was found among his papers after Dr. Edelstein's death (August 16, 1965). In a footnote to the title, he stated: "The paper is now virtually unchanged in substance but is in an expanded form. The footnotes that were added were meant to provide only the indispensable reference to the pertinent literature or to state briefly the difficulties involved in the respective problem. In instances where the subject is highly controversial, I have found it impossible to convey the argument within the limits of a footnote and have, therefore, taken up the discussion in an appendix." No appendix was found; nor had the notes been completed. All the notes must be taken as bibliographical aids rather than the expression of definitive opinions. Up to number 30 they had been worked out in sufficient detail to be utilized, though penciled remarks (most of which had to be disregarded because unclear in intent or illegible) showed that the author had been far from giving them final form. Moreover, some of the references were indicated so vaguely that the editor could not take upon himself the responsibility of giving them a precise interpretation. In such cases it was felt best to drop the reference altogether or, occasionally, to retain it in its vague form as a mere hint to the interested reader. After number 30, the bulk of the notes had to be omitted, since they increasingly took on the character of personal notations. In a few instances, the editor was able to supply missing references for quotations. Because of their fragmentary form, the notes have been placed at the end of the article rather than below the text.

The notation "Loeb" within a reference indicates that the translation in the Loeb Classical Library was used.

[1] M. Pijoan, "Garrison, the teacher," in the "Fielding H. Garrison Memorial Number," *Bull. Inst. Hist. Med.*, 1937, *5:* 371.

[2] H. E. Sigerist, *A History of Medicine*, New York: Oxford Univ. Press, vol. II, 1961, p. 182; see also below, note 3.

[3] In this brief statement I have tried to justify the approach here suggested as seems required in the case of medicine, which is after all an applied science and therefore by definition concerned with human needs. But I would add that in my opinion the historical analysis of all sciences demands that attention be paid to the subjective as well as objective factors involved in the development of knowledge (see L. Edelstein, "Motives and incentives for science in antiquity" in *Scientific Change*, ed. A. C. Crombie, New York: Basic Books, 1963, p. 18 note 42).

[4] It is perhaps exaggerated to claim that "the true picture of the medicine of any particular period is not to be discovered in the medical books, written by contemporary physicians, but rather in the general literature and sociological background of the age" (J. R. Oliver, "Greek medicine and its relation to Greek civilization," *Bull. Inst. Hist. Med.*, 1935, *3:* 623). Yet it is certainly true that in any general evaluation of Greek medicine, non-medical writings are an indispensable source of additional information.

[5] This is true not only of the books that by their very title restrict themselves to the early period—as, for instance, W. A. Heidel, *Hippocratic Medicine*, New York: Columbia Univ. Press, 1941, or the chapter on medicine in André Bonnard, *Greek Civilization*, Vol. II, *From the Antigone to Socrates*, transl. by A. Lytton Sells, New York: Macmillan, 1962—but also of the essay on "Greek Medicine as Paideia," in W. Jaeger, *Paideia*, vol. III, transl. by Gilbert Highet, New York: Oxford Univ. Press, 1944, p. 3 ff. Sigerist's *History of Medicine* unfortunately does not go beyond

Hippocrates, and his pamphlet, *Antike Heilkunde*, München: Heimeran, 1927, deals with post-classical medicine largely as a foil to the classical.

[6] The term "distinctive Hellenism," then, is meant to cover not only those traits which differentiate the Greek achievement from that of the Orient, but also those phenomena which underlie the history of the Greeks as a constant element in their development, what "they were, wanted, thought, saw and were capable of" (J. Burckhardt, *Griechische Kulturgeschichte*, ed. J. Oeri, 3rd ed., n. d., Berlin and Stuttgart: Spemann, vol. I, p. 3).

[7] For the distinction, see O. Temkin, "Greek medicine as science and craft," *Isis*, 1953, *44:* 213 ff., and below note 27.

[8] Sigerist, *Antike Heilkunde, op. cit.*, p. 17.

[9] What is meant by "science" of medicine will be interpreted in more detail later. Here it may suffice to illustrate the difference between (Greek) scientic knowledge and (Oriental) empirical knowledge by the demonstrative proof of the so-called Pythagorean theorem, on the one hand, and the use of the triangle with the sides 3, 4, and 5 for the construction of a right angle, found in Egypt and India, on the other. The formulation of universally valid laws instead of merely phenomenological descriptions of the data is characteristically Greek, see in general H. and H. A. Frankfort, *Before Philosophy*, Pelican Books, 1949, esp. p. 250 ff.; J. A. Wilson, *The Culture of Ancient Egypt*, Chicago: Univ. of Chicago Press, 1951, p. 55 ff.; S. W. Kramer, *History Begins at Sumer*, Garden City, N. Y.: Doubleday Anchor Books, 1958, p. 60 ff. Such a claim is valid irrespective of the question whether Egyptian medicine is "empirico-rational" (Sigerist, *History of Medicine, op. cit.*, vol. I, 1951, pp. 337, 348 ff., 352) and anticipated certain views and methods of the Presocratics (*ibid.*, p. 355) or specific medical categories (R. O. Steuer and J. B. de C. M. Saunders, *Ancient Egyptian and Cnidian Medicine*, Berkeley: Univ. of California Press, 1959 [*perittōma*]). As for India and Greece, I should perhaps state here that I am convinced of the "independent parallel growth" of their medical teachings (H. R. Zimmer, *Hindu Medicine*, ed. L. Edelstein, Baltimore: Johns Hopkins Press, 1948, p. XLVII ff.; also C. Vogel, "Zur Entstehung der Hippokratischen Viersäftelehre," Diss. Marburg, 1956 (p. 18 ff. [*Maschinenschrift*]).

[10] Sigerist, *Antike Heilkunde, op. cit.*, esp. pp. 10 ff., 19 f.; *History of Medicine, op. cit.*, vol. II, pp. 331, 333. His interpretation has become widely accepted, see e.g., W. Müri, *Arzt und Patient bei Hippokrates*, 1936, p. 41 (Beilage zum *Jahresbericht über das Städtische Gymnasium in Bern*); Vogel, *op. cit.*, p. 70, note 158; H. Diller, "Stand und Aufgabe der Hippokratesforschung," *Jahrb. Akad. d. Wissensch. u. d. Literatur*, Mainz, 1959, p. 287.

[11] That Celsus here thinks of scientific, not of philosophical, knowledge is certain, for in his opinion Hippocrates separated medicine from philosophy, see above, p. 373.

[12] The alleged neglect of these particulars on the part of the Methodists (54 ff.)—Empiricists and Dogmatists alike stressed their importance—seems especially objectionable to Celsus (66 f.), who also takes it for granted that hospitals with a great number of patients cannot give attention to the individuality of the sick and therefore have to resort to common characteristics (65). For Hellenistic medicine, see e.g., Celsus 67 (humor in eye; cf. 53); 68 (individuality); 70 (locality; season); and Galen, n. 15, below. The Hippocratic material on the topic has been collected by C. Fredrich, *Hippokratische Untersuchungen* (Philologische Untersuchungen, 15. Heft), Berlin: Weidmann, 1899, p. 6, note 2; see also Edelstein, *Peri aerōn und die Sammlung der Hippokratischen Schriften* (*Problemata*, Heft 4, hereinafter cited as *Problemata*), Berlin: Weidmann, 1931, p. 86 [83*] (On healthy diet, ch. 2); the "fashion" of the diseases is mentioned in *On the nature of man*, ch. 9; the whole doctrine can be

summed up in the statement that the physicians must meet the demands of the occasion, the *kairos* (*Problemata*, p. 114 [109*], VI, p. 338 [Littré]). Under the latter category falls also the difference of countries (*Prognosticon*, end; Rufus says that the difference of countries presents a difficulty for treatment).

[13] On Galen's evaluation of Erasistratus, see Galen *On the natural faculties*, transl. by A. J. Brock; Loeb, p. XXXIV; for his quarrel with the anatomists, *ibid.*, p. XL; for his opposition to the Methodists and the tyranny of names, *ibid.*, pp. XV, XXXII, XXXIX.

[14] On the Galen passage which formulates the principle *individuum est ineffabile*, see Karl Deichgräber, *Die griechische Empirikerschule*, Berlin: Weidmann, 1930, p. 311. (On the principle itself, also Aristotle, *Metaphysics*, VII, 15, 1040 a 8; Boethius, [reference missing]; R. Meissner, "Das Individualprinzip in Skotistischer Schau," *Wissenschaft und Weisheit*, 1934, *1*; Kraus, *Die Lehre des Joh. Scotus von der natura communis*, 1927; "Die Lehre von der realen specifischen Einheit in der älteren Skotistenschule," *Divus Thomas*, Berlin, 1936, *14*). In this sense medicine is an *ars conjecturalis*. But the justifiable opposition to a medicine that treats organs rather than human beings and considers anatomical and scientific insight the most valuable factor in the physician's knowledge and treatment must not obscure the fact of the undoubted value of anatomy and physiology, which had come to be recognized. And that is how the ancients felt.

[15] For Galen, see, *Methodus medendi*, III, 3, vol. 10, p. 181, ed. Kühn. For Aristotle, esp. *Nicomachean ethics*, X, 9. He worked out the problem for the concept of practical knowledge (*phronēsis*) VI, 5, 1140a 24 ff. and juridical wisdom (also V, 14, 1137a 31 ff.); see H.-G. Gadamer, *Wahrheit und Methode*, Tübingen: Mohr, 1960, pp. 19, 301. The problem makes its reappearance in Hobbes (L. Strauss, *The Political Philosophy of Hobbes*, Oxford: Clarendon Press, 1936, p. 85 ff.), Vico, and Shaftesbury (Gadamer, *op. cit.*, pp. 16 ff., 21). Jaeger, *Paideia, op. cit.*, vol. III, p. 24 f., assumes that Aristotle's main ideas are borrowed from medicine. L. F. Heinimann, "Eine vorplatonische Theorie der Technē," *Museum Helveticum*, 1961, *18*: 105 ff., thinks especially of the influence of Protagoras (p. 117 ff.).

[16] That the unity of science was first established by Galen (see L. Edelstein, "Recent trends in the interpretation of ancient science," *J. Hist. Ideas*, 1952, *13*: 573–604 [401*]) seems the personal merit of Galen and not due to any specifically medical considerations. The influence of Rome on the later development of Greek medicine goes of course much further.

[17] The Greek language has no strict equivalents for the terms the modern interpreter must use in his analysis. The words *technē* and *epistēmē* cover the universal aspect of knowledge, at least in Aristotle's philosophy (*Metaphysics*, I, i, 981, a 1 ff.). Experience is the word through which Aristotle denotes the capacity of practical application. In common language *technē* seems often to refer to theoretical and practical knowledge. I do not follow up this linguistic problem (Cicero, *De oratore*, I, 23 presupposes a doctrine according to which art (*ars = technē*) denotes science as well as art (cf. D. L. Clark, *Rhetoric in Greco-Roman Education*, New York: Columbia Univ. Press, 1957, pp. 10, 12). But I should make clear that what I have in mind is an analysis of what Temkin called "scientific medicine," in contrast to leechcraft (see above, note 7), that is, the layer of scientific medicine over the vast body of merely practical applications (Edelstein, "The relation of ancient philosophy to medicine," *Bull. Hist. Med.*, 1952, *26*: 301 [351*]). I need hardly add that my definition does not take in all medicine. The Corpus Hippocraticum shows a one-sided stress on the *nosōn* (*Epidemics*, corrected by Hellenistic writers), and on *hē nosos* or, rather, acute diseases in the prognostic writings (*Problemata*, p. 61), and the Methodists are devotees of names and disease entities. But the victory of the humoral

pathology, of the *krāsis* theory, shows that the harmony of art and science was the *distinctive* feature.

[18] For the theory of political constitutions as attested by Herodotus, III, 80 ff., see Burckhardt, *op. cit.*, p. 282. Polycletus' *Canon* is another example (40 [28]A3 [Diels-Kranz] quoted by Galen).

[19] See Edelstein, "The relation of ancient philosophy to medicine," *op. cit.*, p. 302 [352*]. (K. Sprengel, *Versuch einer pragmatischen Geschichte der Arzneikunde*, vol. 1, 4th ed., Leipzig: Gebauer, 1846, p. 2, rightly speaks of philosophy as "the mother of medicine"). The only strictly speaking medical theories known from the classical centuries are those ascribed in the Meno papyrus to some of the older physicians (though all are variations of the *perissōmata* theory).

[20] The Hippocratic treatise *On the nature of man*, chs. 1–2, indicates, perhaps for the first time, a difference between the knowledge necessary for the philosopher and that sufficient for the physician. In Stoic philosophy the situation is stated unequivocally (Diogenes Laertius, VII, 133), and Chrysippus' research on the seat of the soul bears out the distinction between the medical expert and philosophical critic. Concerning Galen, see Edelstein, "Die Geschichte der Sektion in der Antike," *Quell. u. Stud. z. Gesch. d. Naturwissensch. u. d. Med.*, 1932, *3:* 68, 77, 96 [264*, 272*, 291*].

[21] F. M. Cornford, *Principium sapientiae*, Cambridge: Univ. Press, 1952, p. 42; cf. p. 37 f., also p. 7 f.; also W. H. S. Jones' introductions to his edition of Hippocrates (Loeb Classical Library), vol. II, pp. xlv ff. (war of philosophy over medicine), xliii (sophists, citing Taylor), xxxix, xl, and vol. I, x ff.; also his essay on ancient medicine, *Philosophy and Medicine in Ancient Greece* (Supplements to *Bull. Hist. Med.*, No. 8), Baltimore: The Johns Hopkins Press, 1946; Jaeger, *Paideia, op. cit.*, vol. III, pp. 15–17.

[22] On Protagoras, Edelstein, "Empirie und Skepsis in der griechischen Empirikerschule," *Quell. u. Stud. z. Gesch. d. Naturwissensch. u. d. Med.*, 1933, *3:* 51 [201*]. The literature is so extensive that it cannot be reviewed here. That the book is not post-Platonic, contrary to Diller's assumption, seems now generally agreed (e.g., Heinimann, p. 112, note 32). But the meaning of the theory proposed is still debated. The view prevails that here empiricism is advocated. I still am of the opinion that this empiricism, defeating its own purpose, has turned into skepticism through exaggeration. The simile of letter on which much depends is throughout meant to emphasize skepticism (see the passage quoted in *Problemata, op. cit.*, and also Plato *Republic*, 402 A; *Sophist*, 253 A).

[23] [Concerning the Empirical physicians, see Edelstein, "Empirie und Skepsis in der griechischen Empirikerschule," *op. cit.* (see above, ftn. 22). Ed.] Concerning the Methodists and late skepticism, see Pauli-Wissowa, *Real-Encyclopädie der classischen Altertumswissenschaft*, s. v. Methodiker, Supplement VI, Stuttgart: Metzler, 1935, col. 358 ff. [173*].

[24] Concerning the code of Hamurabbi, see Sigerist, *History of Medicine, op. cit.*, vol. I, pp. 434, 400; also vol. II, p. 203 (on Persia).

[25] For the Greek situation, Antiphon, III, 3, 5 (also Plato, *Laws*, IX, 865 B); for that in Rome, Pliny, XXIX, 8 18. The relation of the Roman law to medical problems has been studied by K. H. Below, *Der Arzt im römischen Recht*, Munich: Beck, 1953, pp. 108 ff. (Münchener Beiträge zur Papyrusforschung und antiken Rechtsgeschichte, 37. Heft.) P. Kibre, "The faculty of medicine at Paris," *Bull. Hist. Med.*, 1953, *27:* 3.

[26] The paradox of Heraclitus, 22 [B 58] Diels-Kranz, alludes to the award which the physician demands though he inflicts pain on the patient.

[27] It is unnecessary here to discuss in detail the various teachings of the Hippocratic writings or of the later schools outlined in every handbook. I merely note that

scientific medicine, most important in this context, never completely replaced the craft of medicine and was in fact a small segment of ancient medical practice. See Edelstein, "The relation of ancient philosophy to medicine," *op. cit.*, pp. 300–302 [350*–351*]; also Temkin, "Greek medicine as science and craft," *op. cit.*, *passim*.

²⁸ The development of medical ethics I have discussed in "The professional ethics of the Greek physician," *Bull. Hist. Med.*, 1956, *30:* 391 ff. [319*]. I have been unable to find in the Oriental material any traces of a professional code of ethics except the remark that certain cases are not to be treated (Sigerist, *History of Medicine, op. cit.*, vol. I, p. 307, for Egypt). Even the famous four questions which the Hindu doctor is taught to ask himself before treating (Zimmer, *op. cit.*, p. 32 ff.) are not ethical questions, nor does the description of the true doctor given by Suśruta (*ibid.*, p. 92) constitute an ethics of medicine. On the other hand, reflection on aims and content of morality are found already in early Greek lyric, and the name of Socrates is connected with the discussion of attitudes fitting the various professions. Here too medicine and philosophy are closely allied, see above.

²⁹ The material on these issues is interpreted in Edelstein, "Greek medicine in its relation to religion and magic," *Bull. Hist. Med.*, 1937, *5:* 201–246 [205*]. On demonology in particular, pp. 216 ff. [219*]. Even if it were true that after the classical centuries, Greek irrationalism increased, this did not influence medical practice. Of an influence of religion on medicine one can talk only in so far as the Greek rationalist sees in the natural a manifestation of the divine, very much in the manner of the seventeenth or eighteenth century rationalists (*ibid.*, p. 211, n. 29 [214*, n. 30]).

³⁰ For Egypt, see H. E. Sigerist, *A History of Medicine, op. cit.*, vol. I, especially p. 314 (316, 347); for Mesopotamia, *ibid.*, esp. p. 464 (472, 483 f., 490, 492); for India, *ibid.*, vol. II, pp. 155, 161 f.; cf. H. Zimmer, *Hindu Medicine, op. cit.*, e.g., p. 107 f. Concerning Greek medicine, see L. Edelstein, "Greek medicine in its relation to religion and magic," *op. cit.;* for the regulation of the Roman law (*Digesta*, L, 13, 1, par. 3), cf. *ibid.*, p. 236, note 108 [237*, n. 109]. That medicine in Greece did not originate in the temples of Asclepius, I have tried to show in vol. II of E. J. Edelstein and L. Edelstein, *Asclepius*, Baltimore: Johns Hopkins Press, 1945.

³¹ Edelstein, *Asclepius, op. cit.*, vol. 1, pp. 263 f. (Testimonies 458 and 459) and 238 f. (T. 425).

³² *Ibid.*, p. 209 f. (T. 416).

³³ See Sigerist, *History of Medicine, op. cit.*, vol. 2, p. 182 f.; Zimmer, *op. cit.*, pp. xiii f. and 71.

³⁴ See L. Edelstein, "Antike Diätetik," *Die Antike*, 1931, *7:* 255–270. [303*].

³⁵ W. Schadewaldt, "Lebenszeit und Greisenalter im frühen Griechentum," *Die Antike*, 1933, *9:* 282–302; also F. Boll, "Die Lebensalter," *Neue Jahrb. f. d. klass. Altertum*, 1913, *16:* 89–145 and A. Dyroff, "Junkos und Ariston von Keos über das Greisenalter," *Rheinisches Museum f. Philologie*, 1937, N. F. *86:* 241–269.

³⁶ See Edelstein, "Antike Diätetik," *op. cit.* [303*].

³⁷ Cf. Rudolf Kassel, *Untersuchungen zur griechischen und römischen Konsolationsliteratur*, München: Beck, 1958 (*Zetemata*, Heft 18).

³⁸ L. Edelstein, *The Hippocratic Oath* (Supplements to *Bull. Hist. Med.*, No. 1), Baltimore: Johns Hopkins Press, 1943 [3*].

³⁹ Galen, *Commentarius IV in Hippocratis Epidem.* VI, c. ix, vol. 17B, p. 145, ed. Kühn.

⁴⁰ Mary Catharine O'Connor, *The Art of Dying Well* (Columbia University Studies in English and Comparative Literature, No. 156), New York: Columbia University Press, 1942, p. 26, who refers to Seneca, *Epistles* XXXI and LIV.

⁴¹ See, e.g., Cicero, *Tusculan Disputations*, I, xlix, 117.

[42] See Galen, *In Hippocratis De medici officina commentarius* I, 8, vol. 18 B, p. 678, ed. Kühn; *The Scriptores historiae Augustae* (Severus Alexander XLIV, 4); Loeb, vol. II, p. 267.

[43] See, e.g., Galen, *De simplicium medicamentorum temperamentis ac facultatibus*, X, 22, vol. 12, p. 299, ed. Kühn.

[44] Aristotle, *Topica*, II, 2, 110a 19, together with *Politica*, VII, 2; 1324 b 30.

[45] Menander, *Phanium* (497K); Loeb, p. 447.

[46] See L. Edelstein, "The professional ethics of the Greek physician," *op. cit.*, pp. 414, ftn. 43, and 416, ftn. 46, where references to Seneca are given [344* and 345*].

PART FOUR

PART FOUR

RECENT TRENDS IN THE INTERPRETATION
OF ANCIENT SCIENCE*

The book by Cohen and Drabkin is a most welcome contribution to the literature on the history of ancient science. No comparable collection illustrating ancient scientific knowledge has ever been attempted. The excerpts brought together by the editors are excellently chosen and set in sharp relief main aspects of the scientific development in antiquity. The English rendering of the texts is wherever possible taken from available translations, but a great number of passages have been translated by Mr. Drabkin (ix), and translated very well indeed.[1] Ample explanatory notes serve to clarify the content and also refer to the modern debate on specific issues; succinct introductions to each of the various fields of science outline the general background. In short, a work of wide scope and of the devoted labor of years has been completed with great skill, full mastery of the diverse literature, accuracy of detail, and with a view to the broader issues.

In examining such a book it would hardly be useful, I think, to concentrate on minutiae. One may of course always raise the question why a certain passage has been selected, while other evidence has not been included, whether or not the interpretation of a certain detail is correct, and so forth.[2] A discussion of this kind would interest merely

---

* *Journal of the History of Ideas*, 1952, vol. 13, pp. 573–604. Reprinted in Philip P. Wiener and Aaron Noland (editors), *Roots of Scientific Thought, A Cultural Perspective*, New York: Basic Books, 1957, pp. 90–121.

A discussion of M. R. Cohen and I. E. Drabkin, *A Source Book in Greek Science* (New York: McGraw-Hill, 1948), pp. xxi, 579; and B. Farrington, *Greek Science*, I, 1944, pp. 154; II, 1949, pp. 181 (Pelican Books).

[1] The translations often amount to a commentary on the text, e.g., the rendering of the passage from Ptolemy (?), *Optics* (271 ff.). Variant readings and other textual difficulties are carefully indicated (e.g., 36,5; 66,1; 169,1; 220,1; 252,1; 253,2; 264,1; 282,2; 337,1; 342,4; 364,3; 496,1). In a reprinting of the book an index of the translated passages should be added so that specific authors could be consulted more easily.

[2] To give some examples: the experiments in acoustics (294 ff.) should perhaps have been illustrated also by Plato, *Republic*, 531A–C, the oldest evidence (cf. 5,1;

the specialist. However, valuable as it is for the specialist, the book is intended mainly for scientists or general historians, so that they may see "something of the original sources on which the historian relies" (vii), or for readers "who wish to achieve some understanding not only of the foundations of modern science, but of a vital element of the humanistic tradition" (viii). The *Source Book* will be used, I trust, in courses on the history of science. Rather than deal with the narrower concerns of the work, it seems appropriate, therefore, to inquire into some of the principles which the editors have followed in compiling the material, to draw attention to general problems on which the evidence here assembled has some bearing, and to discuss some recent interpretations of the history of ancient science as a whole, especially that of B. Farrington, as it is expounded in a number of brilliantly written books which have aroused great interest and have exercised a strong influence. In this way I hope to facilitate the use of the material which has now been put at the disposal of all who are interested in the early beginnings of science.

I. ANCIENT SCIENCE AND MODERN SCIENCE

Since the nineteenth century the great majority of scholars have held that ancient science and modern science are worlds apart. But if one reads through the texts collected in the *Source Book*, he can not but agree with the editors that it is an error to date the rise of natural science in the seventeenth century and to consider the Greeks "mere speculators" (vii). In mathematics (1–88), astronomy and mathematical geography (89–181), physics (182–351), chemistry and chemical technology (352–73), geology and meteorology (374–93), biology (394–466), medicine (467–529), physiological psychology (530–58), in all

---

302,5); the chapter on chemistry ought to include excerpts from Aristotle, *Meteorology*, IV (cf. 374, n. 1). Strabo's account of the tides (cf. 390,1) might have been preferable to that of Pliny (389). For the authorship, etc., of the Ps. Hippocratic treatises *On the Nature of the Child* and *On Diseases*, IV, (453,2; 489,1) J. Ilberg, *Die Schule von Knidos, S. B. Leipzig* (1925), should have been compared. The essay of Theophrastus quoted on p. 392 is hardly genuine; cf. A. Rehm-K. Vogel, *Exakte Wissenschaften*, in Gercke-Norden, *Einleitung in die Altertumswissenschaft* (1933), 46. Not everybody will agree with the comments on Plato, *Timaeus*, 40 B (cf. *Laws*, VII, 822 A–C), concerning the rotation of the earth (98), nor am I certain that the evaluation of number mysticism and astrology in medicine (500,1; 502,1) is correct. The chapter on acoustics and musical theory, an exceedingly difficult subject, might have profited by a more detailed introduction (286 ff.); the remarks on pp. 294 and 302 (notes) do not seem quite sufficient.

these branches of learning the Greeks developed and followed methods that closely approximate, if they do not equal, the standards of modern science. To be sure, the material assembled in these chapters is mostly outdated. What is presented here is not yet modern science. Nevertheless the link between the ancient investigations and those of modern times is obvious.

The quantitative approach to the analysis of phenomena as well as the method of experimentation were well known to the ancients. This is often denied even nowadays; the evidence available should settle the debate once and for all.[3] The most famous example of the quantitative analysis of observations is the work of the Pythagoreans (249 ff.) and of Erasistratus (480; cf. also 239, 280, 312). The experiments known to have been performed are numerous (mechanics: 211, 249–52; optics: 268; acoustics: 294 ff.; physiology: 479). It should also be pointed out that references to experiments are to be found not only in classical and Hellenistic authors, but also in books of the archaistic centuries down to the end of antiquity (e.g., 248). Philoponus investigated the laws of falling bodies in the same manner as Galileo (220).[4] Nor were the ancients unacquainted with the concept of "two sets of experiments," as the editors stress in their comment on an experiment in acoustics (298, n. 1). One statement by Philo, the engineer, seems especially remarkable, because it shows the clear awareness of the necessity of repeated experiments, and, in addition, of the "social conditioning" of such an approach: ". . . the ancients did not succeed in determining this magnitude by test, because their trials were not conducted on the basis of many different types of performance, but merely in connection with the required performance. But the engineers who came later, noting the errors of their predecessors and the results of subsequent experiments, reduced the principle of construction to a single basic element. . . . Success in this work was recently achieved by the Alexandrian engineers, who were heavily subsidized by kings eager for fame and interested in the arts" (318).

The statement just cited is interesting also from another point of

[3] Cf. O. Blüh, "Did the Greeks perform Experiments?," *Amer. Journ. of Physics,* 17 (1949), 384 ff.

[4] That the experiment of Philoponus was known to Renaissance scientists and played an important rôle in the controversy over Galileo's theories has been shown by E. Wohlwill, *Physikalische Zeitschrift,* 7 (1906), 23 ff., 28 ff. Cf. also L. Olschki, *Galilei und seine Zeit, Gesch. d. neusprachlichen wissenschaftlichen Literatur,* III (1927), 160.

view. It formulates the concept of scientific progress. Now it is generally held that ancient scientists were unaware of the idea of progress. Philo's words have been called the only clear expression of this concept, and the value of his testimony has been depreciated, since he was an engineer, a man of practical affairs. The practitioners may have been conscious of the necessity of progress, the true scientists, it is maintained, were not.[5] But is not the intent of Philo's assertion identical with that of Hero, who composed his book in the expectation that from his collection of earlier discoveries, to which he added his own, "much advantage will result to those who shall hereafter devote themselves to the study of mathematics" (249)? And if it is objected that Hero is a mechanician, what about Archimedes, who writes: "I deem it necessary to expound the method . . . because I am persuaded that it will be of no little service to mathematics; for I apprehend that some, either of my contemporaries or of my successors, will, by means of the method when once established, be able to discover other theorems in addition, which have not yet occurred to me" (71)? Is Archimedes' pronouncement basically different from one by Dürer that is considered characteristic of the Renaissance concept of progress: "I know however that he who accepts it [my doctrine] will not only get a good start, but will reach better understanding by daily practice; he will seek farther and find much more than I now indicate"?[6] Many other passages from ancient scientists could be adduced which express the hope that progress will be achieved in the future. Likewise, scientific writings attest that their authors realized their dependence on the work of earlier scientists (e.g., 116, 168 f.). Just as the ancients were familiar with experiments and quantitative analysis, so they knew that scientific progress could be attained solely through the cooperation of successive generations.[7]

Modern science and ancient science, then, are not diametrically opposed. I hasten to add, however, that such a claim can be made good

[5] E. Zilsel, "The Genesis of the Concept of Scientific Progress," pp. 251–275. He considers Ptolemy, *Almagest*, I, 1 (p. 4 Heiberg), as well as Seneca, *Naturales Quaestiones*, VII, 25, 31, exceptional in the extant literature (see specifically p. 253, n. 3; p. 254, n. 4).

[6] Zilsel, *op. cit.*, 334. That the concept of scientific progress originated in the Renaissance is the commonly accepted view. For the general literature on the idea of progress, cf. Zilsel, 325,1. (F. J. Teggart, *The Idea of Progress*, revised ed. by G. H. Hildebrand [1949], deals with the concept of social rather than scientific progress.)

[7] With this problem I intend to deal in detail and to present the pertinent material in a forthcoming essay on *The Influence of Ancient Science on Philosophy*.

only so long as one is willing to do what the editors of the *Source Book* have done, namely to select as evidence that material "which would generally be regarded today as scientific in method, i.e., based, in principle, either on mathematics or on empirical verification" (viii). To put it differently, the impression that ancient science is modern in character is bought at the price of neglecting or omitting all the evidence to the contrary.[8]

The editors, like many other students of antiquity, seem inclined to classify "theories that are now known to be false or even ridiculous" as "magic, superstition, and religion." They speak of " 'pseudo science,' such as astrology and the like," that "can be found in the writings of such sober Greek scientists as Aristotle and Ptolemy" (viii); they refer to "the intrusion of the occult" that is noticeable also in modern scientific writings from Kepler to Eddington (ix). But astrology, the theory of humors, Plato's mathematical scale of music are not "intrusions" in ancient science. Theories like these, which do not pass the muster of modern criticism, constitute in fact the greater part of the preserved material. To the Greeks, they were just as scientific as those other views which happen to seem acceptable to the modern scientist. To be sure, the scientist who says of himself, as Seneca put it, "the day will come when our children will wonder at our ignorance" (*Nat. Quaest.*, VII, 255), may also look in amazement at the ignorance of previous ages. The historian, I think, must try to understand that that which is ridiculous and false in the past is inseparably connected with that which is praiseworthy and true. The errors of the Greeks should teach him as much about their science as do their correct results. What appears to be so "modern" acquires its specific hue only if placed against the setting of the "antiquated."

I should go even one step farther. The "correct" results and methods themselves, if studied more closely, reveal certain implications that are peculiarly their own and are perhaps less correct or modern than one may have supposed at first glance. It is true, empiricism was embraced by many ancient scientists; phenomena were carefully observed and minutely studied (e.g., 122, 134, 283); in many ways, ancient em-

---

[8] In this connection I should emphasize that the chapter headings of the *Source Book* naturally represent the modern divisions of science and were chosen by the editors in the hope that this device "will enable the modern reader concerned with a given special field to find more readily the ancient material that will interest him" (ix).

piricism is identical with modern empiricism. Yet it was the empiricists of antiquity who were the first idolators of books, for it is in books, they claimed, that the empirical knowledge of previous generations is stored up. Further verification of results that were once put down and generally agreed upon thus became superfluous. On the other hand, the empirical approach in antiquity prompted the acceptance of sympathetic and antipathetic effects, which earlier rational and speculative science had disregarded. The experiences of superstitious people were acknowledged as valid, since as experiences they were irrefutable.[9] Again it is true, many scientists experimented in a modern fashion. Yet many others did not experiment to test an hypothesis; rather, they restricted experimental proof to the occasional confirmation of a speculative theory, or they might choose to resort to an experiment in order to refute an opponent. The two attitudes existed side by side in the classical age, as well as in the Hellenistic and archaistic periods. And if some of the ancients clearly saw the advantage of repeated, systematic experimentation, others lacked this insight. No less an anatomist than Galen was unwilling to investigate all phenomena, wherever this did not seem to serve his purpose.[10]

Such differences between the modern and the ancient approach must be emphasized not only for the sake of historical objectivity and accuracy, but also in order to forestall new and unwarranted exaggerations in the appraisal of ancient science. Already it is claimed that all scientific progress in antiquity was due to the fact that the ancients "were prepared to abandon theoretical patterns under the impact of new observations and experiments, performed in order to prove or disprove earlier concepts." If relatively little is known of these experiments, one must remember that "much of their knowledge the Greeks considered as *mysteries*, i.e., as secret knowledge, to be passed on only to a selected few in sacred communities, scientific schools, and trade guilds."[11] I need hardly say that the latter assumption is entirely un-

---

[9] For the book learning of the ancient empiricists, cf. K. Deichgräber, *Die Griechische Empirikerschule* (1930), 298 ff., 317 ff.; for empiricism and the doctrine of sympathy, cf. L. Edelstein, "Greek Medicine in its relation to Religion and Magic," *Bulletin of the Institute of the History of Medicine*, 5 (1937), 229–38 [230*].

[10] For the early history of the experiment, cf. H. Diller, Ὄψις ἀδήλων τὰ φαινόμενα, *Hermes*, 67 (1032), 14 ff. In general cf. O. Regenbogen, "Eine Forschungsmethode antiker Naturwissenschaft," *Quellen u. Studien z. Gesch. der Mathematik, Abt. B, Studien*, I (1930), 131 ff. For Galen, cf. *Opera Omnia*, ed. G. Kühn, II (1821), 286.

[11] Blüh, *op. cit.*, 385, 387.

founded. Enough is known about experiments to warrant the claim that they were widely made, contrary to the assertions of earlier scholars. If the available information about them is still scanty, the reason for this is, in addition to the loss of material, that not all ancient scientists experimented and that in some fields the aim of the work undertaken, as well as its literary recording, differed fundamentally from the aim and the literary expression of later generations. Physics, for instance, which in antiquity remained closely connected with philosophy, was predominantly concerned with the philosophical category of the "why," rather than with the scientific category of the "how." Physicists, therefore, recording their results started with the logical proof, and then added the factual (experimental) proof, which as a superaddition, so-to-say, could be and actually was limited, no matter how many experiments might have preceded the solution of any given problem. They accepted more or less the philosophical style of discourse, the form of the *quaestiones et solutiones*.[12]

The mention of the influence of philosophy on physics brings up the last question I wish to raise in this connection, that of the relation between philosophy and science in general. The editors of the *Source Book* have omitted the "philosophical speculation on cosmology as well as on human affairs," which is easily available; they have drawn a line "between what should be regarded as scientific material and that which would more properly be considered philosophic or speculative," although, as they admit, "such a line must necessarily be arbitrary, since the Greeks themselves did not draw it very sharply" (viii). Indeed, had the editors decided otherwise, their task would have become well-nigh impossible, and they deserve high praise for the adroitness with which they have handled this thorny problem. I simply want to underline the warning given in their preface and to extend it somewhat farther.

It is at least debatable whether the Aristotelian treatises on zoology, which are included, are the work of the philosopher or of the scientist, Aristotle. Theophrastus, whose botanical writings are excerpted, was a philosopher, too. The philosophical discussion of the concept of analogy decisively influenced his scientific studies. His refusal to compare, where comparison seemed unwarranted on general principle, prevented him from recognizing the bisexuality of plants. In anatomy, the

---

[12] Cf. H. Leisegang, *s.v. Physik*, Pauly-Wissowa, *Real-Encyclopädie d. class. Altertumswissenschaft*, XX, 1 (1941), col. 1041.

PART FOUR

same philosophical discussion of the merit of analogies contributed to the discontinuation of animal anatomy in favor of dissection performed on the human cadaver, and even of human vivisection.[13] Similarly many another author, who in the *Source Book* appears as a scientist, was guided in his research also by his philosophical theories. I am not sure that the astronomical hypothesis of Ptolemy can be designated simply as scientific; I doubt that he accepted the geocentric theory merely on scientific grounds, as the editors hold (107 f.). Ptolemy was not averse to using philosophical arguments in proof of scientific data (e.g., 118), and rightly so from his point of view, for in antiquity, science was linked with philosophy much more closely than is true of modern times. It is not by chance that in recent years scholars have paid increasingly more attention to the question as to just when the independent sciences constituted themselves in antiquity, and how far one can speak of such an independence at all.[14]

To repeat, modernity is only one of the components of ancient scientific investigation. Reality is more complex than any generalization, any verdict of "modern" or "antiquated" can indicate. The singling out of those trends in ancient development which resemble or foreshadow modern science, permissible and valuable as this procedure may be, tends to give a picture that necessarily remains one-sided. In fact, evaluating the tension between the various tendencies within ancient science is one of the main problems confronting the historian.

II. ANCIENT SCIENCE AND TECHNOLOGY

It is one of the great merits of the *Source Book* that it includes technological material "that seems either to have been a direct application of Greek scientific theory or to have contributed to its subsequent development" (ix). The examples given are drawn from practically every field of knowledge (84 f., 134–42, 169–81, 307—10, 314–51).

[13] For Theophrastus, cf. Regenbogen, *op. cit.*, 155–57; for the development of anatomy, cf. L. Edelstein, "Die Geschichte der Sektion in der Antike," *Quellen u. Studien z. Gesch. der Naturwissenschaften u. der Medizin*, 3 (1933), 100 ff., 148 f. [247* ff., 293* f.].
[14] E.g., W. Jaeger, *Aristoteles* (1923), 432. F. Solmsen, "Plato and the Unity of Science," *The Philosophical Review*, 49 (1940), 566 ff. The problem demands a more detailed investigation than can be given here. I should at least mention that the principles of physics and physiology always formed part of ancient philosophical doctrines.

The editors also rightly emphasize the fact that in this context the archaeological material, which necessarily had to be excluded from the book, is especially important (182, 314).[15]

That ancient science failed to lead to technological application is another one of those prejudices that die hard. Yet contrary to the assertions repeated over and over again and made the basis of far-reaching generalizations, like those of Spengler, the Greeks were not hostile to technology.[16] Plato, to be sure, blamed the "corrupters and destroyers of the pure excellence of geometry, which thus turned her back upon the incorporeal things of abstract thought and descended to the things of sense, making use, moreover, of objects which required such mean and manual labor" (315). But Plato is not all of antiquity. Archytas, Eudoxus, Menaechmus constructed instruments and machines (Plutarch, *Quaest. Conv.*, VIII, 2, 1, 718e). Aristotle admired mechanical toys (*Politics*, 1340 b 26 f.), Aristoxenus appreciated technical detail.[17] Although Plutarch intimates that Archimedes on account of his "lofty spirit," his "profound soul," that is, on account of his Platonic leanings (cf. 315), did not write on his inventions (317), it still remains true that this "geometrical Briareus," as the Romans called him (*ibid.*), did apply his knowledge to practical ends. The list of his inventions is impressive.[18] Geminus, among others, considered mechanics a branch of that part of mathematics which is "concerned with and applied to things perceived by the senses" (2; cf. 5). Carpus, in the first or second century of our era, was one of the many scientists who did not believe that geometry is "harmed by the association with them [the arts]" (185). Pappus held that the science of mechanics "is justly esteemed by philosophers and is diligently pursued by all who are interested in mathematics" (183).

How far applied science advanced in antiquity is quite another question. The various periods differed in their contributions to tech-

[15] Much of the evidence known from ancient technological writings is discussed by E. Pernice, *Handbuch der Altertumswissenschaft* (*Archaeologie*), VI, 1 (1939), 250 ff. A description of many of the devices used is to be found in G. Childe, *What Happened in History* (1942; Pelican Books), e.g., 235 ff., 250 ff.

[16] Cf. A. Rehm, "Zur Rolle der Technik in der griechisch-römischen Antike," *Archiv f. Kulturgeschichte*, 28 (1938), 135–62, the best and most recent analysis of the subject.

[17] Cf. J. Geffken, "Antiplatonica," *Hermes*, 64 (1929), 92.

[18] Cf. Rehm, *op. cit.*, 146, n. 28; he has also interpreted the various accounts given of Archimedes' attitude, 145, n. 27. Farrington's representation of Archimedes (*Greek Science*, II, 75) does not do justice to the divergencies of the tradition.

nology. In the pre-classical era more was accomplished than in the fifth century B.C.; the early Hellenistic period marked a climax; the Romans made great strides, once the Greeks had prepared the way.[19] On the other hand, ancient technical development, no doubt, never went as far as the available knowledge would have permitted. Especially conspicuous is the absence of any consistent attempt to replace human by non-human energy, an attempt not to be carried out before the late Middle Ages, and at that time based largely on the knowledge inherited from antiquity. And yet, on principle the ancients were quite aware of the fact that ropes and cables are means by which "the motion of living beings may be imitated" (5). Nor was the idea alien to them that "vanquished by nature we become masters through technics" (Ps. Aristotle, *Mechanics*, 847 a 20).[20] The more one studies the astounding technological devices discussed in literature (e.g., 329 ff., 343 ff.) and extant in the archaeological remains, the more one wonders why the ancients did not go farther, why technology did not become more thoroughly integrated into practical life.

The reasons for the relative limitation of ancient technology have been widely debated. As the editors phrase it, "increasing attention has been paid in recent years to the organization of society in antiquity, and in particular the institution of slavery, as affecting the technological development" (314). This problem is of such importance that I feel it necessary to take it up here; naturally it could not be discussed within the scope of the *Source Book* (*ibid.*).

The argument most commonly advanced, and advocated also in the now most widely read histories of ancient science, is that in a slave society labor is cheap; technical improvements therefore were unnecessary in antiquity.[21] Such an oversimplification seems no longer justifiable, for as the investigations of the past few decades have shown, ancient economy can hardly be called a pure slave economy. Especially in the arts and crafts free labor continued to hold its place. In addition

---

[19] Cf. Rehm, *op. cit.*, 136, 138 f., 146, who follows H. Diels' periodization of the history of technology (*Antike Technik* [1914]).

[20] For the interpretation of this statement (=Antiphon, Fr. 4 [Nauck, *Trag. Graec. Frag.*,[2] 793]), cf. Rehm, *op. cit.*, 137; also Farrington, *Greek Science*, II, 46. The progress of mediaeval technology is briefly summarized by Farrington, *op. cit.* II, 168.

[21] Cf., e.g., Diels, *op. cit.*, 35. E. Zilsel, "The Sociological Roots of Science," *The Amer. Journal of Sociology*, 47 (1941/42), 559; Farrington, *Greek Science*, II, 166; F. M. Cornford, *The Unwritten Philosophy and Other Essays* (1950), 93.

to slaves, metics and citizens were employed as artisans during the classical age; in the Roman empire, the ratio of free labor increased even in big factories. Simple reference to ancient society as a slave economy, then, explains nothing.[22] The exact numerical relation of the various components of the laboring class it is difficult to estimate. What is certain is that the number of slaves in antiquity was much smaller than was thought by historians of the nineteenth century, and this is true above all of the classical and Roman ages.[23] However, even assuming that the percentage of slaves was relatively high, slave labor was neither cheap, nor docile, as is evidenced by slave revolts and strikes. To put it in Rostovtzeff's words: "Why then should the employment of slaves prevent an energetic shop-owner from using new technical devices, which would have been a good way of making his products cheaper and better?"[24]

Another argument that has been proffered is that the insufficient demand for goods, the low buying power of the population hampered the rise of technology. Mass production hardly existed in antiquity; big export trades flourished only locally and temporarily; in general, wages were low. Whatever was needed and could be afforded by the consumers

[22] That slave labor never ousted free labor has been stated by Rehm, *op. cit.*, 153. W. L. Westermann, *s.v. Sklaverei, R.E.*, Suppl., VI (1935), cols. 894–1068, deals most extensively with the question of slavery. Concerning the participation of free men, metics and slaves in fifth- and fourth-century crafts and trades, cf., e.g., M. L. W. Laistner, *A Survey of Ancient History* (1929), 289 f.; for conditions in the Roman empire, *ibid.*, 538 ff., esp. 540; M. Rostovtzeff, *The Social and Economic History of the Roman Empire* (1926), 303; also Childe, *op. cit.*, 272, who claims however that in the classical period the slave owners "did not want labour-saving devices" (224). Cf. also T. Frank, *An Economic History of Rome* (1927²), esp. 324 ff. (The Laborer). The material for the Hellenistic period is scarce; in Greece proper, the majority of slaves seem to have worked in the household (Westermann, cols. 934 f.). Factories apparently were manned entirely by slaves (cf. note 24); yet the continuance of free labor is certain.

[23] That the number of slaves in the classical age used to be overestimated, even Rostovtzeff admits, *Social and Economic History of the Hellenistic World*, II (1941), 1258, although he cautions against the tendency to minimize the extent of slave labor in reaction to earlier exaggerations. For the slave trade in Hellenistic times, *ibid.*, 1260 ff. For the decreasing number of slaves in the Roman empire, Laistner, *op. cit.*, 535. Some estimates concerning slaves, metics and freemen are given by A. W. Gomme, *The Population of Athens in the fifth and fourth Centuries B.C.* (1933), 19 ff.; cf. also Childe, *op. cit.*, 272. Rostovtzeff, *Roman Empire*, 178, considers it impossible to state the exact relation between slaves and freedmen.

[24] Rostovtzeff, *Roman Empire*, 303; he adds that "ancient industry reached its highest [technical] level in the Hellenistic period when it was based wholly on slave labour" (*ibid.*).

411

was easily produced without technical apparatus. These and similar considerations may perhaps explain why in the production of commodities like pottery, metal ware and textiles technical progress was slow, even in the Hellenistic centuries, while in building and in the production of war materials, where the demand was great, progress was more rapid.[25] No one will doubt that economic factors have a certain regulative force. Thus even Pliny, discussing the use of mowing machines in agriculture, remarks that the diversity of procedure depends on the size of the harvest and the availability of workmen (*Nat. Hist.*, XVIII, 300). But can economic considerations alone explain why the ancients, who for their elaborate pageants invented automotive carriages and ships much bigger than the size of their usual warships, did not apply their knowledge to their daily needs? That they constructed water clocks, but failed to make effective use of the water mill, which they also knew how to build (*Source Book*, 350), that they employed the wind wheel to play the hydraulic organ (333), but failed to utilize the power of the wind mill, which they likewise invented)?[26]

Moreover, scholars now generally agree that, contrary to earlier views, ancient society was not predominantly a "house economy," but to some extent was also a capitalistic society, no less so at any rate than were some of the societies of the Renaissance. It has been said with regard to the Renaissance artisan that only a man who had "either invented some commercial or technological innovation or who understood the value of the invention of another fellow became a capitalistic manufacturer. Thus the inventive genius of the individual gradually came to the fore."[27] If this were true, it should apply to the ancient craftsman as well. Nor can it be maintained that in antiquity there was no such close cooperation between the scientist and the artisan, as is said to have

---

[25] That industrialization in antiquity remained limited on account of the weakness of the internal market is the thesis of Rostovtzeff, *Roman Empire*, 303 ff. The Hellenistic development he has described in *Hellenistic World*, II, 1205 ff.; 1230 ff. F. M. Heichelheim, *Wirtschaftsgeschichte des Altertums* (1938), 570 ff., seems to be inclined to judge the progress during the Hellenistic period more favorably. Rehm, too, explains the lack of technology through the low cost and ample supply of workers, *op. cit.*, 155, 158 f. In this connection he pays special attention to the number of metics in classical Athens.

[26] For the milling industry, cf. Childe, *op. cit.*, 235, 252. I have borrowed my examples from Rehm, *op. cit.*, 160 f.

[27] Zilsel, "The Genesis of the Concept of Scientific Progress," pp. 251–275. Concerning competitive capitalism in ancient society, cf. Rostovtzeff, *Roman Empire*, 302 f., 482 ff.; also Rehm, *op. cit.*, 146 ff.

stimulated interest in inventions during the Renaissance. Those skilled in the theory and construction of machines, the mechanicians, according to Hero, had to learn at least one craft (184). Vitruvius stresses the important relation between theory and practice (I, 1,2). Inventors were held in high esteem, their names were noted and remembered, whether or not they had written about their subjects or achievements.[28] Social conditions, then, although in some respects they may have retarded the rise of technology, were also favorable to its advancement. Their consideration alone will hardly suffice to explain the limitations of ancient technics; was society really so much better off when in the Middle Ages many of the inventions made in antiquity were put to wider use?

It seems to me that in order to understand the attitude of the ancients toward technology, the basic values underlying ancient life must be considered, the fundamental aims and deep-rooted convictions of those who concerned themselves with inventions. As for the scientist, even where he applied his knowledge to practical matters, his true reward remained the insight he had gained into nature. The "sober drunkenness" of cognition was his highest goal. No ancient scientist, I think, could have said what Pasteur said of himself: "To him who devotes his life to science, nothing can give more happiness than increasing the number of discoveries, but his cup of joy is full when the results of his studies immediately find practical applications."[29] It is rather in the words of Ptolemy that the happiness and joy of the ancient scientist is summarized: "I know that I am mortal, a creature of a day; but when I search into the multitudinous revolving spirals of the stars, my feet no longer rest on the earth, but, standing by Zeus himself, I take my fill of ambrosia, the food of the gods" (*Anthologia Palatina*, IX, 577). His own inner enrichment constituted the celebrated humanism of the ancient scientist. He tried to acquire knowledge for knowledge's sake; he applied it when he was asked to do so in the interest of his city or his king, when an occasion offered itself; he hardly ever sought out such an occasion.

[28] It is usually said that ancient society held the inventor in low regard; cf. e.g., Zilsel, *op. cit.*, *Amer. Journal of Sociology*, 559, and Rehm [*op. cit.*, 161 (cf. 143)] who agrees with Diels, *Antike Technik*, 29 ff. Yet Diels himself quotes even inscriptions recording the names of inventors. Rostovtzeff's appreciation of the position of the inventor, *Hellenistic World*, 1245, is more positive, and rightly so; cf. also Farrington, *Greek Science*, I, 104; II, 48. The evidence has been surveyed by A. O. Lovejoy and G. Boas, *Primitivism and Related Ideas in Antiquity* (1935), 200, 382 ff.

[29] René J. Dubos, *Louis Pasteur* (1950), 85.

Even the work of the mechanician was guided by an unrealistic outlook. To be sure, he propagated inventions, "so that they may be of unlimited usefulness" (351), or in order to "supply the most pressing wants of human life" (249), or to achieve the desired end "without using the laborious and slow method" (342), yet he did not forget the element of wonder, of play or amusement. "The art of those who contrive marvellous devices," "the art of the sphere makers . . . [who] construct a model of the heaven [and operate it] with the help of the uniform circular motion of water," according to Pappus, were subdivisions of mechanics (184). Catoptrics is "clearly a science worthy of study and at the same time produces spectacles which excite wonder in the observer. For with the aid of this science mirrors are constructed which show the right side as the right side, and, similarly the left side as the left side, whereas ordinary mirrors by their nature have the contrary property and show the opposite sides" (262). Sentences like these would hardly figure in a modern textbook on optics.

As for the artisan and the craftsman, in addition to an innate love of invention which he may have possessed, only self-interest could spur him on to go ahead. The artisans of the Renaissance, as is apparent from their own testimony, justified their inventions by reference "to the glory of God and the Saints, of the craft and the workshop—and to the usefulness of their craft and the public benefit."[30] No ancient artisan could have thought of such a justification. It is true, the development of the arts and crafts was generally recognized as an important part of civilization, and therefore as a common good. The invention of tools, of instruments had served to distinguish human life from animal life. Further progress in the arts and crafts could make life more pleasant and more enjoyable. Specialization and division of labor helped to produce more beautiful objects; they bettered the quality of workmanship.[31] But technical improvement to the ancients was not a value in itself; the moral and political order was supreme. Nor would the ancient crafts-

[30] Zilsel, "The Genesis of the Concept of Scientific Progress," pp. 257 f.; for the testimony of Renaissance authors, *ibid.*, 258–71.

[31] For specialization and division of labor, cf. Xenophon, *Cyropaedia*, VIII, 2,4 ff.; Augustine, *De Civitate Dei*, VII, 4, and Rehm's interpretation of these passages (152 f.). That the progress of civilization depended on improvements in the arts was, of course, a commonplace. Contrary to the impression given by J. B. Bury [*The Idea of Progress* (1920), 15 ff.], it was held not only by the Epicureans, but also by the classic philosophers (Plato, *Hipp. Mai.*, 281 D; Aristotle, *N.E.*, 1098a23) and by the Stoics (e.g., Cicero, *De Officiis*, II, 3–4).

man by his inventive genius have enhanced the glory of his art or of his guild. Ancient guilds were private organizations, rather than public institutions; they did not enforce any standards of craftsmanship. The artisan's patron saint was believed by some to have bestowed upon him the knowledge of tools. Yet, while the craftsman owed it to him that he benefited by their use, neither he nor even his god was, in his eyes, a creator rejoicing in ever new manifestations of his creative power. The world was there to live in, not to be used or to be made over.[32]

Among people adhering to such a scheme of values, technological progress, I think, had its natural, its inherent limitations. A change could come and did come about only when another view of the world emerged, when in the later Middle Ages the discrepancy between the two attitudes toward life immanent in Christian thought came to be avowed, when active life began to vie with contemplative life and was finally placed above it, when man at last felt summoned "to participate, in some finite measure, in the creative passion of God, to collaborate consciously in the processes by which the diversity of things, the fullness of the universe, is achieved."[33]

III. Progress and Decay of Ancient Science

Referring to the relation between technology and social factors the editors of the *Source Book* state that social conditions are said to have influenced "possibly also the directions in which science in general developed" (314). The justification of this claim has indeed become the main issue in interpreting ancient science. The various aspects of the problem may conveniently be summed up in the catch phrase "the progress and decay of ancient science."

The expression, of course, is not to be taken too literally. No one

[32] It was characteristic of the ancient craftsman that he was conscious of the limits of human art. This becomes especially clear in the discussion on the art of medicine; cf. L. Edelstein, *Bull. of the Institute of the History of Medicine* (1937), 224 ff. [226* ff.]. The belief in the periodic destruction of the world probably was another hindrance to unlimited progress (Bury, *op. cit.*, 16). Cf. also note 54 below.

[33] A. O. Lovejoy, *The Great Chain of Being* (1948³), 84. In the words quoted Lovejoy describes the opposing tendencies of the Christian dogma. He has also shown how the mediaeval concept of the poet is determined by the Christian concept of creation (86).

will deny that science never became extinct in antiquity, that scientific research was carried on continuously from the turn of the seventh to the sixth century B.C., when scientific studies began, down to the sixth century of our era, when pagan civilization ended and with it what may properly be called Graeco-Roman science. Rather, the terms "progress" and "decay" imply the failure of ancient science "to lead on from its first successes to a continuous growth like that which the modern pioneers of science inaugurated," a failure that "can hardly be attributed to ignorance of scientific method"; or to put it differently, Greek science became sterile, despite the fact that it "had still such vitality that it was capable of a second birth" in the Renaissance.[34] The period of breakdown is variously dated. Some speak of the second century B.C. as the decisive turn; others single out the first century B.C.; still others allow the standstill to have come about only in the second century of our era.[35]

That behind these theories there are facts which need explaining, I readily admit. Ancient science did undergo decisive transformations. After 200 B.C. productive research slowed down; in the second century A.D. the temper of science changed, so that henceforth compilers and commentators usurped the place of original investigators. Needless to add that progress was nevertheless made in the period between 200 B.C. and 200 A.D., and even afterward. The most ardent proponent of the theory of decay would concede this much; he would not deny that Ptolemy and Galen were original scientists, and that the work of Diophantus was of the most far-reaching consequences. Yet generally speaking, the distinctions noted between the various periods seem valid. Can the same be said of the explanations offered?

It is sometimes said that the breakdown of science was due to the "general loss of the spirit of hope and adventure" noticeable throughout ancient society.[36] Even if such a "failure of nerve" had actually occurred, it would be a phenomenon extraneous to science, and I am here concerned only with such factors as could have affected scientific studies specifically. Again, the argument is proposed by some that the decay

[34] The first two quotations are taken from M. Cary, *A History of the Greek World from 323 to 146* (1932), 352 f. (cf. A. J. Toynbee, *A Study of History*, V [1939], 422); the last quotation is from Farrington, *Greek Science*, II, 10 f.

[35] Cary, *loc. cit.*, puts the change in the second century B.C.; so do Farrington [II, 163 f. (but cf. below, note 46)] and Childe, *op. cit.*, 253, although the latter speaks of a decline of practical application of science as early as after 500 B.C. (224).

[36] Thus Cary, *loc. cit.*; Toynbee, in spite of his skepticism as to Cary's dating (*op. cit.*, 422, n. 1), seems to be of the same opinion (cf. also *ibid.*, n. 2).

was accelerated by the lack of precision instruments, an explanation to which the editors of the *Source Book* seem to attribute at least a certain significance (134). The intimate relation between science and technology, which I have discussed before, warrants the guess that scientists would have been provided with all the instruments they needed, had they only asked for them.[37]

The view most widely held, however, is that science decayed because of the existence of slavery, or on account of definite political measures imposed to abridge the freedom of science. The foremost exponent of these views in recent years has been Farrington. As he represents the situation in his *Greek Science*, "it was not . . . only with Ptolemy and Galen that the ancients stood on the threshold of the modern world. By that late date they had already been loitering on the threshold for four hundred years. They had indeed demonstrated conclusively their inability to cross it. . . . When we look for the causes of this paralysis it is obvious that it is not due to any failure of the individual. . . . The failure was a social one. . . . The ancients rigorously organized the logical aspects of science, lifted them out of the body of technical activity in which they had grown or in which they should have found their application, and set them apart from the world of practice and above it. This mischievous separation of the logic from the practice of science was the result of the universal cleavage of society into freeman and slave" (II, 164 f.).[38]

I am not prepared to enter into a discussion of the question whether or not, as Farrington presupposes, science can develop only if it is closely connected with the world of practice and techniques. Others have seen the rise of technology as an unwilled and incidental outcome of the progress of pure science. Yet, although Farrington mentions Bacon, Vico, Hegel, and Marx among those who have seen that "man makes his mental history in the process of conquering the world" (II, 175), a philosophical debate on this issue is here beside the point. As Farrington rightly insists, "the history of science must be really historical" (I, 149). He has written "in the conviction that the better understanding

[37] Cary (*loc. cit.*) stresses the lack of instruments as a subsidiary cause for the stagnation of astronomy, botany, and medicine. Farrington (I, 70 f.) also mentions the absence of instruments of exact measurement.

[38] Of other scholars who see in slavery the reason for the decline of science I mention, e.g., Zilsel, *op. cit.*, *Amer. Journal of Sociology*, 560 f.: "Evidently lack of slave labor is a necessary but not a sufficient condition for the emergence of science"; Childe, *op. cit.*, 253, 258.

of any stage in this long journey [by which man achieves his self-trans-
formation from the animal to the human kingdom] must contribute to
the attainment of the final goal" (II, 175). It is, then, the historical
facts themselves that need careful scrutiny.

Now, why should science after 200 B.C. have been separated from
the world of practice and techniques because of the existence of slavery?
That around 300 B.C. "control of techniques, knowledge of the processes
of which is essential for many branches of science, passed into the hands
of slaves" (II, 8), is merely an assumption which is not borne out by the
evidence. I have already summarized the results of modern studies on
this problem (cf. above, part II), and I do not intend to rehearse the
argument again. Farrington, if I am not mistaken, only once refers to
the fact that "historians of society are still disputing the precise degree
to which the industrial techniques had, by Plato's time, passed into the
hands of slaves." And he adds, "For our purpose it is not necessary to
give a more precise answer to this question than to say that for Plato,
and for Aristotle, the normal and desirable thing was that the citizen
should be exempted from the burden of manual work and even from
direct control of the workers" (I, 141). I agree with Farrington that for
his purpose, namely, an analysis of Plato's and Aristotle's philosophy,
an answer to this question is unnecessary. But can his general assertion
concerning the disastrous influence of slavery on science be accepted,
unless he, or any one who sides with him, first refutes the results of the
sociological investigations which have overturned the very presupposition of his argument? Even after 200 B.C. free men studied and mastered
techniques; even at that time it was not considered improper to work
with one's own hands for scientific purposes; the gentleman-like attitude
of the ancient scholar, so often referred to, did not call for his exclusive
occupation with words.[39]

Yet I should inquire also into the positive side of Farrington's argument. The presupposition of his verdict is, after all, his conviction that
Greek science arose when, in the sixth and fifth centuries B.C., scientists
worked in close cooperation with craftsmen and learned from their techniques. "It was the success with which he applied his techniques that

[39] Farrington speaks of "the more gentlemanly pursuit of theory of numbers and
geometry" (I, 45); of Aristotle he says that "he was not ashamed to use his hands"
at least as a biologist (p. 114). Zilsel, "The Genesis of the Concept of Scientific
Progress," also refers to the gentlemanlike disdain for experimentation and dissection; cf., *idem, Amer. Journ. of Sociology,* 559. The situation has been stated correctly
by Blüh, *Amer. Journ. of Physics* (1949), 387 f.

gave the Ionian natural philosopher his confidence that he understood the workings of nature" (I, 77). Thales turned "primarily on techniques" (33); Anaximander and Anaximenes derived proofs from them, and so did Heraclitus (33–35). Empedocles and Anaxagoras came to the rescue of observational science, which was threatened by the attacks of Parmenides (50 ff.), and they too relied on techniques, as is witnessed by Empedocles' reference to the clepsydra (55) and by Anaxagoras' mention of the same device (58).

Two objections must be raised against such a thesis. First, it can certainly not account for all that the Presocratics called science. Farrington's assumption hardly explains Anaximander's belief in justice as a cosmic force, or Anaxagoras' belief in a divine mind, or Empedocles' mysticism and doctrine of purification, important features of their understanding of the universe, which Farrington fails to mention at all.[40] Secondly, granting that "the doctrine of *Opposite Tension* which Heraclitus applied to the interpretation of nature was derived, as his own words inform us, from his observation of the state of the string in the bow and the lyre" (I, 35), the question arises whether this was properly speaking a scientific procedure. If Heraclitus really based his philosophy on his observations on the tension of the strings and was able to convince others of his conclusions, this was possible only because the universe on speculative grounds was still thought to be uniform, so that everything in it could be compared to everything else. To put it differently, his procedure implies the rather naïve use of analogies. As Farrington himself admits later, the Ionians, "ignorant of the true or even approximate size of the heavenly bodies . . . could argue, without misgiving, from processes going on on earth to processes in the sky; Aristotle felt he could no longer do so" (99–100). Of course, Farrington does not deny that Aristotle was right in refusing to follow the lead of the Presocratics; nor does he deny that this change for the better, by which separate realms of science with specific methods appropriate to their subject matter were constituted, was brought about not by reliance on techniques, but by "the application of mathematics to astronomy" (100; cf. 142).

If, then, it was "the specific originality of the Ionian thinkers . . .

[40] The same criticism applies to Farrington's representation of Anaximander (*Science and Politics*, 19), as Cornford has pointed out: "This statement, no doubt, represents part of the truth; but it fails to account for those features which Mr. Farrington omits" (*Unwritten Philosophy*, 121).

419

that they applied to the interpretation of the motions of the heavenly bodies and all the major phenomena of nature modes of thought derived from their control of techniques" (134), if "the positive content that is decisive" in the Presocratic teaching is "familiarity with a certain range of techniques" (37), this is at the same time the least scientific aspect of their theories. The working model of Anaximander's universe may have been the potter's yard, the smithy, or the kitchen (33). Had subsequent generations not broken away from such analogies and restricted them to their proper scientific use, Greek cosmology might have been free of the influence of the Babylonian god, Marduk, to use a phrase of Farrington (*ibid.*), that is of mythology, but there would hardly have been any science. And what is true of analogies in the field of astronomy and cosmology is equally true of the other branches of knowledge, as Farrington himself indicates (138–40; cf. also II, 123). The contention that science arose in connection with techniques, however important the material which they put at the disposal of the scientist, seems unfounded, and in view of the importance of mathematics in the constitution of science, it seems equally unjustifiable to speak of "the magic wand of Pythagorean mathematics" which "has transformed the natural philosophy of the Ionians into theology" (I, 116).

Even in the later development of science I can find no indication that knowledge of crafts and techniques was a decisive factor. Contrary to the impression one gains from Farrington (II, 27, 30 f.), it is not preoccupation with artisan's skills that accounts for the greatness of the accomplishment of Theophrastus and Strato, the representatives of science around 300 B.C. It is not true that in his *Metaphysics* (8a 19–20) Theophrastus demands that in order to understand the behavior of matter "we must in general proceed by making reference to the crafts and drawing analogies between natural and artificial processes" (27); he rather says that "in general we must understand matter by virtue of an analogy with the arts, or any other similarity that may exist," that is, also by analogies of function or structure and the like (cf. 23). In the complicated system of Theophrastus his references to techniques are but one component; he is an adherent of teleology (22)—of his philosophical discussion of analogy I have spoken before.[41] As for Strato,

---

[41] Cf. p. 407. Farrington's analysis of Theophrastus' system of botany (23), too, is vitiated, I think, by his failure to take into account the difficulties to which Theophrastus' concept of analogy led.

in his mechanical investigations he surely employed analogies drawn from the crafts (30 f., 38). Yet again, this one method does not adequately reflect his general outlook. Strato identified nature with the divine, as an Epicurean critic maintained (Cicero, *De Natura Deorum*, I, 13,35), not "the divine with nature," as Farrington puts it (42). In his doctrine of qualities Strato, despite his acceptance of certain Democritean theories, remained an Aristotelian, just as his concept of nature was derived from Aristotle.[42]

Without depreciating the value of practical knowledge accumulated through the arts and crafts, it is fair to conclude that Greek science did more than "sort out the theoretical implications of this practical knowledge and present the resulting body of knowledge as a logically coherent system" (I, 20). Greek science advocated at all times assumptions about an invisible world of law and order; it was theoretical rather than practical. For better or worse it always was "a relaxation, an adornment, a subject of contemplation" (II, 164), and did not become so simply at the end.[43]

But it is time to turn to the consideration of the second factor which in Farrington's opinion was responsible for the decay of ancient science, namely, political pressure interfering with the freedom of scientific research. This thesis Farrington first set forth in his *Science and Politics in the Ancient World*, where the influence of slavery is mentioned only in passing (165); in his *Greek Science* he has in some measure elaborated the political explanation.[44]

Farrington finds the first signs of political interference with science in Greece. The banishment of Anaxagoras from Athens (61; cf. *Greek Science*, I, 97) was brought about by the masses, though not without the connivance of the upper classes (76 ff.). The conflict between Ionian science and the old-established religion had become evident before in Aeschylus' *Prometheus* (69 ff.; 84; cf. *Science*, I, 135 ff.). It is true, no doubt, that the Athenian democracy was quick in raising the cry of impiety. Yet the banishment of Anaxagoras, the condemnation of Socrates were events that did not halt the progress of science, as Farrington himself admits. After all, in 399, in spite of the trial of Socrates,

[42] For Strato, cf. H. Diels, "Über das physikalische System des Straton," *S. Ber. Berlin* (1893), 112, 116.

[43] Cf. p. 413 f.

[44] The thesis of *Science and Politics* (1939) is expressly taken up in *Greek Science*, II, 113. For Childe's acceptance of Farrington's views, cf. *op. cit.*, 225.

one could buy Anaxagoras' book for one drachma in the market place at Athens (Plato, *Apology*, 26 D–E).[45]

But the situation changed at the end of the fourth century B.C. "In a city-state, where striking inequalities of wealth prevailed and where in consequence civil war was endemic and often violent, the religion of the State tended more and more to be transformed by the ruling-class into an instrument of mental oppression utterly incompatible with the spread of enlightenment. This was the main reason for the slow strangulation of the great speculative movement of natural philosophy that began in Ionia in the sixth century, flourished for about two hundred years, and then slowly died for about another eight centuries" (*Science and Politics*, 164).[46] And how was this strangulation brought about? By disseminating "such ideas as would make the unjust distribution of the rewards and toils of life seem a necessary part of the eternal constitution of things, and [by] suppressing such ideas as might lead to criticism of this view of the universe" (27). It was essential "to foster the belief that the oligarchical nobility were where they were by the will of heaven, and that any effort to dislodge them would be rewarded by condign punishment in this world and the next. Such a programme, of course, never exists in its naked simplicity as the conscious mental attitude of a whole class in society. It reveals itself only in moments of unguarded candour, or when there is a crisis of thought" (225). And since "in the West the rulers of Rome achieved a degree of success in the control of society through superstition that was denied to the Greek oligarchies," the fatal blow was struck with the overthrow of the Roman Republic (231; cf. 202 ff.). "The very understanding that there was such a thing as science, except for a few languishing techniques such as medicine or architecture, almost died out under the Empire" (232).

I have no intention to inquire whether those whom Farrington singles out as the protagonists of this program of the oligarchy—Pindar,

[45] Incidentally, the Plato passage just referred to proves, if proof is needed, the incorrectness of Plutarch's contention that astronomy before Plato was taught only in secret and was tainted with reproach (*Nicias*, 23), a contention in which Farrington seems to put great faith (I, 96 f.). The story obviously is invented in order to explain the persecution of Protagoras, Anaxagoras, and Socrates mentioned by Plutarch. An answer to Farrington's interpretation of the Aeschylean *Prometheus* is given by Cornford, *Unwritten Philosophy*, 123 ff.

[46] The view here expressed slightly differs from Farrington's later assumption that the decay of science began in the second century B.C.; cf. above note 35 and corresponding text.

Plato, Cicero, Virgil, Manilius (225 f.) and Aristotle (e.g., 111)—actually had any such aims. Nor shall I raise the question whether ancient religion, even the state cults, could be used for the purposes for which in Farrington's view they were used, either consciously or unconsciously. In my opinion, Farrington is unconvincing on both these counts, just as he is unconvincing in his indictment of Platonism, which to him is unscientific and antisocial.[47] But again, I wish to scrutinize only the historical facts. Is there any evidence that science was repressed by any political movement that allied itself with religion?

As for Greece, Farrington in his first book alludes in passing to Plato's being prepared "to risk" teaching astronomy (110), to Aristotle's opposing the popular myths "behind [the] closed doors" of the Lyceum (111).[48] But in his *Greek Science* Farrington further develops the thesis that astronomy was the science most widely open to political bias. Plato's and Aristotle's astronomical views were shaped by definite political aims (I, 92–98). The fight over the homocentric hypothesis turned out to be not only a scientific, but also, and primarily, a political issue. The thesis of Heraclides, the "daring innovator," already contained "disturbing suggestions" (II, 78). The heliocentric hypothesis caused a "shock" (79). Cleanthes "expressed the opinion that the Greeks ought to indict Aristarchus on a charge of impiety," and these threats "appear to have involved a real danger to the scientist" (79). The "fear of dislodging the earth from the center of the universe was too great" (87). For "the stability of ancient oligarchical society was bound

[47] Farrington's analysis of Plato has been criticized by Cornford, *op. cit.*, 127 ff.; cf. also P. Shorey, "Platonism and the History of Science," *Proceedings Amer. Philosophical Society*, 66 (1927), 159–82. It is rather strange that Plato, who in the nineteenth century was heralded as the prophet of socialism, as the only one to have fought against the unjust distribution of wealth, and to have advocated mixed government as the sole remedy for the class system, should now be considered the protagonist of reaction. In regard to Farrington's view on religion I should at least mention that even those among the ancient philosophers who distinguished between political and philosophical religion (*Greek Science*, II, 113) did not deny the existence of a deity; they merely distinguished between two different ways of understanding the same truth. To speak of a "police function of religion," which the Epicureans alone abolished (*Science and Politics*, 160; cf. *Science*, II, 113), is quite misleading. Certainly religion in antiquity was sometimes misused for political purposes, by democrats and aristocrats alike. But generally religion held no worldly power over men. And Lucretius' poem, which to Farrington is a source of true and unimpeachable information, attests clearly that aristocrats and masses, in the opinion of the Epicureans, were under the sway of religious beliefs. If the ancient oligarchs tried to deceive the masses by religious means, they were indeed deceived deceivers.

[48] Concerning the risk of teaching astronomy, cf. p. 422, n. 45.

up with a particular view of astronomy [namely, the homocentric or geocentric one]. To hold other views was not a scientific error but a heresy. Astronomy in antiquity was as thorny a subject as biblical criticism in modern times. Observational astronomy was subjected to anxious scrutiny and careful management . . . The astronomers themselves were often torn between two loyalties, like modern historians of religion. They had scientific consciences, but they knew that they were trespassing on a field where opinion involved political and social consequences" (88).

Excepting Duhem's speculations about the accusations of impiety "that ancient Paganism *would* have levelled" against the proponents of a heliocentric theory (88; cf. 79), Farrington does not adduce any evidence in proof of his views. In fact, nothing happened to Aristarchus, or to any one who sided with him. As is well known, trials for impiety became almost extinct after 300 B.C.[49] Hipparchus rejected the heliocentric hypothesis as unscientific, because to him it did not seem to square with observations that had been made. Posidonius opposed Heraclides on the ground that the choice of an astronomical hypothesis lies within the province of philosophy. Others chose to adhere to their respective views because they "had a prejudice in favour of the system which arranges all the spheres concentrically about the centre of the Universe," as Sosigenes suggested, who being himself a Peripatetic accused Eudoxus and his followers of having neglected the data known even to them (86). This explanation apparently is unconvincing to Farrington (cf. 87 f., 89). Yet the fact that philosophical prejudices can hamper insight into truth seems very clear in the case of Epicurus and the Epicureans. To Farrington, they were the only ones in antiquity not to hold "two doctrines," that is, one by which to deceive the ruled and another one for the rulers (*Science and Politics*, 17). Through science they tried to liberate men, not to oppress them. They upheld what was the counterposition to oligarchic religion, insisting as they did that believers in unorthodox opinions on the heavenly bodies "were not in danger of being damned for them" either here or in the hereafter (*Science*, II, 89). Nevertheless, they too refused to accept the heliocentric hypothesis. Obviously it did not fit in with their notion of true knowledge.

All the facts, then, militate against Farrington's claim that political

---

[49] Cf. A. B. Drachmann, *Atheism in Pagan Antiquity* (1922), 7 ff. The skeptic Carneades, for instance, held high political offices.

reasons can be made responsible for the rejection of correct astronomical views, that they "checked mechanical and chemical speculation on the motion and substance of the heavenly bodies" (II, 89). The silence of ancient writers on this point is the more significant, since they were by no means unaware of a possible conflict between truth and political exigency. Despite some fervent pleas for the rulers' support of science and research, the suspicion remained that the court was not the place where studies would flourish. Not only did the life of the courtier scholar seem insecure on account of the "irrational wrath" of the tyrant—and occasional expulsions of scholars are known to have occurred in Hellenistic times (II, 100)—it was clearly realized that dependence on governments may jeopardize intellectual integrity and freedom of research. This awareness comes out in a general way in the never-ceasing debate about the question whether or not the philosopher should and could live at the court of a tyrant, or even have any intercourse with prominent political figures. The historian's task, it was said, calls for life in a free city and for independent means; the geographer in the service of the mighty, it was feared, would feel obliged to falsify facts in order to please their whims and ambitions. That rhetoric can survive only in a democracy, while it is bound to decay in an oligarchy, was a commonplace.[50] And yet, it is not attested that strictly scientific opinions were made a matter of persecution, that astronomers or physicists were afraid to hold certain views on the universe.

As for political interference with science under the Roman empire, Farrington, as far as I can see, does not adduce any specific instances. It is indeed hard to imagine how the Roman oligarchy could have put its supposed program into practice. Roman law left it to the gods to punish those who had sinned against them; even the Christians, after all, could be persecuted only as offenders against the emperor. No censorship of publications existed; if at times books were burnt, these were historical or political pamphlets put out by the opposition to the monarchy.[51] It is true, Tiberius ordered the execution of an architect and inventor who had aroused his displeasure and did not even allow

[50] The general discussion of these topics is summarized by Plutarch, *Maxime cum principibus philosophandum esse*. The ideal conditions for historical research are outlined by Lucian, *Quomodo Historia Conscribenda*. The falsification of geographical facts in order to enhance the glory of political leaders is implied in Posidonius' stricture of Polybius, Strabo, III, 4, 13.

[51] Cf. F. H. Cramer, "Bookburning and Censorship in Ancient Rome," *Journal of the History of Ideas*, 6 (1945), 157 ff.

his name to be recorded (Dio Cassius, LVII, 21). Vettius Valens in the second century bewailed the fact that he had not the good fortune "to live in those spacious days [of old] and to breathe the fresh air of their spiritual freedom for research"; since he is thinking of the days when even "kings and despots . . . were enthusiasts for the science [of astrology]" (*Anthologiae*, VI, Introd.), one can hardly take his testimony at face value.[52] At any rate, Sosigenes in the same century did attack the homocentric hypothesis in favor of the more modern theory of eccentric circles and epicycles, as did the later Peripatetics in general. And although the Roman attitude toward death and burial probably contributed to the decline of human anatomy, nobody objected to Galen's dissections of apes which most closely resembled human beings.[53] It seems fair, then, to say that in Greece as well as in Rome scientists were free to follow the bent of their minds. The decay of science can hardly be attributed to any political conditions that abridged freedom of thought.

Nor can one say with Farrington, I think, that in society as it emerged under the reign of Augustus, resting on Stoicism which itself continued the Platonic tradition, "science . . . was doomed" (*Science and Politics*, 219); that it was incompatible with "the tone and temper" of this society (229). In the first century B.C. the members of the Epicurean school "almost alone, . . . fought to rid nature and history of the arbitrary interference of supernatural forces" (*Greek Science*, II, 111). "Wherever men studied nature, not as a manifestation of the mind of a benevolent providence, but as a non-human environment by the control of which men had laid the foundations of civilized life; wherever men studied history, not to trace in it the mysterious intentions of the gods, but as a record of the trials and errors of mankind; wherever men thought of society as a sphere in which man by the exercise of his political or technical inventiveness might improve his conditions of life; wherever human nature was studied as a basis for a rational control of the instinctive life; there the teaching of Epicurus was likely to be at the root of it" (II, 109 f.). But the Epicureans were "the defeated party in ancient philosophy" (II, 119), defeated because they did not serve the desired political ends.

[52] The first reference I owe to Rehm, *op. cit.*, 161, the second to Toynbee, *op. cit.*, V, 423, whose translation I have reproduced.
[53] Cf. Galen, *Opera Omnia*, ed. Kühn, II, 222, and in general Edelstein, *Quellen u. Studien z. Gesch. der Naturwiss. u. d. Medizin*, III, 136 ff., 150 [281* ff., 295*].

Farrington's praise of Epicurus as the "first champion of popular enlightenment" (*Science and Politics*, 129) does not call for my criticism. It has already been pointed out that Epicurus was not a reformer, he had no interest in politics; great ethical teacher that he was, he wanted to improve man rather than social conditions.[54] I wish to urge, however, that Epicureanism was not conducive to scientific research. In recent years, the picture of an Epicurus utterly ignorant of science has rightly been abandoned. To go to the other extreme now and to consider Epicurus the protagonist of science is in my opinion equally erroneous.

The fact that atomism has become the basis of progress in modern science should not make one forget the fundamental differences between the ancient and the modern atomic theory. Epicurus' atoms were the elements of rational philosophy, not the working hypothesis of empirical science. The neglect of mathematics in the field of physics is another characteristic of his unscientific approach.[55] More important still, Epicurus' belief in the "diversity" of causes makes it impossible to establish that astronomical and mechanical science, the absence of which Farrington laments and attributes to political conditions (II, 89). While in regard to the atoms one cause alone is to be considered (*Epistula* I, Diogenes Laert., X, 78), in astronomy and meteorology, Epicurus holds, as in "all that is unknown, we must take into account the variety of ways in which analogous occurrences happen within our experience" (*ibid.*, 80; cf. *Epistula* II, *ibid.*, 94, 96). "If then we think that an event could happen in one or other particular way out of several, we shall be as tranquil when we recognize that it actually comes about in more ways than one as if we knew that it happens in this particular way" (*Epistula* I, *ibid.*, 80). Has the quest of science not always been the search for the

---

[54] Cf. Cornford, *op. cit.*, 93 f. (first published in *Background to Modern Science*, ed. J. Needham and W. Pagel [1938]); the tendency to identify progress with Epicureanism can be traced at least to the nineteenth century (*ibid.*, 90). Rostovtzeff, *Hellenistic World*, III, 1128 ff., has dealt with the general failure of ancient philosophical thought to advocate social reform. It is fair, however, to underline the fact that so far as philosophy became active in politics, it was the Platonists and the [The rest of the sentence reads: "science, is in my opinion equally erroneous." This is an obvious typographical error, repeating part of a line of the text.—Ed.].

[55] For the difference between Epicurus' theory and that of modern science, cf., e.g., W. C. Dampier, *From Aristotle to Galileo* (*Background to Modern Science*, 25 f.); also Cornford, *op. cit.*, 122 f. For Epicurus' relation to mathematics, I. E. Drabkin, "Notes on Epicurean Kinetics," *Transactions Amer. Philological Ass.*, 69 (1938), 373 f. Epicurus' dogmatism, evidenced by his insistence that his pupils should learn his teachings by heart (*Ep.* I, Init.; II, Init.), likewise can hardly be considered a stimulus to further research.

specific explanation of any given phenomenon?[56] And Epicurus' condemnation of specific causality in matters which "are only seen at a distance" (*ibid.*) was not abandoned even by those among his followers who in the first century B.C. scrutinized the structure of empirical science and elaborated the doctrine of inference from observed facts. For they considered this inference applicable only to painting, grammar, rhetoric, music, poetry, as well as to medicine, navigation and mathematics; astronomy and the other natural sciences were not included.[57]

It is therefore not astonishing that Farrington in his history of science, excepting the assertion that the Epicureans were "the best anthropologists of the ancient world" (*Greek Science*, II, 43), cannot name even one Epicurean scientist of note, or one outstanding scientific discovery made within the Epicurean school. Epicureanism during more than five hundred years in which it had devoted adherents made no contributions to science.[58] Wherever atomism as such played a rôle in Greek science, it was after it had been integrated into other systems and considerably modified, as for instance in the case of Strato (II, 41), or Heraclides of Pontus, or Asclepiades, the physician of the first century B.C. Those who furthered research, as far as they belonged to any philosophical sect, were Platonists, Aristotelians, or Stoics, members of those schools which to Farrington represent the unscientific spirit. The achievement of the philosophical dogmatists was even more important than that of the philosophical empiricists or skeptics. When skepticism,

---

[56] The Epicurean principle of causation is exemplified in *Ep.* 2; e.g., "Snow may be formed when a fine rain issues from the clouds . . . or again by congelation in clouds . . . And there are other ways in which snow might be formed" (*Diog. Laert.*, X, 107 f.). From this, one must distinguish the recognition of a possible multiplicity of causes (*Ep.* II, 96); cf. C. Bailey, *Epicurus, The extant Remains* (1926), 296. For Lucretius' application of the thesis that "all explanations are true and correspond to existing facts, which are not contradicted by phenomena," cf. C. Bailey, *Lucretius, De Rerum Natura* I (1947), 57 ff. Even the attempt to find in Epicurus a concept of order that is fundamentally biological (F. Solmsen, "Epicurus and Cosmological Heresies," *Amer. Journ. of Philology*, 72 [1951], 18 ff.) leads to the recognition that "the application of the concept of cosmic matters remains problematical" (21).

[57] Cf. Ph. H. De Lacy and E. A. De Lacy, *Philodemus on Methods of Inference* (1941), 136, 152. Appreciation of the method of inference and of the importance which the arguments of Philodemus acquired later, when they were rectified and further worked out, should not deceive one about the shortcomings inherent in the original discussion.

[58] Lucretius' description of the development of civilization is based on Democritus, cf. Farrington, II, 115; by the way, this is not different in principle from that given by the Stoics (cf. above, note 31). Whether Epicurean anthropology should be called the best ever formulated by the ancients (Farrington, II, 43) depends on the point of view of the interpreter.

which generally withheld all judgment and was hostile to all investigation, at one time allied itself with medical theory, every attempt at generalization was given up and there remained only the observation of individual phenomena.[59]

In every respect, then, Farrington's explanation of the development of ancient science seems to be untenable. His books have done much to arouse interest in the subject. The thesis which they advocate is vitiated however by what, in my opinion, is the basic error in many of the recent evaluations of ancient science, namely, the misapplication of historical analogies. Conditions in antiquity are seen in the light of subsequent events. The conflict between science and religion, which characterized later ages, is injected into the ancient world. Progress and decay of Greek and Roman science are judged by the standards of modern science.

Such an approach not only tends to distort the reconstruction of the actual happenings, it also loses sight of the peculiar problems and solutions which were characteristic of antiquity. The history of ancient science is not merely a history of the more or less correct answers to scientific questions. The very attempt to constitute a scientific view of the universe was beset with difficulties that had to be met. The reaction of society to this attempt, the position of the scientists within the social order, in short, the organization of science had an essential part in shaping the particular way in which science was tackled by the ancients. The achievement of the Greeks, their scientific merit, can be judged more adequately and fairly only if seen within its own setting. Even the various phases of ancient science, the rapid progress at first, the stagnation which set in after the second century of our era and is usually regarded as decay, acquire a meaning of their own if the categories of interpretation are derived from an analysis of the particular and unique historical situation. It is some of these neglected aspects that I propose to discuss in concluding my survey of recent studies.

IV. THE ORGANIZATION OF ANCIENT SCIENCE

The question when science began may at first glance seem as meaningless as the question when poetry and art had their beginning. Yet

[59] For skepticism and science, cf. Edelstein, *Quellen u. Studien z. Gesch. d. Naturwiss. u. d. Medizin*, III, 253 ff. [195* ff.]; *idem, s.v. Methodiker, R.E.*, Suppl. VI, cols. 367 ff. [184* ff.]. For Heraclides and Asclepiades, cf. K. Lasswitz, *Geschichte der Atomistik*, I (1890), 211 ff.

provided that by science one does not understand just any kind of
knowledge or technical skill, however highly developed, but a consistently rational explanation of phenomena, the question is meaningful
and allows of an answer. It was with the Presocratic thinkers that such a
science came into existence, as the Greeks themselves were well aware.
To be sure, there were those who saw in Homer the father of science, of
astronomy, geography and history, and who consequently made science
coeval with Greek history. But they could make good their claim only
by applying to the poet's work the method of allegorical interpretation,
that is, by translating his thought, concealed as they believed in poetical
language, into the scientific categories of a later period. However, in
general it was agreed that a new attitude toward the comprehension of
facts began to arise after the heroic age had vanished. On the basis of
the hypothesis that the world can be understood by reason some men in
Ionia in the early sixth century created a world that reason understands.[60]

Of this new and unprecedented vision society at first took hardly
any notice. Xenophanes' angry denunciations of the rewards bestowed
on others while he and his kin remained without recognition (21 B 2
Diels) are typical of the situation. In his devotion to learning and insight
into nature the scientist was isolated and on his own. A hitherto unknown ideal of human existence—symbolized in Democritus' saying
that to find an etiology is greater gain than to become king of Persia
(68 B 118 Diels)—challenged the old established ideals of a political or
agonistic or acquisitive life. Unrecognized by his contemporaries the
scientist found himself outside the confines of the social order. There
were no jobs for him; science was not a career. He had to have independent means with which to carry out his investigations or to travel
for the sake of his geographical studies. Society had a place for the practicing physician, but not for the biologist. The architect could earn a
living; in the builder's workshop mathematical knowledge developed
incidentally and empirically; but there was no position for the theoretical mathematician. As interest increased in knowledge as such, the
scientist began to teach others who wanted to know about his subject.

[60] The ancient doxographical tradition unanimously attests the Ionian origin
of philosophy and science. Here I need not discuss the question whether the Orient
had an influence on the beginnings of the Greek development; cf. J. Burnet, *Early
Greek Philosophy* (1948⁴), 15 ff. For Homer, cf. F. Wehrli, *Zur Geschichte der alle-
gorischen Deutung Homers im Altertum*, Diss. (Basel, 1928).

Occasionally he found a protector who provided for his livelihood. On the whole, even in the classical centuries everything was left to the initiative and courage and determination of individuals, who pursued their studies at their own expense and at their own risk. Athens forced her citizens to pay for producing the plays of Aeschylus, Sophocles and Euripides. At the great festivals everywhere, poets and musicians competed for rewards and prizes; no similar opportunity existed for scientists.[61]

In the Hellenistic age a few research centers were established, notably Alexandria and Pergamum. Some of the kings gave support to scientific investigations, especially to such as were likely to bear practical fruit, further their own interests and enhance their own fame. Yet it was a very limited circle of scholars who profited by royal munificence, who received pay for their work, who were offered the facilities of a library or the resources of scientific collections.[62] In the free cities where the great majority of researchers lived, they still failed to get any help or employment; even public collections of books were rarely at their disposal. The philosophical schools no less than the scientific ones were private organizations, maintained entirely by private contributions. For the acquisition of instruments and all other implements of research the scientists were still forced to fall back on their own resources.[63]

The sober truth, then, is that in the early stages of science, society, far from interfering with the scientist's work, on the whole remained completely indifferent to its value. To the modern interpreter, Greek science may seem to be one of the greatest achievements of the ancients. To the Greeks of the classical and Hellenistic centuries, it was of little

[61] That it is characteristic of Greek scientific and philosophical achievement that the work was done by individuals without the support of society has been emphasized most strongly by J. Burckhardt, *Über das wissenschaftliche Verdienst der Griechen, Vorträge* 1844–1887, ed. E. Dürr (1919[4]), 140 ff. Even if one is inclined to speak with Burnet (*op. cit.*, 28 ff.) of philosophical schools at the time of the Presocratics, one must admit that these schools were private organizations.

[62] For the organization of the Museion, cf. *s.v. Museion, R.E.*, XVI, 1 (1933), cols. 807 ff. That even the support given by Alexander the Great to scientists has been exaggerated by recent scholars has been shown by O. Regenbogen, *s.v. Theophrastos, R.E., Supplement*, VII (1950), cols. 1459 ff.

[63] For the rare occurrence of public libraries in free cities, cf. W. Christ-W. Schmid, *Geschichte der griech. Literatur*, II, 1 (1920), 19. Concerning the philosophical schools after Plato, cf. U. v. Wilamowitz, *Antigonos von Karystos, Philologische Untersuchungen*, IV (1881), 263 ff.

consequence. The progress that was accomplished was brought about by individuals fighting against almost insuperable odds. They took up their studies without any proper training in their youth. For even the educational system was impervious to the advance of scientific thought. The instruction of children, a matter left in the hands of parents and private teachers, was concentrated mainly on poetry, music, and gymnastics. The teaching of scientific subjects was rudimentary.[64] Once the scholar had overcome the initial difficulties in acquiring the elementary knowledge which he needed, he could not devote himself exclusively to his work. The constant demands made upon him by the community in the interest of public life curtailed his leisure and diverted much of his energy. Finally, since under the existing conditions only a few were willing or could afford to choose science as their profession, the number engaged in scientific investigations was small indeed. It was a handful of people who had to carry the burden.[65]

That this was the situation and that it impaired the effectiveness of whatever inquiries were made, the ancients realized themselves. "Inasmuch as no city holds [solid geometry] in honor," Plato says (*Republic*, 528 B), "these inquiries are languidly pursued," and he suggests that if the state superintended and honored such studies, "continuous and strenuous investigation would bring out the truth." The historian Diodorus, comparing Greek science with that of the Chaldaeans (II, 29), gives a more comprehensive picture of the state of affairs, which also shows that even in his time no essential improvement had been brought about. In Babylon, he says, knowledge is handed on from father to son; the pupils "are bred in these teachings from childhood up"; afterward they are "relieved of all other services to the state." In Greece, on the contrary, the student "who takes up a large number of subjects without preparation turns to the higher studies only quite late, and then, after laboring upon them to some extent, gives them up, being distracted by the necessity of earning a livelihood; and but a few here and there really strive for the higher studies and continue in the pursuit of them as a profit making business, and these are always trying

[64] Cf. H. J. Marrou, *Histoire de l'éducation dans l'antiquité* (1948), esp. 160 ff., 225 ff., 243 ff.

[65] The importance of this fact has been underlined by O. Neugebauer, *Exact Sciences in Antiquity* (*Studies in Civilization*, University of Pennsylvania Bicentennial Conference [1941], 25), and pointed out as one of the reasons for the rapid decline of science. Cf. also below, n. 70.

to make innovations in connection with the most important doctrines instead of following in the path of their predecessors."[66]

It is true, Diodorus is an idolator of the Chaldaeans and Egyptians. In the caste system he finds the explanation of the superiority of the Orientals. One may well wonder whether Greek science could have arisen at all, had Greek life been fettered by similar traditions, had Greek society not left it to its members to do whatever they wanted, even if they could not count on the support of their fellow citizens. The admiration for the greatness of Greek scientific achievement should be enhanced by the realization that everything depended on the effort of the individual, unaided by the world in which he lived. Nevertheless, it remains true that what on the one hand constitutes the glory of Greek science, on the other hand accounts for certain of its limitations. Progress necessarily was slowed down and limited by the scarcity of scholars and their insufficient preparation. The lack of social recognition and the consequent lack of permanent and stable forms of organization had a decisive influence, I think, also on the course which science took during the initial phases of its history.

At the outset a few general traits may be emphasized reflecting the insecurity of science within the social order, which was aggravated by the philosophical skepticism concerning the possibility of gaining true knowledge. Such treatises as the Ps. Hippocratic essay *On the Art* inveigh against the detractors of science. The physician who here defends the actual existence of a medical art is well aware of the fact that all the other arts and sciences are also threatened and expects their representatives to come forth in rebuttal of the attacks made upon them. Obviously written for the élite interested in the new sophistic movement, the treatise shows how the craftsman who intends to be a scientist is fighting for the recognition of his novel aspiration.[67] Nor are later writings devoid of such justifications of the existence and truth of knowledge, its value and usefulness, coupled again with a rejection of the philosophical skepticism that undermined science from within. The rhetorical character of many scientific books is an indirect indication of the insecurity of the position of science. One writes with an eye on the public who must be convinced and propagandized. Since the state or the community in

[66] Strictly speaking Diodorus' comparison of Greeks and Chaldaeans concerns their philosophy, but this quite obviously includes the sciences.

[67] Cf. L. Edelstein, Περὶ ἀέρων und die Sammlung der hippokratischen Schriften, *Problemata*, IV (1931), 105 ff. [101* ff.].

no way supervises science and its application—no examinations, no system of licensing existed—the physician for instance develops a technique by which he can convince the layman that he is truly a doctor and not a mere pretender. The greater part of ancient medical prognostic serves this social purpose rather than a scientific one.[68] And it is likely that the insistence on the impressiveness of mechanical devices, the constant emphasis on the marvelous and the astounding, to which I have referred above, is determined also by the wish to gain the approval of public opinion. Thus, a considerable amount of what is, strictly speaking, unscientific matter is integrated into the body of science, naturally to the detriment of more important and strictly scientific features. Finally, no satisfactory solution of the relative position of expert and layman was found. Just as in education no heed was paid to scientific progress, so ancient life in general remained untouched by the results of a scientific understanding of the world. The myth continued to be the prevailing power. In the fifth century B.C. the Athenian general Nicias took an eclipse of the sun for a bad omen; Roman generals or noblemen of the first century A.D. were wont to react similarly. The fundamentals of scientific knowledge were no prerequisite for an official, for the scientific analysis of facts had no authority. The astronomical and geographical views even of the upper strata of society fell far behind the available information, and their lack of knowledge was no matter of reproach. Nowhere did the expert play a rôle or have a clearly defined place in public affairs.[69]

To turn now to questions more intrinsically connected with science proper, I suggest that the failure of the empirical trend to establish itself securely was in great measure due to the lack of a social integration of science. Collecting a vast mass of information presupposes stabilized institutions. Individual effort at assembling data necessarily is limited. To be sure, the Aristotelian school and its members achieved a great deal, and so did the Museion in Egypt. But these were rare exceptions.

[68] Cf. Edelstein, *op. cit.*, 60 ff. [65* ff.]. It is in this way, I think, that one must explain "the tendency to popularize science in accordance with the taste of the ruling class," noted by Neugebauer, *loc. cit.*, and regarded by him as the second element responsible for the decay of science. But there is no attempt "to adapt [science] to the teaching level of the schools," *ibid.*; cf. above, note 64 and corresponding text.

[69] Here I have rephrased some of Burckhardt's arguments, *op. cit.*, 146 f. The ancients, even in scientific matters, were wont to subordinate the expert's opinion to the judgment of the free citizen, or in Plato's words, to "the user's art" (*Republic*, 601 D). How far the individual wished to go in accepting scientific knowledge, was up to him.

Historical and geographical studies were hampered by the scholars' tendency to avoid political entanglement and to live as private citizens (cf. above, p. 430). Astonishing though it is how much was accomplished, how documents were assembled and facts were compiled, still the researcher had only as much material at his disposal as he could lay hands on himself. The experimental sciences labored under similar handicaps. No close collaboration in laboratories developed; records were hardly kept beyond the lifetime of the individual scientist. The isolation of the individual and of the private schools was intensified by the difficulties of communication. One seldom knew what other men in the same field were doing. Results gained at one time were forgotten again or not referred to because they were not generally available.[70]

However, the fact that science had originated as an individual endeavor and continued to depend on private initiative even in the Hellenistic centuries had a still more serious consequence: no agreement existed among scientists about the fundamental tenets of science. Science was not yet an aggregate of opinions on which all scientists must and do agree. Of course, there are always periods when revolutionary changes take place in science, so that disagreement may exist for some time. But after the discussion has settled down, unanimity about the basic principles and approaches is reestablished. In its essentials, science in America, England, France, Germany is alike. A very different situation prevailed throughout the early phases of ancient science.

For science as it was elaborated by the various Presocratic philosophers or scientists of the classical age really expressed their individual conviction, which was true in the opinion of its respective proponent and his pupils, but of no validity for anyone else. The evolution of nature as conceived by Anaximander or Anaxagoras had no persuasive power for a Democritean. The physics of Diogenes of Apollonia was anathema to an Empedoclean. There were almost as many kinds of science as there were scientists. The *Corpus Hippocraticum*, the only large bulk of scientific writings preserved from that epoch, illustrates the infinite variety of definitions considered scientific as regards so basic a concept as the etiology of diseases.[71] The Hellenistic age witnessed a gradual

---

[70] Neugebauer, *loc. cit.*, has suggested that "the number of scholars in the ancient world was by far too small to undertake any kind of program based on systematic organized collaboration." I should consider this factor as only one among others that were responsible for the failure of empiricism.

[71] Edelstein, *op. cit.*, 154 ff.

change. Not only did schools or organizations now come into existence—thought itself became more uniform. The number of individualistic formulations of science was reduced. Methods and systems that found a wider following coalesced. Still, there remained a great variety of doctrines, and adherence to any one of them was optional, as it were. There was dogmatic and empirical science, the one aiming at establishing causes, the other renouncing the search for an explanation of hidden phenomena. The geography of Polybius differed from that of Eratosthenes not only as regards factual data, but also as regards the basic approach: Polybius, for the sake of the usefulness of geography to the political leader, abandoned the standards of mathematics. Aristarchus and Hipparchus disagreed not only about the heliocentric hypothesis, but also about the principles governing the formulation of astronomical laws. Others doubted the possibility of applying mathematics to astronomy. The debate about the foundation of geometry—whether it was rational or empirical knowledge—jeopardized even the progress of that science which naturally had always been comparatively free of dissension. The medicine of Erasistratus and of Herophilus on the one hand and empirical medicine on the other were as much at cross-purposes, as were Stoic and Epicurean physics. And these divergencies did not imply a distinction between science and non-science; they merely characterized rival systems of thought which continued to exist side by side.[72]

It is this still unreconciled dissension among scientific outlooks which explains why, studying the remains of classical and Hellenistic science, we can detect one type of scientific argument strikingly similar to modern science, while a vast amount of other material, though scientific to the Greeks, does not strike the modern interpreter as scientific at all. Moreover, it should be noted that the reign of rival systems lasted down to the second century A.D. Galen's *Introduction to Medicine*, addressed to beginners, places before them the theories of the three medi-

---

[72] The ancients certainly were well aware of the dissension among scientists, cf., e.g., Diodorus, II, 29, and below, n. 74. Modern scholars, if they pay any attention at all to the phenomenon in question, consider it typical of Greek science generally. Thus Zilsel says, on p. 253, ". . . it would be an overstatement to characterize scientific activity in classical antiquity as a merely individualistic undertaking. Classical science had rather reached, approximately, that degree of continuity and cooperation which in our era is characteristic of philosophy." But as will be shown, this does not apply to the last phase of the ancient development.

cal sects which at that time competed with one another, that of the Dogmatists, of the Empiricists, and of the Methodists, and the young student is asked to make a choice among them; otherwise he would be at a loss with whom to study.

However, in the same second century—at which time, according to most historians, the decay of ancient science became complete—the confusion of opinions gradually began to disappear. The knowledge gained by previous generations was collected, criticized and, with the addition of new material, synthesized. Such a tendency can be observed in all fields of learning, in grammar, metrics and literary history, no less than in geography, optics, astronomy, algebra and medicine.[73] That it is not by chance that so many works of the new type were composed in this second century, that they were instigated by a conscious effort to dispense with the bewildering diversity of approaches characteristic of earlier periods, follows, I think, from the program which one of these authors, Galen, outlines in his work *On Scientific Demonstration* and in many others of his writings. Oppressed by the "wide dissension" that existed, he wished not to defend any sectarian dogma but to show to the physician or to any other scientist how one can establish "the best sect." The doctrine of such a sect in Galen's opinion was to stand above all doctrines and to acknowledge as its criterion not the opinion of any one school, but of truth alone. The method of Euclidean geometry, in praise of which all philosophers agreed, he considered the model of the method of the new science.[74] In other words, as the merely individual views of the Presocratic scientists had been superseded by the more comprehensive Hellenistic systems, so these divergent systems themselves were now to be integrated into a uniform science. It is true, the authors of the second century added relatively little to the knowledge already available. Yet they took a step that had not been taken, they accomplished

[73] For the work of the ancient grammarians and historians of literature, cf. U. v. Wilamowitz, *Euripides Herakles*, I (1889), 179 (*Einleitung in die Tragödie*). It was in the second century too that the classical tragedies and comedies which have survived were selected for use in school.

[74] The fragments of Galen's treatise *On Scientific Demonstration* have been collected by J. v. Müller, "Über Galens Werk vom wissenschaftlichen Beweis," *Abh. Akad. München*, XX (1894), 405 ff., who in his introduction has also surveyed Galen's statements on "the best sect" he contemplated. The specific passages I have referred to are to be found *Opera Omnia*, X, 469 (Müller, 419, n. 17); I, 81 (420, n. 19), 225; *Scripta Minora*, ed. J. v. Müller, II (1891), 117. I should add that in late antiquity and in the Middle Ages Galen was held to be the foremost theoretician of science.

a task that had not been accomplished before, they solved a problem that called for a solution, if science was to be science. It is their merit to have created the *scientia aeterna*, a science in which all scientists equally share. That is why their books soon became canonical, why they were used, commented upon and excerpted by later generations, while the works of the classical and Hellenistic ages were hardly accorded further study. The scholasticism of late antiquity with its rigid rules for instruction and study, its limitation to certain authors is but the working out of the new ideal of a unified science.[75]

This is not the place to inquire how far certain trends of eclecticism, noticeable even before the second century, or the Roman interest in encyclopedic summaries of knowledge prepared the way for the work done by men like Galen, Ptolemy, and others. One cannot help feeling that they were inspired also by the political unification of the world. It is surely of significance that Galen prided himself on having unified medicine, just as Trajan had unified Italy by means of the roads that he had built (X, 632 f. Kühn). At any rate, the ascendance of the new vision of science was considerably aided by social factors. In the Roman empire the educational system as well as the attitude of society toward science underwent revolutionary changes. The state provided educational facilities. Public schools were founded, universities sprang up. Professorships were endowed, examinations for scholars were introduced. Instruction in the schools all over the empire became standardized. Alexandria, Rome, Massilia, Athens were all part of the same political structure, and consequently also representative of the same science. The varied ancient democracies corresponded to the individualistic systems of science in the classical age; the various Hellenistic kingdoms

[75] Wilamowitz, *loc. cit.*, claimed that it was due to the weakness and unoriginality of later generations that the second-century authors became canonical, and he considered it the task of historical scholarship to "eliminate the predominance of these men, in order to lay bare the truly scientific and equally important work of the [earlier] Greeks." It is in this spirit that most of the work on ancient science has been undertaken during the past decades, and rightly, in so far as it is only through the work of the later compilers that the content of Hellenistic science and a good deal even of classical science can be recovered. Yet in making such an attempt one should not forget that these later writings also have a value of their own, that their authors with good reason were regarded as great scientists in late antiquity, during the Middle Ages, and even down to the eighteenth century. The unification of science was only one of their merits. For ancient scholasticism in philosophy, cf. K. Praechter, *Byzantinische Zeitschrift*, 18 (1909) 516 ff.; in medicine, O. Temkin, "Studies on late Alexandrian Medicine," *Bull. of the Institute of the Hist. of Medicine*, III (1935), 405 ff.

corresponded to the several schools; the uniform Roman empire came to have one science only.[76]

I am not arguing that these considerations fully explain the course of ancient science. If we wish to understand the development of scientific thought in antiquity, we shall have to take into account a great many other factors, the relationship between philosophy and science, the specific concepts of scientific methods, certain presuppositions that were never challenged, unscientific though they were. Thus in the history of ancient astronomy the prejudice in favor of rest as opposed to motion was as decisive as it was later in the controversy between Galileo and his contemporaries. In the history of ancient physics, the prejudice in favor of the circle as the more beautiful and perfect geometrical form precluded the acceptance of other, more correct views.[77] Theories like these were also responsible for the stagnation of research. Nor am I arguing that ancient science did not suffer through the process of scholastic unification. Progress was retarded; there was a loss of fibre. The "sober drunkenness" which had inspired earlier investigations no longer prevailed; scientists became specialists and officials. I am arguing only that it is incorrect simply to speak of the "decay" of ancient science. Even at the end there was progress, for it was in the final stage of the development that ancient scientists for the first time succeeded in bringing about a satisfactory organization of scientific endeavor. This gain made by the archaistic generation exercised as much influence on all subsequent scientific research as did the discoveries of classical and Hellenistic scientists.

[76] For educational institutions in the Roman empire, cf. Marrou, *op. cit.*, 398 ff. The importance of the Roman reforms for the whole intellectual development has been succinctly analyzed by W. Dilthey, *Pädagogik, Ges. Schriften,* IX (1934), 72 ff.

[77] Cf. E. Goldbeck, "Der Untergang des kosmischen Weltbildes der Antike," *Die Antike,* I (1925), 72 ff.; A. E. Haas, *Archiv für Geschichte d. Philosophie,* XXII (1909), 80 ff. For other considerations, cf. A. Reymond, *History of the Sciences in Greco-Roman Antiquity* (Engl. ed., 1927), 222 ff.; Cornford, *Unwritten Philosophy,* 87.

ANDREAS VESALIUS, THE HUMANIST*

Vesalius' relation to the humanism of his time has been given scant attention by modern historians. Of course, it is generally recognized that the great scientist was a classicist by education; that he knew Greek and Latin to perfection; that he zealously studied the ancient authors and extolled them to the skies. In this sense it is a commonplace to speak of Vesalius as a humanist. Does not even the Oxford Dictionary say that a humanist is "one of the scholars who at the Revival of Learning in the fourteenth, fifteenth, and sixteenth centuries, devoted themselves to the study of the language, literature, and antiquities of Rome, and afterwards of Greece?"[1] But with all due respect to the authority of the Oxford Dictionary and of those who agree with its definition of the term "humanist"—it is no longer possible to maintain that the knowledge of Greek and Latin and the study of old books suffice to make a humanist. During the past few years it has become more and more evident that the humanists, beyond their predilection for antiquity, upheld other ideals which were peculiarly their own; that they adhered to certain aesthetic, historical and philosophical views which were distinctly different from those accepted by most of their contemporaries.[2] Vesalius, therefore, can justly be called a humanist only if, in addition to his formal training in the classics, he also shared those general principles which underlay the humanist movement.

Now, no direct testimony survives that might decide whether or not Vesalius approved of the humanist dogma. Yet, in my opinion, one can conclude from his main work, the *De Fabrica*, what was his attitude toward humanism. Evidence to this effect is afforded even by the pecu-

* *Bulletin of the History of Medicine*, 1943, vol. 14, pp. 547–61.

[1] Cf. *A New English Dictionary*, ed. by J. A. H. Murray, V, 1, 1901, *s.v.* Humanist, 3. Literary Hist. For Vesalius' classical studies, cf. M. Roth, *Andreas Vesalius Bruxellensis*, 1892, esp. pp. 61 ff., and in general also Wm. H. Welch, The Times of Vesalius, *The Johns Hopkins Hospital Bulletin*, XXVI, 1915, pp. 118 ff.

[2] Concerning the new interpretation of the humanist movement, cf. especially K. Burdach, *Reformation, Renaissance, Humanismus*, 1926[2]; E. Cassirer, Individuum und Kosmos in der Philosophie der Renaissance, *Studien der Bibliothek Warburg*, X, 1927. Cf. also the note of P. O. Kristeller, The Place of Classical Humanism in Renaissance Thought, *Journal of the History of Ideas*, IV, 1943, pp. 59 ff.

liar language in which the book is written. When I say "peculiar language," naturally I do not mean the fact that the *De Fabrica* is composed in Latin. Hardly any scientist of the sixteenth century would have presented his findings in the vernacular. But Vesalius renounced the Latin that was spoken and written by scholars of his time; he purified the common stock of words; he abandoned the simple colloquial prose style, the logical sequence of thought characteristic of the scientific literature of that period. Instead, Vesalius reintroduced the terminology of a time long past; he adopted a stately and rhythmical style, a rhetorical word order, in short, he imitated the periodic Latin, the "artistic prose" of Cicero, and he was the first anatomist to do so.[3] That this innovation was motivated by any arbitrary preference or by mere whim I cannot believe. I rather think that Vesalius wrote like Cicero because he wanted to write like a humanist. A few years previous to the time in which the manuscript of the *De Fabrica* was prepared, a bitter fight had raged in the humanist camp. The issue was whether Cicero was the only true model of correct Latin, or whether it was permissible to write a Latinity of one's own which integrated the changes brought about by the varying tastes and needs of the centuries.[4] Scaliger, the great philologist, had been the leader of the archaists; Erasmus, the profound scholar, had been the spokesman of the neoterics. The outcome of the struggle was that Scaliger won, while Erasmus was defeated. Learning vanquished erudition; the Ciceronians, as they were called, gradually gained ascendancy. Henceforth, a humanist who set store by himself in style and vocabulary never deviated from Cicero. But scientists, for decades, continued to write the Latin that they thought fit.[5]

[3] This has been recognized by L. Olschki, *Geschichte der neusprachlichen wissenschaftlichen Literatur*, II, 1922, pp. 81 ff.; 98 ff. I differ with Olschki only in so far as I classify Vesalius' style not simply as "Kunstprosa," cf. *op. cit.*, p. 98, of which there are many kinds, but more definitely as Ciceronian "Kunstprosa," which it undoubtedly must be in Olschki's opinion, too; cf. his analysis, *op. cit.*, p. 99. Incidentally, Celsus, whose work *De Medicina*, for Vesalius as well as for other Renaissance authors, was the most important source of their new medical terminology (cf. C. Singer, *The Evolution of Anatomy*, 1925, pp. 104, 117), was the only ancient author to apply the rules of Ciceronian "Kunstprosa" to the composition of medical writings; cf. J. Ilberg, A. Cornelius Celsus und die Medizin in Rom, *Neue Jahrbücher für das Klassische Altertum*, X, 1907, p. 378; pp. 387 f. Cf. below, n. 6.

[4] For details of this debate, cf. E. Norden, *Die antike Kunstprosa vom VI. Jahrhundert v. Chr. bis in die Zeit der Renaissance*, II[4], 1923, pp. 773 ff.

[5] Concerning Erasmus and Scaliger as the protagonists in this fight, cf. J. Burckhardt, *Die Kultur der Renaissance in Italien*, ed. W. Goetz, 1925[16], p. 232; J. Huizinga, *Erasmus*, 1928, pp. 180 ff.; p. 183. Norden's remark, *op. cit.*, p. 778, that the discus-

Vesalius, then, by subscribing to the Ciceronian ideal clearly ranged himself with the humanists. In every sentence which he composed, in every word which he chose, he attested his dependence on their newly established aesthetic theory.[6]

The classical Latin style in which Vesalius ventured to formulate his findings made it rather difficult for the average physician of his day to understand the content of the *De Fabrica*. Many a contemporary reader must have wondered why Vesalius took this risk; he must have found it meaningless, if not ridiculous, that the great anatomist should have labored to veil his discoveries, the results of his empirical investigations, in the garb of so artificial a language.[7] But to a humanist, this

sion between Ciceronians and anti-Ciceronians lasted until the second third of the seventeenth century does not imply that for the majority of the humanists the issue had not been decided long before that time, cf. F. Skutsch, Die Lateinische Sprache, *Die Kultur der Gegenwart*, I, 8, 1905, p. 446. The anti-Ciceronian position taken by such men as Lipsius (cf. Norden, *op. cit.*, p. 775) was exceptional. For the style of later anatomists, cf. Olschki, *op. cit.*, II, p. 101. Vesalius' humanist tendencies taken into account, it does not seem fortuitous that he twice attacks Erasmus because of his having used a faulty Latin term, *De Fabrica*, I, 31, p. 140, l. 19; I, 23, p. 107, l. 18; Roth, *op. cit.*, p. 149; Vesalius rarely quotes writers of his time, especially non-medical authors; cf. L. Thorndike, *A History of Magic and Experimental Science*, V, 1941, pp. 523 ff. Another echo of Vesalius' stand regarding the question of proper Latinity I find in Scaliger's high praise of Vesalius, cf. *Prima Scaligerana*, 1670, p. 99; Roth, *op. cit.*, p. 301, n. 8.

[6] Olschki, the first to see the problem presented by Vesalius' Latin, suggests, *op. cit.*, p. 99, that the style of the *De Fabrica* was developed from that of Vesalius' lectures. But even if this were so, the question would still remain why Vesalius spoke and wrote Ciceronian Latin. Vesalius' achievement in introducing a new scientific language, for which he had a model in Celsus' work alone, cf. above, n. 4, is great indeed. When he speaks of his own style as *ieiuna et parum exercitata*, *De Fabrica*, praefatio, p. 4v, ll. 9–10, cf. also Roth, *op. cit.*, p. 180, n. 2, one can interpret this statement only as an expression of modesty in a young author (cf. *ibid.*, p. 4r, l. 43: *iuvenile hoc meum studium*), whether it be genuine or demanded by literary cant. It should be noted that even in his early writings Vesalius showed a keen interest in stylistic matters. In his edition of Rhazes, which appeared in 1537, he condemned the Arabic style as coarse and showed a fine appreciation of the classical style, its beauty, harmony, elegance and conciseness; the *Letter on Bloodletting*, 1539, is a masterpiece, embodying all those qualities which Vesalius admired in the ancients; the same seems true of the *Letter on the China Root*, 1546; cf. Roth, *op. cit.*, pp. 76, 98 f., 216, who also notes the changes in grammar and punctuation which Vesalius made in the second edition of the *De Fabrica*, *op. cit.*, p. 232. [When this was already in proof there appeared H. Cushing, *A Bio-Bibliography of Andreas Vesalius*, 1943, which contains an English rendering of the prefatory letter to Vesalius' translation of Rhazes (pp. 4 ff.) and of the Postscript (pp. 6 f.) outlining his stylistic views referred to in this note.]

[7] Olschki, *op. cit.*, p. 99, is right, I think, in maintaining that it was on account of the complicated Latin of the *De Fabrica* that a German translation, "dem ge-

procedure was a necessity. He believed that by recovering true and correct speech the road was opened to the recovery of true and correct knowledge. If Cicero set the standard of accurate Latin, it was necessary for the humanist to acquire the faculty of expressing himself in Cicero's language. In that famous manifesto of humanism, the preface to his book on the elegance of Latin, Valla gave voice to the conviction that inspired all humanists as regards their task and privilege: "Unhappy were the earlier centuries in which no erudite man was ever found; the more are we to be congratulated, for among us, if we exert our strength a little farther, then I trust the Roman language will soon flower even more than the city of Rome and together with the language all disciplines will be restored."[8] Under this supposition, it was only by writing Latin as he did that Vesalius was able properly to pursue science, to approach the aim which he had set for himself—the resurrection of anatomy.

For there can be no doubt: however revolutionary Vesalius' achievement may seem to the modern historian, for him it was only the revival of the work of ancient anatomists. Anatomy, he says, "should be recalled from the dead, so that if it did not achieve with us a greater perfection than at any other place or time among the old teachers of anatomy, it might at least reach such a point that one could with confidence assert that our modern science of anatomy was equal to that of old, and that in this age anatomy was unique both in the level to which it had sunk and in the completeness of its subsequent restoration."[9] And he rejoices because "there is ground for hope that anatomy will ere long be

meinen Mann zu gut," was published in the same year in which the *De Fabrica* appeared; for the translation itself, cf. Roth, *op. cit.*, pp. 134 f.

[8] Cf. L. Valla, *Elegantiae Linguae Latinae*, 1480 (Rome), praefatio: "Superiora tempora infelicia fuere quibus homo nemo inventus est eruditus: eo plus his nostris gratulandum est: in quibus si paulo amplius annitamur confido propediem linguam Romanam vere plus quam urbem et cum ea disciplinas omnes iri restitutum"; for the significance of the document, cf. J. Huizinga, Das Problem der Renaissance, *Wege der Kulturgeschichte*, 1930, p. 92. Valla, perhaps not yet a fullfledged Ciceronian, though a follower of Quintilian, the apostle of Cicero, cf. G. Voigt, *Die Wiederbelebung des classischen Altertums*, I³, 1893, pp. 463–64, believes that the Latin language was corrupted by the Goths, cf. *Elegantiae*, III, praefatio, and Norden, *op. cit.*, p. 770, n. 1. For Vesalius' agreement with such an explanation of the decay of ancient grandeur, cf. below, p. 448. The interrelationship between the restoration of language and the rise of science is nicely illustrated in Rabelais' *Gargantua*, II, 8, a passage to which my attention was drawn by Prof. L. Spitzer.

[9] Cf. *De Fabrica*, praefatio, p. 3r, ll. 22 ff.: ". . . hoc naturalis philosophiae membrum ita ab inferis revocandum putavi, ut si non absolutius apud nos, quam alias

cultivated in all our academies as it was of old in Alexandria."[10] Restoration of the dead past to a new life; Padua, the universities, a new Alexandria—this is the typical humanist concept of the rebirth of learning. The humanists were not "Mirnachs" like Paracelsus or Telesio or Cardano, they did not constantly shout "I say," "I have discovered for the first time." Their slogan was: "The truth was long since found, and has united noble spirits, do but grasp the ancient truth."[11] Once the Greeks had been in possession of the truth; now truth and perfection were reborn, they came to light again. This is the way in which the humanists, starting with Villani, viewed the contemporary development of art and literature. Michelangelo, for whom all Italy had become a new Greece, maintained in regard to modern artistic endeavor: "Our art is that of ancient Greece." Shortly before Vesalius, Vives methodically applied the concept of renaissance to the study of science as well.[12] Nor was Vesalius merely theorizing when he extended the same category to include anatomy. He knew from Cicero and from Celsus that the

---

unquam apud priscos dissectionum professores versaretur, eo tamen pertingeret, ut aliquando haud puderet asserere, hanc dissectionis rationem cum antiqua illa conferri posse: nostraque hac tempestate nihil simul ita collapsum, moxque integritati restitutum, ac Anatomen fuisse." (The translation of quotations from Vesalius' preface, given here and in the following, is that of B. Farrington, The Preface of Andreas Vesalius to the De Fabrica Corporis Humani 1543, *Proceedings of the Royal Society of Medicine*, XXV, 1932, pp. 1357 ff.).

[10] Cf. *De Fabrica*, praefatio, p. 3v, ll. 30 ff.: ". . . ut spes sit, hanc brevi in omnibus Academiis ita excolendam, quemadmodum . . . in Alexandria olim exerceri consuevit." To the importance which the concept of renaissance has for Vesalius—cf. e.g., praefatio, p. 3r, l. 30: ". . . medicinam prospere renasci vidimus . . ."—attention has been drawn by M. H. Fisch, Vesalius and his book, *Bulletin of the Medical Library Association*, XXXI, 1943, pp. 214 ff. But cf. below, n. 13.

[11] Cf. Goethe, *Vermächtnis*, ll. 7–9: "Das Wahre war schon längst gefunden, / Hat edle Geisterschaft verbunden, / Das alte Wahre fass es an!" / For the egotistic component in the philosophy of nature as evolved by Paracelsus and the others referred to here, cf. E. Cassirer, Die Antike und die Entstehung der exakten Wissenschaft, *Die Antike*, VIII, 1932, pp. 287 ff. Cassirer, in a recent article, Giovanni Pico della Mirandola, *Journal of the History of Ideas*, III, 1942, p. 124, has also quoted the lines from Goethe as an appropriate motto for Pico's philosophy. It seems to me that they may well be taken as characteristic of humanism in general.

[12] Cf. in general W. K. Ferguson, Humanist Views of the Renaissance, *The American Historical Review*, XLV, 1939, pp. 1 ff.; and for Villani in particular, *ibid.*, pp. 19 f. For Michelangelo, cf. H. Grimm, *Leben Michelangelo's*, II[5], 1879, p. 306; his statement has been transmitted by F. de Hollanda, Vier Gespräche über die Malerei, Geführt zu Rom 1538, verfasst 1548. *Quellenschriften für Kunstgeschichte*, Neue Folge, IX, 1899. For the influence of humanist philosophy on Michelangelo, cf. Cassirer, *Individuum und Kosmos*, p. 143. Concerning Vives' *De Disciplinis* [1532] the first section of which (*De corruptis artibus*) deals with the history of scientific

ancients had dissected human bodies; he learned from Galen that Alexandria had been the center of ancient anatomical research. Modern anatomy was indeed the resurrection of ancient anatomy.[13]

But why did the knowledge that men had possessed of old deteriorate at all, and when did the decline begin? Vesalius dwells on these questions at some length. He opens his book with a survey of the history of medicine, or rather with an evaluation of those factors which are apt to retard progress in other sciences as well as in medicine. Isolation of the various branches of learning he considers disastrous; specialization, to him, means the impairment of knowledge; if theory and practice are divorced, nothing worthwhile can be accomplished. Such a thesis certainly was not new. Cicero, Celsus, Galen had been preaching in the same vein.[14] Nor was it in any way a novelty that Vesalius attributed the decay of medicine and of anatomy in particular to the fact that physicians had ceased to perform dissections and had given up the practice of surgery. Galen, in almost the same words, had accused his con-

endeavor, cf. W. Rehm, Der Untergang Roms im abendländischen Denken, *Das Erbe der Alten*, XVIII, 1930, p. 68. Vives' importance for the development of Renaissance thought has been outlined by W. Dilthey, Weltanschauung und Analyse des Menschen seit Renaissance und Reformation, *Gesammelte Schriften*, II, 1923, pp. 423 ff.

[13] Cf. Cicero, *Academica*, II, 122; Celsus, praefatio, 23 ff. [Marx], and for Alexandria as the center of ancient anatomical studies, e.g., Galen, *Opera*, ed. G. Kühn, II, 1821, p. 220. Vesalius in four passages enumerates the names of the great Hellenistic anatomists in accordance with Galen's testimony, cf. Roth, *op. cit.*, p. 148, n. 5. Even Vesalius' interest in vivisection (cf. *De Fabrica* VII, chap. 19, Roth, *op. cit.*, p. 152)—the illustrations of the book, too, aim at representing the anatomy of the living body, cf. e.g., C. Singer, *From Magic to Science*, 1928, p. 108—has a parallel in the insistence of the Greek Dogmatists that vivisection is superior to dissection practiced on the dead body, cf. Celsus, praefatio, 23 ff. [Marx]. Modern scholars have sometimes doubted that the ancient testimonies concerning dissections are reliable. I do not see any reason for doing so, cf. L. Edelstein, The Development of Greek Anatomy, *Bulletin of the Institute of the History of Medicine*, III, 1935, pp. 235 ff. At any rate, in Vesalius' sources dissections of the human body were attested, and he was therefore justified in believing that his undertaking was nothing but the revival of the work of the ancients. That is why I cannot agree with Fisch, *op. cit.*, pp. 214–215, who says: ". . . he (*sc.* Vesalius) imagined for himself a pre-Galenic anatomy based on dissection of the human body . . . Thus it was still possible for Vesalius to preserve his reverence for antiquity and to regard his reformation of anatomy as a renaissance."

[14] Cf. Cicero, *De oratore*, III, 132; Celsus, praefatio, 47 [Marx], and Ilberg, *op. cit.*, p. 389; Galen, VI, p. 368 K., XIII, p. 604 K., and for the interpretation of these passages, cf. J. Ilberg, Aus Galens Praxis, *Neue Jahrbücher f. das Klassische Altertum*, XV, 1905, pp. 311 f.; 284.

temporaries of endangering the pursuit of medicine. After Galen other physicians had used similar arguments.[15] The destructive tendencies to which Vesalius refers had long been operative in the history of science. But at a certain moment they were allowed free play and thus brought about ruin, "In bygone times," Vesalius asserts, "that is to say [in the West] after the Gothic deluge and [in the East] after the reign of Mansor at Bochara in Persia . . . medicine began to be sore distempered."[16] Does Vesalius propose this chronological fixation on the basis of his own investigations into history, or at least into the history of ancient and medieval medicine? From his medical studies he may have derived the notion that the Arabs up to the time of Mansor, that is up to the ninth century, remained in possession of true knowledge.[17] Yet his explanation of this fact immediately reveals the humanist bent of his thought. The Arabs, he contends, were able to stave off the downfall of medicine for such a long time because under Mansor they "still lived as was right on terms of familiarity with the Greeks."[18] In exactly this manner Ghiberti had traced the greatness of Cimabue's achievements to his painting in the *maniera Greca*, and from then on it became the watchword of the humanists that to do things perfectly meant to do them in the Greek fashion.[19] On the other hand, in dating the misfortunes of Western medicine from the invasion of Italy by the Goths, Vesalius merely adopted

[15] Cf. Galen, X, p. 455; XVIII A, p. 346; XIII, p. 604 K., and in general, Ilberg, *op. cit.*, pp. 283; 307. For more immediate precursors of Vesalius, cf. Roth, *op. cit.*, esp. pp. 9 ff.; 37 ff.

[16] Cf. *De Fabrica*, praefatio, p. 2r, ll. 18 ff.: ". . . quod aliquando, et praecipue post Gotthorum illuviem, Mansoremque Bocharae in Persia regem . . . medicina eousque lacerari cepit . . . ," cf. also, *ibid.*, l. 41: "maxime post Gotthorum vastationem."

[17] That the Mansor referred to by Vesalius is the king whom Rhazes treated I have learned from O. Temkin. Vesalius edited Rhazes' *ad Almansorem* shortly before the publication of the *De Fabrica*, cf. above, n. 6.

[18] Cf. *De Fabrica*, praefatio, p. 2r, l. 19: ". . . sub quo Arabes nobis adhuc cum Graecis merito familiares vigebant . . ."

[19] For Ghiberti, cf. Rehm, *op. cit.*, p. 68. There is a curious parallel between Vesalius' high estimation of the time of Mansor and Biondo's praise of the time of Charlemagne when, he thinks, a revival of the arts took place, cf. Ferguson, *op. cit.*, p. 13; for Biondo, cf. also following note. The humanists in general, of course, paid little attention to the development of culture among the Arabs. But such men as Pico della Mirandola, whose influence on Vesalius seems certain, cf. below, p. 452, gave heed to the Arabs, cf. Burckhardt, *op. cit.*, pp. 184 f., who also stresses the specific concern of the physicians with Arabic studies. With Pico, Vesalius also shared an interest in Hebrew knowledge, cf. Singer, *Evolution of Anatomy*, p. 117; Cassirer, *Journal of the History of Ideas*, 1942, p. 125.

the chronology which the Florentine humanist Biondo had introduced into historical writing. Biondo explained the decline of ancient culture not through political changes such as the fall of the Republic and the rise of the Imperial regime, but rather through one historical event and its fateful consequences for mankind—the sack of Rome by the Goths.[20] In the time of Vesalius this opinion came to be generally accepted by the humanists. Based upon the division of history into Antiquity, Middle Ages and a New Age, it formed an integral part of the humanist teaching, while outside that orbit students kept on writing world history according to the periods marked off by the succession of the Four World Monarchies.[21] No doubt, the views of Biondo reflect what nowadays is often called the humanist bias against the Middle Ages as the time of darkness, and on these grounds one might aver that Vesalius only re-

[20] Cf. Rehm, *op. cit.*, pp. 50 ff., and in general E. Fueter, *Geschichte der neueren Historiographie*, 1911, pp. 106 ff. Some of Biondo's views have now been traced to Petrarch, cf. T. E. Mommsen, Petrarch's Conception of "The Dark Ages," *Speculum*, XVII, 1942, p. 239. For the dependence of the humanists on Biondo's work, cf. Fueter, *op. cit.*, p. 109.

[21] Cf. Fueter, *op. cit.*, pp. 182 ff. This fact is important because it proves that Vesalius consciously chose the side of the Italian humanists and rejected other theories still in vogue in his time. Incidentally, before Vesalius, Vives, in his description of the breakdown of ancient science, had made use of the humanist periodization of history, cf. Rehm, *op. cit.*, p. 68, and above, n. 12. The interpretation of Vesalius' views given here is at variance with that of B. Farrington, Vesalius on the Ruin of Ancient Medicine, *The Modern Quarterly*, I, 1938, pp. 23 ff. According to him, Vesalius blames the decay of anatomy on "the aristocratic prejudice against manual labour," on "the prejudices of a slave-owning aristocracy" (*op. cit.*, pp. 25, 27). True, Vesalius considers it detrimental that medicine once was divided between physicians and slaves in such a way that the latter performed all manual tasks (*De Fabrica*, praefatio, p. 2r, l. 44). But this was not the necessary consequence of ancient slave economy—for centuries physicians had practiced surgery and performed dissections—it was the concomitant result of the invasion of Italy by the Goths, "when all the sciences, which before had flourished gloriously and were practised as was fitting, went to ruin" (praefatio, p. 2r, l. 42). Vesalius' words, then, have "social significance" (Farrington, *op. cit.*, p. 23), but "the cause" (*ibid.*, p. 25) of the ruin of ancient anatomy does not lie in social factors. Moreover, the humanist Vesalius naturally compared the attitude toward medicine arising after the sack of Rome to that of the ancient Romans. Tradition had it that they fought wars and tilled the soil but left all handicrafts to slaves and foreigners (cf. Dionysius of Halicarnassus, *Antiquitates Romanae*, II, 28, 1-2). Only in those centuries in which the Romans, just as the Arabs (cf. above, n. 18), "lived on terms of familiarity with the Greeks," was the condemnation of arts abandoned. Again, the final decay of medicine started in Italy and extended only gradually to the other parts of the world (praefatio, p. 2r, ll. 43 ff.), because the devastation of Rome and the destruction of ancient culture first made itself felt in Italy. In all these instances, it seems to me, Vesalius reasons as a thorough humanist, not as a social thinker or a historian in his own right as Farrington contends.

peats the prejudices held by his friends.[22] But one should not forget that
the humanist periodization of history had been a liberating deed. The
condemnation of the centuries immediately preceding their own implied
high hopes for human progress and human happiness in the "Golden
Age" in which men were now living. Vesalius, too, speaks of his time as
a "felicitous age," and the optimistic view of the present and even of the
future which pervades his utterances is, I think, to some extent the
result of his humanist philosophy of history.[23]

The fulfillment of Vesalius' dreams necessitated courageous opposition to the traditional authorities, above all to the predominance of
Galen. Vesalius was well aware of this fact, and even those who were
wont to defend Galen, he jubilates, "drawn by the love of truth, gradually abandon that attitude and, growing less emphatic, begin to put
faith in their own not ineffectual sight and powers of reason rather than
in the writings of Galen. These true paradoxes, won not by slavish reliance on the efforts of others, nor supported merely by masses of authorities, they eagerly communicate . . . to their friends."[24] In his endeavor
to restore anatomy to its old glory, Vesalius, then, relied on original
research, on observation and investigation. He did not take refuge in
books, he intended to read nothing but "the book of the human body
that cannot lie."[25] To be sure no writings were preserved which he could
follow. The works of the ancient anatomists who had dissected human

[22] Thus Thorndike, *op. cit.*, p. 523, says: ". . . shouldering the blame [for them]
upon the preceding mediaeval period, concerning which he seems to have had more
humanistic prejudice than accurate knowledge."

[23] Cf. *De Fabrica*, praefatio, p. 3r, ll. 15–16: huius seculi . . . foelicitate, and for
the concept of the "Golden Age" in Renaissance humanism, Burdach, *op. cit.*, pp.
105 f. It is true, the humanists often were "Kulturpessimisten," that is, they expected a new decay to follow their own achievements (cf. in general, Rehm, *op cit.*,
pp. 68 ff., and Michelangelo's gloomy prediction in his conversation with Francesco
de Hollanda, *op. cit.*, p. 307). But apart from the fact that their fears concerned not
their own generation but those to come, they were based on a theory which explained
the past by the inevitable cycle from democracy to tyranny; in other words they
presupposed Villani's concept of history, not that of Biondo, which was shared by
Vesalius, cf. above, p. 448. Still, catastrophes like the sack of Rome must not necessarily recur and culture, therefore, may not be drawn into another cataclysm.

[24] Cf. *De Fabrica*, praefatio, p. 3v, ll. 26 ff.: ". . . hi veritatis amore ducti, paula-
tim inde mitescant, suisque oculis ac rationibus non inefficacibus plus fidei, quam
Galeni scriptis adhibeant, haec vere paradoxa non ab aliis autoribus emendicata,
neque autoritatum congerie tantum firmata, . . . ad amicos sedulo perscribentes . . ."

[25] Cf. *De Fabrica*, p. 600, l. 42: ". . . paradoxa ex hominis haud mendaci libro
deprompta . . ."; cf. Roth, *op. cit.*, p. 117, n. 5. The expression "book of nature" appears before Vesalius, cf. Roth, p. 68, n. 5; 125, n. 3. But the term "book of the
human body" seems original with him.

cadavers were lost; as Vesalius maintains, they were destroyed by envious people who grudged later generations the enjoyment of the truth.[26] Yet it is not a subterfuge which the humanist Vesalius is using when he recommends the study of nature. On the contrary, it is precisely by asking men to employ their own faculties that Vesalius proves himself to be a true humanist. Not because Cimabue had imitated Greek paintings did Ghiberti call him the reviver of art, the painter who had restored the *maniera Greca*—no Greek pictures existed which Cimabue could have copied. Nor did Michelangelo say of Italian art that it equaled the artistic skill of the Greeks because he and his contemporaries imitated the statues excavated in the gardens of the Vatican.[27] Ghiberti, the theorist, and Michelangelo, the creative genius, founded their judgment on the fact that Cimabue and all the other Italian artists had studied and followed Nature, who had also been the teacher of the Greeks, that like the Greeks they had trusted "their own not ineffectual sight and powers of reasoning." Humanism was a call to self-reliance.[28] The rôle of the Greeks was only that of giving encouragement through their example. If such support is needed by everybody who dares to be independent, it was especially longed for by that generation which, after centuries of bondage, for the first time ventured to shake off the yoke of authority. Thus Copernicus in the same year in which Vesalius published the *De Fabrica* confessed in his book *De Revolutionibus* that, dissatisfied with the system of Ptolemy, he eagerly read the ancient authors to see whether any of them had proposed other theories. When he found mention of the Pythagorean doctrine, according to which the earth was moving whereas the sun was at rest, he began to ponder over such a possibility because "to others before him had been given the same liberty."[29] The reversal of anatomical studies no less than the reversal of astronomical research was instigated by scientists who in the emulation of others found their own freedom.

But humanism did not only rid men of the dust of books, it did not

[26] Cf. *De Fabrica*, praefatio, p. 3r, ll. 51 ff.

[27] For Ghiberti, cf. above, n. 19; for Michelangelo, cf. also A. Hekler, Michelangelo und die Antike, *Wiener Jahrbuch für Kunstgeschichte*, VII, 1930, pp. 201 f.

[28] Burdach, *op. cit.*, pp. 164 f., has pointed out most clearly that humanism does not mean imitation but study of the objects themselves.

[29] Cf. Copernicus, *De Revolutionibus*, praefatio (Thorn, 1873), p. 6, ll. 16–17: ". . . quia sciebam aliis ante me hanc concessam libertatem . . ." Note that the works of the mathematicians with whose theories Copernicus concerned himself were lost, as were the books of the ancient anatomists whom Vesalius admired.

only open their eyes to the world, it also made them see man and the world as nobody before had ever done. How strongly Vesalius was influenced by this new attitude seems evidenced by the novel meaning which he gave to anatomical studies. Of course, in his opinion, too, anatomical findings are principally of concern to the physician. Medicine without anatomy cannot flourish. The physician who does not know the structure of the human body cannot succeed in healing diseases, as the ancient Dogmatists had already claimed.[30] Besides, anatomy is important for the philosopher and the theologian. Vesalius is conscious of the fact that in antiquity philosophers had investigated cadavers, and he notes the attention paid to his science by philosophers and divines of his time.[31] But it is not only for the physician and the philosopher and the doctor of theology that he intends to write. Addressing Charles V in the preface of the *De Fabrica*, he takes it for granted that the Emperor will find delight in the anatomical book that is dedicated to him. Charles had always been fond of mathematics and especially of astronomy. So great was his interest "that it can hardly be but that as you are attracted in an unique degree by the science of the universe, so also you should at times delight in considering the most perfectly constructed among all created things, and should take pleasure in considering what is the temporary dwelling-place and instrument of the immortal soul. For this in many particulars exhibits a marvellous correspondence with the universe, and for that reason was by them of old not inappropriately styled 'a little universe.' "[32] Yet Vesalius goes farther. "I am of opinion," he says, "that out of the whole Apolline discipline, and indeed out of the whole philosophy of nature, nothing could be fashioned more pleasing or more acceptable to Your Majesty than an account from which we

[30] Compare *De Fabrica*, praefatio, p. 2v, ll. 46 ff., with Celsus, praefatio, 23 [Marx].

[31] Cf. *De Fabrica*, praefatio, p. 4v, l. 6. For the interest of ancient philosophers in anatomy, cf. L. Edelstein, Die Geschichte der Sektion in der Antike, *Quellen u. Studien z. Geschichte d. Naturwissenschaften u. d. Medizin*, III, 1932, pp. 67 ff. [264* ff.]. Thorndike, *op. cit.*, p. 526, understands Vesalius' remark about the theologians, *De Fabrica*, p. 531, ll. 22–23, as an "unkind cut." But the problem of generation was a main topic of Aristotle's and Galen's biological studies and a legitimate subject of theological speculation. Even Dante, *Purgatorio*, XXV, 37 ff., does not refrain from such discussions, cf. Olschki, *op. cit.*, p. 100, n. 2.

[32] Cf. *De Fabrica*, praefatio, p. 4v, ll. 1 ff.: ". . . quin ut mundi scientia unice teneris, ita etiam aliquando omnium creaturarum absolutissimae fabricatione expendenda delecteris, et immortalis animae diversorio ac instrumento considerando voluptatem capias: quod domicilium, quia permultis nominibus mundo egregie correspondet, veteribus haud ab re microcosmus nuncupabatur."

451

learn of the body and of the mind and furthermore of a certain divine
power consisting of the harmony of both, in sum, of ourselves, whom to
know is man's proper study."[33] And though Vesalius has decided that
this is not the place for glorifying a knowledge of the structure of the
human body he cannot refrain from adding that it is "the knowledge
most worthy of man and in itself by far the most commendable for
him."[34] Not astronomy, not the world, but man, the worthiest object of
human inquiry, the proper concern of every human being—hardly
anyone but a humanist of the Renaissance could have made this assertion; it seems understandable only within the framework of humanist
philosophy and its concept of the dignity of man.[35]

True, just as the ancients and as men of the Middle Ages, so the
humanists, and with them Vesalius, call man a microcosm. Pico della
Mirandola himself says: "It is a commonplace of the schools that man
is a little world in which we may discern a body mingled of earthly elements, and ethereal breath, and the vegetable life of plants, and the
senses of the lower animals, and reason and the intelligence of the angels,
and a likeness of God."[36] But for Pico and the humanists, the idea of
man as a microcosm acquires a more exalted meaning. Man is no longer
a link in a chain that stretches from heaven to earth. God and angels no
longer rank above him, nor are animals and plants beneath him—he is
apart from everything. For man is not to be compared with other beings,

[33] Cf. *De Fabrica*, praefatio, p. 4r, ll. 47 ff.: ". . . augurer, ex universa Apollinea
disciplina, adeoque tota naturali philosophia, nihil tuae Maiestati gratius acceptius
ve procudi posse, historia, qua corpus et animum, ac praeterea divinum quoddam
numen ex utriusque symphonia, et nosmetipsos denique (quod vere hominis est)
cognoscimus."

[34] Cf. *De Fabrica*, praefatio, p. 4v, ll. 4–5: ". . . uti modo homini dignissimam sui
corporis structurae cognitionem, per se longe commendatissimam, . . ." Farrington
translates this passage as follows: "worthy as it is of the attention of man, and in
itself to be commended above all others." But such a rendering, it seems to me, does
not do full justice to the peculiar flavor of the words.

[35] At least as far as I am aware, the motivations for a study of the human body
as given in antiquity and in the Middle Ages are different. They are derived from
scientific or philosophical considerations, cf. above, n. 30 and 31, or from a natural
interest of man in his body, cf. L. Edelstein, *op. cit.*, pp. 65 ff. [261* ff.], or from a
certain standard of education similar to that set up even by Melanchthon who says:
Turpe est homini prorsus ignorare sui corporis (ut ita dicam) aedificium; *De anima*,
Basil. 1543, p. 423; Roth, *op. cit.*, p. 244, n. 4.

[36] Cf. Pico della Mirandola, *De dignitate hominis:* "Tritum est in scholis esse
hominem minorem mundum, in quo mixtum ex elementis corpus et spiritus coelestis
et plantarum anima vegetalis et brutorum sensus et ratio et angelica mens et Dei
similitudo conspicitur." I quote from W. Pater, *The Renaissance*, 1910, p. 40 (Pico

he is his own free creator and conqueror, he alone is endowed with development, with growing according to his own free will, he has in himself the seeds of an omnific life, and this pre-eminence constitutes his unique dignity.[37] Consequent to such a belief, the representation of man became the supreme task of Renaissance art. Sculptors and painters vied in forming the likeness of the new Prometheus, because he was the subject most deserving of their skill. Philosophers and scientists wrote about the dignity of man, and even in the structure of his body they discovered not so much the providence of God, but rather the excellence of the human being.[38] In the same vein Vesalius declared the study of the human body to be the proper task of man, the worthiest study of all that can be pursued by him. This saying aphoristically summarizes the humanist philosophy. It is symbolic of the pride of that generation, of its belief in the "empire of man," who finds his destiny in himself, not in God.[39]

---

della Mirandola). The translation given in the text is also that of Pater. For Vesalius cf. *De Fabrica*, praefatio, p. 4v, l. 4: microcosmus; p. 636, ll. 29–30: ". . . quod nobis rationalem animam, quam cum angelis (ut Plato etiam male tractatorum philosophorum haud immememor innuebat) communem habemus, largitus fuerit (*sc.* Deus rerum omnium opifex)." Roth, *op. cit.*, p. 179, and Olschki, *op. cit.*, p. 98, n. 1, on account of the latter statement, consider Vesalius a Platonist. But this he is only in so far as Platonism is integrated into Pico's philosophy and Renaissance thought in general.

[37] Cf. Pico, *op. cit.* The importance of the passage referred to here for the Renaissance concept of man was first recognized by Burckhardt, *op. cit.*, pp. 330 f. The philosophical implications of Pico's oration have been discussed in more detail by Cassirer, *Individuum und Kosmos*, pp. 88 f.; cf. also Burdach, *op. cit.*, pp. 168 f.

[38] Concerning Renaissance art and the ideal of the new Prometheus, cf. Burdach, *op. cit.*, pp. 166 f. For reflections of the humanist evaluation of man's position in scientific inquiry, cf. such books as that of Magnus Hundt, *Antropologium de hominis dignitate natura et proprietatibus de elementis, partibus et membris humani corporis*, 1501, and G. Manetti, *De dignitate et excellentia hominis*, written in 1452 and published in 1532; the significance of the latter book in the development of Renaissance thought has been pointed out by G. Gentile, *Giordano Bruno e il pensiero del Rinascimento*, 1920, pp. 154 ff. The second book of Manetti's treatise deals with the fabric of the human body, cf. Gentile, *op. cit.*, p. 166; for Manetti, cf. also Cassirer, *Individuum und Kosmos*, p. 88.

[39] I am not sufficiently familiar with Renaissance literature to say with assurance that no such phrase as that used by Vesalius may be found in books written before the *De Fabrica*. At any rate, Vesalius' statement ought to be considered another modification of that feeling which was first expressed in Socrates' ἀνθρώπινα λέγειν, cf. Xenophon, *Memorabilia*, I, 1, 11 ff., and became immortalized in Pope's lines: "Know then thyself, presume not God to scan, / The proper study of mankind is man," An Essay on Man, *Epist.*, II, 1–2. The commentaries on Pope, cf. *The Works of A. Pope*, ed. by J. W. Croker and W. Elwin, II, 1871, *ad loc.*, and the

I trust I do not overstate my case when I maintain that Vesalius was not only a classical scholar, that he did not only wear the robe of the humanist, but that he also professed the main articles of the humanist faith. The *De Fabrica*, whatever it may be in other respects, is also a living testimony to the fact that the scientist Vesalius had joined the fellowship of the humanists.

thesauri, cf., e.g., *A Dictionary of Quotations from Authors Old and New*, Everyman's Library, I, p. 187, give as "sources" only Charron, *De la sagesse*, 1601, I. chap. 1: la vraye science et le vray étude de l'homme c'est l'homme, and Pascal: . . . l'étude de l'homme, et que c'est la vraie étude qui lui est propre, *Pensées*, ed. by L. Brunschvicg, II, 1904, p. 71, section II, 144. To the Socratic resignation shared by Pope; to Pascal's humility in rejecting science in favor of a search into the human heart; to the passion of truth by which Charron is inspired; Vesalius' formula adds the Renaissance ethos of confidence in man's value and the scientist's admiration for the perceptible matter in which the human spirit dwells.

SYDENHAM AND CERVANTES*

Blackmore, a physician and poet of great renown in the times of Queen Anne and George I, but soon afterward forgotten or belittled, in one of his treatises poses the question whether experience or learning is more important for the acquisition of medical knowledge.[1] His answer is that if one must choose between the two, experience is by far to be preferred. "For it is very evident," says Blackmore, "that a Man of good Sense, Vivacity, and Spirit, may arrive to the highest Rank of Physicians, without the Assistance of great Erudition and the Knowledge of Books: And this was the Case of Dr. Sydenham abovementioned, who became an able and eminent Physician, though he never designed to take up the Profession till the civil Wars were composed, and then being a disbanded Officer, he entred upon it for a Maintenance, without any Learning properly preparatory for the Undertaking of it." But while experience thus is superior to learning, it is the possession of both these "armours" which in Blackmore's opinion makes the perfect physician. Sydenham, however, Blackmore holds, took the opposite stand; he despised learning. In proof of this thesis Blackmore continues: "And to shew the Reader what Contempt he had for Writings in Physick, when one Day I asked him to advise me what Books I should read to qualify me for Practice, he replied, Read *Don Quixot*, it is a very good Book, I read it still. So low an Opinion had this celebrated Man of the Learning collected out of the Authors, his Predecessors."

Sydenham's bon mot on Cervantes has become very famous, and it has usually been understood in the same way in which it was interpreted by Blackmore. Though few go as far as he did and claim that Sydenham vilified learning of which he was no master "and perhaps for that reason,"[2] most people conclude from Sydenham's remark that he was opposed to book learning, his maxim being: "Read what you like; reading books will never make a doctor"; or that he was contemptuous

* *Supplement to the Bulletin of the History of Medicine*, no. 3, Baltimore: The Johns Hopkins Press, 1944, pp. 55–61.
[1] Cf. Sir Richard Blackmore, *A Treatise upon the Small Pox*, 1723, pp. xi–xii.
[2] Cf. Blackmore, *ibid.*, p. xii.

455

at least of contemporary learning.[3] Yet long ago Samuel Johnson commented on Sydenham's saying: "Whatsoever was his meaning . . . it is
certain that Sydenham did not think it impossible to write usefully on
medicine, because he has himself written upon it; and it is not probable
that he carried his vanity so far, as to imagine no man had ever acquired
the same qualifications besides himself."[4] Moreover, Sydenham wor-
shiped Hippocrates, the Romulus of the physicians as he calls him. He
read and reread the writings of the "divine old man," from which he believed the main principles of his doctrines had been derived. He expressly acknowledged that the Hippocratic treatises and the works of
other authors, small as their number may be, contained not only the
seeds of truth but truth itself.[5] Nor can Sydenham have discounted the
value of contemporary erudition. He was closely attached to Locke; he
was a friend of Boyle. Both these men he praised highly in the dedica-
tions prefixed to his essays.[6] Sydenham then, although he gave first
place to the study of phenomena, was in fact not a detractor of learning,
nor was he an enemy of all scientific literature.

Johnson, realizing the improbability of Blackmore's interpretation
of Sydenham's cryptic reply, tentatively proposed that Blackmore was
misled by "that self-love which dazzles all mankind" from discovering
that Sydenham perhaps merely intended to say that Blackmore would
never become a good doctor, whatever he might read.[7] This explanation,
however, Johnson can give only *ex eventu*. Sydenham knew Blackmore
apparently as a student or as a young man who had just started on his
career. It would have required the gifts of a prophet to foresee at that
time the shortcomings of the future physician, of the "famous Modern,"
at whom Swift pokes fun in the *Battle of the Books*.[8] Again it has been
maintained that Sydenham simply intended to ridicule Blackmore, the

[3] For the former interpretation, cf. e.g., J. F. Payne, *Thomas Sydenham*, 1900,
p. 191; for the latter, cf. K. Faber, *Nosography*, second ed., 1930, p. 11.

[4] Lives of Sundry Eminent Persons [Sydenham], *The Works of Samuel Johnson*,
XII, 1810, p. 183.

[5] Cf. Thomas Sydenham, *Opera Omnia*, ed. G. A. Greenhill, 1844, pp. 13; 14;
307; and in general concerning Sydenham's relation to Hippocrates, cf. Payne, *op.
cit.*, pp. 222 ff.; O. Temkin, Die Krankheitsauffassung von Hippokrates und Sydenham in ihren Epidemien, *Archiv f. Geschichte der Medizin*, XX, 1928, pp. 327 ff.

[6] Cf. Sydenham, *op. cit.*, pp. 6; 7. Cf. also Payne, *op. cit.*, pp. 236 ff.

[7] Cf. Johnson, *op. cit.*, pp. 182–183.

[8] Cf. Payne, *op. cit.*, pp. 192 f. The question put to Sydenham by Blackmore
would be quite meaningless had he been already well established in his calling. For
Swift's mention of Blackmore, cf. *The Prose Works of Jonathan Swift*, ed. H. Davis,

"pedant and prig." Yet, the poetical works of Blackmore which made him the "butt of all the 'wits'" were published after Sydenham's death.[9] All attempts to find in Sydenham's statement an innuendo at Blackmore's character or achievements therefore are unconvincing.

Thus one feels almost driven to accept Johnson's final verdict and to regard Sydenham's recommendation of the *Don Quixote* as "a transient sally of an imagination warmed with gaiety, or the negligent effusion of a mind intent upon some other employment, and in haste to dismiss a troublesome intruder." And under this supposition one can hardly refrain from complaining, again with Johnson: "The perverseness of mankind makes it often mischievous in men of eminence to give way to merriment. The idle and the illiterate will long shelter themselves under this foolish apophthegm."[10] For indeed, inconsistent as it might be with his true opinion, does Sydenham not seem to encourage disdain for medical literature when he directs Blackmore to the reading of a novel rather than to the reading of scientific books? But before the historian and the critic dismiss Sydenham's remark as a dangerous jest, before those who are too lazy to study console themselves with what they call Sydenham's contempt for books and protest his example as an excuse for their weakness, they may find it worth their while at last to take Sydenham's words as they stand and not to impute to them any hidden meaning. After all, he did not advise against the reading of books or against any study. Asked by Blackmore what books he should read to perfect himself in practice, Sydenham referred him to a book, the *Don Quixote*. He affirmed that he liked this book, that he was still reading it in his mature years, and he counseled Blackmore to read this work if he aspired to become a good doctor. Apparently Sydenham considered the *Don Quixote* a piece of art worthy of the attention and praise of the physician. There must have been some reason for his delight in the novel of Cervantes. Besides, granted that he spoke in a jocular mood and somewhat out of tune when he recommended to Blackmore the *Don Quixote* instead of the treatises of Hippocrates, the question arises why he chose this work of fiction and not any other; what, in his opinion,

I, 1939, p. 158; for Blackmore's life and the rôle which he played in his time, cf. T. N. Toomey, Sir Richard Blackmore, M. D., *Annals of Medical History*, IV, 1922, pp. 180 ff.

[9] Cf. Payne, *op. cit.*, p. 192.

[10] Cf. Johnson, *op. cit.*, p. 182; the same, *Lives of the English Poets*, ed. G. B. Hill, II, 1905, p. 236 [Blackmore].

a physician could possibly learn from the adventures of the Knight of the Mancha. If one heeds Sydenham's injunction; if one peruses the *Don Quixote* and reflects, as a thoughtful reader ought to do, on the method employed by the author in writing his work and on the purpose to which he devotes it, then the true import of Sydenham's puzzling words will perhaps become apparent.

Cervantes, in the introduction to his immortal story, pretends that for some time he was hesitant about publishing it. Once, he says, he even arrived at the decision that his manuscript should never see the light of day; for it seemed to him to be lacking in scholarly trimmings. But then, he continues, a friend of his persuaded him to change his mind. He pointed out that long quotations from learned authors, the whole paraphernalia of erudition, were quite useless for this history of the valorous and witty knight-errant: "Onely it hath neede to helpe it selfe with imitation, for by how much the more it shall excell therein, by so much the more will the worke bee esteemed."[11] Cervantes, in other words, was intent on representing reality as it was, on imitating nature. Nor did Sydenham's contemporaries fail to notice the realistic background of Cervantes' work. Locke wrote: "Of all the books of fiction, I know none that equals 'Cervantes's History of Don Quixote,' in usefulness, pleasantry, and a constant decorum. And indeed no writings can be pleasant, which have not nature at the bottom, and are not drawn after her copy."[12] Now Sydenham, for whom the apprehension of the nature of diseases was the main task of medical inquiry, demanded that "in writing the history of a disease . . . the clear and natural phenomena of the disease should be noted—these, and these only. They should be noted accurately, and in all their minuteness; in imitation of the exquisite industry of those painters who represent in their portraits the smallest moles and the faintest spots."[13] Under these circumstances,

---

[11] Cf. *The History of Don Quixote of the Mancha, translated by Thomas Shelton,* ed. J. Fitzmaurice-Kelly, I, 1896, p. 10 [The Tudor Translations, XIII]. I am quoting Shelton's translation which Sydenham must have used—the second English translation of the *Don Quixote* made by J. Philips, 1687 (cf. J. Fitzmaurice-Kelly, *The Life of Miguel de Cervantes Saavedra,* 1892, p. 340) appeared only two years before Sydenham died—because I do not want to read into Cervantes' text a meaning which Sydenham would not have known.

[12] Cf. Some Thoughts concerning Reading and Study for a Gentleman, *The Works of John Locke,* III, tenth ed., 1801, p. 275.

[13] Cf. *The Works of Thomas Sydenham,* translated by R. G. Latham, I, 1848, p. 14 [The Sydenham Society]. Cf. also O. Temkin, Thomas Sydenham und der Naturbegriff des 17. Jahrhunderts, *Neuburger Festschrift,* 1928, pp. 1 ff.

is it astonishing that Sydenham should have called the *Don Quixote* a good book? What he himself tried to do in his writings, Cervantes, the poet, had accomplished in his work: he had portrayed nature without omitting the smallest detail. There was a natural affinity between the two authors, in their aims no less than in their methods and even in their language. Well may Sydenham have said of his treatises what Cervantes says of his tale: "Onely endeavour to deliver with significant, plaine, honest and welordred words thy . . . discourse, expressing as neere as thou maiest possibly thy intention, making thy conceites cleare, and not intricate or dark."[14]

If thus it is easy to discern why Sydenham was fond of the *Don Quixote*, it seems no less understandable that, given his point of view concerning medicine, he should never have ceased to read Cervantes' novel and should have admonished other physicians to read this book as a means of preparation for their own task. What Sydenham detested most in the study of diseases was the intrusion of theories. In the same moment in which he demands from the investigator that he cling to the simple and complete description, or rather copying of nature, he urges upon him: "In writing the history of a disease, every philosophical hypothesis whatsoever, that has previously occupied the mind of the author, should lie in abeyance. . . . No man can state the errors that have been occasioned by these physiological hypotheses. Writers, whose minds have taken a false colour under their influence, have saddled diseases with phenomena which existed in their own brains only; but which would have been clear and visible to the whole world had the assumed hypothesis been true. Add to this, that if by chance some symptom really coincide accurately with their hypothesis, and occur in the disease whereof they would describe the character, they magnify it beyond all measure and moderation; they make it all and in all; the molehill becomes a mountain; whilst, if it fail to tally with the said hypothesis, they pass it over either in perfect silence or with only an incidental mention, unless, by means of some philosophical subtlety, they can enlist it in their service, or else, by fair means or foul, accommodate it in some way or other to their doctrines."[15]

Now Don Quixote, as Cervantes says in the very beginning of his story, was in the habit of plunging himself deeply into the reading of books. "His fantasie was filled with those things that he read. . . . And

[14] Don Quixote, *op. cit.*, p. 11.
[15] Sydenham, *op. cit.*, p. 14.

these toyes did so firmely possesse his imagination with an infallible opinion, that all that Machina of dreamed inventions which he read was true, as he accounted no History in the world to be so certaine and sincere as they were." Consequently, when for the first time he ventured out into the world, "our Knight Errant esteemed all which he thought, saw, or imagined, was done or did really passe in the very same forme, as he had read the like in his bookes."[16] This is the reason why he fights with windmills. It is because for him "dreams are facts and facts are dreams,"[17] because for him everything takes on the color of his imagination, of the fancies of his brain, that he constantly mistakes reality. He overlooks all instances which speak against him, or fits them, as best he can, into his vagaries, just as do the believers in windy hypotheses against whom Sydenham inveighs. And pitifully he suffers shipwreck in his undertaking just as, in Sydenham's opinion, the adherents of physiological theories are bound to do when they attempt to understand nature.[18]

Only at the end of his life does Don Quixote realize what a fool he was. Nothing remains for him but to praise the mercy of God through whom he has at last, though much too late for this life, regained "a free and cleere judgement, and nothing overshadowed with the mysty clouds of ignorance, which the continuall reading and plodding on bookes of Chivalry had over-cast mee withall."[19] The reader of Cervantes' book is supposed to experience the same conversion, but while there is still time to charter a new course. Thus Cervantes' friend says in the introduction to the *Don Quixote:* "Let thy project be to overthrow the ill compiled Machina, and bulke of those Knightly Bookes, abhorred by many, but applauded by more. For if thou bring this to passe, thou hast not atchieved a small matter." Thus the poet reiterates in closing his account: "I never desired any other thing, then that men would utterly abhor the fabulous impertinent and extravagant bookes of Chivalries: And to say truth, by meanes of my true Don Quixote, they begin already

[16] Don Quixote, *op. cit.*, pp. 25; 31.

[17] J. Fitzmaurice-Kelly, *The Life of Cervantes*, p. 271.

[18] As far as I am aware, John D. Comrie, *Selected Works of Thomas Sydenham*, 1922, p. 2, is the only one who has in any way connected Sydenham's remark with the meaning of the Don Quixote. He says that the words in question indicate "at once his contempt for the medical literature of the time and the knowledge to be gained from Cervantes's romance as to the foibles of mankind." I do not believe that Sydenham was indulging in such generalities but rather that he thought of the physician and his specific task.

[19] Cf. Don Quixote, *op. cit.*, IV, p. 270.

to stagger; for, undoubtedly such fables and flim-flam tales will shortly faile, and I hope shall never rise againe."[20]

I suggest then that Sydenham read the *Don Quixote* as a kind of cathartic and preventive medicine for the physician and that he wanted others to read the book to the same end. Whether the masterpiece of Cervantes is but the biography of a madman who through bitter trial comes to his senses as one is led to believe by the poet's words; whether the *fabula docet* of the well-nigh fathomless story is different from what it purports to be or something more in addition, this is not the place to argue. It suffices that the book can be understood as Sydenham seems to have understood it and that it was generally understood in this way in Sydenham's time.[21] Locke expressed his astonishment that "after the pattern Dr. Sydenham has set them of a better way, men should return again to the romance way of physic." And he added: "I see it is easier and more natural for men to build castles in the air of their own than to survey well those that are to be found standing."[22] It is this human instinct for self-deception against which Sydenham warned Blackmore, an inclination particularly dangerous for the physician. Beware of your imagination, he wants to say; get rid of your fancies; let facts be facts; do not view nature in the light of your preconceived ideas; otherwise you will be all your life a Quixote, a "Knight of the Woeful Countenance."

[20] Cf. Don Quixote, *op. cit.*, I, p. 11; IV, p. 278.

[21] For the history of the interpretation of the Don Quixote, cf. e.g., W. J. Entwhistle, *Cervantes*, 1940, pp. 147 ff. For Cervantes in England, cf. G. Becker, Die Aufnahme des Don Quijote in die englische Literatur, *Palaestra*, XIII, 1906; R. Schevill, On the Influence of Spanish Literature upon English in the Early 17th Century, *Romanische Forschungen*, XX, 1907, pp. 604 ff.; also J. Fitzmaurice-Kelly, Cervantes in England, *Proceedings of the British Academy*, vol. II, 1905.

[22] Locke to Thomas Molyneux, 20. January, 1692–3; cf. H. R. Fox Bourne, *The Life of John Locke*, II, 1876, p. 243.

MEDICAL HISTORIOGRAPHY IN 1847*

A characterization of medical historiography of a hundred years ago is made difficult by the fact that little work has so far been done on the subject of historical writing in the nineteenth century. Only German historiography of the period between 1800 and 1846 has been carefully investigated.[1] The few observations which I shall venture to present are based on a chance acquaintance with the material rather than on a methodical study of the pertinent literature. I can but hope that I shall not draw too badly the broad outlines of the situation as it prevailed around the year 1847.[2]

Although my survey aims at a general picture of the work done in historiography by scholars everywhere, I shall take the various countries one by one. In the nineteenth century, the attitude toward historical studies was no longer uniform. National ideologies began to play a rôle in the interpretation of the past. Then, again, I shall have at times to touch upon questions that lie beyond the pale of historiography proper. By 1847 the task of the historian implied more, or less, than the actual writing of history. Finally, if those who discussed medicine in 1847 were forced occasionally to overstep their date line, I am afraid I shall have to make use of this license even more liberally. What history means at a particular moment often becomes clear only if viewed in the perspective of some decades before or after.

* Bulletin of the History of Medicine, 1947, vol. 21, pp. 495–511. [This article was part of a symposium, "One Hundred Years Ago," presented by the Johns Hopkins Institute of the History of Medicine.]
    [1] E. Heischkel, Die Deutsche Medizingeschichtschreibung in der ersten Hälfte des 19. Jahrhunderts, *Klinische Wochenschrift*, XII, 1933, pp. 714 ff.; Hans von Seemen, Zur Kenntnis der Medizinhistorie in der deutschen Romantik, *Beiträge zur Geschichte der Medizin*, III, 1926. For writings on historiography in general, cf. O. Temkin, An Essay on the Usefulness of Medical History for Medicine, *Bulletin of the History of Medicine*, XIX, 1946, p. 9, n. 1.
    [2] Haeser's remarks on "Bearbeitung der Geschichte der Medicin und der Volkskrankheiten," *Lehrbuch der Geschichte der Medicin*, II³, 1881, pp. 1086 ff., were of some help. However, I am especially indebted to the generous advice of my colleagues.

Now to start with the state of affairs in America, some work of
course was being done in the history of American medicine. Thacher's
American Medical Biography (1828) had focused attention on this
theme. He had written lest "the recollection of the most splendid and
noble achievements of a meritorious life be consigned to irremediable
oblivion," lest "the brightest examples of piety, of patriotism and
philanthropy be lost to posterity" (I, p. v); he had provided models
"worthy of imitation by the physician, the christian, the patriot and
philanthropist" (p. vi). In 1845, Stephen W. Williams published a four
hundred page continuation of Thacher's dictionary, "writing in a manner most satisfactory to the student of early medicine and at the same
time showing a more careful regard for facts than Thacher."[3] And at the
meeting of the American Medical Association in 1848 "Dr. J. R. W.
Dunbar read a letter from Dr. Stephen H. Williams, of Deerfield, Mass.,
on the propriety of taking measures for preserving a record of the lives
of the eminent physicians of the United States." But when Dunbar
subsequently submitted the proposal: "*Resolved*, That . . . a permanent
committee be appointed on Medical History and Biography," no action
was taken. The motion, as the Minutes laconically state, was "laid
over."[4]

The unwillingness of the Medical Association to support Williams'
project at first seems astonishing, the more so since research in American
history was much en vogue at that time. By 1848 *The American Archives*
of P. Force, that gigantic collection of documents, was in its fifth series.
Three volumes of Bancroft's *History of the United States* had already
appeared; three volumes of Hildreth's history on the same topic were to
appear in 1849.[5] Yet the stand taken by the members of the Medical
Association is perhaps more revealing and characteristic of the attitude
of physicians than is that of Williams. Granted that there were a number

[3] Cf. *A Cyclopedia of American Medical Biography*, by H. A. Kelly, II, 1912,
p. 512.

[4] *The Transactions of the American Medical Association*, I, 1848, p. 45. The
passage was brought to my attention by Miss Genevieve Miller. It evidently escaped
the notice of the writer of Williams' biography in the *Cyclopedia*. But cf. H. A.
Kelly and W. L. Burrage, *Dictionary of American Biography*, 1928, pp. 1308 f. (In
the *Transactions* the initials of Williams are incorrect.)

[5] Cf. J. Spencer Bassett, Writers on American History, 1753–1850 in *The Cambridge History of American Literature*, II, 1944, pp. 120, 108, 112. For Sparks' *American Biography*, cf. *op. cit.*, p. 117. I need not detail here the rise of historical societies
in the first half of the nineteenth century, cf. in general Bassett, *op. cit.*, III, pp.
172 f.

of people like him, that much of their work vanished with the day for which it was destined, as did Williams' address on the "Medical History of the County of Franklin in the Commonwealth of Massachusetts" delivered before the Massachusetts Medical Society in 1842[6]—one does not gain the impression that medical men were greatly concerned with the history of their profession, be it American history or history at large. A review of American medical literature from 1797 to 1848, written by Heusinger for *Janus*, does not mention any strictly historical papers. At best it refers to articles dealing with certain diseases or epidemics that had just been observed, to the sort of articles, that is, which Henschel, the editor of *Janus*, somewhat contemptuously calls "Tagesgeschichte," material for future historians.[7] Nor did the generation of Prescott and Motley produce a single great historian of medicine. Dunglison's lectures on the history of medicine, held at the University of Virginia from 1824 to 1833, show little originality and were the only American venture in the subject. Their printing had to wait until 1872. Even then there hardly existed "a convenient congenial work on the history of medicine" to which students could have access and the study of this topic, therefore, was "usually wholly neglected" (p, iv).[8]

It is merely in regard to one aspect of general medical history that I am able to find an outstanding contribution of an American: I have in mind J. R. Coxe's *The Writings of Hippocrates and Galen* (1846). The book contains abstracts of the Hippocratic and Galenic treatises which Coxe had made thirty years earlier for his own personal convenience (p. vi). They are still valuable and constitute even today the only sur-

[6] Cf. *Cyclopedia*, II, p. 512. Of course, one should not forget such studies as that of D. Drake on the diseases of the Mississippi Valley (1850) which takes into consideration historical factors.

[7] Dr. Heusinger, Die medicinischen Zeitschriften der amerikanischen Freistaaten, *Janus*, N. F. I, 1851, pp. 149 ff. (ed. K. Sudhoff, 1931). The article is based on and adds to the enumeration given in *The Transactions of the American Medical Association* in 1848 and 1849. To be sure, it is not Heusinger's intention to note the historical literature in particular. Yet it seems a fair assumption that writing for *Janus*, the first organ of medical history (cf. below, p. 474 f.), he would have mentioned any historical articles which he might have found. For Henschel's views, cf. *Janus*, N. F. I, pp. 1 ff.

[8] Note that Dunglison's *History of Medicine* was based mainly on Freind and Sprengel (p. iv); it was out of date even when it appeared (cf. also below n. 22). Incidentally, the example set by Dunglison's lectures found no following until 1897, when Roswell Park delivered lectures at the University of Buffalo, cf. E. F. Cordell, The Study of the History of Medicine, *Medical Library and Historical Journal*, II, 1904, p. 272.

vey that is at hand of the most important works of Hippocrates and of Galen. As Coxe says in his introduction, "the names of both these great men are familiar to our ears, as though they were the daily companions of our medical researches. Our teachers refer to them ex cathedra; our books continually quote them" (p. iii). One will consider his assertions less trustworthy if one remembers that Coxe was forced to retire from the chair of materia medica and pharmacy because his teaching was too conservative; "the doctrines and opinions of the earlier fathers of Physic had so superior a value in his estimation as to lead to too exclusive an exposition of them in his lectures."[9] Moreover, Coxe himself candidly admits that not "one in a hundred of the Profession, at least in America, have ever seen them [the works of Hippocrates and of Galen], and if interrogated, could not inform us of what they treat." Few copies, either in the original Greek or in Latin translations, were then available in America; no English translations did as yet exist (p. iv). Coxe's outlines, to which a short essay on the theories of Hippocrates and Galen was added (pp. 17–39), therefore, should have proved helpful. However, they hardly made a great impression on his contemporaries or achieved wide circulation.

What were the reasons for the lack of historical production in the United States? Were American scientists of the era under consideration generally experiencing the antagonism which many of their European colleagues felt toward history, the splendid progress of historical research notwithstanding? Did they sense that the American approach to historiography, if it was to be of value, had to be reformed by the scientific trend of the midcentury, a reform that actually took place after 1850?[10] The answer to these questions must await further investigation. Only this much is certain: the lack of American publications in the history of medicine was partly due to the fact that the country was still dependent on the work done abroad, as it was, according to Holmes, on foreign medical research, especially in regard to the more theoretical and less practical branches.[11] Americans relied on European literature,

[9] Cf. *Dictionary of American Biography*, IV, 1930, p. 487. Coxe studied in England, and later under Benjamin Rush. He was the editor of the *Medical Museum* (1805–11).

[10] For the opposition of European scientists to history, cf. A. W. E. Th. Henschel, Ist die Geschichte der Medicin an der Zeit? *Janus*, N. F. I, pp. 9 ff. For the change of American historiography from "elevated sentiment" to detached objectivity, cf. Bassett, *op. cit.*, III, pp. 171 f.

[11] *The Transactions of the American Medical Association*, I, 1848, pp. 286 ff.

most of all on English literature, to the consideration of which I now turn.

If the American happened to open *The British and Foreign Medical Review* of 1847, he found a lengthy article (XXIII, pp. 521 ff.) that drew his attention to one of the greatest accomplishments of English scholarship of the time, the discovery of Hindu medicine.[12] H. H. Wilson (1823) and J. F. Royle (1837) had inaugurated the study of the subject; T. A. Wise's *Commentary on the Hindu System of Medicine* (1845) gave the first complete survey. Before the investigations of these men, Indian thought had received but scant attention from medical historians. Sprengel devoted only eight pages of his work to India; Haeser in 1845 wrote no more than two; Renouard, whose history appeared in 1846, still considered the Hindus an inferior race.[13] Now it was realized that the Hindus had a scientific medical system of their own (p. 525). The old picture of world history consequently was bound to change; the question of the interdependence of medical thought was bound to be put on a new basis. The reviewer of Wise's treatise is well aware of these implications of the recent studies of Hindu medicine. He compares them to the revolutionary results of Assyrian excavations, of the deciphering of Persian cuneiform inscriptions which were reported in 1846 (pp. 521 f.). He points out that Whewell, in his *History of the Inductive Sciences*, denying that the Greeks owed anything to the Egyptians, had already asked whether they might not be indebted to India (p. 523). Indeed, the historical horizon of Europe began to broaden. Far Eastern culture was opened to the inquiring mind. In these studies, too, the English were leading: in 1846 J. Wilson gave a detailed description of Chinese medicine.[14]

On the other hand, the England of 1847 reached an unprecedented height in editing and translating old familiar source material according to the new standards and methods of historical research. W. A. Greenhill finished in 1847 and published in 1848 his translation of Rhazes' *Treatise on the Small-Pox and Measles*, the first English translation and the first translation into a European language from the original Arabic (p. 9). Thus, material concerning which Haeser still had to ask the advice of the Orientalists was made generally accessible by a scholar who

[12] The reference to the *British and Foreign Medical Review* I owe to Dr. Sanford Larkey.

[13] For Haeser, cf. below, p. 475 f.; for Renouard, cf. below, p. 471 f.

[14] Cf. Heusinger's summary of Wilson's book in *Janus*, III,. 193 ff.

was an Arabist and a physician and medical historian at the same time.[15] A few years earlier Greenhill's *Theophilus* (1842) and his *Sydenham* (1844 and 1846) had appeared. The last volume of Adams' translation of Paulus of Aegina came out in 1847. It was followed a few years later by his *Hippocrates* (1849) and his *Aretaeus* (1856). All these books were supported by the Sydenham Society which was founded in 1843.

It is fair to say that with their publication of sources the English medical historians were in advance of the other historians of their country. The *Rolls Series*, the first great collection of general historical material, was inaugurated only in 1847; English historical scholarship lagged behind that of France and Germany. Greenhill and Adams worked in close cooperation with their French and German colleagues and probably were stimulated by their methods.[16] They also agreed with them in doing historical research for the sake of the physician. The translations which they made were meant for "any well-educated member of the profession at the present day" (Adams, *Hippocrates*, I, p. v; cf. Greenhill, *Rhazes*, pp. v f.). With Adams it was perhaps the erudition resulting from historical studies that counted most; in addition to being a physician he was a friend of learning, a man with a "classical bent."[17] Greenhill, a more active and politically minded personality, seems to have believed in the exemplary value of history. He was a pupil of Thomas Arnold, for whom the history of Greece and Rome was "not an idle inquiry about remote ages and forgotten institutions, but a living picture of things present, fitted not so much for the curiosity of the scholar, as the instruction of the statesman and the citizen."[18]

But while England was leading in Oriental studies and was progressive in the opening up of sources, she remained backward in the study of the history of medicine as a whole. To be sure, Adams' translations, with their elaborate notes and introductions, amount to a

[15] For Haeser, cf. his *Lehrbuch der Geschichte der Medicin und der Volkskrankheiten*, 1845, p. viii. The foundation of the study of Arabic medicine had been laid by Wüstenfeld's *Geschichte der arabischen Aerzte und Naturforscher* (1840).

[16] For the state of historical studies in England until the middle of the nineteenth century, cf. J. W. Thompson, *A History of Historical Writing*, II, 1942, p. 281. Adams was influenced by the work of Littré, Malgaigne and Ermerins (*Hippocrates*, I, p. vi); Greenhill was a frequent contributor to *Janus*.

[17] For Adams cf. Charles Singer, A Great Country Doctor: Francis Adams of Banchory (1796–1861), *Bulletin of the History of Medicine*, XII, 1942, pp. 1 ff.

[18] For Thomas Arnold, cf. Thompson, *op. cit.*, II, p. 490. For Greenhill, cf. *Asclepiad*, XI, 1894–95, pp. 165 ff.; *Lancet*, II, 1894, p. 948; *British Medical Journal*, II, 1894, p. 734.

scrutiny of Greek medicine and its transmission by the Arabs. Green-hill's comments on Rhazes show the encyclopedic range of his knowledge; the articles on Greek physicians and Greek medicine which he contributed to Smith's *Dictionary of Greek and Roman Antiquities*, appearing in its second edition in 1848, are models of original historical research.[19] Nevertheless, the Englishman of 1847 who wished to read a general history of medicine was forced to turn to books that contained faulty and second-hand material and that were outmoded in their point of view.

Thus W. Hamilton's comprehensive *History of Medicine, Surgery, and Anatomy, from the Creation of the World to the Commencement of the Nineteenth Century* (I–II, 1831), with its mixture of high moral convictions and of low critical standards, is a quaint book indeed. To Hamilton, history of medicine is "the history of peace and good will, of endless harmony, and unceasing philanthropy." It does not record "the desolations of war, and the growth of immorality . . . her province is to note the diminution of mortal suffering; and the only triumphs which she records are those obtained over sickness, death, and sorrow" (I, p. v). But progress was slow. After Hippocrates had driven out superstition, after early Christianity had shed a new light, darkness followed again "till, at length, the discovery of the art of Printing unbarred afresh the gates of Heaven, and let in that flood of light, of knowledge, and of wisdom, which enabled men to emancipate themselves again from the slavery of superstition . . . and prove themselves to be—as the Almighty himself originally formed them—inferior only to the Angels" (I, p. vii). While a humanist of the Renaissance might have written these words, it is ancient and modern enlightenment that determines the final summing up of the development of the human faculties that came about "with the occasional interruptions and fluctuations which it experienced in proportion as the human mind was left more or less free from the shackles of arbitrary power or spiritual despotism" (II, pp. 307 f.). And without any apparent feeling of contradiction there goes together with such views the steadfast belief in the Bible: "Our blessed Redeemer himself, indisputably the first authority in all such questions, expressly discountenances, in more than one passage in the Gospels, the idea of any other interposition than by the natural operation of those causes

[19] I should also mention Greenhills' project of a dictionary of Greek medical terms, for which he gathered material in various articles in *The British and Foreign Medico-Chirurgical Review*.

which were ordained from the beginning, except in cases in which the Almighty so clearly manifests his intention as to prevent its being misunderstood" (I, p. 23).[20]

Compared with Hamilton's book, J. Bostock's *Sketch of the History of Medicine from its Origin to the Commencement of the Nineteenth Century* (1835) in some respects seems superior. Bostock has some sense of criticism; he starts with medicine in Egypt, not with the time before the Flood. Yet Bostock, too, copies facts and dates from older works; he does not make use of source material that had become available in the meantime; he neglects the new historical perspectives.[21] And his views are rather narrow and old-fashioned. Aiming at a history of practical medicine, he considers theories only because "the direct details of experience are, with a few exceptions, deeply tinged with the prevailing doctrines of the day, or with the individual speculations of the writer" (p. 2). One must, however, try to separate facts from hypotheses; otherwise medicine cannot become science, and "it will be a special object of attention, in the following pages, to endeavour to point out the limits between practice and theory, between facts, and the opinions that have been deduced from them" (*ibid.*). One believes to hear the voice of Sydenham, for whom Bostock had the highest admiration (pp. 159 f.). Nor do the lessons drawn from history breathe a less skeptical spirit (pp. 237 ff.). The results achieved so far seem hardly adequate to the labor of so many generations. What, then, is to be done in the light of history? The "strong avidity for the marvellous" must be overcome by a more careful exposition of facts. Facts, moreover, ought not to be accepted "upon the authority of a single individual"; scientific societies ought to pass on their accuracy. Only the generalization of the facts properly substantiated should be left to the individual, to his judgment and sagacity. In addition, it is indispensable that medicine acquire a good technical and scientific terminology; many controversies of the past were fights about words. Last but not least, there is required of the

---

[20] Cf. p. vi: "Of the years before the Flood, we can catch but those rare and partial glimpses which Omnipotence has been pleased to reveal in the writings of Moses—glimpses which are hardly sufficient for the construction of a plausible hypothesis, or the foundation of a probable conjecture." The other authorities quoted by Hamilton are LeClerc, Schulze, Freind; Sprengel it seems is never mentioned. I have been unable to find any biographical sketch of Hamilton.

[21] Cf. *Dictionary of National Biography*, II, 1908, p. 885: "The work shows small acquaintance with medical books, and has no merit of originality." Incidentally, Bostock was a friend of Roscoe, the editor of Poe, and obviously had literary ambitions.

physician a mind disposed to the reception of the truth, a "high sense of moral obligation"; the medical profession "is a deposit placed in his hands for the benefit of mankind."[22]

Hamilton's and Bostock's histories being the only ones in the English tongue to which the English and American readers of 1847 could resort, it is not astonishing that the more progressive students should eagerly search for new foreign books. It looked as if France had provided for their needs with P. V. Renouard's *Histoire de la Médecine* (I–II), that appeared in 1846 and was enthusiastically welcomed in *The British and Foreign Medical Review* of 1847 (XXIII, pp. 86 ff.) which I quoted before.[23] Renouard's work, dealing with nosology, therapeutics, hygiene, phrenology, and other sciences, doubtless has its merits, and is written from an original point of view. The author is interested in the history of medicine because from it the physician can derive certainty, the patient confidence. Why is this so? First of all, as history shows, the medical art is not a product of degeneration but a natural need. Moreover, it grows steadily instead of remaining stationary. Sprengel's skepticism as to the value of theories is to be rejected. Doubt, though necessary as a preliminary attitude, must and can be resolved into conviction, especially required for medical practice; one must and can detect the right theories. In attempting to prove this thesis, Renouard shows interest in biographical questions, for the personal example is important (I, p. 9); he is aware of the influence of the general state of society on medicine (p. 10); he considers not only the strictly medical teaching but also philosophical speculation (p. 11). But progressive as Renouard is in his general approach, he still shares Hamilton's and Bostock's disdain for the early Middle Ages; he completely neglects Oriental medicine. His

[22] It is not without interest to compare Bostock with Dunglison (cf. above, pp. 465 f.). For the latter, the study of history leads to the deduction "that we ought to be very tardy in embracing any sect or system" (pp. 274 f.). Observation and reflection are the true means for the improvement of medical science. Systems detract from observation. And yet, from every system something useful can be culled by the philosophical inquirer. The adoption of an exclusive theory makes man more notorious, but eclecticism is truer. And there is hope of achieving the goal. Great stupidity lies behind us. "As the physical and moral sciences pursue their onward progress, and as the means of observation and experiment are augmented and facilitated, our own noble science may attain a pitch of perfection, of which at the present time we can form no adequate conception, shedding light where all is now obscurity, and tending to dispel doubt and difficulty wherever existent" (pp. 275 f.).

[23] The German reviewer, Thierfelder (*Schmidt's Jahrbücher*, LVI, 1847, pp. 365 ff.), was less enthusiastic, cf. below p. 475. This review was brought to my attention by Dr. Owsei Temkin.

book, too, leans heavily on the authority of others, foremost among them that of Sprengel. He fails to go back to the source material.

The first truly modern history of medicine representative of the historical school was that of Daremberg, the first part of which appeared in 1847. Its title was *Cours sur l'histoire et la littérature des sciences médicales* (1–5 leçon), and it comprised the development from the beginning down to the school of Alexandria. The work was finished in 1870. As Daremberg then said,[24] the medical historian at the end of the seventeenth and in the beginning of the eighteenth century, had been concerned with names rather than with facts; he wrote the history of the kings and noblemen of medicine. Toward the end of the eighteenth century medical history suffered from the prejudices of the encyclopedists. Hecker, whose work was published in 1822, was the first, though still imperfect, writer of the historical school which is intent on studying the whole material, on scrutinizing all the sources, on dealing objectively and equally with every phase of the past. Among the general historians in France, the protagonists of this all-embracing method, of this "histoire des gens du tiers," were Guizot and Thierry. The latter's *Histoire de la conquête de l'Angleterre par les Normands* (1825) set the model. Guizot, even in 1811, had consulted the original documents for a lecture course which he was then delivering; he was one of the founders of the Société de l'Histoire de France which, starting in 1835, published the most important texts, memoirs, chronicles, and letters concerning the history of France.[25] It is the example of these two writers by which the method of the French medical historian was determined.

On the other hand, Daremberg intended to carry out to the letter the intentions of his master, Littré, who contemplated writing a history of medicine but was prevented from doing so by other duties. For Littré, medicine without history remains a mere craft, a métier. The task of the historian is that of following the development of the human spirit in the realm of time; he must show the link between past and present, for the thought of today is ripened by contact with the thought of yesterday. With this conviction, Littré edited the works of Hippocrates, the fifth volume of which appeared in 1846.[26] Moreover, as a pupil and friend of Comte, Littré was bent on finding "determined laws" in order to under-

---

[24] I am following his account in *Histoire des Sciences Médicales*, I, 1870, p. 66.

[25] For Thierry, cf. Thompson, *op. cit.*, II, pp. 230 f.; for Guizot, II, pp. 258–60.

[26] Cf. *Oeuvres complètes d' Hippocrate*, I, 1839, p. xiv. For Littré's view on medical history in general, cf. Daremberg, *Histoire*, I, dedication.

stand society, and history provides the raw material for the analysis of social phenomena. It is in Littré's and Comte's spirit that Daremberg worked out his history of medical sciences and tried to discover the common law that explains progress and decay. In such a knowledge he saw the value and usefulness of his research.[27]

But as I pointed out before, by 1847 Daremberg's *Histoire* was still in its beginning. Only the preparatory work was going ahead in great strides. After his dissertation on Galen's anatomy, physiology and pathology of the nervous system (1841), and after his translation of Hippocrates (1843) and his report on his manuscript studies in Germany, England, and Belgium (1845), Daremberg in 1847 announced his greatest plan, in which the program of the historical school found its most poignant expression: the publication of a *Bibliotheca medicorum classicorum Graecorum atque Latinorum*. All Greek and Latin authors were to be edited on the basis of the best manuscripts that were extant. Littré endorsed the project in a memorandum which he wrote for the Institut de France; the Académie de Médecine approved of it. Both documents were printed together with Daremberg's outlines and a sample of Bussemaker's new edition of Oribasius. And Daremberg, who had just succeeded in persuading the authorities of the Collège de France to announce the first official course on the history of medicine, also convinced Guérin, the editor of the *Gazette Médicale*, to devote sixteen pages of his journal to reviewing the history and literature of medicine.[28]

From all that I have said about France, it will be evident that by 1847 she was a center of historical investigation. She seems to have been superior even to England in that the French scholars attempted a more constructive interpretation of history as a whole. France's only other rival was Germany. But before turning to this country, the last to be considered in my survey, I should at least mention that the smaller European nations were not inactive in the field of medical history. Holland was especially prominent. I have already referred to Bussemaker's share in Daremberg's enterprise. F. Z. Ermerins was another Dutch

---

[27] *Histoire*, I, p. 15. For Comte, cf. Thompson, *op. cit.*, II, pp. 445 f.

[28] A good report on Daremberg's activities is given in *Janus*, III, pp. 833 f.; cf. also 815 f., and II, p. 399. In 1847 Daremberg published his *Notices sur l'antiquité et l'endémicité de la peste en Orient et particulièrement en Egypte;* in 1848 he brought out Galen's commentary on the *Timaeus*. I should also mention at least Malgaigne's edition of Ambroise Paré (1840) which contains an excellent introduction, outlining the various periods of medical history. For the problem of periodization of history, cf. Daremberg, *Histoire*, I, pp. 29 ff.

scholar of great merit. His work on Greek medicine was outstanding.[29] Generally speaking, it was the study of the various national achievements that flourished in the smaller states of Europe. Between 1837 and 1849 the histories of Belgian, Dutch, Italian and Spanish medicine were carefully investigated in a number of comprehensive books.[30] The question as to whether one could speak of a national system of medicine was widely discussed at the time; it is perhaps the Romantic movement that is echoed in these debates. But even Holmes was inclined to contrast the American mind with the attitude of the English, the French and the Germans, and he thought that "the American climate remoulds the European, and casts a new die of humanity—will it not generate causes of disease different from those of the Old World?"[31]

And now Germany. Here the foremost event of the year 1847 doubtless was the publication of the second volume of *Janus*, itself the first journal devoted exclusively to studies in the history of medicine. The main aim of *Janus* was the furtherance of special investigations. Individual historical phenomena were to be explained pragmatically, to be evaluated in relation to their time, with due attention to the data of politics, of arts and sciences, of religion, of national life.[32] To put it differently, German scholarship had reached the stage of "Quellenforschung." It had definitely given up philosophical history, as it had been written by Damerow, Kieser, Leupoldt, Isensee and Lessing. Harless had been the first to criticize the philosophical bias of his countrymen. His censure, voiced in 1842, had been reiterated the following year by Quitzmann. Ranke and his school probably made medical historians in general realize the importance of the study of the sources.[33]

[29] For Ermerins, cf. Ch. Daremberg, Notices sur la vie et les écrits du docteur Ermerins, *Union médicale*, 1872, No. 1 (Haeser, *op. cit.*, II³, 1881, p. 1095).

[30] Cf. Daremberg, *Histoire*, I, p. 65. He refers to Broeckx, Chinchilla, Morejon and De Renzi; cf. also Manfre (*op. cit.*, 59; and *Janus*, II, pp. 609 ff.).

[31] *The Transactions of the American Medical Association*, I, 1848, p. 287. For the view of the Romanticists, cf. B. Hirschel, Über die Herrschaft des nationalen Elements in der Medicin, *Biedermann's Monatschrift*, February 1842; the same, *Geschichte der Medicin*, 1843, p. 9, note.

[32] Cf. p. 6 of the prospectus dated 1845, which announced the publication of *Janus*, and which appears at the beginning of the 1931 reprint edition of the first volume of *Janus*. Cf. in general G. Rosen, Janus 1846–1946, *Journal of the History of Medicine and Allied Sciences*, II, 1947, pp. 5 ff.

[33] Cf. Heischkel, *op. cit.* (above, note 1). But one must not forget that the *Monumenta Germaniae Historica* started in 1826, that Böckh's *Corpus Inscriptionum* started in 1825; cf. Thompson, II, 166 f.; 157. The study of sources began even before the influence of Ranke made itself felt.

It should be stressed, however, that the founding of *Janus* was only the final victory of a movement that had long been noticeable. Almost all the co-editors of *Janus*, men like Choulant, Henschel, Spiess and Wüstenfeld, to single out but a few, had done important work in special fields, quite undisturbed by the metaphysical ambitions of their contemporaries.[34] And after all, in 1845 H. Haeser had published his *Lehrbuch der Geschichte der Medicin und der Volkskrankheiten.* He emphatically renounced philosophical history for his own work (p. vii); he turned back to the works of Sprengel and Hecker (pp. v f.). He wished to give facts, and he addressed himself to those who did not know the facts. Moreover, he saw clearly that the facts, in many instances, had not yet been uncovered. That is why he himself searched the sources, except where he could depend on reliable and exhaustive research of others (p. viii). Arabic medicine, the teaching of the Middle Ages, the doctrines of Vesalius, of Harvey, and of all later physicians were represented by Haeser on the basis of his own investigation of the material (pp. viii f.).[35]

It is true, Haeser's book is not a complete history of medicine; it is a "Lehrbuch," a textbook, in the strict sense of the term. It selects the important data, that which is significant (pp. xi ff.), and thus differs fundamentally from Daremberg's history of the "gens du tiers." Haeser modestly admits that, given the modern standards of criticism, it would be beyond his power to present a survey of the entire development. He even doubts that any one author could achieve such a task (p. xii). In this, Haeser is in agreement with Thierfelder, who in his review of Renouard's history, published in *Schmidt's Jahrbücher* of 1847, stressed the impossibility of writing at that moment a perfect study in accordance with the new ideals. In Thierfelder's opinion, it would be necessary to distribute the various subjects among different scholars, to institute a "Verein" of co-workers. Thus, and thus only, could the way be prepared for an adequate interpretation of the manifold events of the past (LVI, pp. 365 ff.). But even if Haeser, and the others too, fell short of the highest goal, in what he did he anticipated and put into practice the principles sponsored by *Janus*. The first organ of medical history did not mark a complete break with earlier tendencies, it merely reinforced them and secured their general acceptance.

[34] I have selected names to which Haeser refers, pp. viii; cf. also ix f. Eble's, Kopps' and Siebold's histories of anatomy and physiology, chemistry and obstetrics had already appeared. For Wüstenfeld, cf. above, n. 15.

[35] For Haeser, cf. Pagel in *Allgemeine Deutsche Biographie*, L, 1905, pp. 53 f.

It is also noteworthy that the opposition of the German historical school to the philosophical historiography of its predecessors was, in many respects, an opposition in name rather than in fact. Even Haeser considers a philosophy of history the proper and most elevated achievement of the historian (*Lehrbuch*, p. vii). The prospectus of *Janus* invites the cooperation of those who with deeper insight and philosophical acumen know how to elicit the spirit from historical matter (p. 6). Henschel ("Ein Blick auf das Ganze der Geschichte der Medicin," *Janus*, III, pp. 1 ff.) wonders whether the development of medicine is determined by a law, a hidden plan, a constant, secret sort of progress (p. 1). He regards the history of medicine as a science, inductive-intuitive, reflective, in part constructive, to a certain extent transcendent, though not transcendental (p. 18). In historical phenomena there is observable the eternal triad, the organic soul of history (p. 23). The organism of the history of medicine, organic moments, organic epochs—these three concepts express demonstrable verities (p. 27). It is history thus understood in which truth appears even in falsehood, in which a spiral movement predominates (*Janus*, N. F., I, pp. 20 f.). And when Henschel advocates historical studies for his own day, when he expects from them that just as in the time of Döring and Sennert, of Leclerc and Freind, in other words, just as in previous periods of uncertainty, reflection on the past will show what is good, what is certain, and where we are bound (p. 17), then he does not think of a simple interpretation of facts, he thinks of a philosophical analysis of the data assembled.

The French representatives of the historical school likewise aspired to ascertain the laws of history. But Littré and Daremberg were followers of Comte, while behind the concepts of Henschel and Haeser one still senses the categories of the Hegelian system. I do not feel under obligation to decide the issue whether both Comte's positivism and Hegel's idealism are metaphysical syntheses. There is, at any rate, a marked difference between the two philosophies, as far as facts and their evaluation are concerned. To Daremberg, German historiography as a whole seemed mythical.[36] One will find his verdict exaggerated in view of the results achieved by individual scholars; one will find it decidedly unfair to Haeser, although he, too, inclined toward an organic view. Nevertheless it contains a kernel of truth as regards the work of the German historical school and its most cherished ambitions.

[36] *Histoire*, I, p. 66.

In summing up my fragmentary conclusions I may say that in 1847 the history of medicine had constituted itself as it is cultivated even today by medical historians. The fundamental methods had been evolved, the range of subjects to be considered had been outlined, the importance of historical research for the practice and theory of medicine had been realized. I should add that, although the history of medicine was still written by physicians and for physicians, its importance for the non-professionals was beginning to be understood as well. In 1848, Virchow emphatically asserted that the history of epidemics forms an inseparable part of the cultural history of mankind. It presents warnings which no statesman can leave unheeded. Long before Virchow, Niebuhr had stressed the fact that a study of Greek medicine was essential for a correct appreciation of Greek history.[37] In 1839, Ranke in his *History of the Popes* dealt with the history of science as an integral part of the historical situation. In 1858, he pleaded before the Bavarian Academy that it was impossible to write the history of a nation without taking account of the scientific development. He wished for specialists to work on this subject, for which the general historian was unqualified through lack of training.[38] In short, everything that is promising in the present historical approach was implicit in the approach of the generation of a hundred years ago. No less obvious were the pitfalls of the historical method. The effort of the individual became insufficient for the understanding of the whole; the whole became lost in the maze of detail. If a hundred years hence medical historiography of 1947 is reviewed, may the critic be able to say that the advantages of the past were guarded faithfully, while the shortcomings were successfully overcome!

[37] For Virchow, cf. O. Temkin, *Bulletin of the History of Medicine*, XIX, 1946, pp. 31 f.; for Niebuhr, cf. *Vorträge über alte Geschichte*, II, 1848, p. 78. The lectures were published seventeen years after Niebuhr's death.

[38] For Ranke, cf. *Sämmtliche Werke*, LI–LII, 1881, pp. 490, 551, and Thompson, *op. cit.*, II, p. 444.

INDEX

Abortion: attitudes toward, 9–20, 26, 340, 343
Academicians, 197n, 198, 199, 200, 202n, 213, 232, 241n, 315, 352, 374
Acoustics, 403
Acumenus, 160n
Acute diseases: prognosis of, 67–68
Adams, F., 22n, 122, 134n, 468
Adoption of pupils, 40–48, 57n
Adultery: attitudes toward, 35n
Aenesidemean Skepticism, ix, 186, 187, 202n, 374
Aeschylus, 421, 422n, 431
Aesculapius, 195n, 205n
Aesop, 383, 384
Aetius, 231n
Agathon, 154, 155, 161, 162n, 163, 164, 169
Age: affecting therapy, 83n, 180, 188, 304; views on old age, 381–82
Aglaion, 252
Air: taken into body, 112, 114, 115, 116, 137, 140, 141
Aischines, 87n
Akron of Agrigentum, 195, 196
Alcibiades, 163–64, 169, 170
Alcmaeon of Croton, 24n, 256
Alexander of Aphrodiseas, 238n
Alexander the Great, 431n
Alexander of Tralles, 233n, 235, 239n
Alexandria: medicine in, 26; medical ethics in, 58; anatomy studies in, 247, 270, 281, 285, 293, 300–1, 445; research centers in, 431. *See also* Egypt
Alexis, 38n
Allbutt, T. Clifford, 205n
Alterations: constitutional, 83–84
Aly, W., 16n

America: historiography in, 464–67
American Medical Association, 464
Amman, I. C., 230n
Ammianus Marcellinus, 239n
Ammonius, 26n
Amulets, 232–33
Analogical thinking, 292–94, 407–8, 419
Anankē, 109
Anatomy: and Hippocratic medicine, 151, 247, 253–59, 270, 292, 370; dissection in Alexandria, 247, 250–51, 270, 281, 283, 285, 293, 300–1; history in Antiquity, 247–301; in Homeric medicine, 252–53; animal and human organs compared, 254, 295, 353, 372, 408; textbooks on, 257, 294–95; and interest in human body, 261–64; interest of philosophers, 264, 272; Christian attitude toward, 265; Dogmatic views on, 268, 274, 275, 280, 282, 286, 290–91, 299; Empiricist views on, 269–70, 274, 280, 282, 286, 290–91, 299; Galen's doctrine on, 271; and ideas of death, 273–85; and religion and magic, 279, 295, 297; Roman views on dissection, 281–83, 426; purpose of dissections, 286–97; and analogical thinking, 292–94; bodies for vivisection, 297; cadavers for dissection, 298–300; plastic anatomy, 299n; revival by Vesalius, 444–46; importance of, 451. *See also* Dissection; Vivisection
Anaxagoras, 118, 126, 208, 210, 212n, 280n, 419, 421, 422, 435
Anaximander, 264, 419, 420, 435
Anaximenes, 126, 419
Ancient science: interpretation of, 401–39; and modern science, 402–8; and

479

481

226–27; on incantations, 238; on
human body, 264; on death, 275–77,
279, 290*n*; on medicine, 313, 354; on
self-interest, 325; on health, 359, 391;
on desires of soul, 362; values of, 364,
365; comments on, 402*n*; on geometry,
409; on labor, 418; on astronomy,
422*n*, 423; analysis of, 423*n*
Pleistonicus, 231
Pleurisy, 68
Pliny, 11*n*, 12*n*, 146, 149, 176, 177, 190,
195, 222*n*, 224, 230, 235*n*, 239, 245*n*,
263, 344*n*, 375, 395, 412
Plotinus, 221
Plouthygieia, 387
Plutarch, 43*n*, 45*n*, 211*n*, 212*n*, 223,
224*n*, 225, 231*n*, 245*n*, 359, 382, 386,
390, 391, 409, 422*n*, 425*n*
Pneuma, 105*n*
Pneumonia, 68
Pohlenz, M., x, 32*n*, 111–20, 133, 134,
135, 136, 137, 138*n*, 140, 141, 142,
143*n*, 144*n*, 201*n*, 327*n*, 332*n*, 336*n*,
339*n*, 341*n*
Poison: rules concerning, in Oath, 9–20,
26, 63, 64
Political interference with science, 421–
26
Polybius, 140*n*, 425*n*, 436
Polycletus, 395
Polyhistor, Alexander, 19
Pope, A., 453*n*
Porphyry, 19*n*, 30*n*, 32*n*, 52*n*, 57*n*, 225*n*,
226*n*
Posidonius, 219, 223, 343*n*, 424, 425*n*
Powell, I. U., 51*n*
Praechter, K., 21*n*, 32*n*, 34*n*, 56*n*, 57*n*,
58*n*, 234*n*, 438*n*
Praxagoras, 231
Prayers: attitudes toward, 239–41, 378
Preisendanz, K., 232*n*, 235*n*
Prescott, 465
Presocratics, 354, 372, 419, 430, 435, 437
Priscianus, Theodorus, 235
Professional ethics. *See* Ethics
Professions: concepts of, 341–43
Prognosis: Hippocratic, 65–85, 434;
significance for treatment, 66, 75; for
acute diseases, 67–68; meaning in
Hippocratic medicine, 69–70; mantic,
70, 82; interpretation of writings, 70–
82; seasons affecting, 71, 72, 74, 77,

83; communication of, 76; and public
recognition, 76–77; objective interpre-
tation of, 79–80; patients impressed
by, 81–82; misuse of, 82; for healthy
persons, 83–85; for athletes, 85
Proklos, 173
Prometheus: ideal of, 453
Prosper Alpinus, 191
Protagoras, 167*n*, 201, 212*n*, 373, 394,
395, 422*n*
Pseudo-Galenic writing, 173, 174, 178,
179, 180, 181, 182, 184, 191
Ptolemy, 401*n*, 404*n*, 408, 413, 416, 417,
438, 450
Pupil-teacher relationship, 40–48, 57*n*
Purgatives: use of, 83, 200
Purification: use of, 224
Purity: concept of, 15, 20, 32, 35*n*, 37*n*,
50*n*, 59, 340*n*
Puschmann, 65*n*, 233*n*, 235*n*
Pyrrho, 352–53
Pyrrhonist skepticism, 198*n*, 202, 203
Pythagoras, x, 61, 236*n*, 241*n*, 329
Pythagoreans: attitude toward suicide,
17; attitude toward abortion, 18–20;
Plato influenced by, 20*n*, 57*n*, 61;
doctrines compared with Hippocratic
Oath, 20–39; and dietetics, 26; taboos
of, 32*n*; and teacher-pupil relation-
ships, 43–48; Oath of, 48*n*; invoking of
deities, 50; desire for glory, 52; attitude
toward vows, 53; transmission of doctrine, 58; development of doctrine,
58; medical ethics of, 59; compared
with Christians, 63–64; doctrine of,
160*n*, 233*n*, 276, 327, 340*n*, 362, 389,
403, 450

Quintilian, 346*n*, 444*n*
Quitzmann, 474

Rabelais, 444*n*
Ranke, 474, 477
Records: scientific, 434–35
Regenbogen, Otto, viii, ix, 133*n*, 234*n*,
293*n*, 294*n*, 328*n*, 406*n*, 408*n*, 431*n*
Regimen: in days of crisis, 78; for healthy
persons, 83–84; moist, of Methodists,
181–83, 186, 190. *See also* Hippocratic
writings (individual), *On regimen*
Reginos, 173

Designed by Gerard A. Valerio

Composed in Monotype Binney 21 EFG by Monotype Composition Company

Printed offset by Universal Lithographers, Inc. on 50 lb., Olde Forge F, S

Bound by Moore and Company in Bradford Buckram and Bolton